Political and Economic Implications of Blockchain Technology in Business and Healthcare

Dário de Oliveira Rodrigues
Instituto Politécnico de Santarém, Portugal

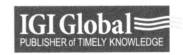

A volume in the Advances in Data Mining and
Database Management (ADMDM) Book Series

Published in the United States of America by
   IGI Global
   Business Science Reference (an imprint of IGI Global)
   701 E. Chocolate Avenue
   Hershey PA, USA 17033
   Tel: 717-533-8845
   Fax: 717-533-8661
   E-mail: cust@igi-global.com
   Web site: http://www.igi-global.com

Library of Congress Cataloging-in-Publication Data

Names: Rodrigues, Dario de Oliveira, 1963- editor.
Title: Political and economic implications of blockchain technology in
  business and healthcare / Dario de Oliveira Rodrigues, editor.
Description: Hershey, PA : Business Science Reference, [2021] | Includes
  bibliographical references and index. | Summary: "This book provides
  relevant theoretical frameworks on the political and economic impact of
  blockchain technology, which is thought to be able to redesign human
  interactions concerning transactions"-- Provided by publisher.
Identifiers: LCCN 2021005801 (print) | LCCN 2021005802 (ebook) | ISBN
  9781799873631 (hardcover) | ISBN 9781799873648 (paperback) | ISBN
  9781799873655 (ebook)
Subjects: LCSH: Technological innovations--Economic aspects. | Blockchains
  (Databases)--Industrial applications. | Blockchains
  (Databases)--Economic aspects.
Classification: LCC HC79.T4 P649 2021 (print) | LCC HC79.T4 (ebook) | DDC
  338/.064--dc23
LC record available at https://lccn.loc.gov/2021005801
LC ebook record available at https://lccn.loc.gov/2021005802

This book is published in the IGI Global book series Advances in Data Mining and Database Management (ADMDM) (ISSN: 2327-1981; eISSN: 2327-199X)

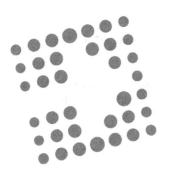

Advances in Data Mining and Database Management (ADMDM) Book Series

David Taniar
Monash University, Australia

ISSN:2327-1981
EISSN:2327-199X

MISSION

With the large amounts of information available to organizations in today's digital world, there is a need for continual research surrounding emerging methods and tools for collecting, analyzing, and storing data.

The **Advances in Data Mining & Database Management (ADMDM)** series aims to bring together research in information retrieval, data analysis, data warehousing, and related areas in order to become an ideal resource for those working and studying in these fields. IT professionals, software engineers, academicians and upper-level students will find titles within the ADMDM book series particularly useful for staying up-to-date on emerging research, theories, and applications in the fields of data mining and database management.

COVERAGE

- Enterprise Systems
- Data Analysis
- Data Warehousing
- Customer Analytics
- Predictive Analysis
- Data Mining
- Neural Networks
- Quantitative Structure–Activity Relationship
- Text Mining
- Cluster Analysis

IGI Global is currently accepting manuscripts for publication within this series. To submit a proposal for a volume in this series, please contact our Acquisition Editors at Acquisitions@igi-global.com or visit: http://www.igi-global.com/publish/.

Titles in this Series

For a list of additional titles in this series, please visit:
http://www.igi-global.com/book-series/advances-data-mining-database-management/37146

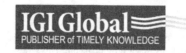

701 East Chocolate Avenue, Hershey, PA 17033, USA
Tel: 717-533-8845 x100 • Fax: 717-533-8661
E-Mail: cust@igi-global.com • www.igi-global.com

Table of Contents

Section 3
Blockchain Healthcare

Detailed Table of Contents

Section 1
Blockchain Ethics

The new developing ethical framework.

Chapter 1

    Dario de Oliveira Rodrigues, Instituto Politécnico de Santarém, Portugal

By cutting transaction costs and streamlining agreements' execution via "smart contracts," blockchain technology (BT) turns decentralization into an economic advantage and an antidote against politically harsh decisions that can obliterate privacy, freedom, and democracy. Although BT's ethical bottom line is still uncertain, its use can smooth out the trade-off between privacy and convenience, reconciling both. BT can also help reconfigure the compromise between intellectual property rights and the common good, opening more ethical routes to the diffusion of innovation. BT's data security can be translated into straightforward access to information. On the one hand, this signals new inclusion routes for "identityless" and unbanked people, and on the other, it releases society from biased information and fake news providing access to trusted data. BT guarantees contents precision, distributing a consensual tamper-proof "hyperledger" proving transactions' authenticity and data's integrity. As consensus should be plural, BT's decentralization is thought to be a must in ethical terms.

Section 2
Blockchain Society

Blockchain political-economic implications for citizens and consumers.

Chapter 2

    João Pedro Vieira, University of Lisbon, Portugal
    Cátia Neves Sousa, University of Lisbon, Portugal

Trust is vital to the sustained existence of money. No currency can prevail without it. However, following the international crisis of 2008, the liability-side of trust became increasingly apparent. Blockchain and cryptocurrencies challenged the need to trust and proposed an alternative "trustless" system. In the context of rising interest and concern about cryptocurrencies, the authors intend to discuss the role of trust in the evolution of money, from ancient Mesopotamia to modern sovereign fiat currencies and cryptocurrencies, and whether cryptocurrencies are prompting a shift in the paradigm of money or not.

Chapter 3

Dario de Oliveira Rodrigues, Instituto Politécnico de Santarém, Portugal

Blockchain technology is changing the world incentive system, making programmable money. This kind of money is only fruitful and democratically livable in a transparent political environment. Otherwise, instead of unleashing innovation and collective action with the market's visible hand of qualified money, the new internet of value will deliver a digital money with the same algorithmic fate that social media met on the previous internet. The latter allows digitizing users' data and has been used to manipulate consumers and public opinion (possibly in the last two U.S. Presidential elections). Similarly, the former will let states and corporatocracy cross-reference social media and digital money's data, hurting privacy even more. As blockchains disseminate, having the crucial economic advantage of reducing transaction costs, only free-market competition between private and public blockchains guarantee transparency and democracy. Blockchain technology is the real McCoy, and decentralizing digital money is the free world's best shot, especially in the new normal triggered by COVID-19.

Chapter 4

Dario de Oliveira Rodrigues, Instituto Politécnico de Santarém, Portugal
Pedro Santana Lopes, GlobalLawyers, Portugal

There has been a fundamental change in the genesis of political-economic trust, with the arrival of a decentralized but structured way to reach consensuses and automatically implementing decisions through self-executable contracts. Blockchain technology (BT) is a distributed, consensus-based, and secure way for individuals to make enforceable censorship-resistant quantifiable agreements. Every vote is a transaction, and BT is paving the way for decentralizing politics, defending privacy, and streamlining voting procedures. It has the potential to provide much more granular governance that hopefully will preserve freedom and defend democracy. However, especially in an embarrassing post-COVID-19 world, BT's centralization can, instead, pave the way for citizens' control, turning cryptographic protocols into an authoritarian digital corset tightened by some to menace the privacy and freedom of many.

Chapter 5

Mitchell Loureiro, Immunefi, Portugal
Ana Pêgo, Centro de Estudos de Doenças Crónicas (CEDOC), NOVA Medical School,
*   Universidade NOVA de Lisboa, Lisbon, Portugal*
Inês Graça Raposo, ISEG Executive Education, Lisbon School of Economics and
*   Management, University of Lisbon, Portugal*

The single critical output of a blockchain is creating trust where previously impossible. While this feature delivers compelling value for many use cases (bitcoin for money, standards setting and data sharing for permissioned blockchains, audit trails and protection against liability in supply chains), the most novel use case has been something unexpected: the birth of a new type of social structure to provide goods and services. The early examples of this new type of social structure have shown themselves to be incredibly effective at providing those services to their users.

Chapter 6

The internet and digital transformation have changed our relations with the market. These technologies have been developing continuously, creating opportunities for new business models, and e-commerce has grown overwhelmingly worldwide, changing the consumption process of a large part of the world's population. Companies are increasingly using blockchain technology to improve and create new global trading business models. Blockchain had its first application in cryptocurrencies, but it has quickly become a major solution in all sorts of activity sectors, providing increased security in commercial transactions. An important question is how the blockchain can leverage e-commerce in solving problems and improving business results. It was concluded that blockchain could leverage e-commerce in the four fundamental areas of (1) e-commerce financial transactions, (2) e-commerce supply chain management, (3) e-commerce forecasting and contractual relations, and (4) e-commerce transactions systems' trust and credibility.

Section 3
Blockchain Healthcare

Blockchain political-economic implications for patients and providers.

Chapter 7

The COVID-19 pandemic has disrupted healthcare worldwide and laid several fundamental problems that will have to be tackled to ensure high-quality healthcare services. This pandemic has represented an unparalleled challenge for healthcare systems and poses an opportunity to innovate and implement new solutions. Digital transformation within healthcare organizations has started and is reshaping healthcare. Technologies such as blockchain and IoT can bring about a revolution in healthcare and help solve many of the problems associated with healthcare systems that the COVID-19 crisis has exacerbated. In this chapter, IoT and blockchain technologies were discussed, focusing on their main characteristics, integration benefits, and limitations, identifying the challenges to be addressed soon. The authors further explored its potential in describing concrete cases and possible applications for healthcare in general and specifically for COVID-19.

Chapter 8

The electronic health records (EHR) patient portals are an integrated eHealth technology that combines an EHR system and a patient portal, giving patients access to their medical records, exam results, and services, such as appointment scheduling, notification systems, and e-mail access to their physician. EHR patient portals empower patients to carry out self-management activities and facilitate communication with healthcare providers, enabling the patient and healthcare provider to access the medical information quickly. Worldwide governmental initiatives have aimed to promote the use of EHR patient portals. The implementation of EHR patient portals encompasses several challenges, including security, confidentiality concerns, and interoperability between systems. New technological approaches like blockchain could address these issues and enable a successful worldwide implementation of EHR patient portals.

Chapter 9

Blockchain is being explored as a potential solution to many problems in areas other than the one created initially: cryptocurrency. Blockchain technology allows the authenticity of data, security in transactions, and privacy without the need for a third party. For that main reason, one of the growing interests concerns its application in healthcare, namely in clinical research. Multiple pain points of clinical research might benefit from the implementation of blockchain technology. This chapter shows some examples in which this technology is already implemented, identifying the advantages of its use. One of those advantages is clinical research, with the possibility of the patients managing their own clinical data and being properly rewarded for that. Research about clinical data monetization for patients is currently limited, and this chapter also proposes a hypothetical scenario of health data monetization workflow.

Blockchain technology in a clinical trial setting is a valuable asset due to decentralization, immutability, transparency, and traceability features. For this chapter, a literature review was conducted to map the current utilization of blockchain systems in clinical trials, particularly data security managing systems and their characteristics, such as applicability, interests of use, limitations, and issues. The advantages of data security are producing a more transparent and tamper-proof clinical trial by providing accurate, validated data, therefore producing a more reliable and credible clinical trial. On the other hand, data integrity is a critical issue since data obtained from trials are not instantly made public to all participants. Work needs to be done to establish the significant implications in security data when applying blockchain technology in a real-world clinical trial setting and generalized conditions of use to establish its security.

Ana Pêgo, Centro de Estudos de Doenças Crónicas (CEDOC), NOVA Medical School,
Universidade NOVA de Lisboa, Lisbon, Portugal
Inês Graça Raposo, ISEG Executive Education, Lisbon School of Economics and
Management, University of Lisbon, Portugal
Mitchell Loureiro, Immunefi, Portugal

Clinical research evolved side-by-side with technology, leading to exponential data generation contributing to social and economic development. Nevertheless, data storage, integrity, and privacy concerns have emerged, raising trust issues regarding data sharing. This chapter will demonstrate how blockchain technology (BT) can address these problems and help optimizing processes, minimize costs, and monetize data. It will explain why these models are not fully explored and how cryptocurrencies are advantageous compared to traditional currency. Worldwide examples of companies developing network infrastructures that rely on private players will be provided, and European cases, where consortium models that count with different partners to build health blockchain infrastructures are being developed, will be discussed. Considering the business models to be addressed under the European Union (EU) jurisdiction, a hypothetical BT-based healthcare model with potential application in the EU scenario will also be highlighted.

Rafael Duarte Pinto, ISEG, Lisbon School of Economics and Management, University of
Lisbon, Portugal
Diana Madaleno Ferreira, ISEG, Lisbon School of Economics and Management, University
of Lisbon, Portugal
Maria Teresa Barbosa, ISEG, Lisbon School of Economics and Management, University of
Lisbon, Portugal
Margarida Chinita Nieto, ISEG, Lisbon School of Economics and Management, University
of Lisbon, Portugal
Ana Filipa Funenga, ISEG, Lisbon School of Economics and Management, University of
Lisbon, Portugal
Marta Sousa da Silva, ISEG, Lisbon School of Economics and Management, University of
Lisbon, Portugal
Pedro Picaluga Nevado, ISEG, Lisbon School of Economics and Management, University of
Lisbon, Portugal

Blockchain is a decentralized digital ledger of transactions shared amongst all participating web nodes, over which every data is recorded. Since the first blockchain was conceptualized in 2008, much research has been done to expand its applications to non-financial purposes. Dentacoin is the first cryptocurrency ever created worldwide that strives to create a dental industry community by rewarding people with a given token—Dentacoin cryptocurrency—for specific actions that have a desirable effect on the Dentacoin ecosystem. This concept aims to improve the global dental market by applying blockchain technology advantages and promoting intelligent prevention in dental healthcare. The purpose of this chapter is to review the concept of blockchain-based Dentacoin ecosystem, as it is expected that, in the future, this method will significantly improve dental health and oral hygiene habits, thus improving the quality of life for individuals resulting in overall health enhancement and increased longevity.

Chapter 13

   Francisco Ribeiro de Sousa, ISEG, Lisbon School of Economics and Management,
      University of Lisbon, Portugal

Blockchain, a distributed ledger technology (DLT) that sustained the creation of the first digital currency, Bitcoin, crosses many business areas, including healthcare, to promise better economic solutions. Blockchain generalized implementation is already a reality in Estonia, perhaps the most digitally advanced country globally, with proven healthcare results for its citizens. From a pharmaceutical industry perspective, blockchain offers solutions as diverse as the structuring of clinical trial protocols, the traceability of medicines along the supply chain, and intellectual property rights. Additionally, the DLT's cryptographic protocol, whose main characteristics are immutability, consensus, security, and transparency, may support both the web's decentralization and the transition to a Semantic Web, which is recognized by many as highly recommended.

Preface

Everything changed after users' data were made public on the Internet and privately traded by Big Tech companies, and nothing will be the same once such data are made private on the Internet and publicly transacted by their rightful owners.

Blockchain Technology (BT) leverages the disruptive capacity of the Internet in what is thought to be an inflection point for humanity. The dawn of the *Blockchain Era* coincides with a *post-Covid-19 new normal* that mixes health and economic problems, unleashing an even faster transition to digital society. Knowing that money and health are crucial factors in peoples' lives and the two greatest human aspirations besides love, Business and Healthcare are natural choices to envision BT's impact on society.

In the first phase of the Internet, information sharing, and social media economics led to decentralization that stood well below expectations. Instead of Internet democratization made by the people and for the people, the disintermediation envisioned by some has resulted in the fastest reintermediation and personal enrichment processes in business history. Such a successful business reengineering sacrificed traditional editors and old media publishers while, paradoxically, despite Internet's potential to democratize accessing information, new digital business models rather centralized users' data without any further consideration.

Again, disintermediating and re-intermediating processes will be inexorable. Moreover, this time it will not be just about sharing and monetizing users' data. Now, it will be about users' transactions. Indeed, opting for democratizing (public blockchains) or segregate (private blockchains) transaction procedures will have further implications on privacy, free initiative, and even democracy. In the Blockchain Era, not only the users' profiles but also their money will be processed digitally on the Internet. The blockchain's digital functionalities are proven, and it is necessary to choose who will be allowed to use them and whether transparently. Hence, as both economic media went digital (social media and digital money), a redoubled Internet impact on people's lives is expected. This book looks into the political-economic consequences of such impact in the new digital paradigm triggered by blockchain protocols.

It is known that money talks, but it is challenging to realize that digital money is multilingual. Contrary to what one would think possible, money's universal language is changing because the universe of money is now a multiverse—the multiverse of digital tokens. Cryptocurrencies and other crypto-assets can express a wide range of innovative value propositions made possible by blockchain cryptographic techniques.

Digital tokens should not be understood as amounts kept in virtual wallets but as keys that allow exercising ownership by transferring assets and rights. The so-called wallets are, in fact, keychains, which keep private cryptographic keys safe. These keys allow acknowledging tokens' ownership and ciphering the rights to record specific immutable transactions in tamper-proof global digital ledgers or *hyperledgers*. Transferable rights may be related to an increasingly vast array of fungible and non-fungible assets such as money, votes, bonds, collectibles, and many other goods and services. Hence, personal rights on the Internet can be guaranteed by using private cryptographic keys to access public blockchains, while transactions carried out on private blockchains stay dependent on third parties who have their master keys. In other words, some blockchains decentralize power, and others do the opposite.

Central Bank Digital Currencies (CBDC) can be politicized using particular types of blockchains. For instance, when created by authoritarian governments or totalitarian political regimes, such currencies can even be transformed into globalized rationing tickets tailored to each citizen's political profile, with no private cryptographic keys available whatsoever. Thus, as seen in Chapters 1 and 4, only some blockchains guarantee privacy and freedom of choice in transacting, making it possible to defend private initiative and democracy in a challenging Blockchain Era.

The purpose of this book is to contribute to a discussion of BT's political and economic implications. It is not aimed at discussing buzzwords nor the ups and downs of cryptocurrency prices. While such volatility can impress some and attract the attention of others on the still universal scale of traditional money, this book has more to do with the opportunities and threats raised in the new multiverse of money. It is believed that traditional uni-dimensional money is being replaced by multidimensional programmable money that will enter the financial mainstream perhaps soon than expected. The non-programmable traditional money reduces all the tradable value to just one dimension and limits the spectrum of financial incentives for humanity. However, to freedom advocates, even such uni-dimensional money may be remembered as bearable if digital money becomes a monopoly of the state and corporatocracy. Thus, in this book, it is argued that BT should remain open to free initiative and permeable to human ingenuity so that cryptocurrencies and other digital tokens can be designed and programmed transparently both by governments and companies and by civil society and communities as well. This evolution will extend to many areas besides finance and politics. One of these areas is Healthcare.

Governments are regarding the digitalization of the Healthcare sector as a topic of the utmost importance, especially in developing countries. Although developed countries are driving the digitalization of health, many emerging countries are also implementing digital health programs. Due to its efficiency, these programs enable such limited national economies to make better healthcare investments.

Usually, people only relate Blockchain to digital currency and the investment sector. However, not considering the importance of Blockchain in the Healthcare sector can be misleading because this is one of the areas that may benefit the most. Digital Health is enabling a more patient-centric approach to healthcare. The limited ability of traditional information systems architectures to manage big data quickly, open, secure, and reliable makes BT critical. The privileged use of Blockchain in Healthcare starts at the clinical trial level, moves through the exchange of data between healthcare professionals and healthcare industries, and finally gets to the exchange of information between patients and the other healthcare stakeholders. No other existing technology can manage the very complex inter-relations in healthcare as Blockchain does.

The book's third section covers how vital Blockchain is in different healthcare issues. When considering national and multi-country projects that require a massive amount of sensitive data to be shared, like the COVID-19 vaccination passport, transparency, decentralization, immutability, and auditability, it turns out that Blockchain can be the most reliable and safe approach. This global convenience is no surprise as Blockchain can be crucial to connect communities, countries, healthcare providers, and patients in a decentralized, safe, and tamper-proof manner.

The following lines present a panoramic view of how the book contents are organized.

The book's first section presents the new ethical framework in the light of BT, which is explained throughout this section in relation to Business and Healthcare.

The first chapter, entitled "Blockchanging Trust: Ethical Metamorphosis in Business and Healthcare," opens the book because BT is neither good nor bad, nor by no means neutral. A systematization of the ethical dilemmas in cyberspace, proposed in 2012 by the same author, is now used as a starting explanatory model of the new *distributed trust* ethical consequences. BT changed the trust paradigm for humanity, which requires, above all, a thoughtful, ethical approach. Hence, in this first chapter, it will be seen why BT modifies the technical specifications of the trade-off between privacy and convenience, also changing the compromise between ownership and public rights. In Chapters 1, 3, and 4, it will be argued that the financial incentives and many kinds of transactions can now enjoy transparency and privacy simultaneously, two concepts brought together for the first time in history. BT also seems to allow catalyzing access to information and facilitating digital inclusion, benefiting citizenship and financial literacy. Several new ethical possibilities will be observed as BT offers tamper-proof solutions to certify data accuracy and content precision, which can be a crucial civilizational advantage in a time of *fake news* and political distrust. Throughout the chapter, it is highlighted why BT is a double-edged sword, which can either inaugurate a trustworthy openness era or, on the contrary, reinforce data centralization and feed a lust for power, perhaps pushing society into a worrisome non-democratic path.

The second section of this book (chapters 2 to 6) focuses on the impact of BT on society in general and on business in particular, analyzing the respective political and economic implications.

Chapter 2 is entitled "The Evolution of Trust in Money: A Historical Approach from Clay Tablets to Blockchain." This chapter makes a thoughtful review of the trust evolution underlying the history of money. For many centuries or even millennia, the reckless monetary policies of kings and emperors, often to finance wars (both in east and west), contributed to high inflation periods. Distrust in the economic and financial soundness of currency value foundations boosted money metallization, with emphasis on silver and gold standards, as a way to reinforce currency credibility. However, human greed resulted in seigniorage costs and speculation leading to successive cycles of devaluation in which the bad currency tends to expel the good currency from the market, as stated in Gresham's law. This pragmatic monetary course is justified because people save the most reliable money, withdrawing it from the market, preferentially using the one offering more devaluation perspectives. For decades, the world witnessed the widespread use of the so-called *fiat* currencies, which are not backed by anything else than confidence in the states' ability to finance themselves by collecting taxes. Nevertheless, as explained in this chapter, when the nominal value of currencies is essentially determined by authorities and is not related to its intrinsic value, money's value has been historically interrupted whenever the lack of confidence in money's issuers is so blatant that fiduciary trust ceases its effect. Over the centuries, a vicious circle of measures and countermeasures motivated by inflation and greed formed a spiral that persisted in the last century (*e.g.*, World War I and II) and reached this century with a financial crisis (2008-2009) that was not a good omen. Right at the beginning of the second decade of the 21st century, a severe pandemic further eroded confidence reminding that the specter of inflation or even hyperinflation always lurks. Chapter 2 also shows that, at least for the past 500 years, there have been financial instruments, such as the Bill-Of-Exchange and the Scriptural-Money issued by banks, that have provided economic agents, like merchants, companies, and banks with valuable networking information on the financial position and commitments of the parties involved in commercial transactions. For centuries, these documents were *paper tokens* registering financial movements in ledgers shared on the economic agents' networks, making international trade much more dynamic. Such *paper tokens* can be considered somehow *equiva-*

lent to the current digital tokens, inscribing precisely the same type of valuable information in a global digital ledger (hyperledger) to ensure safe transactions carried out on blockchain networks. The chapter's journey through money's underlying trust finally reaches the 21st century with the advent of cryptocurrencies, which are viewed with some skepticism, although tempered by recognizing their important role in the evolution of trust.

Chapter 3 is entitled "Blockchanging Money: Reengineering the Free World Incentive System." It begins by discussing money's essence, arguing that cryptocurrencies can be genuinely considered, from a market perspective, as being real money despite having no intrinsic value. Hence, it is explained why, for centuries, the so-called *stone money* of the Yap Islands in Micronesia was perfectly handled even though each one of such coins could weigh several tons. This *stone money* is a weighty argument against the assumption that intrinsic value is an indispensable currency's attribute because a stone's value is practically null. Instead, the value of *stone money* was due to its costly production (which was responsible for their scarcity) and to the fact that such stones were tokens playing an essential role in double-entry bookkeeping thanks to the oral ledger of Yap's natives' collective memory. According to several authors, this oral ledger can be considered a precursor of BT's *hyperledger*, and *stone money* can be compared to Bitcoin. This case serves both to illustrate the nature of money and to show how erroneous intrinsic value can be when one is assessing the economic potential of cryptocurrencies. This chapter acknowledges programmable money's political-economic potential, emphasizing how crucial its governance will be keeping freedom and democracy safe (the political question is further detailed in chapter 4). As seen throughout the chapter, digital tokens bring together all the characteristics and technical attributes of money (most of them with comparative advantages). However, the story does not end just like that. Unlike traditional currencies, cryptocurrencies and other digital tokens can be programmed to incorporate *labor* and *capital*, integrating both productive factors in the same unit of account for the first time in history. This financial chimera puts humankind on the verge of a multidimensional monetary system where cryptocurrencies can integrate social and individual incentives. A new architecture of financial incentives, which will be discussed throughout the chapter, may induce socially desired behaviors in producers and consumers. The author thinks that the new *crypto economy* will make it possible to use digital tokens to foster collective action in a decentralized way (without resemblances with collectivism). By endowing the free market's invisible hand with blockchain cryptographic credentials, it will be possible to shake that hand, making it visible to society, promoting the alignment between human ingenuity, ambition, and merit on the one hand, and ethical entrepreneurship socially endorsed by human values on the other. As seen in this chapter, private cryptographic keys will code free initiative in a liberal political scenario, protecting privacy to openly catalyze innovation, unleashing a myriad of cryptocurrencies integrating private financial incentives with the public interest, not only creatively incentivizing and rewarding individuals but nurturing social synergies in sustainable community ecosystems.

Chapter 4 is political, and one should acknowledge that it is framed by a liberal reformist political perspective and written in co-authorship with a Former Prime-Minister of Portugal and Former Mayor of Lisbon whose political positions are also well known. Entitled "Blockchanging Politics: Opening a Trustworthy but Hazardous Reforming Era," this chapter argues that digital centralization should not be a political option for free societies in the Blockchain Era. It presents political solutions and recommendations that figuratively can be equivalent to a vaccine against the ideological virus of single-thought because BT can also be used in a particularly virulent way. In the authors' opinion, for the worst scenario to materialize, it is enough that law-abiding citizens be prohibited from using private cryptographic keys to protect data's property and defend their privacy. As discussed throughout the chapter, such personal secret keys are digital passports to free initiative, privacy, and democracy. They are like *digital masks* that will protect citizens against contagions digitally spread in economic media vectors (social media and digital currencies) by authoritarian governments, especially when the centralized digital currencies enter the global financial mainstream. Probably, this will be the case of Digital Yuan, which is already booming in China. In this chapter, Digital Yuan and Bitcoin are comparatively watched, anticipating the clash between *surveillance money* and *money that sets people free*. It is thought that this confrontation will be much more than a financial dispute, introducing what probably will be the most crucial political dichotomy in the following decades: open/decentralized vs. closed/centralized. Blockchain cryptographic technologies are paving the way for establishing decentralized and transparent governance models based on community consensus. As seen in this chapter, transparency allows more auditable and granular governance models that will provide secure information through *public blockchains*. On the other hand, thanks to *smart contracts*, digital tokens can make citizens' will more actionable and be used as votes scrutinizing the government often, if there is the freedom to do so. However, unfortunately, instead of giving people a voice, BT can be used to do just the opposite, which should be a matter of great political concern. Indeed, digital money protocols can be used to serve society in good and evil ways, and this chapter discusses how to take political advantage of BT possibilities to increase governance transparency, which is anticipated as something truly essential in the Blockchain Era.

Chapter 5 is entitled "The Real Blockchain Game Changer: Protocols and DAOs for Coordinating Work to Provide Goods and Services." After the hierarchical organizations that drove institutions for thousands of years, followed by digital platforms that increasingly streamlined the creation of value in many areas in the last three decades, it is now time for *protocols* creating value in a new decentralized way. BT protocols make it possible to develop ecosystems and synergies between people by integrating the productive factors *labor* and *capital* in a way only possible thanks to advanced cryptographic techniques. Thus, creating new decentralized forms of governance is viable either in politics or other areas of social and economic interest through Autonomous Decentralized Organizations (DAO). This chapter explains DAOs straightforwardly and compellingly, presenting use cases that include decentralized finance projects (Defi). Although pioneer DAOs like Yearn (yearn.finance) presents competitive financial solutions, one should understand that money is just the beginning, and probably many other DAOs and decentralized apps (*dApps*) will thrive, delivering a vast array of products and services. DAOs protocols ensure growth by promoting a synergistic alignment between consumers who are also producers (*prosumers*) that add value, primarily through their intellect, and the required capital to start the projects, integrating it with the necessary *labor* to provide products and services. Four concrete DAO cases are presented: (i) censorship-resistant money; (ii) trustless operating system; (iii) permissionless hedge fund; (iv) trustworthy data feeds to decentralized applications.

Section 2 ends studying how BT can leverage e-commerce. As is well known, commerce has been a fundamental wealth generator for humanity, which justifies relating BT and e-commerce. The *pre-blockchain* Internet was endowed with significantly simplified information sharing protocols, and the business models have adapted accordingly: given the impossibility of charging for the consumption of content copied at practically zero cost, business models reengineering sought indirect and sophisticated profitable approaches extracting value from the very human tendency to share information to satisfy affiliation, self-esteem, and self-fulfilling needs, especially if there are no payments involved. Thus, "freemium" business models and tactics that artificially exacerbated market segmentation (deceptive marketing) have emerged using controversial biased algorithms to monetize users' data (see Chapter 1). However, direct commercial exchanges between people, *i.e.*, the simple purchase and sale of products and services, have always been the mainstay of human progress and economic development. Today, as BT's cryptographic protocols make it possible to preserve the originality of data transmitted on the Internet, it is possible to simplify and speed up digital transactions, which can now be carried out in decentralized markets, between individuals, and without intermediaries (see Chapter 3). It is thought that such democratization can take e-commerce to a higher level, justifying Chapter 6.

Chapter 6 is entitled "Combining E-Commerce and Blockchain Technologies to Solve Problems and Improve Business Results: A Literature Review." It presents a comprehensive and in-depth assessment on how BT can leverage *e-commerce*, identifying the advantages of combining blockchain and e-commerce, and raising foundation grounds for future research in this regard. Through thoughtful thematic analysis, this chapter points the spotlight to scientifically illuminate a way of leveraging e-commerce that is expected can be taken by humanity in favor of progress and wealth creation.

The third section of the book (Chapters 7 to 13) discusses BT's political and economic implications in *Healthcare*, covering how vital Blockchain is in different health issues, enabling a more *patient-centric* approach to Healthcare.

Chapter 7 is entitled "Application of Technology in Healthcare: Tackling COVID-19 Challenge: The Integration of Blockchain and Internet of Things." This chapter discusses the importance of blockchain and IoT technologies in the healthcare system. The number of medical devices that allow data collection and remotely interconnection increases exponentially every year, and the security problems due to the IoT architecture must be handled to ensure better privacy and security. A synergy between BT and IoT will help overcome these issues. The three cases explored in this article show the potential of integrating these two technologies in the healthcare sector, focusing on possible applications to face the COVID-19 crisis and its aftermath, making industries more resilient and help the public health systems cut costs improving healthcare.

Chapter 8 is entitled "Electronic Health Record Patient Portals and the BT." *Electronic Health Record Patient Portals* play a significant role in promoting *patient-centric* digital Health. Thanks to digital Health, patients can access their medical records, book appointments, and ask for prescription refills. *EHR Patient Portals* manage complex and sensitive patient data and should be able to support the transfer of data between different systems. Interoperability, confidentiality, and data consistency are critical features that should be embedded in the logic of *EHR Patient Portals*. BT comprises all these characteristics and should be used to support *EHR Patient Portals*.

Chapter 9 is entitled "A Concrete Way to Develop Clinical Research in a Fair Way to the Users/Patients Using BT." Combining the incorruptibility of BT with clinical research might be a powerful tool to re-establish trust in clinical data. Moreover, the introduction of this technology may allow patients to possess their clinical data and decide to share it in exchange for tokens representing financial gains and other benefits. Hence, this chapter describes how to develop clinical research fairly using BT, discussing the main advantages of blockchain-based technologies in this particular, focusing on some examples and the challenges of their implementation. On the other hand, it explores *patient-centric data monetization* using *smart contracts*.

Chapter 10 is entitled "Data Security in Clinical Trials Using BT." Clinical Trials are technically very complex studies that have to manage pharmaceutical drugs and patient data. Another challenge is connected with the fact that clinical trials often use multiple clinical sites and multi-country approaches. Concerns with security and data integrity in clinical trials encourage the use of BT, which comprises characteristics that include traceability, decentralization, immutability, and auditability critical to the success of clinical trial data management. This chapter maps the current use of blockchain systems in clinical trials, particularly data security managing systems, and their characteristics. It concludes that BT can produce a more transparent and tamper-proofing clinical trial by providing accurate, validated data, producing more reliable and credible outcomes in clinical trial research.

Chapter 11 is entitled "Blockchain and Clinical Data Economics: The Tokenization of Clinical Research in the EU." In this chapter, next-generation technologies in clinical research are presented, and innovative solutions are identified given their potential to accelerate biomedical research and give patients new tools to take control and monetize their data. Specifically, the current status of BT in the EU is presented, observing how it can impact the development of clinical research going forward. Several examples to put personal health data in the hands of the patient also be shown. This chapter enlightens the primary goal of using BT, which is to facilitate the interaction between organizations and individual data-owners, although blockchain integration in healthcare systems creates some technical challenges. Not less important are the misperceptions of different players (researchers, patients, funders) about BT, making it difficult to embrace this technology.

Chapter 12 is entitled "Dentacoin: A Blockchain-Based Concept for Dental Healthcare." Dentacoin is an excellent example of a community-based ecosystem (in the dentistry area) whose existence is only possible due to BT. After discussing BT and the new token economy, the chapter follows observing the case of Dentacoin, both a customer-centric and an industry-centric solution whose primary purpose is to improve dental care worldwide and make it affordable by reducing the costs and increasing the benefits for all participants. As more and more people earn Dentacoin (DCN) and use them in various ways, the value of the cryptocurrency can rise, which would give more freedom and trust to the Dentacoin Community. Indeed, the idea behind Dentacoin is a revolutionary technology, and it is thought that it will only be a matter of time before it reaches other areas of the healthcare industry once that Dentacoin numbers of users and partners are growing each day.

The book's third section ends with Chapter 13, entitled "Blockchain Pharma: A Prospective Overview." BT is at the epicenter of a progressive digital revolution which includes the pharmaceutical industry, where BT is changing the supply chain, clinical trials, and research, offering more transparency, traceability, and security. As it is highlighted in this last chapter, BT aggravates the dilemma between data centralization and the original vision of a decentralized Internet, namely because it provides the necessary confidence to transact value on the Internet even in the absence of intermediaries, and this disintermediation can be used predominantly in favor of patients or be focused on increasing other stakeholders' privileges. Throughout this chapter, the aim is to examine the eventual shift towards a health system where the patients are the legitimate owners of their medical records. As it will be seen, Estonia, perhaps the most digital country worldwide, stands out as an example of health systems modernization. This chapter discusses blockchain's structural characteristics and competitive advantages (immutability, transparency, and security) that it is thought will justify its wide use by the pharmaceutical industry. In the pursuit of greater process rationality and simplification, blockchain is applied in diverse areas as supply chain, clinical trials, and R&D. The author will present existing solutions that allow the end consumer to verify provenance and authenticity using a simple smartphone *app*. Finally, it will be observed how BT plays a crucial role in R&D, notably protecting intellectual property rights.

As of last remarks, the editor emphasizes that this book intends to convey that humanity is experiencing one of the most important, if not the most, inflection points in its social, political, and economic history.

If freedom prevails, which is not guaranteed, especially when times are tough, BT will allow taking advantage of the most remarkable reduction in transaction costs of human history, a value created by the new *distributed trust*. This historic landmark constitutes a unique opportunity to foster ethical entrepreneurship and sustainable human development.

As digital tokens are tradable without intermediaries and may carry specific workloads by integrating *labor* and *capital* valences (and not just capital like traditional money), money becomes a means of expressing other types of value in addition to the financial value in the restricted sense, and one must start reasoning upon monetary value in a broader sense. The new *multiverse of money* can now serve to express political, economic, and social wishes. Digital tokens are programmable and can be used to vote for achieving specific outcomes through self-executable contracts (*smart contracts*) that articulate resources in a decentralized, although structured way, allowing people to take options, make deals, and trigger deeds in many different areas, as explained throughout this book.

Dario de Oliveira Rodrigues
Instituto Politécnico de Santarém, Portugal

Section 1
Blockchain Ethics

The new developing ethical framework.

Chapter 1
Blockchanging Trust:
Ethical Metamorphosis in Business and Healthcare

Dario de Oliveira Rodrigues
https://orcid.org/0000-0002-2817-5115
Instituto Politécnico de Santarém, Portugal

ABSTRACT

By cutting transaction costs and streamlining agreements' execution via "smart contracts," blockchain technology (BT) turns decentralization into an economic advantage and an antidote against politically harsh decisions that can obliterate privacy, freedom, and democracy. Although BT's ethical bottom line is still uncertain, its use can smooth out the trade-off between privacy and convenience, reconciling both. BT can also help reconfigure the compromise between intellectual property rights and the common good, opening more ethical routes to the diffusion of innovation. BT's data security can be translated into straightforward access to information. On the one hand, this signals new inclusion routes for "identityless" and unbanked people, and on the other, it releases society from biased information and fake news providing access to trusted data. BT guarantees contents precision, distributing a consensual tamper-proof "hyperledger" proving transactions' authenticity and data's integrity. As consensus should be plural, BT's decentralization is thought to be a must in ethical terms.

INTRODUCTION

"Technology is neither good nor bad, nor is it neutral" (Kranzberg, 1986). Kranzberg's First Law

This chapter's main objective is to show why an ethical reform can be expected in a *new normal* (Berwick, 2020; Tam, 2021) time of shaken confidence, perhaps even more shaken than in the last financial crisis (2007-2008). Hence, the ethical impact of Blockchain Technology (BT) on the *Cyberethics-mix* will be considered, entailing four fundamental ethical issues to cope with in the cyberspace: (i) *Privacy*

DOI: 10.4018/978-1-7998-7363-1.ch001

of Personal Data; (ii) *Property Rights on Digital Data*; (iii) *Possibility of Accessing Information*; (iv) *Precision of Digital Content* (Rodrigues, 2012).

BT is a data management technology (Alcazar, 2017, p. 93) for distributed databases, which can be seen as an institutional or social technology for coordination (Davidson et al., 2016; Swan, 2015) that creates a "secure, robust, and transparent distributed ledger able to leverage resources within a global peer-to-peer network by building algorithmic trust" (Narayan, 2020, p. 121442).

Seeking to understand the political-economic implications of a new trust mechanism underlying human transactions that it is thought will profoundly change society, this chapter relates Internet evolution with the referred four ethical issues, especially noting business and healthcare.

First, it should be mentioned that this chapter emphasizes the author's liberal perspective. The chosen investigation method was based on qualitative research, using the literature review research methodology, which is considered adequate to overview several thematic areas on a given topic. Among the literature reviews available, the most used for business studies are systematic review, semi-systematic review, and integrative review (Snyder, 2019). Considering the need to carry out a synthesis to envision the intended ethical repercussions of BT, the author used the integrative literature review, which is indicated to frame a study from new perspectives, especially when it comes to research themes and topics little explored (Torraco, 2005), as is the case as far as the author was able to observe.

This chapter is sequentially organized to accomplish four specific objectives. The first one is to shed light on the evolving trade-off between privacy and convenience, highlighting that BT's protocol makes it possible to overcome secular privacy limitations and emphasizing that its innovative features eventually can be restrained by misinformed or mistaken (to say the least) political decisions. The chapter's second specific objective is to observe the trade-off evolution or the changing compromise between self-controlling personal data and public interest. The chapter's third specific objective is to remark how BT can catalyze access to information and digital inclusion (*e.g.*, access to financial services), assuring information integrity and avoiding a silo mentality usually justified by privacy constraints. It is also discussed why BT is a double-edged sword, which also can reinforce data centralization and the lust for power, pushing society into a worrisome non-democratic path. The chapter's fourth and last specific objective is to highlight the ethical importance of content precision and accurate information in a time of fake news and political distrust, showing that BT can deliver transparency and trust, eventually inspiring the wake of a Truth Age. Finally, the author presents solutions and recommendations, observes some technical limitations, advocates research priorities, and concludes.

BACKGROUND

Business Ethics and Trust

Defining business ethics, Somerville & Wood (2008) pointed out that "[it] focuses on how we use and should use traditional ethical views to evaluate how institutions orchestrate human behavior" (p. 143). It is known that ethics focuses on studying human conduct, but when it has to do with business, it is also essential to assess how institutions impact humans. Hence, it is crucial not losing sight of what is next, considering that Blockchain Technology (BT) allows even strangers to transact without intermediaries.

The blockchain protocol, which is based on a set of cryptographic techniques, ignited a second phase of the Internet, the definitive "Internet of Value" (Twesige, 2015), a decentralized operating system powered by BT that people can also use to transact value directly with each other and not only to share information as they did so far.

Enabled by blockchain technology, entrepreneurs and innovators have recognized the possibilities of creating an open financial system that has limited or no involvement from financial institutions. (...) Although this movement is still at its early stages, it showcases the potential of blockchain technology in spawning a new set of business models that are centered around decentralization and disintermediation. If this movement continues to gain momentum, it may start to disrupt existing industries and create new opportunities for entrepreneurship and innovation. (Chen & Bellavitis, 2020, p. 152)

It is known that decentralization avoids the vulnerability (*e.g.*, hacker attacks) inherent to the "single points of failure" from which trust is often conveyed over a network (Liu et al., 2018). "[There is] no single point of failure [when] records are on many computers and devices that hold identical information" (Kshetri, 2017, p. 70). However, decentralization comes with a problem: the lack of trust resulting from eventual disagreements between parties on every transaction. During millennia, such mistrust has relegated peer-to-peer (P2P) transactions to the reliable but small context of a family or a local group of trusted friends (*e.g.*, ancient tribes). Later on, such lack of trust was mitigated by relying upon trusted intermediaries, as will be seen next. Remarkably, this trust limitation was finally solved early this century (Nakamoto, 2008), with the invention of a new kind of trust based on consensus among peers.

As referred by Turkanović et al. (2018), "a blockchain node is any computer that has the core blockchain client installed and operates a full copy of the blockchain ledger" (p. 5115). The output of such ubiquitous data's replication is the so-called *distributed trust* (Bellini et al., 2020), which results from maintaining a unique, unmistakably, immutable, and verifiable timestamp of all transactions in a network, *i.e.*, an "hyperledger" (Nakamoto, 2008).

No bonds nor trust between business parties are needed anymore for contractual ties being established and settled between strangers, which the continuous trade of cryptocurrencies has shown for more than a decade. This distributed trust is also of paramount importance when using self-executable contracts ("smart contracts") in blockchain networks such as Ethereum (Hartel et al., 2019). It is essential to understand that BT empowers the Internet both to share information and transact value peer-to-peer. In other words, data can now also represent digital assets on the Internet. Thus, it is thought that such tokenized data will change the world financially, economically, and politically (precisely in this exact order).

[Tokenization] is the process of converting a piece of data into a random string of characters known as a token. Tokenization protects sensitive data by [replacing it with] non-confidential data. The token serves merely as a reference to the original data, but cannot be utilized to determine those values. (...) tokenization in essence allows you to compartmentalize personal data and manage them across different users simply and effectively. That data can therefore only be accessed by an entity who has the correct token. The information is secure and completely portable since the personal data is controlled by the individual and shared with permission, a stark difference to data that are being utilized currently. (Morrow & Zarrebini, 2019, pp. 221-222)

It is not surprising that BT's first application has been a cryptocurrency. Bitcoin has attracted attention and led to financial speculation, eventually distracting people from BT's true meaning, which is no less than altering the genesis of trust. Hence, the general understanding of what it can represent politically and economically was postponed.

The real promise of BT, then, is not that it could make you a billionaire overnight or give you a way to shield your financial activities from nosy governments. It's that it could drastically reduce the cost of trust by means of a radical, decentralized approach to accounting—and, by extension, create a new way to structure economic organizations. (Casey & Vigna, 2018, p.5)

BT's adoption brings a change in trust's very genesis (Casey & Vigna, 2018). This change is significant because "systems that alter the scope of trust change society" (Werbach, 2018). Before this technology was known, there were only three types of trust available:

1. Trust between peers (Schneier, 2012): held between family and friends, it is a kind of tribal trust only useful among groups with less than 150 individuals (Dunbar, 2010).
2. Confidence in the "rule of law": based on the social contract between the individual and the nation-state, giving the latter the institutional power to enforce agreements (Hobbes, 1914).
3. Trust in intermediaries: based on the dependence on centralized entities, like banks, that manage the trust necessary to ensure the smooth running of transactions (Datta & Chatterjee, 2008).

Nowadays, a fourth type of trust becomes available: *distributed trust.* As stated by Werbach (2018), "Bitcoin's blockchain mechanism just might have launched a revolution in trust." (p. 17). Over more than 30 years, the world witnessed the exponential growth of information shared by Internet users who have emancipated from traditional media thanks to a vibrant social media ecosystem. Social networks, blogs, and other applications (e.g., torrents) enabled social media and P2P sharing information. Drawing a parallel with the onset of the Internet's first economic media (social media), one can consider that humanity is now entering the second phase of the Internet, the moment in time when users started to carry out transactions with each other due to the onset of another economic media: the digital money (Beller, 2020). Thus, conveying both economic media when it encompasses information and money for the first time, the Internet contemplates both types of value (use and exchange value), becoming either ground-breaking or disruptive and entailing several ethical consequences.

Economic thinking has long distinguished "value-of-use" from "value-of-exchange" (Smith, 1937). "[Value is a word that] has two different meanings, and sometimes expresses the value of [using] some object, and sometimes [expresses] the power of purchasing other goods that the possession of that object conveys" (Smith, 1989, p. 47). In its first phase, the Internet's usefulness resulted from sharing information between users at a level never seen in human history. This sharing of information, nowadays mostly done through the services of a few giant multinationals (e.g., Facebook) that concentrate user's data and effectively control the Internet (Lopez et al., 2019), has made the *Internet of Information* an instrument of choice to provide a kind of value that users could not sell but have been using to fulfill human affiliation and self-esteem needs (Maslow, 1943). Significantly, during this process, users' data have been captured and *monetized* by digital media intermediaries who have obtained an enormous economic advantage in capturing the value of data extracted from users (Lopez et al., 2019). So, the product sold by Facebook to third parties has been precisely the same one that users have not been able to monetize themselves. Although this limitation is still endured on the Internet by billions of people, it is already technically solved, and things will probably be very different in the more or less near future, hopefully for the best if ethics, privacy, and freedom prevail.

Empowered by BT, the Internet entered the second phase of its existence. This second phase is also the last because there are only two types of economic value, and both are now served as economic media on the Internet: social media and digital currencies. Hence, besides sharing information, users can now directly trade digital assets on the Internet, transacting data with each other in the absence of intermediaries. In other words, the Internet is becoming an instrument of choice to decentralize data, democratize trade and let payments be made directly among users (P2P). As stated by Bergeron et al. (2020), "the blockchain is a brilliant concept for democratizing currency exchange and has been fully realized in many cryptocurrency implementations" (p. 51). Thus, according to several authors (Antonopoulos, 2017; Tapscott & Euchner, 2019; Visconti, 2020), this is the beginning of the so-called "Internet of Value" (IoV) where the middleman is not needed anymore.

Just like the internet that was introduced in the 1960s and late 1970s, is a communications protocol that governs the rules and regulations for information exchange over the network of networks, [blockchain] is a protocol that governs the rules and regulations for value exchange. One is the internet of information, while the other is the IoV. Internet is a communications protocol and Blockchain is value exchange protocol. With value being broadly defined. (Twesige, 2015, p. 3)

As the digital *copy-paste* procedure has no marginal costs, sharing data became a no-brain operation. Whoever shares digital information still will keep such's information utility, abdicating nothing. Therefore, digital sharing does not involve trust requirements (because there is no trade involved). On the other side, transacting is entirely different. Unlike sharing, trading implies giving up something and relying on the other parties' ability to respect deals. Transacting requires trust, which is equivalent to social capital, creating *reserves of goodwill* that facilitate business networking and optimize social relationships, thus increasing society's wealth (Werbach, 2018).

In the first phase of the Internet, the FTP-IP and HTTP protocols made it possible to democratize information sharing and bypass traditional media. Hence, the new digital media tycoons disintermediated the mass media sharing information process and re-intermediated it in an entirely new way. More recently, BT industrialized the generation of trust between peers (Berg et al., 2017), inaugurating an "Internet of Money" (Antonopoulos, 2016) and paving the way to democratize transactions, perhaps driving complete disintermediation of both economic media. If it is so, it is thought that this time things can change for good.

[Blockchain] could enable a new era of the Internet usage called the Internet of Value (IoV) in which any types of assets such as intellectual and digital properties, equity and wealth can be digitized and transferred in an automated, secure, and convenient manner. (Truong et al. 2018).

The same reasons that made and still make the internet a success, are the same ones that will make the Block Chain thrive. For example, its fast, public, open to anyone, cheap and easy to utilize, transparent and programmable. Just like how the internet made it possible to transfer information instantaneously from any part of the world, the Block Chain technology lets the users transfer value globally. (Twesige, 2015, p. 3)

It is thought that BT will be ubiquitous, and eventually, the IoV will notoriously impact society. After all, "if you look back at history, every time there was a big expansion in the world's economic activity, it was generally induced by the creation of a new form of trust." (Berg et al., 2019, p.4).

Concerning healthcare, it is thought that patient-centric applications powered by BT will play a decisive role in enabling more ethical healthcare businesses. Patient data is now "big data," and it turns out that BT allows a seamless health data integration without compromising security and confidentiality. Hence, BT can provide trust in real-time, data for predictive modeling and the generation of insights, ultimately improving patient involvement and satisfaction.

BT will reform the relationship with providers by offering solutions that safeguard data's integrity and privacy. Considering the current patients' inconvenience when accessing clinical data and health records, one can anticipate that BT will be highly transformative in healthcare. For example, in clinical trials, guaranteeing data's integrity is a fundamental professional and ethical obligation to protect patients and produce reliable results that can lead to new treatments and save lives. Observing the Estonian pioneer case, Heston (2017) stated that "the success of the Estonian medical record blockchain project will depend upon its ability to keep medical records private while at the same time widely available to medical providers [pharmaceutical companies,] and insurance companies.".

The world is witnessing a global implosion of trust with "public distrust of government, business, media, and NGOs" (Edelman 2017), and it is unlikely that the SARS CoVid-19 pandemic will contribute to reverse such tendency. Thus, trust is needed, and the author considers BT to be a game-changer in altering the rationale that justifies human conduct from an ethical point of view, implying a metamorphosis of the "cyberethics-mix" (Rodrigues, 2012). This ethical evolution will be covered in the following pages, just after a brief explanation of BT.

Blockchain Technology

On October 31, 2008, a white paper showed how to institute a protocol to distribute trust through a digital network (Nakamoto, 2008). This protocol is called *blockchain*, a set of cryptographic techniques that ensures data's authenticity, confidentiality, and integrity. The two former qualities are guaranteed by a digital signature system that uses a public and a private key mechanism called asymmetric encryption. It should be acknowledged that "encryption is said to be asymmetric because the key for encryption is different from the key for decryption (Martins, 2018, p. 24). Both keys only work in pairs: by signing a transaction with his private key, the sender guarantees data's authenticity as the recipient will only be able to decrypt data if he uses the sender's public key. In turn, by signing a transaction with the recipient's public key, the sender guarantees data confidentiality because only the recipient will be able to decrypt that data using his private key.

The digital signature system usually consists of two parts: a signature algorithm and a verification algorithm. The signature algorithm is used to generate a digital signature on the message, the signature is usually controlled by the signature key, the signature algorithm or the signature key is kept secret and is controlled by the signer. The verification algorithm is used to verify the digital signature of the message, and the message can be verified according to the signature effectively. The verification algorithm is usually controlled by the verification key, but the verification algorithm and the verification key are public, so the person who needs to verify the signature can easily verify it. (Zhai et al. 2019, p. 6)

Regarding the third quality of BT's protocol, data integrity, it can be guaranteed thanks to an algorithm called *hash*. The *hash function* transforms any data set, with variable size (there is a theoretical maximum size of 2'091'752 terabytes which in practice is unattainable), into a short sequence of characters with fixed size (a string of 256 bits in the case of bitcoin). Applying the hash function consecutively to a given data set whose integrity persists always results in the same hash string. It is easier to compare small sets of data, which means that comparing *hash values* is a safe way to check the data set's integrity without making exhaustive (perhaps unfeasible) comparisons. The *hash function* is not reversible, and even knowing the *hash value* of a given data set, there is no logical way to reconstitute that data set backward. Hence, the *hash function* allows both to safely check data's integrity and increase privacy concerning sensitive data (Nakamoto, 2008).

The hash algorithm is a function that maps a sequence of messages of any length to a shorter fixed-length value, and is characterized by susceptibility, unidirectionality, collision resistance, and high sensitivity. Hash usually used to ensure data integrity, that is, to verify the data has been illegally tampered with. When the data tested changes, its hash value also changes correspondingly. Therefore, even if the data is in an unsafe environment, the integrity of the data can be detected based on the hash value of the data. (Zhai et al. 2019, p. 3)

Therefore, blockchain cryptographic techniques guarantee data's authenticity, confidentiality, and integrity (Yaga et al., 2019), and blockchain-based decentralized distributed ledgers have shown to be viable (Berg et al., 2017). Hence, such *cryptographic cocktail* can be used for coordinating activity in a distributed economy (Davidson et al., 2016),

CYBERETHICS METAMORPHOSIS

Data Privacy

Privacy risks are associated with the uncontrolled disclosure of personal information (AICPA., 2020). The right to personal and family privacy has been considered one of the most fundamental rights of individuals. For decades it is consecrated as a human right (UN, 1948). The European General Data Protection Regulation also recognizes privacy as a right to which every person is entitled (GDPR, 2018). The philosopher Bertrand Russell (1931) considered that technology consists of a change from the contemplation of nature to its manipulation, and such a change carries risk (Marturano, 2002). Hence, given the extraordinary development of Information and Communication Technologies (ICT) and nowadays digital pervasiveness, it is understandable why privacy violation has become a preoccupying ethical concern.

ICT progress makes it necessary to employ fewer and fewer people in surveillance efforts, and limits to controlling citizens are no longer guaranteed by the numerical need to employ a significant part of the population in doing so, which opens the way for abuses and disproportionality in such monitoring (Brown & Korff, 2009). For this very reason, attacking the privacy of many people or even that of an entire population has never been easier than it is today. As Rodrigues (2012) pointed out, "it is important to mention the loss of some privacy as a tolerable downside of getting and securing a greater convenience [and] one could think that the fundamental ethical objective is to achieve a balance between the "need to know" and the "right not to divulge" (pp. 329, 330). However, ICT progress aggravated the privacy loss, and it seems reasonable to ask whether the present trade-off is justifiable, for instance in healthcare.

Decades ago, before computers came into widespread use, IMS [(Intercontinental Medical Statistics)] field agents photographed thousands of prescription records at pharmacies for hundreds of clerks to transcribe—a slow and costly process. Nowadays IMS automatically receives petabytes (1015 bytes or more) of data from the computerized records held by pharmacies, insurance companies and other medical organizations—including federal and many state health departments. Three quarters of all retail pharmacies in the U.S. send some portion of their electronic records to IMS. All told, the company says it has assembled half a billion dossiers on individual patients from the U.S. to Australia. (Tanner, 2016, p.26)

Privacy on the Internet of Information

As mentioned above, the first phase of the Internet was characterized by the then-new and disruptive possibility of sharing information between peers. Some companies early recognized the inherent value of this new reality, namely the Internet's potential to increase the marketing benefits of personalized products and services and how new digital resources could facilitate the job (Kotler, 1999; Kotler et al., 2016). As stated by Rodrigues (2012), "the possession of detailed information about customers allows companies to create personal profiles that lead to a better service rendering. This way, companies can provide consumers personalized offers." (p. 330).

Understanding that the exponential progress of ICT has been changing the game rules, tilting the marketing playfield so much that privacy can be overturned, the author mentioned, still in 2012, the disadvantage for privacy resulting from using social networks:

It is crucial the professional commitment of those who are responsible for social networks, which must be governed by its own code of ethics and promote a self-regulation that encourages an ethical participation of all users. After all, without a moral responsibility capable of accepting the sacred nature of the right of individuals to the privacy of their private lives and to the information they wish will remain confidential, the business practice on the Internet will constitute a continuing threat from an ethical point of view, always subsisting the risk of someone invading the privacy of others. (Rodrigues, 2012)

Some years later, taking a notorious example of privacy loss, one can say that the indignation caused by the Cambridge Analytica & Facebook scandal was justified by the unexpected exposure of about 50 million Facebook users' profiles (Cadwalladr et al., 2018), showing how deceptive can be the use of personal data by third parties. After all, even with recent stringent data protection laws in Europe and the USA, namely the General Data Protection Regulation (GPDR) and the California Consumer Privacy Act (CCPA), many companies still feed their business models with personal data to sell advertisements (Lopez et al., 2020).

A documentary shown in 2020 by cable TV operator NETFLIX presented the pungent testimony of former employees of some of the leading ICT multinational companies, increasing the awareness of privacy issues by denouncing that social media users have their data processed by algorithms that feed ethically doubtful business models (O'Neil, 2017). As mentioned by Rodrigues (2020), "[whistle-blowers explained] that these gigantic multinationals use artificial intelligence and sophisticated algorithms to become very rich, at an unprecedented pace, profiting from the emotions and opinions expressed by social media users."

According to Petrescu & Krishen (2020), such companies monetize personal information following "business models based on algorithms that encourage addiction and privacy breaches as features of social media platforms" (p.187). This encouragement can make sense from a business point of view, as it allows those digital platforms to make a strongly targeted segmentation of their users, increasing their appetite for specific ads. This because better-delineated segments are more valuable and reach higher prices for the advertising space disputed in online auctions. (Rodrigues, 2020).

To make things worse for users, there is a so-called privacy paradox identified by Barnes (2006), "according to which people often state to care about privacy, but at the same time freely relinquishes private information online" (Bleier et al. 2020, p. 26).

Known as the privacy paradox, it is a documented fact that users have a tendency towards privacy-compromising behavior online which eventually results in a dichotomy between privacy attitudes and actual behavior (...) Although users are aware of privacy risks on the internet, they tend to share private information in exchange for retail value and personalized services (Barth & De Jong, 2017, p. 1039)

This psychological vulnerability reaches worrying proportions in social networks. Ubiquitous digital platforms let users satisfy a long-time known hierarchy of needs (Maslow, 1943). Very profitable business models wisely predict that users do not need to be compensated for their loss of privacy other than by obtaining successive opportunities to climb a hierarchy of needs whose top is unreachable (King, 2009).

Instead of working to decrease consumers' privacy concerns, firms might therefore also aim to attenuate the negative effects of such perceptions by providing increased value in exchange, for instance through better service or lower prices - although that is admittedly tough if the price is already zero. (Bleier et al. 2020, p. 26).

For users, the trade-off is losing privacy in exchange for a so-called "better service." However, that service seems to have a never-ending exchange value, namely because users cannot monetize (and so, cannot perceive) the value of the data they give in exchange for losing privacy. Hence, monetizing data has been an extremely profitable business, especially for some ICT multinational companies (*e.g.*, Facebook) that set up an oligopoly or even a monopoly since "they grow very fast and that, in the end, often one winner remains" (Van der Aalst et al. 2019). Also, Taplin (2017) stated that this kind of business model seems to collide with privacy, freedom, and democracy.

As will be seen in the next sections, such an ethically reprehensible business reality can now change and should so. Blockchain Technology (BT) offers new possibilities concerning data ownership and business transactions on the Internet. After all, it may be time for data monetization to start working both ways, reverting as well to users and not only to "the giants of the internet [that] expanding into every corner of the economy, politics and our lives." (Alleman, 2018).

Concerning healthcare, ICT development makes choosing between privacy and convenience more complicated. As referred by Wildman et al. (2019), "Sweeney (2015) was able to match patient names to publicly available anonymized health data. [His studies] show that the claim that anonymized data poses no threat to privacy is dubious at best. (p. 35)

Currently, much of the open data available is spatial (geographic or satellite) data, which is relatively unproblematic to post online as it poses minimal privacy risks. However, for the full benefits of open data to be gained, this spatial data needs to be supplemented with information on welfare payments, hospital admission rates, income tax assessments and other potentially sensitive areas of government policy and administration which could drive innovation. As more and more datasets from these disparate policy areas are posted online, the greater the risk that individuals may be reidentified and their personal details exposed. (Hardy & Maurushat 2017, p.33).

Once upon a time, simply removing a person's name, address, and Social Security number from a medical record may well have protected anonymity. Not so today. Straightforward data-mining tools can rummage through multiple databases containing anonymized and non-anonymized data to reidentify the individuals from their ostensibly private medical records. (Tanner, 2016, p.27)

A particularly threatening tool that menace privacy rights is thought to be applications (apps) for smartphones and other mobile devices. Given the need to deal with an increasing volume of information, it is foreseeable that future apps will be equivalent to "digital prostheses" that will inevitably be part of everyday life. Accordingly, privacy issues will become more worrisome.

The apps that can help, for instance, to avoid humans' physical presence quickly proved to be indispensable in a pandemic. Hence, privacy concerns will probably grow. For example, in monitoring contagious diseases, the mandatory installation of such apps, advocated by certain politicians, has increased the controversy surrounding protecting privacy. As stated by Bengio et al. (2020), "the advent of the coronavirus disease 2019 (COVID-19) pandemic has seen widespread interest in the potential utility of automatic tracing apps, as well as concern over their potential negative effects on individual privacy" (p.1).

Other authors take their concern even further, considering freedom itself threatened. According to Rowe et al. (2020, p.1), "if the app is imposed, individuals will feel they are being surveilled, which raises immediate ethical concerns and may signal authoritarian regimes."

Seeking to obtain a comparative overview of various apps' privacy vulnerabilities, Wen et al. (2020) conducted a study of covid-19 contact tracing apps by performing a cross-platform comparison on 41 apps (26 Android and 15 iOS) "having obtained significant privacy concerning findings, including broadcasting users' fingerprints, tracking a specific individual, and collecting other mobile device information." (p. 14).

After observing some privacy concerns on the *Internet of Information*, the focus on privacy will now be shifted to the new *Internet of Value*.

Privacy on the Internet of Value (IoV)

The cryptographic resourceful blockchain technology (BT) both allows keeping the originality of digital information over the Internet (and consequently the value resulting from such exclusivity) and simultaneously overcoming severe limitations concerning privacy.

While the traditional privacy model limits personal data's public visibility, it does not prevent service providers from accessing that same data. However, the privacy model based on the blockchain protocol separates personal data from data owners' identities (see Figure 1). Separating people's identities from their data is now possible, "because metadata [*e.g.*, *hash values*] such as patient identity, visit ID, provider

ID, payer ID, etc. can be kept on a Blockchain, but the current [sensitive] records should be stored in a separate universal health cloud" (Karafiloski & Mishey, 2017, p. 767).

Figure 1. The privacy model metamorphosis overview (pre-blockchain & post-blockchain)

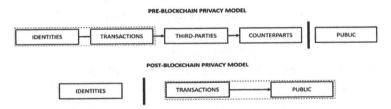

As mentioned in the previous section, digital interactivity facilitates consumers' profiling, and such knowledge allows the adaptation of products and services (Kotler et al., 2016). Meanwhile, most companies want to focus their businesses on distinctive competencies, gladly dispensing the burden of possessing data not relevant to their core business, mainly when this ownership implies liabilities in safeguarding customers' privacy under penalty of not comply with the law. These companies want to streamline their business processes and reduce their transaction costs (Coase, 1993). Therefore, there is a coincidence of interest between most companies and their customers regarding privacy issues, being that personal data control made by customers and data protection laws are no problem at all for most companies.

With the introduction of the General Data Protection Regulation (GDPR), the European Commission has provided a legal framework that aims to empower individuals in taking control of their personal information. Such control is not necessarily a disadvantage to parties processing personal information: when used properly, GDPR can actually facilitate data flows that used to be much more complicated. (Buyle et al., 2019, p.346)

There are not real reasons for personalization and privacy to be antagonists; good governance and regulation are the starting points that will allow the right controls to be in place for data to be collected in a meaningful and ethical way. Privacy, online and offline, is not about sharing information or leaving people alone, but about transparency on the methods used and the purposes sought. It is about each person's right to decide, free from commercial and governmental pressures and interests. (Garcia-Rivadulla, 2016, p.235)

However, although this ethical stance favoring privacy, there are significant exceptions in the ICT sector, as is the case for the largest multinationals responsible for a worrying asymmetry of information in society (Neitz, 2019). Thus, instead of being under citizens' control, information about people's lives is channeled to these powerful companies. Meanwhile, data centralization is probably happening in totalitarian states, as authoritarian political regimes try to collect data and concentrate information about their citizens seeking complete political control.

The reality is bleak: centralization is reigning in the cyberspace, with huge technological corporations controlling our data, and re-intermediation and control are stronger than ever in the so-called" sharing "economy. The Internet is also fragmented by countries, with many states imposing heavy controls to information and communication services. (Lopez et al., 2020, p. 901)

In this worrying ethical framework, the blockchain protocol may emerge to public eyes as *a trust-distributing formula* that endows the Internet with a functional language to transact value and not just to share information. It turns out that this change can result in both good and evil (Kewell et al., 2017), increasing ethical dilemmas.

Centralizing and controlling the ability to share information about user's preferences in social media raises ethical concerns, but the idea of combining that ability with the new BT features that make it possible to control consumers' digital transactions is even more worrisome. Centralized digital currencies can do this workload easily, either at the state level (Peters et al. 2020) or privately (Gerard, 2020). After all, everyone is a consumer, and it is not only privacy that eventually will be threatened but also the freedom of choice and democracy (see the same book, Chapter 4 - *Blockchanging Politics: Opening a Trustworthy But Hazardous Reforming Era*).

Some say that Central Banks Digital Currency is not cryptocurrency (Insight, 2021). However, it is indeed cryptocurrency, although centralized (Echarte Fernández et al., 2021), and there is a trade-off between privacy and accountability in any traceable digital currency as is the case of CBCD, which is "managed on a permissioned blockchain, i.e., only authorized entities are involved in transactions verification" (Barki & Gouget, p. 1).

A CBDC will also in some way need to address an innate tension between privacy and transparency, protecting user data from abuse while selectively permitting data mining for end-user services, policymakers, and law enforcement investigations and interventions. [...] This is typically achieved using advanced cryptographic primitives known as zero-knowledge proofs. [...] To reap the benefits of zero-knowledge proofs, participants must be able to generate and validate transactions containing encrypted data. (Allen et al., 2020, p. 2)

CBDC is programmable money, and "regulators and central banks are right to be cautious" (Ali & Narula, 2020, p. 13). However, citizens must be cautious because money is essential and digitally controlling it is not a question of minor importance. One should have in mind that "power corrupts and the absolute power corrupts absolutely" (Dewing, 2021, p. 74). As referred to by Bichler & Nitzan (2021), "the quest for capitalized power - and more and more of it - is the key driving force of modern capitalism." These authors stated the further warning that "U.S. subjects are likely to hear much more about the benefits of [many] processes that, they will be told, require them to accept ever-larger corporations and a much more authoritarian society" (Bichler & Nitzan, 2021). Furthermore, CBDC can also be issued by authoritarian governments, let alone the perils of a *post-Covid-19 new normal* (Berwick, 2020) corset influence even in democratic states.

[Although] programmability seems like a promising avenue (...) enabling privacy and auditability through cryptographic techniques will be necessary to reduce the risk of financial surveillance and misuse of data. [The question is] who will develop this system? Will it be an upstart cryptocurrency-based stable coin, or a coalition led by a large company like Facebook which already connects with billions of users globally? [...] In this case, exercising caution means understanding what the technology can and cannot do, whether by staffing up internally or partnering with technical organizations, and preparing for an

uncertain future. The industry is moving fast; the most perilous path of all is inaction. (Ali & Narula, 2020, p. 13)

Considering what is at stake in terms of citizens' privacy and freedom, transparency in handling digital currencies is a new ethical fundamental aspect of democracy. If it is true that such transparency is ensured in the case of data transmitted in *permissionless-blockchains* such as the Bitcoin network, the same cannot be said concerning the *permissioned-blockchains* where CBDC will be processed. Thus, CBDC blockchain protocols must be equipped with "advanced cryptographic primitives known as zero-knowledge proofs" (Allen et al., p. 43) and techniques such as "homomorphic cryptography" (Liu et al., p. 296) that can also have an essential role in securing electronic voting and protecting democracy. It is thought that these and other programming details should be open-sourced to guarantee "a traceable, transferable and divisible digital currency system that protects user's privacy while enabling the retrieval of user's identity in case of suspicious transactions, e.g., suspicion of fraud or money laundering activities" (Barki & Gouget, 2021).

This being said, hopefully decentralization brought about by BT may contribute to defending citizens' privacy rights, reducing the growing threat that hangs over freedom itself. After all, ciphered data can decisively contribute to optimizing the trade-off between "Privacy" and "Convenience," allowing new privacy standards by letting users own and control their data.

The blockchain recognizes the users as the owners of their personal data. Companies, in turn, can focus on utilizing data without being overly concerned about properly securing and compartmentalizing them. (…) [With such a] decentralized platform, making legal and regulatory decisions about collecting, storing and sharing sensitive data should be simpler. Moreover, laws and regulations could be programmed into the blockchain itself, so that they are enforced automatically. (Zyskind & Nathan, 2015)

It should be noted that these privacy guarantees also translate into competitive advantages for companies. As Bleier et al. (2020) pointed out, "consumers are more willing to permit marketers to use their information when the firm treats their information fairly" (p. 30), and "firms catering to consumers' privacy concerns may obtain a favorable market positioning relative to others who pay little attention to such concerns. Privacy can create opportunities." (p. 30). Governments could also benefit from such guarantees. According to Karafilovsky & Mishey (2017), "[blockchain] will help governments and other enterprises be liberated from the liability that data is becoming." (p. 767). For instance, the Estonian government has harness BT's potential In recent years (Meier et al. 2020).

The ethical concern with privacy protection is of paramount importance in healthcare. Data has value, and health data have enormous value. A multi-billion-dollar industry is currently built around data brokers that buy patients' health data from doctors and hospitals, anonymize it, and sell it to other firms to guide their pharma investments or better target their advertising (Tanner, 2016).

The possibilities opened by BT are changing the trade-off between privacy and convenience, making it possible to establish new privacy standards that let patients own and control their data. For instance, BT can be used to manage personal data and identities (Mainelli, 2017), facilitating the process of assessing individuals for enrolment to specific clinical trials (Bergeron et al. 2020) and transacting personal data such as Electronic Medical Records (Liu et al. 2018a, p.6)

[Distributed ledgers] can help you keep relevant health or qualification records at your fingertips. Using "smart" ledgers, you can forward your documentation to people who need to see it, while keeping control of access, including whether another party can forward the information. You can even revoke someone's access to the information in the future. (Mainelli, 2017, p.4)

As stated by Karafiloski & Mishey (2017), "losing control of privacy is what happens when social media networks are constantly collecting users' data, actions and habits" (p. 764), both in the case of social media and in the case of mobile apps. Concerning the so-called "contact tracing applications," it has been noticed that current solutions do not offer absolute privacy guarantees (Dehaye & Reardon, 2020). When using these apps, almost always the only way for a user to revoke access to personal data is to uninstall the application itself. Still, there is no guarantee that personal data will not exist forever on the companies' central servers that own this application or not will be transferred to third parties.

Users lose total control of what happens with the data afterwards and they cannot withdraw the permissions. Usually there is a privacy setting page on most of the social media sites, where users can limit what other people see about them. What they cannot control and configure is what the social media corporation sees. (Karafiloski & Mishev, 2017, p. 764)

One major concern with mobile applications is that users are required to grant a set of permissions upon sign-up. These permissions are granted indefinitely and the only way to alter the agreement is by opting-out. (Zyskind & Nathan, 2015, p.181)

There are also healthcare applications that use pseudo-anonymized data, sometimes presented as a guarantee of privacy. However, several studies point to the fact that this is not a way to ensure privacy, as such data can be combined and end up revealing personal information.

It was recently used to show that individuals in a simply anonymized mobile phone data set are re-identifiable from only four pieces of outside information. Outside information could be a tweet that positions a user at an approximate time for a mobility data set or a publicly available movie review for the Netflix data set. Unicity quantifies how much outside information one would need, on average, to reidentify a specific and known user in a simply anonymized data set. The higher a data set's unicity is, the more re-identifiable it is. It consequently also quantifies the ease with which a simply anonymized data set could be merged with another. (De Montjoye et al. 2015, p. 538)

Some authors mention several encryption techniques to reinforce BT's privacy guarantees. As stated by Hassan et al. (2019), "modern differential privacy algorithms in conjunction with blockchain, can eradicate the issue of privacy loss (p. 762).

Another promising technique is homomorphic encryption. Although it is "still not efficient enough for real-time applications" (Moore et al. 2014, p. 2793), homomorphic encryption "shows that stronger and cost-effective encryption schemes are possible to be added to blockchain technology to make it more suitable to security and privacy-based applications, specifically using artificial intelligence" (Yaji et al. 2018, p.85).

One can use homomorphic encryption techniques to store data over the blockchain with no significant changes in the blockchain properties. This ensures that the data on the blockchain will be encrypted, addressing the privacy concerns associated with public blockchains. The use of homomorphic encryption technique offers privacy protection and allows ready access to encrypted data over public blockchain for auditing and other purposes, such as managing employee expenses. Ethereum smart contracts provide homomorphic encryption on data stored in blockchain for greater control and privacy. (Zhang et al. 2019, p. 28)

Finally, it should be noted that BT has revealed, in practice, sufficiency in assuring privacy because asymmetrical encryption guarantees confidentiality, and the hash algorithm makes it impractical to reverse the encrypted data (Nakamoto, 2008). BT also has revealed to ensure convenience. As stated by Liu et al. (2018), "by implementing [blockchain based privacy-preserving data sharing, [the patients] can have complete control over their EMRs [(electronic medical records)] and the users or institutions can use data conveniently without any risk on patients' privacy." (p. 6)

Thus, it can be said that BT's cryptographic properties open a very promising avenue in terms of privacy protection. Hopefully, it will translate into increased individual autonomy, which can substantially impact politics, the economy, and healthcare.

Data Ownership

The ethical dilemma of choosing between protecting intellectual property rights or defending the public interest has been heightened in the digital age. Technological innovations and the creation of new products and services require substantial effort (time and money), so the desire to obtain some return on investment (ROI) is ethically defensible. On the other hand, considering the public convenience of disseminating innovations (*e.g.*, an essential vaccine), it becomes necessary to optimize the trade-off between intellectual property rights and the public interest.

There is no single answer to determine whether innovative ideas have an owner or whether only the expression of those ideas can be considered as belonging to a particular individual. Some will give more credit to the merit of intellectual creation, while others will judge that those creators did nothing more than use and express society's accumulated knowledge, often counting on others' work before him. If this answer makes a difference in people's lives, then this is an ethical dilemma, indeed. However, if this is not the case, it is just an ideological matter of opinion. To clarify which is the case, one should investigate the Blockchain Technology (BT) enabling role in the upcoming "Augmented Internet" (Dai, 2020).

Until recently, digital data ownership was not like physical ownership. The latter can be held and transferred indefinitely, while the former only works in specific contexts, and moving its value around on the Internet has not been possible without trustable intermediaries.

Indeed, sharing digital information does not require much effort because the marginal cost of doing *copy-paste* on the Internet is practically zero, so digital copies quickly become abundant. As a result of such immediate convenience, original data lose their exchange value as soon as shared on the Internet. Even if shared information keeps its usefulness, price instantly falls to zero (Anderson, 2009). Therefore, it becomes practically impossible to prevent someone (even anonymously) from making unauthorized copies and spreading them over the Internet, diminishing the value of the original pieces of information. As stated by Romer (2002), "technological change has substantially undermined the effective protection offered by copyright" (p. 213)

Although the *pre-blockchain Internet* was still incomplete and unable to endure peer-to-peer trade, its sharing features were competitive enough to create a digital economy that started to change the world right away. Hence, the first phase of the Internet brought difficult times to authors and data ownership. As such, since those days, a few powerful intermediaries took full advantage of the digital *status quo.*

Artists, designers and creative workers can share easily on the Internet, but keeping the right with proper attribution or getting fairly compensated has proven difficult in the digital world that we know. There is not a transparent way to own something that can be so easily copied and fully replicated, with no sign of the original. (...) Once the work is put online, or even sold online, the author loses control. (Karafiloski & Mishev, 2017, p. 766).

Ownership on the Internet of Information

The first stage of the Internet highlighted the competitive importance of networks (Castells, 2011). As referred by Power & Phillips-Wren (2011), "the value of a telecommunications network is proportional to the square of the number of connected users of the system" (p. 254). Success calls for creativity and cross-fertilization of projects and ideas from different minds and owners in such a competitive environment. Therefore, restrictive copyright laws are not flexible enough to allow creators to innovate and be competitive. Unfortunately, for many editors, the *free web content's paradise* became a living hell for many scarcity-based business models. Indeed, the traditional *copyright licenses* seemed to help neither authors nor consumers. Some less restrictive approaches paved their way, as is the case of *Creative Commons Licenses*, a legal framework that pursues competitiveness on behalf of authors by freeing creativity and innovation (Flew, 2005).

[Creative Commons] attempts to build on existing copyright law by offering a set of "some rights re-served" licenses designed primarily for authors and artists. Copyright owners who choose to release their work under a Creative Commons license disclaim some part of the default protection that attaches under statutory law. (...) Essentially, users of these types of licenses are reframing their "property right" protected by federal law into a contract right ordered by the terms of the agreement. (Goss, 2007, p. 964)

On the *Internet of Information*, the great enemy of authors and other digital producers was not piracy as it may seem, but instead obscurity. After all, popularity can be easily monetized on the Internet through advertising (Anderson, 2009). For instance, the Creative Commons type of licenses and the so-called *freemium* business models have been successful in the *pre-blockchain* phase of the Internet (Anderson, 2009; Günzel-Jensen & Holm, 2015).

As will be seen in the following section, Creative Commons Licenses can be articulated with BT, opening avenues for the transaction of digital assets (tokens) and streamlining business through "smart ledgers" (Mainelli, 2017) and "smart contracts" (Hartel et al. 2019).

During the past thirty years, data has become increasingly valuable (Jørgensen, 2020). The advances in ICT made it possible to massify data collection, storage, analysis, and application to the resolution of many problems, including in healthcare:

A growing number of companies specialize in gathering longitudinal information from hundreds of millions of hospitals' and doctors' records, as well as from prescription and insurance claims and laboratory tests. Pooling all these data turns them into a valuable commodity. Other businesses are willing to pay for the insights that they can glean from such collections to guide their investments in the pharmaceutical industry, for example, or more precisely tailor an advertising campaign promoting a new drug. (Tanner, 2016, p. 26)

The value of the clinical data used for clinical trial development only exceptionally reverts in favor of those who originate that same data. For instance, when such individuals have the chance to benefit as patients in those clinical trials directly and that is it. One cannot doubt that this redistributive system is unfair to those who have been information sources for years or decades without being paid.

For decades researchers have run longitudinal studies to gain new insights into health and illness. By regularly recording information about the same individuals' medical history and care over many years, they have, for example, shown that lead from peeling paint damages children's brains and bodies and have demonstrated that high blood pressure and cholesterol levels contribute to heart disease and stroke. To this day, some of the original (and now at least 95-year-old) participants in the famous Framingham Heart Study, which began in 1948, still provide health information to study investigators. (Tanner, 2016)

Tanner (2017) pointed out that "after a person gets medical care, pharmacies, insurers, labs, electronic record systems, and the middlemen connecting all these entities, automatically transmit patient data directly to what is, in effect, a big health data bazaar" (p. 2). One can notice that the numbers are getting more significant: "the data market in healthcare was estimated $14.25 billion in 2017 and is estimated to grow over $68.75 billion by the end of 2025." (Rooney et al., 2019, p. 19).

There is no doubt that clinical data is most profitable for some healthcare stakeholders that are almost exclusively information intermediaries, and the correspondent value can now be disputed by patients thanks to BT. As will be seen in the next section, BT opens an entirely new digital ownership world and data management permissions. As such, an "Augmented Internet" (Dai, 2020) is fitted to process *smart contract* operations nurturing *peer-to-peer* (P2P) trade among healthcare stakeholders, including patients. Moreover, this new digital reality is reaching and embracing the physical world, like it is happening in the energy sector (Bao et al., 2020).

Some P2P energy trading markets based on blockchain mainly use blockchain to realize market auction mechanism. The work in [Mengelkamp et al., 2018] proposed a decentralized market platform for consumers and prosumers in local energy markets based on the private blockchain. A central intermediary is never needed to manage local energy transactions. (Bao et al., 2020, p.5)

Ownership on the Internet of Value (IoV)

Empowered by BT, the Internet facilitates and makes the transaction of digital tokens ubiquitous. Tokens are units that quantify value, and they can represent digital assets (see Chapters 3 and 4). There are also tokens whose properties allow representing non-fungible assets.

Non-fungible tokens (NFT) are a class of tokens introduced in late 2017 with the ERC-721 standard. While fungibility – the ability to be substituted in place of one another – is an essential feature of any currency, non-fungibility is the opposite as every token is distinguishable and thus also cannot be di-

vided or merged. This also has implications for tracking the ownership of tokens as each NFT needs to be tracked separately. (Regner et al. 2019, p. 4)

[A non-fungible asset] is not equal to its counterparts. The most tangible example of a non-fungible asset is any sort of collectible. A baseball is just a baseball until it is signed by Babe Ruth. Then, it gains additional value and becomes a non-fungible asset, valued differently than all other baseballs out there. Non-fungible assets generally have a greater scarcity than fungible ones, and therefore hold more intrinsic and unique value. With scarcity and value now measurable in the digital realm through blockchain and distributed ledgers, we are just beginning to see the potential of non-fungible digital assets. (Muzzy, 2018)

The distinct properties of NFTs have opened a new type of digital representation of value, namely allowing the tokenization of individualized assets, a function prohibited to fungible tokens, which cannot digitally represent the exclusivity of assets such as physical ones.

According to the ERC-721 standard, each NFT has a unique identification, is transferable, and includes metadata (Entriken et al., 2018).

ERCs [see Key Terms and Definitions] are predefined rules developed using Smart Contracts for implementing token measures in Ethereum Blockchain. ERC-20 can define by providing the contract address and availability of tokens. (…) ERC-721 token standard supports Non Fungible Tokens. It makes these tokens have a unique value and identity. Tokens are attached to digital objects using metadata to help off-chain rendering or storage (Muthe et al. 2020, p. 75)

NFT's specific purpose is to represent the ownership of physical assets, such as houses or works of art, and digital assets such as music or exclusive photos. Therefore ERC-721 tokens cannot be divided because they represent an entire and indivisible asset. These tokens can be used in exchanges, but their value results from each one's uniqueness or singularity. They can also represent *negative value assets*, such as loan debts and other liabilities. This faculty is possible because NFT are distinguishable from each other, and it is possible to trace any of them (Entriken et al., 2018). As happens with so many other aspects related to the democratization of value transfers made possible by *blockchain cryptographic protocols*, it is believed that NFTs will contribute to the political-economic disintermediation making individuals more autonomous in managing their assets without resorting to intermediaries.

NFTs will change the market. The collectibles market has always been centralized. Topps made the money, not the baseball players. The same is happening again, with sports leagues like the NBA minting money on NFT videos. But that's just in the short term. Big companies will always make money, but expect more players and artists to get in on the action. The rise of NFTs holds the power to tear down some of those walled gardens and put power back in the hands of the creators and the athletes. (Jeffries, 2021)

The above-mentioned Creative Commons Licenses can now be fully integrated in a self-executable manner through *smart contracts*. This new operational granularity allows for more resourceful and innovative transactions to be carried out, eventually matching entrepreneurship and sustainable human development. As stated by Helbing (2017), "to benefit from the digital revolution, we need an entirely new approach. [...] We need to build an ecosystem of socio-economic activities, where each new idea, product, and service creates opportunities for further ideas, products, and services." (p. 316).

Therefore, the Creative Commons' flexible type of property rights license makes sense in the digital era, especially in the light of BT; as was described by Savelyev (2018), "it is possible to combine the simplicity of using open source/creative commons licenses with receipt of a licensee fee by the licensor. It can be facilitated by a set of standardized smart contracts, the terms of which can be described in a comprehensible language ("laymen code")" (p. 6).

Tokenization processes show a digital reality that was understood more than 25 years ago: the digital world has much more *elasticity* than the physical world (Negroponte, 1995), and such versatility is now reaching the financial world. This *digital plasticity* is now cryptographically encoded, conferring additional features to the one-dimensional money of the *pre-blockchain* era. It is believed that this is a historical shifting fact that soon will change, by this order, finance and economy (see the same book, Chapter 3 - *Blockchanging Money: Reengineering the Free World Incentive System*, and Chapter 4).

By allowing its users to trade fungible assets directly with each other and adding unique properties to non-fungible assets (changing the way one relates to these assets), BT increases individual autonomy and commercial dynamics, making it possible for everyone to transact globally in the absence of intermediaries.

When you are the sole owner of your personal data on purchases, online browsing history, or mobile data, you can also choose whether or not to "sell" your own data, with rights and restrictions using smart ledgers. This could shift the power of (and profit from) data management from big, established firms back to individual users. (...) Mutual distributed ledger systems have the potential to provide us with identity and activity management, even permitting us to make a market selling information about ourselves, taking control and cash back from companies (Mainelli, 2017, p.5)

In healthcare, clinical data eventually will contribute to a revenue redistribution, shifting value from shareholders to stakeholders (*e.g.*, patients). When everyone guarantees their health data's absolute ownership, any person can stipulate the conditions for aggregating their health data with other individuals, such as patient organizations and other health-related communities. As such, individuals will release and monetize data in the proportions agreed between themselves. *This type of collective action has nothing to do with collectivism because it is based on the decisive role of individual economic incentives.* Hence, incentives can now work according to community interests, paving the way for more public utility coming from civil society.

BT can be used to level the economic playing field, allowing individuals to gain bargaining power in the face of organizations that usually get patients' data without giving any financial consideration (although clinical data is precious, as seen above). Such bargaining power will come from a consensus on aggregated data's fair value, leading to balanced business agreements.

It must be mentioned that to understand the new "cryptoeconomy" (Buterin, 2017), one should know that collective action results from individual incentives, and that has nothing to do with collectivism (see Chapters 3 and 4).

Blockchains are generally positioned to disrupt processes reliant on centralized mediation or trust-based operations. Blockchains interoperating with end-user applications for managing personal medical data, i.e., medical data vaults, have been envisioned as effective mechanisms for individuals to share their medical data with researchers and receive tangible rewards, such as cryptocurrency payments, for such data sharing. (Bergeron et al. 2020, p. 45)

While privacy regulation alone can lead to a decrease in planning and operational health information exchanges, when coupled with incentives [cryptocurrencies], privacy regulation with requirements for patient consent can actually have positive effects on the development of health information exchanges efforts. (Bleier et al. 2020, p. 28)

In a blockchain society, public knowledge of transactions no longer has to imply bargaining to keep the underlying information private. So, it increases individual autonomy by allowing individuals to manage and store their digital identities. This way, it is possible to transact personal data in the absence of intermediaries and safely. Hopefully, disintermediation in healthcare will eventually lead to a more ethical distribution of wealth derived from patients' valuable data.

Data Accessibility

The ubiquity of ICT can and must make the world more human. Computers and the Internet are precious resources in the pursuit of individual and organizational goals. Therefore, access to such resources is fundamental, and it is crucial, from an ethical point of view, to observe how they should be distributed in society.

Individuals with access to an instrument as powerful as the Internet, will always be in a better position to achieve their objectives. Indeed, one concern regarding the social effects of computers is the fact that they could increase the cleavage between the more and the less favored individuals, and the gap between "have" and "not to have" may become the abyss between the "knowing" and "not knowing. (Rodrigues, 2012, p. 326)

According to World Bank statistics, there are currently one billion people without legal identity documentation worldwide (Allan & Mortensen, 2020). This exclusion hurts not only those persons but also the economy as a whole. Several authors have described that expeditious access to data is a fundamental condition for individuals' competitiveness. According to Bleier et al. (2020), citing Martin and Murphy (2017), "a competitive advantage may then not only materialize in terms of higher sales or market share but also increased access to consumer data" (p. 30).

Accessibility of data requires trust in whoever accesses it, whereby a way to solve the lack of trust raised on the Internet before the current transition for the *blockchain* era will now be discussed.

Accessibility on the Internet of Information

Even during the first phase of the Internet, the possibility of accessing information has been a controversial issue. The Internet was made technically possible by joining two inventions: the TCP / IP suite protocol, developed almost 50 years ago by the Defense Advanced Research Projects Agency - DARPA (Clark, 1988), thanks to their creators, Vinton Cerf and Robert Kanh (Leiner et al., 2009), and the HTTP protocol, developed more than 20 years later by Sir Tim Berners-Lee (Berners-Lee et al. 1996). The latter provided the Internet with "the lightness and speed necessary for distributed, collaborative, hypermedia information systems" (Berners-Lee et al. 1996, p. 1). Therefore, it was a joint effort, separated by more than two decades, that gave rise to the Internet.

The controversy about accessing the information on the Internet still exists; while updating or correcting detected data errors seems ethically irreproachable, the need to guarantee the integrity of the information and prevent, for example, the possibility of an individual falsifying his own identity advises to limiting access to information (Rodrigues, 2012).

The limitations due to privacy protection have contributed to maintaining a large volume of data in silos, making it difficult to interconnect and elaborate the ontologies necessary to develop a semantic web that aims to "making web content interpretable" (Euzenat & Rousset, 2020, p. 181). As referred in Sfetcu (2019) an ontology is a description (like a formal specification of a program) of the concepts and relationships that can exist for an agent or a community of agents, and Koufakis et al. (2020), citing Feilmayr and Wöß (2016), refined the definition of ontology stating that "An ontology is a formal, explicit specification of a shared conceptualization that is characterized by high semantic expressiveness required for increased complexity." (p. 3)

Today, there is an appeal for constructing the so-called *linked data*, an effort on a global scale sponsored by the World Wide Web founder, Sir Tim Berners-Lee. Disagreeing with the Internet's centralized path, he is trying to reverse such a situation with its "Solid" project (Buyle et al., 2019). His discomfort with the current data centralization on the Internet is understandable because it goes against the original idea mentioned by Leiner et al. (2009) regarding the creation of the Internet in the early 70s: "The Internet as we now know it embodies a key underlying technical idea, namely that of open-architecture networking" (p. 2).

Thus, not surprisingly, several authors propose to combine the new protocol developed by Berners-Lee for his latest project with the blockchain protocol, allowing users to maintain ownership and control of their data in a truly decentralized environment.

Combining Solid Pods and distributed ledgers in introducing complete decentralisation of data with total user-control, keeping the integrity of the stored information intact through Blockchain-based verification (…) These configurations introduce new dimensions on the Web and mobile applications' data storage that developers can benefit from building Distributed Applications (DApps) in a complete decentralised environment. (Ramachandran et al. 2020, p. 645)

It is thought that by freeing economic agents from the burden of protecting privacy, BT can streamline the data linkage process and the ontology engineering necessary for semantic web development.

As will be seen in the next section, the blockchain protocol optimizes the trade-off between the freedom to access information and the risks that this possibility entails. In healthcare, this risk limits patients' access to their health records and clinical data, but things can be different in the blockchain era.

Accessibility on the Internet of Value (IoV)

In the recently created IoV, which encompasses both *economic media* (social media and digital money), the possibility of accessing information will be more critical than ever before. The transaction costs reduction that BT made possible, especially by avoiding the cost of distrust (Davidson et al., 2018; Berg et al., 2019), should result in more straightforward digital information access. Such efficiency can help to ethically tackle global financial challenges, including those created by more than two billion people who have a mobile phone but no bank account (Bhyer & Lee, 2019), and at least one billion *identityless* individuals that cannot exercise citizenship. Hopefully, both these large groups of people will significantly benefit from *blockchain-based* proof-of-identity applications.

[Blockchain] allow the almost instantaneous transfer of digital tokens, if not at zero cost then at a significantly cheaper rate than established services. This makes the transfer of small amounts of currency economically viable, enabling new actors to enter the field and new opportunities (…) It might be anticipated, then, that reductions in the cost of financial transactions through DLTs [(Distributed Ledger Technologies)] will result in widening financial inclusion. (Kweel et al. 2017, pp. 19, 20)

By combining the decentralized blockchain principle with identity verification, a digital ID can be created that would act as a digital watermark which can be assigned to every online transaction. The solution can help the organizations to check the identity on every transaction in real time, hence, eliminating rate of fraud. Consumers will be able to login and verify payments without having to enter any of the traditional username and password information. (…) [An app] will store their encrypted identity, allowing them to share their data with companies and manage it on their own terms. (Jacobovitz, 2016, p. 3)

Decentralized apps (Dapps) eventually free many people who depend almost exclusively on social media oligopoly to communicate. Hopefully, they will help to avoid the politically dangerous "polarization, and dehumanization" (Hartel et al. 2020) derived from continuous social media's "fragmentation and polarization of audiences" (Hart et al. 2009; Sunstein, 2009).

Influential selection biases, indicating that citizens do not merely seek for congruence on the content level, but that sources and negativity biases also drive people's motivation to consolidate digital spaces that reassure consistent image of the self and potentially result in distorted and fragmented worldviews on the individual level. (Van der Meer, et. al, 2020, p. 958)

Today, healthcare data goes almost entirely to providers and intermediaries' databases. One of the reasons for this high centralization level is that privacy requirements limit information sharing by stakeholders. Thus, most patients rarely can access their health records directly.

By adopting blockchain networks that interconnect the various players in the health sector, patients will be able to access their own clinical and personal data, ensuring their confidentiality without resorting to intermediaries (Yaeger et al., 2019). This confidence is possible because the blockchain protocol provides an assignment to everyone, which lets patients take total control over access permissions and share their clinical data with complete security. Clinical data is aggregated to the individual and always accessible instead of being transmitted through intermediaries (Goldwater, 2016).

Furthermore, everyone's health data can be collected and added to the blockchain through the so-called *oracles* (see Chapter 3) bridging blockchains and the external world. It is thought that many *oracles* will be integrated into more and more mobile devices and *wearable interfaces,* such as glasses and bracelets equipped with biometric sensors, that will be part of the so-called *Internet of Things* (IoT).

In healthcare, IoT devices have the ability to provide real-time sensory data from patients to be processed and analyzed. Collected IoT data are subjected to centralized computation, processing, and storage. Such centralization can be problematic, as it can be a single point of failure, mistrust, data manipulation and tampering, and privacy evasion. Blockchain can solve such serious problems by providing decentralized computation and storage for IoT data. (Ray et al., 2020)

Using cryptographic keys, the patient obtains full control over the permissions necessary to share or transact his data with total security. The only necessary mediation will be provided by sensors and *oracles* that will be part of the IoT.

A blockchain oracle is a mechanism that fetches data from the external world to include it in the isolated execution environment of a blockchain. (…) Blockchain oracles are needed to bridge blockchains and the external world because of unique characteristics of blockchain. Some kinds of data in the external world are inherently unable to be independently validated by multiple distributed parties, for example because the data has restricted access, or is transient sensor data. Oracles import this kind of data as transactions into a blockchain. (Lo et al., 2020, p. 10658)

Finally, it should be added that governments can also benefit their social capital by increasing healthcare digital access, namely instituting government transparency and giving patients open access to healthcare information. For example, this openness and transparency already occur in Estonia, where e-health systems have been operational for over 20 years. As Metsallik et al. (2018) refer, "The main success factors for the e-health system in Estonia are clear governance, legal clarity, a mature ecosystem, agreement about access rights, and standardization of medical data and data exchange rules." (p. 1).

For the past decade, the Estonian government has been focusing on BT to increase government transparency and secure citizens' access to information. For example, "the Estonian eHealth Foundation started a new era in securing healthcare data by safeguarding off-chain stored EHRs [(Electronic Health Records)] using a blockchain protocol that logs all data access activities" (Einaste, 2018).

The blockchain ensures that users own and control their personal data. Our system respects the fact that the user owns the data and only gives access to the data to healthcare professionals after approval by the user. The access control is fine-grained, thus strengthening compliance with data privacy and data security. For example, users can revoke access authorizations at any time or grant one-time access only. Moreover, the accesses are logged transparently and traceably. (Meier et al. 2020, p. 2)

It is expected that BT will provide data accessibility and transparency to fulfill the ethical principles of free societies and democratic regimes. One should notice that the opposite direction, towards data centralization, appears to be ethically reprehensible and politically dangerous (Chapter 4).

Precision of Content

The progress of ICT has led to a situation where it has never been easier to access or distribute information. Unfortunately, data sharing on the Internet makes it easier to obtain and disclose false or incorrect information and, also, to manipulate or be manipulated even by correct information if tailored and repeatedly presented.

The author already mentioned the economic interest in signaling well-defined segments of users on social networks. This market segmentation aims to increase advertising performance, thanks to business models tunned to selling ads that become more profitable in case of user's profiles are well outlined.

There are reports that an artificially exacerbated market segmentation (deceptive marketing) and subsequent targeting practices lead to an information bias determined by algorithms that are "telling lies" (O'Neil, 2017. p.7). The ethical implications and practical consequences of such *fake news* and *biased content* are very harmful. The information interactively and iteratively conveyed in social media may persist as an erroneous and surreptitious input on users' decision-making processes on politics, economy, and healthcare.

[Algorithms] are merely "opinions embedded in mathematics" and reflect subjective goals and ideologies (…) Creators of said algorithms, unintentionally (or intentionally) weave "human prejudice, misunderstanding, and bias" into their models (…) The welfare of society depends on the benevolent use of data. (…) Algorithms filter, curate, and dictate the information consumed by the public, profoundly, "shap(ing) lives and outcomes as a consequence" (Berry, 2020, pp. 93, 94)

First, while mistakes may be unintentional, ignoring or even fostering mistakes is unethical. Second, by creating inscrutable algorithms, which are difficult to understand or govern in use, developers may voluntarily take on accountability for the role of the algorithm in a decision (…) algorithms are a less visible part of the decision and often less accessible to question—even being held secret. (Martin, 2019, pp. 129, 136)

Precision of Content on the Internet of Information

In the *pre-blockchain* stage of the Internet, besides critical user thinking, several indicators were already available about the authority, reliability, and credibility of content providers. These indicators came from "trusted third parties" (*e.g.*, Verisign) or the users themselves.

[Surowiecki's "crowd wisdom" (2005)] can quickly show each user the popularity and the level of acceptance of particular web content. This democratic criterion of popular validation is [integrated] in algorithms such as the Google company's PageRank, which uses [attention and reputation indicators] to determine [content] relevance (Rodrigues, 2012).

As stated by Kraft & Donovan (2020), "both people and platforms play roles in disinformation spreading" (p. 196), and there are many humans and sources of information on the Internet. After all, even a reckless child can post information, write a comment, or even make a website. As still pointed out by Kraft & Donovan (2020), "disinformation relates to the fragmentation of conversational contexts across platforms" (p. 196), and despite institutional seals, high levels of disinformation have been diminishing the confidence raised on the Internet.

Moreover, unlike traditional media, Internet sources can be anonymous or have only a virtual identity. Also, most content producers are small in size, not benefiting in any way from the credibility associated with the scale and reputation of traditional mass media, like TV channels, the press, and other gatekeepers of information in the industrial age.

Therefore, each time becomes more difficult for individuals to distinguish the important from the trivial on the Internet. As if all this were not enough, predatory business models and actors who take advantage of new digital possibilities with the deliberate intention of centralizing, compartmentalizing, and manipulating information aggravate the ethical problem of contents' imprecision.

Till now, the Internet was and still is very different from traditional mass media, and digital inter-activity is mostly responsible for this difference, shifting power from the emitter to the receptor, from broadcasting to narrowcasting (Hirst, et al., 2014), *i.e.*, from antennas and TV cables to the computers, smartphones, and other user's devices. Such interactivity turned consumers into "prosumers," who are not mere information recipients. "Prosumers" are both consumers and producers (Toffler & Alvin, 1980), and it is thought that in the same way that they share data on the Internet of Information today, they will trade every time more tokens on the Internet of Value in the years ahead.

Of course, when it is about business transactions, for instance, in the energy sector, data accuracy and content precision will become even a more critical factor than when it was just about data sharing.

Today, many households and office buildings have solar panels installed on their premises, and this allows them to be producers capable of selling surplus energy to others. This fostered the P2P concept of energy trading, by encouraging consumers to become prosumers (i.e., capable of both producing and selling surplus energy). This means that more energy is available, and consequently reduces overall energy costs. (…) Applying blockchain for energy trading has the potential to increase efficiency and security. (Ali et al., 2020, p. 2)

For all these reasons, it is increasingly important to investigate new ways to increase content's preci-sion on the Internet, considering that the use of new decentralized ways of doing so is likely to provide guarantees of plurality and exemption that are practically impossible to obtain when the legitimacy of the information is centrally dictated.

Here is where Blockchain Technology (BT) comes in, obviating the need to trust intermediaries and central specifications thanks to a new kind of legitimacy defined by consensus. In a blockchain, there is virtually no risk of someone changing previously validated information or delete it. As will be seen in the next section, when distrust and polarization induced by social media content reach unprecedented limits (*e.g.*, US Presidential Elections and Washington Riots), it is believed that the precision provided by BT applications will have an essential ethical role in modern society.

Precision of Content on the Internet of Value (IoV)

Blockchain Technology brought value to the Internet and empowered its users. This was possible be-cause blockchains work by widely distributing a consensual ledger on the web, which has proved to be an immutable source of truth, auditable by stakeholders, and capable of guaranteeing the authenticity and integrity of transactions carried out in cyberspace. Thus, this *smart ledger* was soon called an "hip-erledger" (Salem et al., 2008)

Traditional secure network design vests trust-relationship management and gatekeeping roles in a central actor with complete authority within the hierarchy of the network. Blockchain removes the re-quirements for centralized authority by removing the need for the trust management middleman role. (…) Its game-changing design secures and inscribes data, protecting it from tampering and corruption (Alcazar, 2017, pp. 92, 93)

As stated by Kewell et al. (2017), "a blockchain is a ledger of transactions of digital assets: of who owns what, who transacts what, of what is transacted and when" (p. 9), and therefore blockchains are known as "smart ledgers" which "allow for the storage and future execution of computer programs, so-called smart contracts" (Carter, 2018, p. 8).

Blockchains are ledgers (or databases) and anything that can be coded into a ledger can be recorded on a blockchain. The most obvious data are numbers recording units of account. But strings of numbers can be used to represent identities, or programs, and in this way, ledgers can become units of computation. (…) What blockchains bring to the internet are public ledger protocols. What this does, in effect, is to turn the internet into a 'public computer', or a 'world computer.' (Davidson et al. 2017)

Blockchain Technology (BT) is a powerful "trust machine" (Economist, 2015). It will have profound implications for society, especially by allowing the execution of *smart contracts*, which applications are not limited to the financial sector, going from the detection of *fake news* and *deepfake*, to the creation of a new type of political confidence based on cryptography.

It is crucial to have techniques to detect, fight, and combat "deepfake" digital content that may include fake videos, images, paintings, audios, and so on. Achieving this purpose is not difficult if there is a credible, secure, and trusted way to trace the history of digital content. Users should be given access to a trusted data provenance of the digital content, and be able to track back an item in history to prove its originality and authenticity (Hasan & Salah, 2019, p. 41596)

The application of the blockchain protocol to ensure data's accuracy is a mark to the economy. As mentioned above, BT makes it possible to create tokens that certify fungible assets (*e.g.*, guaranteeing their provenance) or prove non-fungible ones' genuineness (*e.g.*, artwork uniqueness). Not least, tokens will streamline transactions. For example, the fungible tokens can perform speedy transactions with no middleman (Grover et al., 2019), and the non-fungible ones can allow partial ownership of expensive items that are yet illiquid because of their price tag so that many more individuals can own them and transact them (Dai, 2020).

Blockchain is like a register that stores transactions in an accruable, safe, transparent, and traceable way. As a secure and distributed register of transactions, blockchain is being explored as a means of reliably certifying the origins and history of particular products: whether in terms of securing food supply chains, or in recording the many linked acts of creation and ownership that define the provenance of an artwork. In the future, we may adopt the same solution wherever there is a need to ensure (or establish) the originality and authenticity of some artefact, be it a written document, a photo, a video or a painting. (Floridi, 2018, p. 321)

Smart-contracts can specify business terms, including those necessary to assure content precision. In a few words, *smart-contracts* remove distrust not only from business equations but also from digital interactions in general. For instance, they can be used to authenticate a video and avoid *deep fakes*, *i.e.*, "hyper-realistic videos that apply artificial intelligence (AI) to depict someone say and do things that never happened" (Westerlund, 2019, p. 39). In this case, the *smart-contract* may include attributes and variables to register the video's details and its owner's data.

Smart contracts typically codify the business logic of a blockchain application. For example, a lottery contract contains logic that decides when the player wins the jackpot, and what percentage of each bet will go to the owner of the lottery. (…) Millions of smart contracts have already been deployed on Ethereum. Consistent with all human endeavour, the developers of smart contracts are striving for success. (Hartel et al. 2019, p. 177539)

Smart contracts can also have parameters that include the editing and distribution permissions of a video according to contractual clauses. This convenient integration is done through code and math, and the entire execution of the contract is immediately registered, being that the *hash* of the video will forever seal its authenticity. Therefore, if a user wants to track a video to its source, he can easily do that. This blockchain's method is a remarkable way to verify *contents' pedigree*, and it works well with data stored in any digital format, as is the case of decentralized files storing systems:

We provide a solution [using] smart contracts to trace and track the provenance and history of digital content to its original source even if the digital content is copied multiple times. The smart contract utilizes the hashes of the Inter-Planetary File System (IPFS) used to store digital content and its metadata. (…) IPFS generates a unique hash which is the address of a bundle of files containing the video content and its metadata. The hash address is used to locate and access the bundle of files stored on the IPFS network. (Hasan & Salah, 2019, pp. 41596, 41598)

Stored files can also be bundled with property rights agreements and deployed in "smart-contracts, and "[that] bundle can include a file containing the terms and conditions agreement of copying and editing in case the video [or any other data format] to be copied to create [or remix] different content by other authors or artists." (Hasan & Salah, 2019, p. 41598)

It is thought that *smart-contracts* will be very relevant in healthcare. For example, they can determine which specific health data will be shared with researchers accredited by the university A or instead by paying the amount X. They also can be executed on a specific date or if blood test results have a particular value. In the first case, the smart-contract would be executed by unblocking a payment when calendar date Y arrived, while in the second case, the *smart-contract* would be fulfilled by sending a medical prescription when the blood test reached a Z level. In yet another example, a researcher can hire N participants for clinical trials, doing so based on a quantification of a given variable, for instance, genetic (Gn), therapeutic (Tn), or demographic criteria (Dn). It should be noted that researchers must be able to stipulate contractual conditions without having access to the patients' identity. On the contrary, as long as patient data belong to intermediaries, clinical trial participants will continue not to be *hired* but instead recruited. This usual terminology can be quite revealing of the interests at hand, namely showing the absence of financial compensation for the *recruited* ones. In summary, *smart-contracts* guarantee precision to clinical research while ensuring that patients themselves will control their clinical data (Srinivasan, 2017).

Finally, BT also makes it possible to eliminate counterfeit medicines, ensure knowledge of provenance, and track the pharmaceutical industry's supply chain. This provenance checking is essential, directly impacting a patient's health and augmenting consumer trust. Among many other applications, BT can be used to check medical records (*e.g.*, vaccination bulletins) or manage safe transactions with stakeholders, for example, insurance companies (IEEE, 2018).

SOLUTIONS AND RECOMMENDATIONS

As stated by Kranzberg (1986), "technology is neither good nor bad; nor is it neutral" (p. 545), and it is the way technology is used that dictates the respective outcomes, both for good and evil. Thus, technological innovations dispense *a priori* ethical justifications. As referred by Keweel et al. (2017), "innovations are morally and ethically instantiated" (p. 429). Nonetheless, although it does not make sense from an ethical point of view to evaluate a technology innovation by itself, it is worth evaluating it in terms of its effectiveness and transformative potential. In the case of Blockchain Technology (BT), "study shows that there are huge potentials to use blockchain technology" (Lorne et al. 2018, p. 107), and this is a potentially disruptive technology (Frizzo-Barker et al. 2020).

Data's centralization is being promoted by "tech giants as data-driven intellectual monopolies" (Rikapp & Lundvall, 2020, p. 2). Sure, these colossal data silos organize their innovation activities but can delay data sharing and compromise privacy and complicate data linkage, preventing ontologies from being made to create a fully semantic web. As those data silos are too big, it also can perish competition and the free market. Only when information is securely shared, cross-fertilization of ideas can occur, and innovation can thrive. Therefore, openness is considered an ethical solution, which is why BT, "as a data management technology" (Alcazar, 2017, p.93), should be recommended.

As it is known, the electronic health records (EHR) repository is fragmented across healthcare providers and other stakeholders. Decentralized tamper-proof data repositories can be combined with a data management system to avoid patient data leakage and arbitrary modifications on personal clinical data. Such modifications should not be done by anyone other than the patients themselves or whoever delegated by them (*e.g.*, clinicians). Therefore BT-based data management solutions can be the right choice aiming at safety and convenience.

Sharing and transacting health data is crucial to improving healthcare service (including self-service) and reducing medical costs. Hence, distributed BT-based networks can facilitate patient data collection by creating a reliable environment for a secure data exchange and eliminating the privacy problem. This environment can solve, for example, ethical-legal problems in running clinical trials. BT also should be considered to create supply chain traceability solutions, letting patients have access to information about the provenance and validity of medicines, increasing consumer confidence and safety.

Finally, by implementing secure blockchain networks in healthcare services, patients regain ownership of their health data. Being in control of own data is required to share or transact it safely to satisfy patients 'needs and their communities' healthcare goals. Finally, it is thought that this rationale generally applies to other sectors of society.

LIMITATIONS AND FUTURE RESEARCH DIRECTIONS

There are limitations inherent to the Internet itself that can prevent Blockchain Technology (BT) from ethically fulfilling its democratizing potential. Internet basic functionalities depend on very few service providers, and the Internet is controlled by only a few multinational companies (Jensen, 2020). As stated by Lopez et al. (2019), "Even though the Internet design is inherently decentralized, in practice, key functionalities rely on a very few service providers, who support and thus may effectively control the Internet." (p. 1901). Hopefully, BT will decentralize the political-economic playing field, mostly when user-friendly decentralized apps (dApps) become available, reducing the costs of trust and empowering users with the cryptographic resources needed to use blockchains without losing their privacy (see Chapter 4). Therefore, the investigation of such dApps is crucial for ethical reasons, allowing building more competitive solutions to lower transaction costs, which most economic agents will appreciate.

There are also technical limitations in the blockchains themselves. According to Qin & Gervais (2018), *the scaling trilemma* dictates that blockchains can have at most two of the following three properties: *decentralization*, *scalability*, and *security*. This technical trade-off is related to performance aspects, such as the slow rate of transactions featured on *public-permissionless blockchains*, which are freely accessible. These blockchains have no hierarchical constraints to work, and although such absence of authoritative parts eventually makes them function too slow as more computation tasks are required, that is the price to pay for having a *trustless* system just based on sophisticated math, namely a *cocktail* of cryptographic functions.

The governance of *public-permissionless blockchains* is entirely decentralized, which can be advantageous, but their programming and maintenance, in charge of the so-called *core developers*, is complex. Without getting into technical specifications, which are out of this chapter's scope, there are reasons to believe that more agile and versatile solutions will arise from using better algorithms and *hybrid blockchains*. There are at least two hybrid solutions to optimize the trade-off mentioned above: *private-permissionless blockchains*, which allow more privacy by restricting transactions log viewers and more security by extending consensus participants, as well as *public-permissioned blockchains*, which allow gaining speed by restricting consensus participants, and more transparency by extending log viewers. The latter combines transparency and scalability gains with the privacy and security limitations inherent to centralization, sacrificing the *non-censorship resistance* as authoritative nodes can override/delete any commands. The former combines privacy and security gains with the scalability limitations of consensus (Neitz, 2019). It is thought that these and other BT technical limitations (some inflated as is the case of alleged electricity excessive consumption dealt with in the homonymous section of Chapter 4) will be overcome because its protocols are evolutionary and are being improved since its creation. This improvement effort has already produced alternative consensus protocols (*e.g.*, *proof-of-stake*), which can validate and record transactions more efficiently (Irresberger et al., 2020). As such, BT's Research and Development (R&D) should focus on the trade-off between network speed, scalability, and privacy on the one hand and the consensuses' transparency and security on the other.

Finally, one should notice that if more than half of the blockchain networks' computer nodes accept incorrect information as legit, this information will become the network accepted truth. Such a problem is called *the 51% attack*, and "adversaries controlling more than half of the total hashing power of a [blockchain] network can perform this attack" (Sayeed & Marco-Gisbert, 2019, p. 1788). Hence, the R&D of trustable consensus mechanisms is crucial to reducing transaction costs by improving BT's efficiency and safety. Thus, this is a top research priority, and the referred *cyberethics-mix* will benefit from improved blockchain governance (see Chapter 4). Hopefully, such governance will be decentralized to safeguard citizens' privacy, property accessing rights, content precision, transparency, plurality, and democracy.

CONCLUSION

On the one hand, blockchain technology (BT) allows democratizing several political-economic prerogatives once exclusively used by public and private intermediaries. On the other hand, BT grants centralizing governance even further, and Central Bank Digital Currency (CBDC) is a good example of that. Such ambivalence raises ethical dilemmas as a new confidence-building mechanism unleashes distributed trust on the new Internet of Value decisively changing the political power dynamics.

Thanks to blockchain protocols, Internet users can share and transact *zero-knowledge proofs* (see *Key Terms and Definitions*) about which data is valid and who stands for that validity without revealing the data itself. In this way, identity owners do not need to store private data or personal information on a blockchain network to use and transact that same data. What is stored is just cryptographic code that represents the data but hides sensitive information. This way, for the first time, people can have the best of two worlds: privacy and convenience.

Enabling data interoperability without compromising its security and confidentiality, BT is changing the data management paradigm. Blockchain-powered *decentralized apps* (see *Key Terms and Definitions*) will make it possible to store the consumers' encrypted identities, solving personal data management's ethical constraints hampering the stipulation of business terms, especially for privacy reasons.

Data accuracy can be used to prove data genuineness. Such precision allows creating *smart contracts*, which are self-executable and can be used to automate business transactions, making them irrevocable, assuring transparency, and guaranteeing accountability. Smart contracts can also ensure privacy and data ownership rights, being widely applicable in many situations. For example, they can be used to prove data authenticity (*e.g.,* clearing fake news) and guarantee government accountability, for instance, binding political promises to electoral results. This blind trust is possible because smart contracts deliver immutable budget allocation (see Chapter 4).

BT also reduces complexity and costs in healthcare, making it possible for patients to become the sole owners of their data. Once released from privacy constraints, patient communities will be able, for example, to aggregate and monetize individual health records according to their collective interests, such as participating or not in specific clinical trials.

Supposing that free-market prevails, one can expect that user-friendly decentralized applications (*dApps*) will change healthcare, including pharmaceutical research and development (R&D). Aggregated data increases the bargaining power of patients' communities facing healthcare intermediaries. Thus, blockchain-enabled business networks can induce a redistribution of value, transferring it from shareholders to stakeholders. BT will also make it possible to eliminate counterfeit medicines, safely check medical records (*e.g.,* vaccination certificates) and guarantee safe transactions with other stakeholders (*e.g.,* insurance companies), among many other applications.

BT can change the data management paradigm decentralizing transactions and redistributing wealth by democratizing value transfer prerogatives, paving the way to a more ethical society. In 2012, the author figuratively referred to the need for an ethical computer engineer to apply the appropriate digital technologies to safeguard people's rights in the digital era. Hopefully, there will be political discernment in the present decade to unleash the new distributed trust so that people themselves can play the role of that ethical engineer.

REFERENCES

AICPA. (2020). *Privacy Risk Management*. Available online at: https://www.aicpa.org/interestareas/informationtechnology/resources/privacy-risk-management.html

Alcazar, C. V. (2017). Data you can trust. *Air and Space Power Journal, 31*(2), 91–101.

Ali, F., Aloqaily, M., Alfandi, O., & Ozkasap, O. (2020). *Peer-to-Peer Blockchain based Energy Trading*. arXiv preprint arXiv:2001.00746.

Ali, R., & Narula, N. (2020). *Redesigning digital money: What can we learn from a decade of cryptocurrencies. Digital Currency Iniative (DCI)*. MIT Media Lab.

Allan, K., & Mortensen, J. (2020). Legal Identity Documenting in Disasters: Perpetuating Systems of Injustice. In Natural Hazards and Disaster Justice (pp. 261-278). Palgrave Macmillan.

Alleman, J. (2018). Threat of Internet Platforms: Facebook, Google, etc. In *29th European Regional Conference of the International Telecommunications Society (ITS): "Towards a Digital Future: Turning Technology into Markets?"*. Trento, Italy: International Telecommunications Society (ITS).

Allen, S., Čapkun, S., Eyal, I., Fanti, G., Ford, B. A., Grimmelmann, J., & Zhang, F. (2020). *Design Choices for Central Bank Digital Currency: Policy and Technical Considerations (No. w27634)*. National Bureau of Economic Research. doi:10.3386/w27634

Anderson, C. (2009). *Free: The future of a radical price*. Random House.

Antonopoulos, A. M. (2016). *The internet of money* (Vol. 1). Merkle Bloom LLC.

Antonopoulos, A. M. (2017). *Mastering Bitcoin: Programming the open blockchain*. O'Reilly Media, Inc.

Bao, J., He, D., Luo, M., & Choo, K. K. R. (2020). A survey of blockchain applications in the energy sector. *IEEE Systems Journal*, 1–12. doi:10.1109/JSYST.2020.2998791

Barki, A., & Gouget, A. (2020). *Achieving privacy and accountability in traceable digital currency*. Cryptology ePrint Archive, Report 2020/1565.

Barnes, S. B. (2006). A privacy paradox: Social networking in the united states. *First Monday, 11*(9). Advance online publication. doi:10.5210/fm.v11i9.1394

Barth, S., & De Jong, M. D. (2017). The privacy paradox–Investigating discrepancies between expressed privacy concerns and actual online behavior–A systematic literature review. *Telematics and Informatics, 34*(7), 1038–1058. doi:10.1016/j.tele.2017.04.013

Beller, J. (2020). Economic Media: Crypto and the Myth of Total Liquidity. *Australian Humanities Review, 66*, 215–225.

Bellini, E., Iraqi, Y., & Damiani, E. (2020). Blockchain-based distributed trust and reputation management systems: A survey. *IEEE Access: Practical Innovations, Open Solutions, 8*, 21127–21151. doi:10.1109/ACCESS.2020.2969820

Bengio, Y., Ippolito, D., Janda, R., Jarvie, M., Prud'homme, B., Rousseau, J. F., ... Yu, Y. W. (2020). Inherent privacy limitations of decentralized contact tracing apps. *Journal of the American Medical Informatics Association: JAMIA*. Advance online publication. doi:10.1093/jamia/ocaa153 PMID:32584990

BergC.DavidsonS.PottsJ. (2017). Blockchains industrialise trust. Available at SSRN 3074070.

Berg, C., Davidson, S., & Potts, J. (2019). BT as economic infrastructure: Revisiting the electronic markets hypothesis. *Frontiers in Blockchain, 2*, 22. doi:10.3389/fbloc.2019.00022

Bergeron, J., Nguyen, A., Alt, C., Brewster, N., Krohn, T., Luong, V., ... Moss-Pultz, S. (2020). Simulating patient matching to clinical trials using a property rights blockchain. *Digital Medicine, 6*(1), 44. doi:10.4103/digm.digm_30_19

Berners-Lee, T. Fielding, R. & Frystyk, H. (1996). *Hypertext transfer protocol--HTTP/1.0*. Academic Press.

Berry, P. (2020). Troubleshooting algorithms: A book review of Weapons of Math Destruction by Cathy O'Neil. *The McMaster Journal of Communication, 12*(2), 91–96. doi:10.15173/mjc.v12i2.2450

Berwick, D. M. (2020). Choices for the "new normal". *Journal of the American Medical Association, 323*(21), 2125–2126. doi:10.1001/jama.2020.6949 PMID:32364589

Bichler, S., & Nitzan, J. (2021). *Corporate Power and the Future of US Capitalism*. Real-World Economics Review Blog.

Bleier, A., Goldfarb, A., & Tuckerc, C. (2020). Consumer privacy and the future of data-based innovation and marketing. *International Journal of Research in Marketing, 37*(3), 466–480. doi:10.1016/j.ijresmar.2020.03.006

Brown, I., & Korff, D. (2009). Terrorism and the proportionality of internet surveillance. *European Journal of Criminology, 6*(2), 119–134. doi:10.1177/1477370808100541

Buterin, V. (2017). *Introduction to Cryptoeconomics*. Paper presented to Ethereum Foundation.

Buyle, R., Taelman, R., Mostaert, K., Joris, G., Mannens, E., Verborgh, R., & Berners-Lee, T. (2019, November). Streamlining governmental processes by putting citizens in control of their personal data. In *International Conference on Electronic Governance and Open Society: Challenges in Eurasia* (pp. 346-359). Springer.

Cadwalladr, C., & Graham-Harrison, E. (2018). Revealed: 50 million Facebook profiles harvested for Cambridge Analytica in major data breach. *The Guardian, 17*, 22.

Carter, S. (2018). *Timestamping Smart Ledgers: Comparable, Universal, Traceable, Immune*. Timestamping Smart Ledgers-Long Finance.

Casey, M. J., & Vigna, P. (2018). In blockchain we trust. *MIT's Technology Review, 121*(3), 10–16.

Castells, M. (2011). *The rise of the network society* (Vol. 12). John Wiley & Sons.

Chen, Y., & Bellavitis, C. (2020). Blockchain disruption and decentralized finance: The rise of decentralized business models. *Journal of Business Venturing Insights, 13*, e00151. doi:10.1016/j.jbvi.2019.e00151

Clark, D. (1988, August). The design philosophy of the DARPA Internet protocols. In *Symposium proceedings on Communications architectures and protocols* (pp. 106-114) 10.1145/52324.52336

Coase, R. H. (1993). *The nature of the firm: origins, evolution, and development.* Oxford University Press.

Dai, C. (2020). DEX: A DApp for the Decentralized Marketplace. In *Blockchain and Crypt Currency* (pp. 95–106). Springer. doi:10.1007/978-981-15-3376-1_6

Datta, P., & Chatterjee, S. (2008). The economics and psychology of consumer trust in intermediaries in electronic markets: The EM-Trust Framework. *European Journal of Information Systems, 17*(1), 12–28. doi:10.1057/palgrave.ejis.3000729

DavidsonS.De FilippiP.PottsJ. (2016). Disrupting governance: The new institutional economics of distributed ledger technology. Available at SSRN 2811995. doi:10.2139srn.2811995

Davidson, S., De Filippi, P., & Potts, J. (2017). Blockchains and the economic institutions of capitalism. *Journal of Institutional Economics, 14*(4), 639–658. doi:10.1017/S1744137417000200

DavidsonS.NovakM.PottsJ. (2018). The cost of trust: a pilot study. Available at SSRN 3218761.

De Montjoye, Y. A., Radaelli, L., Singh, V. K., & Pentland, A. S. (2015). Unique in the shopping mall: On the reidentifiability of credit card metadata. *Science, 347*(6221), 536–539. doi:10.1126cience.1256297 PMID:25635097

Dehaye, P. O., & Reardon, J. (2020, November). Proximity Tracing in an Ecosystem of Surveillance Capitalism. In *Proceedings of the 19th Workshop on Privacy in the Electronic Society* (pp. 191-203). 10.1145/3411497.3420219

Dewing, M. (2021). Combining Social & Legal Constructions: Constitutional Reformations for the Future. *FAU Undergraduate Law Journal*, 57-79.

Dunbar, R. (2010). *How many friends does one person need? Dunbar's number and other evolutionary quirks.* Faber & Faber.

Echarte Fernández, M. Á., Náñez Alonso, S. L., Jorge-Vázquez, J., & Reier Forradellas, R. F. (2021). Central Banks' Monetary Policy in the Face of the COVID-19 Economic Crisis: Monetary Stimulus and the Emergence of CBDCs. *Sustainability, 13*(8), 4242. doi:10.3390u13084242

Economist. (2015). The promise of the blockchain: The trust machine'. *The Economist, 31*, 27.

Einaste, T. (2018). *Blockchain and healthcare: the Estonian experience—e-Estonia.* https://eestonia.com/blockchain-healthcare-estonian-experience/

Entriken, Evans, & Sachs. (2018). *ERC-721 Non-Fungible Token Standard.* Retrieved from https://eips.ethereum.org/EIPS/eip-721

Euzenat, J., & Rousset, M. C. (2020). Semantic web. In *A Guided Tour of Artificial Intelligence Research* (pp. 181–207). Springer. doi:10.1007/978-3-030-06170-8_6

Feilmayr, C., & Wolfram, W. (2016). An Analysis of Ontologies and Their Success Factors for Application to Business. *Data & Knowledge Engineering, 101*, 1–23. doi:10.1016/j.datak.2015.11.003

Flew, T. (2005). Creative Commons and the creative industries. *Media and Arts Law Review*, *10*(4), 257–264.

Floridi, L. (2018). Artificial intelligence, deepfakes and a future of ectypes. *Philosophy & Technology*, *31*(3), 317–321. doi:10.100713347-018-0325-3

Frizzo-Barker, J., Chow-White, P. A., Adams, P. R., Mentanko, J., Ha, D., & Green, S. (2020). Blockchain as a disruptive technology for business: A systematic review. *International Journal of Information Management*, *51*, 102029. doi:10.1016/j.ijinfomgt.2019.10.014

Garcia-Rivadulla, S. (2016). Personalization vs. privacy: An inevitable trade-off? *IFLA Journal*, *42*(3), 227–238. doi:10.1177/0340035216662890

GDPR. (2018). *General data protection regulation (GDPR)*. Intersoft Consulting.

Gerard, D. (2020). *Libra Shrugged: How Facebook Tried to Take Over the Money*. David Gerard.

Goldwater, J. (2016). The use of a blockchain to foster the development of patient-reported outcome measures. In *ONC/NIST Use of Blockchain for Healthcare and Research Workshop*. Gaithersburg, MD: ONC/NIST.

Goss, A. K. (2007). Codifying a commons: Copyright, copyleft, and the Creative Commons project. Chi.-. *Kent L. Rev.*, *82*, 963.

Grover, P., Kar, A. K., Janssen, M., & Ilavarasan, P. V. (2019). Perceived usefulness, ease of use and user acceptance of blockchain technology for digital transactions–insights from user-generated content on Twitter. *Enterprise Information Systems*, *13*(6), 771–800. doi:10.1080/17517575.2019.1599446

Günzel-Jensen, F. & Holm, A. B. (2015). Freemium Business Models as the Foundation for Growing an E-Business Venture: A Multiple Case Study of Industry Leaders. *Journal of Entrepreneurship, Management and Innovation, 10*.

Hardy, K., & Maurushat, A. (2017). Opening up government data for Big Data analysis and public benefit. *Computer Law & Security Review*, *33*(1), 30–37. doi:10.1016/j.clsr.2016.11.003

Harel, T. O., Jameson, J. K., & Maoz, I. (2020). The Normalization of Hatred: Identity, Affective Polarization, and Dehumanization on Facebook in the Context of Intractable Political Conflict. *Social Media + Society*, *6*(2). doi:10.1177/2056305120913983

Hart, W., Albarracín, D., Eagly, A. H., Brechan, I., Lindberg, M. J., & Merrill, L. (2009). Feeling validated versus being correct: A meta-analysis of selective exposure to information. *Psychological Bulletin*, *135*(4), 555–588. doi:10.1037/a0015701 PMID:19586162

Hartel, P., Homoliak, I., & Reijsbergen, D. (2019). An Empirical Study Into the Success of Listed Smart Contracts in Ethereum. *IEEE Access: Practical Innovations, Open Solutions*, *7*, 177539–177555. doi:10.1109/ACCESS.2019.2957284

Hasan, H. R., & Salah, K. (2019). Combating deepfake videos using blockchain and smart contracts. *IEEE Access: Practical Innovations, Open Solutions*, *7*, 41596–41606. doi:10.1109/ACCESS.2019.2905689

Hassan, M. U., Rehmani, M. H., & Chen, J. (2019). Differential privacy techniques for cyber physical systems: A survey. *IEEE Communications Surveys and Tutorials*, 22(1), 746–789. doi:10.1109/COMST.2019.2944748

Helbing, D. (2017). From remote-controlled to self-controlled citizens. *The European Physical Journal. Special Topics*, 226(2), 313–320. doi:10.1140/epjst/e2016-60372-1

Heston, T. (2017). *A case study in blockchain healthcare innovation*. Academic Press.

Hirst, M., Harrison, J., & Mazepa, P. (2014). *Communication and new media: From broadcast to narrowcast*. Oxford University Press.

Hobbes, T. (1914). *Leviathan*. Dent.

IEEE SA Beyond Standards. (2018). *Leveraging Blockchain for Clinical Trials/Research*. Available at: https://beyondstandards.ieee.org/leveraging-blockchain-clinical-trials-research/

Insight, A. (2021, May 30). *Digital Currency v/s Cryptocurrency: Brief Overview for Beginners*. Retrieved May 30, 2021, from https://www.analyticsinsight.net/digital-currency-v-s-cryptocurrency-brief-overview-for-beginners/

IrresbergerF.JohnK.SalehF. (2020). The Public Blockchain Ecosystem: An Empirical Analysis. Available at SSRN. doi:10.2139srn.3592849

Jacobovitz, O. (2016). *Blockchain for identity management*. The Lynne and William Frankel Center for Computer Science Department of Computer Science. Ben-Gurion University.

Jeffries, D. (2021, May 21). *Dan Jeffries: It's 2031. This Is the World That Crypto Created*. Retrieved May 22, 2021, from https://www.coindesk.com/its-2031-this-is-the-world-that-crypto-created

Jensen, J. L. (2020). *The Medieval Internet: Power, politics and participation in the digital age*. Emerald Group Publishing.

Jørgensen, R. F. (2020). The right to privacy under pressure. *Nordicom Review*, 37(s1), 165–170. doi:10.1515/nor-2016-0030

Karafiloski, E., & Mishev, A. (2017, July). Blockchain solutions for big data challenges: A literature review. In *IEEE EUROCON 2017-17th International Conference on Smart Technologies* (pp. 763-768). IEEE. 10.1109/EUROCON.2017.8011213

Kewell, B., Adams, R., & Parry, G. (2017). Blockchain for good? *Strategic Change*, 26(5), 429–437. doi:10.1002/jsc.2143

King, P. W. (2009). *Climbing Maslow's pyramid*. Troubador Publishing Ltd.

Kotler, P. (1999). *Marketing management: The millennium edition* (Vol. 199). Prentice Hall.

Kotler, P., Kartajaya, H., & Setiawan, I. (2016). *Marketing 4.0: Moving from traditional to digital*. John Wiley & Sons.

Koufakis, A., Chatzakou, D., Meditskos, G., Tsikrika, T., Vrochidis, S., & Kompatsiaris, I. (2020). *Invited keynote on IOT4SAFE 2020: Semantic Web Technologies in Fighting Crime and Terrorism: The CONNEXIONs Approach.* Academic Press.

Krafft, P. M., & Donovan, J. (2020). Disinformation by design: The use of evidence collages and platform filtering in a media manipulation campaign. *Political Communication, 37*(2), 194–214. doi:10.10 80/10584609.2019.1686094

Kranzberg, M. (1986). Technology and History:" Kranzberg's Laws. *Technology and Culture, 27*(3), 544–560. doi:10.2307/3105385

Kshetri, N. (2017). Can blockchain strengthen the internet of things? *IT Professional, 19*(4), 68–72. doi:10.1109/MITP.2017.3051335

Leiner, B. M., Cerf, V. G., Clark, D. D., Kahn, R. E., Kleinrock, L., Lynch, D. C., ... Wolff, S. (2009). A brief history of the Internet. *Computer Communication Review, 39*(5), 22–31.

Liu, J., Li, X., Ye, L., Zhang, H., Du, X., & Guizani, M. (2018a, December). BPDS: A blockchain based privacy-preserving data sharing for electronic medical records. In *2018 IEEE Global Communications Conference (GLOBECOM)* (pp. 1-6). IEEE.

Liu, J., Li, B., Chen, L., Hou, M., Xiang, F., & Wang, P. (2018, June). A data storage method based on blockchain for decentralization DNS. In *2018 IEEE Third International Conference on Data Science in Cyberspace (DSC)* (pp. 189-196). IEEE.

Liu, T., Cui, Z., Du, H., & Wu, Z. (2021). Privacy-Preserving and Verifiable Electronic Voting Scheme Based on Smart Contract of Blockchain. *International Journal of Network Security, 23*(2), 296–304.

Lo, S. K., Xu, X., Staples, M., & Yao, L. (2020). Reliability analysis for blockchain oracles R. *Computers & Electrical Engineering, 83*(10658), 2.

Lopez, P. G., Montresor, A., & Datta, A. (2019, July). Please, do not decentralize the Internet with (permissionless) blockchains! In *2019 IEEE 39th International Conference on Distributed Computing Systems (ICDCS)* (pp. 1901-1911). IEEE.

Lorne, F. T., Daram, S., Frantz, R., Kumar, N., Mohammed, A., & Muley, A. (2018). Blockchain Economics and Marketing. *Journal of Computer and Communications, 6*(12), 107–117.

Magyar, G. (2017, November). Blockchain: Solving the privacy and research availability tradeoff for EHR data: A new disruptive technology in health data management. In *2017 IEEE 30th Neumann Colloquium (NC)* (pp. 135-140). IEEE.

Mainelli, M. (2017). Blockchain could help us reclaim control of our personal data. *Harvard Business Review Digital Articles*, 2-5.

Martin & Murphy. (2017). The role of data privacy in marketing. *Journal of the Academy of Marketing Science, 45*(2), 135-155.

Martin, K. (2019). Designing Ethical Algorithms. *MIS Quarterly Executive, 18*(2).

Martins, P. (2018). *Introdução à Blockchain.* FCA-Editora de Informática, Lda.

Marturano, A. (2002). The role of metaethics and the future of computer ethics. *Ethics and Information Technology*, *4*(1), 71–78.

Maslow, A. H. (1943). A Theory of Human Motivation. *Psychological Review*, *50*, 370–396.

Meier, P., Beinke, J. H., Fitte, C., & Teuteberg, F. (2020). Generating design knowledge for blockchain-based access control to personal health records. *Information Systems and e-Business Management*, ●●●, 1–29.

Mengelkamp, E., Notheisen, B., Beer, C., Dauer, D., & Weinhardt, C. (2018). "A blockchain-based smart grid: Towards sustainable local energy markets," Comput. Sci.-. *Research for Development*, *33*(1-2), 207–214.

Metcalfe, B. (1995). Metcalfe's law: A network becomes more valuable as it reaches more users. *InfoWorld*, *17*(40), 53–54.

Metsallik, J., Ross, P., Draheim, D., & Piho, G. (2018). Ten Years of the e-Health System in Estonia. CEUR Workshop Proceedings.

Monkiewicz, J. (2020). New Finance: In Search for Analytical Framework. Academic Press.

Moore, C., O'Neill, M., O'Sullivan, E., Doröz, Y., & Sunar, B. (2014, June). Practical homomorphic encryption: A survey. In *2014 IEEE International Symposium on Circuits and Systems (ISCAS)* (pp. 2792-2795). IEEE.

Morrow, M. J., & Zarrebini, M. (2019). Blockchain and the Tokenization of the Individual: Societal Implications. *Future Internet*, *11*(10), 220.

Muthe, K. B., Sharma, K., & Sri, K. E. N. (2020, November). A Blockchain Based Decentralized Computing And NFT Infrastructure For Game Networks. In *2020 Second International Conference on Blockchain Computing and Applications (BCCA)* (pp. 73-77). IEEE.

Muzzy, E. (2018). *CryptoKitties Isn't About the Cats*. Retrieved from https://medium.com/@everett. muzzy/cryptokitties-isnt-about-the-cats-aef47bcde92d

Nakamoto, S. (2008). *A peer-to-peer electronic cash system*. Bitcoin. https://bitcoin.org/bitcoin.pdf

Nakamura, Y., Zhang, Y., Sasabe, M., & Kasahara, S. (2020). Exploiting smart contracts for capability-based access control in the Internet of Things. *Sensors (Basel)*, *20*(6), 1793.

Narayan, R., & Tidström, A. (2020). Tokenizing coopetition in a blockchain for a transition to circular economy. *Journal of Cleaner Production*, *263*, 121437.

Negroponte, N. (1995). *Being Digital–A Book (P) review*. Wired.com, 3.

Neitz, M. B. (2019). The Influencers: Facebook's Libra, Public Blockchains, and the Ethical Considerations of Centralization. *NCJL & Tech.*, *21*, 41.

O'Neil, C. (2017). How can we stop algorithms telling lies? *The Guardian*, 7-16.

Peters, M. A. Green, B. & Yang, H. (2020). *Cryptocurrencies, China's sovereign digital currency (DCEP) and the US dollar system*. Academic Press.

Petrescu, M., & Krishen, A. S. (2020). The dilemma of social media algorithms and analytics. *J Market Anal, 8,* 187–188. https://doi.org/10.1057/s41270-020-00094-4

Power, D. J., & Phillips-Wren, G. (2011). Impact of social media and Web 2.0 on decision-making. *Journal of Decision Systems, 20*(3), 249–261.

Ramachandran, M., Chowdhury, N., Third, A., Domingue, J., Quick, K., & Bachler, M. (2020, April). Towards Complete Decentralised Verification of Data with Confidentiality: Different ways to connect Solid Pods and Blockchain. In *Companion Proceedings of the Web Conference 2020* (pp. 645-649). Academic Press.

Ray, P. P., Dash, D., Salah, K., & Kumar, N. (2020). Blockchain for IoT-Based Healthcare: Background, Consensus, Platforms, and Use Cases. *IEEE Systems Journal.*

Regner, F. Urbach, N. & Schweizer, A. (2019). *NFTs in Practice–Non-Fungible Tokens as Core Component of a Blockchain-based Event Ticketing Application.* Academic Press.

Rikap, C., & Lundvall, B. Å. (2020). Big tech, knowledge predation and the implications for development. *Innovation and Development,* 1-28.

Rodrigues, D. (2012). Cyberethics of Business Social Networking. In E-Marketing: Concepts, Methodologies, Tools, and Applications (pp. 756-780). IGI Global.

Rodrigues, D. (2020, October 29). *The Dangerous Business Model of Social Networks.* Observador. https://observador.pt/opiniao/o-perigoso-modelo-de-negocio-das-redes-sociais/

Romer, P. (2002). When should we use intellectual property rights? *The American Economic Review, 92*(2), 213–216.

Rooney, L., Rimpiläinen, S., Morrison, C., & Nielsen, S. L. (2019). *Review of emerging trends in digital health and care.* A report by the Digital Health and Care Institute.

Rowe, F., Ngwenyama, O., & Richet, J. L. (2020). Contact-tracing apps and alienation in the age of COVID-19. *European Journal of Information Systems,* 1–18.

Salem, A. O., Safeia, M. T. A., & Siam, S. M. (2008). *Report of Blockchain Techniques and Applications.* Academic Press.

Savelyev, A. (2018). Copyright in the blockchain era: Promises and challenges. *Computer Law & Security Review, 34*(3), 550–561.

Sayeed, S., & Marco-Gisbert, H. (2019). Assessing blockchain consensus and security mechanisms against the 51% attack. *Applied Sciences (Basel, Switzerland), 9*(9), 1788.

Schneier, B. (2012). *Liars and outliers: enabling the trust that society needs to thrive.* John Wiley & Sons.

Sfetcu, N. (2019, February 17). *Blockchain Design and Modelling.* SetThings. https://www.setthings.com/en/blockchain-design-and-modelling/

Smith, A. (1937). *The wealth of nations.* Academic Press. (Original publication 1776)

Smith, A. (1989). Of the Origin and Use of Money. In General Equilibrium Models of Monetary Economies (pp. 47-53). Academic Press.

Somerville, I., & Wood, E. (2008). Business ethics, public relations and corporate social responsibility. In *The public relations handbook* (pp. 143–160). Routledge.

Srinivasan, P. (2017, November 9). *Healthcare Blockchain: How smart contracts could revolutionize care delivery*. Prolifics.

Sunstein, C. R. (2009). *Going to extremes: How like minds unite and divide*. Oxford University Press.

Surowiecki, J. (2005). *The wisdom of crowds*. Anchor.

Sweeney, L. (2015). Only you, your doctor, and many others may know. *Technology Science*, *2015092903*(9), 29.

Szabo, N. (2002). *The Origins of Money (No. 0211005)*. University Library of Munich.

Tam, K. P. (2021). The new normal of social psychology in the face of the COVID-19 pandemic: Insights and advice from leaders in the field. *Asian Journal of Social Psychology*, *24*(1), 8.

Tanner, A. (2016). For Sale: Your Medical Records. *Scientific American*, *314*(2), 26–27. Retrieved November 30, 2020, from https://www.scientificamerican.com/article/how-data-brokers-make-money-off-your-medical-records/

Tanner, A. (2017). *Strengthening protection of patient medical data*. The Century Foundation.

Taplin, J. (2017). *Move fast and break things: How Facebook, Google, and Amazon have cornered culture and what it means for all of us*. Pan Macmillan.

Tapscott, D., & Euchner, J. (2019). Blockchain and the IoV: An Interview with Don Tapscott Don Tapscott talks with Jim Euchner about blockchain, the IoV, and the next Internet revolution. *Research Technology Management*, *62*(1), 12–19.

Toffler, A., & Alvin, T. (1980). *The third wave* (Vol. 484). Bantam books.

Truong, N. B., Um, T. W., Zhou, B., & Lee, G. M. (2018, May). Strengthening the blockchain-based IoV with trust. In *2018 IEEE International Conference on Communications (ICC)* (pp. 1-7). IEEE.

Turkanović, M., Hölbl, M., Košič, K., Heričko, M., & Kamišalić, A. (2018). EduCTX: A blockchain-based higher education credit platform. *IEEE Access: Practical Innovations, Open Solutions*, *6*, 5112–5127.

Twesige, R. (2015). *A simple explanation of Bitcoin and Block Chain technology*. https://www.researchgate.net/profile/Richard-Twesige 2/publication/270287317_Bitcoin_A_simple_explanation_of_Bitcoin_and_Block_Chain_technology_JANUARY_2015_RICHARD_LEE_TWESIGE/links/54a7836f0cf267bdb90a0ee6/Bitcoin-A-simple-explanation-of-Bitcoin-and-Block-Chain-technology-JANUARY-2015-RICHARD-LEE-TWESIGE.pdf

United Nations General Assembly. (1948). Universal declaration of human rights. United Nations.

Van der Aalst, W., Hinz, O., & Weinhardt, C. (2019). *Big digital platforms*. Academic Press.

Van der Meer, T. G., Hameleers, M., & Kroon, A. C. (2020). Crafting our own biased media diets: The effects of confirmation, source, and negativity bias on selective attendance to online news. *Mass Communication & Society, 23*(6), 937–967.

Visconti, R. M. (2020). Blockchain Valuation: IoV and Smart Transactions. In The Valuation of Digital Intangibles (pp. 401-422). Palgrave Macmillan.

Wen, H. (2020). A study of the privacy of covid-19 contact tracing apps. *International Conference on Security and Privacy in Communication Networks.*

Werbach, K. (2018). *The blockchain and the new architecture of trust.* MIT Press.

Westerlund, M. (2019). The emergence of deepfake technology: A review. *Technology Innovation Management Review, 9*(11).

Wildman, N., Archer, A., Brouwer, H. M., & Cawston, A. (2019). *The ethics of data acquisition: Protecting Privacy and Autonomy While Harnessing the Potential of Big Data.* Academic Press.

Yaeger, K., Martini, M., Rasouli, J., & Costa, A. (2019). Emerging BT solutions for modern healthcare infrastructure. *Journal of Scientific Innovation in Medicine, 2*(1).

Yaga, D., Mell, P., Roby, N., & Scarfone, K. (2019). *Blockchain technology overview.* arXiv preprint arXiv:1906.11078.

Yaji, S., Bangera, K., & Neelima, B. (2018). Privacy Preserving in Blockchain Based on Partial Homomorphic Encryption System for Ai Applications. *IEEE 25th International Conference on High Performance Computing Workshops (HiPCW)*, 81-85. doi: 10.1109/HiPCW.2018.8634280

Zhai, S., Yang, Y., Li, J., Qiu, C., & Zhao, J. (2019). Research on the Application of Cryptography on the Blockchain. *Journal of Physics: Conference Series, 1168*, 032077.

Zhang, R., Xue, R., & Liu, L. (2019). Security and privacy on blockchain. *ACM Computing Surveys, 52*(3), 1–34.

Zyskind, G., & Nathan, O. (2015, May). Decentralizing privacy: Using blockchain to protect personal data. In *2015 IEEE Security and Privacy Workshops* (pp. 180-184). IEEE.

KEY TERMS AND DEFINITIONS

Consensus: A group decision-making process in which group members develop and agree to support a decision in the best interest of the whole.

Decentralized Apps (DAPPS): Digital applications or programs that exist and run on a blockchain or P2P network of computers (instead of a single computer) and are outside the purview and control of a single authority.

Ethereum Request for Comments (ERC): A token standard that implements an Application Programming Interface (API) for tokens within *smart contracts*. It provides functionalities like transferring tokens from one account to another, to get the current token balance of an account, and the total supply of the token available on the network.

Smart Contract: A smart contract is a piece of code implementing arbitrary rules on a computer with distributed consensus (a blockchain), such that when the code is live it cannot be changed. Smart contracts are business logic that runs on a code that no one party controls or can turn off.

Token: A unit of value secured by cryptography that represents an asset or a specific use or functionality. It is created on top of a blockchain by using *smart contracts*.

Zero-Knowledge Proof: A cryptographic way of proofing that a statement is true without revealing anything beyond the veracity of that statement.

Section 2
Blockchain Society

Blockchain political-economic implications for citizens and consumers.

Chapter 2
The Evolution of Trust in Money:
A Historical Approach From Clay Tablets to Blockchain

João Pedro Vieira

https://orcid.org/0000-0002-0318-9297

University of Lisbon, Portugal

Cátia Neves Sousa

University of Lisbon, Portugal

ABSTRACT

Trust is vital to the sustained existence of money. No currency can prevail without it. However, following the international crisis of 2008, the liability-side of trust became increasingly apparent. Blockchain and cryptocurrencies challenged the need to trust and proposed an alternative "trustless" system. In the context of rising interest and concern about cryptocurrencies, the authors intend to discuss the role of trust in the evolution of money, from ancient Mesopotamia to modern sovereign fiat currencies and cryptocurrencies, and whether cryptocurrencies are prompting a shift in the paradigm of money or not.

INTRODUCTION

In recent years, there has been a surge in the interest in blockchain and cryptocurrencies. Blockchain, cryptocurrency, bitcoin, altcoin, token, ICO (Initial Coin Offering), DLT (Distributed Ledger Technology), and other expressions are part of a broader and specialized vocabulary that has come to the fore worldwide in all kinds of media. Many people felt that an underground or silent revolution of money had been underway for some years. However, for many others, cryptocurrencies had become a real "fountain of fortune" in the face of the staggering capitalization of some cryptocurrencies: in less than

DOI: 10.4018/978-1-7998-7363-1.ch002

a year, bitcoin's price has skyrocketed, surpassing US $41,500 on 8 January 2021, even if for a short while (CoinDesk, n.d.).

Blockchain already proved it is here to stay, with manifold applications, from supply-chain monitoring, authentication systems, and land registration to smart contracts and cryptocurrencies. For their part, cryptocurrencies are making their way, despite serious criticism and even rejection by monetary and political authorities. Some even believe that cryptocurrencies will eventually gather enough support and power to overthrow sovereign fiat currencies. Nevertheless, unlike all other forms of money, past or present, cryptocurrency's creators often claim that trust has no role in the functioning of blockchain-powered cryptocurrencies: they are supposedly built on a "trustless" system.

Such a claim calls for serious attention and raises several questions. Is it possible to create a successful currency without trust? What is the role of trust as money is concerned? What can the history of money tell about the role of trust? Are blockchain and cryptocurrencies disposing of trust for good? And after all, what does it mean "to trust"? These are some of the questions addressed in the present chapter. The authors will start by revisiting the concept of trust and its correlatives. This will provide the necessary conceptual background for addressing the history of money and the role played by trust across the centuries. Within this all-encompassing timespan, the analysis and discussion will focus on some of the most relevant evolutionary steps of money, hopefully contributing to dispel common historical oversimplifications and misconceptions (sometimes ideologically biased) and demonstrate that money cannot endure without some kind of trust.

THE NATURE OF TRUST

Trust is vital in human relationships and interactions. It is part of human nature to be able to trust and being trusted. It seems evident that trust is the cornerstone of society and its survival but understanding what it involves seems difficult to achieve. Everyone can distinguish people they trust. However, if several individuals were asked to define trust with certainty, a consensual definition would not be obtained. Still, one would probably get several common key aspects of such a complex concept.

The concept of trust has been studied in such disciplines as psychology, philosophy, sociology, business or political science, and conceptualised according to different theories, frameworks and approaches. Some authors have studied its development since early childhood (Erikson, 1982), in the organizational environment and performance (Bencsik, Jakubik, & Juhasz, 2020), others have studied trust in customer-salesmen interaction (Mangus, Jones, Folse, & Sridhar, 2020), healthcare context (Peters & Bilton, 2018), and many other areas of human interaction. Because of the extent of the concept, it is nearly impossible to find a consensual definition of it, even in the field of science.

Trust seems to have a brain processing dimension, in which a semantic pointer is nurtured by bindings of the self, the person trusted, the situation and emotion, which in turn bounds to other bindings representing information. Trust and mistrust emerge from the result of processing this entire network of interconnections (Thagard, 2019). However, to reach a more holistic understanding of the concept it is crucial to examine it from other perspectives.

Besides its processing dimension, interpersonal trust can be viewed as "the willingness of a party to be vulnerable to the actions of another party based on the expectation that the other will perform a particular action important to the trustor, irrespective of the ability to monitor or control that other party" (Mayer, Davis, & Schoorman, 1995, p. 712). Consequently, trust has always an inherent dimension of vulnerability, that is, the trustor is willing to assume risk (Mayer et al., 1995). The amount of risk that one is willing to take is indicative of the level of trust (Schoorman, Mayer, & Davis, 2007). In this estimation of risk (that is, in the assessment of trustworthiness), besides the trustor's propensity to trust, crucial variables must be taken into account, namely the ability, benevolence and integrity of the trustee. Ability refers to skills and competencies to do what is trusted to do, while benevolence assigns to the perceived motivation of a trustee to do good to the trustor, and integrity to the acceptance of the set of principles perceived in the trustee. The willingness to trust increases as the perception of each of these factors increases. (Mayer et al., 1995). Therefore, trust as an interpersonal phenomenon, which exists in a context of exchange and risk, has a potential to be harmful, since there is a possibility of betrayal, as the trustee has the freedom to correspond or not to expectations (McLeod, 2020).

A control system can be suggested to control risk and convey trust. However, if there is a strong control of the risk, there is no need to trust, and the trustee's actions may be perceived as responses to the control instead of being driven by benevolence or integrity, which are seen as conditions of trustworthiness (Schoorman et al., 2007). It does not mean that the absence of trust involves distrust. Trust as confident positive expectations regarding another's conduct, and distrust as confident negative expectations regarding another's conduct are not necessarily opposite concepts. Moreover, these constructs can be viewed as two separate but linked dimensions. As such, they are not opposite ends of a single continuum. According to this point of view, positive predictors of trust would not be negative predictors of distrust (Lewicki, McAllister, & Bies, 1998). Additionally, trust and distrust are not positive or negative by themselves. In fact, under some conditions, higher trust levels can be harmful (Langfred, 2004) and distrust can be productive and functional (Lewicki et al., 1998), and beneficial (Lowry, Schuetzler, Giboney & Gregory, 2015).

In everyday life, one trusts people, such as a coworker or a friend, and institutions such as a bank or an online business. Trust is visible across different levels and referents. Based on research review on organizational trust, Fulmer and Gelfand (2012) conceptualised a multilevel-multireferent framework of trust, that distinguishes between trust at a level of analysis and trust in a referent, that is the target of trust. The authors identified three levels — individual, team and organizational —, and three referents — interpersonal, team, and organization. At an individual level, trust stands for an individual's degree of trust, whereas at the higher levels denotes a degree of a collective sense of trust shared within a unit. Within each level, the entity can trust in a specific other, in "a collectivity of interdependent people pursuing a shared goal with inherently unique dynamics" (p. 1174), or in an institutional entity. This conceptualisation of trust makes it possible to understand and distinguish different interrelated forms of trust within a context.

Trust increases economic efficiency by reducing transaction costs, thus it is expected that groups exhibiting a higher degree of trust to be more economically efficient (Fukuyama, 1995). This is expected to be seen within different trust architectures, that is, distinct institutional structures that developed over time reflecting social complexity. The earliest architecture is peer-to-peer trust. This kind of interpersonal trust manifested on direct social interaction among families and clans predated the emergence of state and is vital even today. Peer-to-peer trust is based on mutual commitments and has a relatively small radius, meaning that trust is directed to specific tasks. The second architecture, named Leviathan trust, rose to maintain a baseline level of trust on more complex social interaction. It developed with the rise of state and is the state that operates to prevent others from imposing their will and endanger social order and stability. The state performs that via law enforcement with the legal system and military force. Another system of trust that raised with social complexity is the intermediary trust. Within this architecture, the intermediaries are a vital authority for trust to which individuals hand over power or control. Here trust is delegated on the intermediary because it provides valuable services, and the trustor give up some freedom to gain the benefits of trust. Therefore, this kind of trust is characteristically asymmetrical as for power and information distribution.

In 2008, after thousands of years of socio-economic complexification and evolution of trust systems, blockchain apparently gave rise to a new structure of trust, which helps to overcome the limitations of interpersonal, authority and intermediary trust, that is, "trustless trust". This is an intangible but valuable concept of trust. Here one trusts the network blockchain is based on, in a distributed machine without trusting any individual, authority or intermediary. In this context, economic incentives (cryptoeconomic security) and a consensus mechanism generate trust in the network without the need to trust on individuals or intermediaries (Werbach, 2018). Doing so, blockchain reduces friction, transaction costs and risks of intermediary trust, supporting "models of peer-to-peer mass collaboration". It makes it possible for parties who may not even know each other to make transactions and forge agreements without intermediation (Tapscott & Tapscott, 2017).

TRUST, RELIANCE, CONFIDENCE AND PREDICTABILITY

Does trust mean reliance? Philosophers agree that trust and reliance are distinct phenomena, yet what differentiates them is a matter of some controversy. It is widely accepted that trust is a kind of reliance with an important moral dimension. However, it is not consensual how this moral component is expressed. One can rely on something (objects, behaviours, natural phenomena and even people) without fully believing (not disbelief) that it will lead to the expected result. For example, one can rely on the alarm clock based on the supposition that the alarm clock has always rang without fully believing that it is really going to happen again. When relying on something, if one is let down, one is not going to feel resentment or betrayal, instead one might feel disappointment or sadness. Reliance does not involve the need of one being aware that is relying on something, nor the need for the relied-upon object to be aware of being relied upon (Goldberg, 2020).

Does trust and confidence refer to the same phenomena? Both concepts refer to expectations though they are distinct. Trust presupposes a situation of risk, involves recognizing and assuming risk, involves a choice despite the possibility of being disappointed. Confidence has no risk assumed, because there are no other alternatives available except to live in a state of uncertainty without expectations and anything else to replace them. Therefore, there is more dependency in confidence than on trusting relations. When confidence is disappointed one tends to attribute it to external forces, while when it is the case with trust, one has to consider internal factors (Luhmann, 1988).

Trust is also distinct from predictability. Although both are means to reduce uncertainty (Lewis & Weigert as cited in Mayer et al., 1995), being predictable is not the same as being trustworthy, since trust involves willingness to be vulnerable and predictability does not. Finally, it is important to distinguish between trust and cooperation, because although trust can lead to cooperative behaviour, there can be cooperation without trust. This can happen when there is external control and punishment for deceitful behaviour or when it does not exist vulnerability to the trustor (Mayer et al., 1995).

AN HISTORICAL APPROACH TO MONEY AND TRUST

Nobody really knows how money was created, nor when did it first appeared. Its origins are buried deep in history, most likely beyond the reach of any historical or archaeological enquiry. Nevertheless, the extant evidence and historical interpretations about the development of complex societies dating from approximately 5,000 years ago, as well as speculative theoretical approaches from the fields of anthropology and economic theory, do provide relevant insights on what may have been the possible origins of such a crucial instrument in human cultures.

Trust may not have been there on the inception of money, depending on how one accounts for its origins, but it appears to have been crucial to the sustained existence and development of money, in its vast array of historical forms, for at least 5,000 years (Graeber, 2011). One thing seems clear: nothing can become money and fulfill the main functions of money unless a significant number of members of a given community recognise it and accept it as such. And this cannot be done without a certain amount of consensus and some kind of trust. Yet, most of the times, money also implies the use of authority and force over individuals.

The following sections will be devoted to highlighting some of the most important steps and developments in the history of money until the affirmation and widespread use of the so-called fiat currencies. Although often implicit, the role of trust, trustworthiness, credibility and expectations should become increasingly clear along the narrative.

CONCEPTIONS OF MONEY

In the history of money, there are traditionally two opposing conceptions about the nature of money. One is the metallist conception, according to which the nominal value of money derives essentially from the intrinsic or market value of its material. As the name itself suggests, metal — and above all precious metals — are the ideal substance of currencies, regardless of their exact material shape. In fact, most historical monetary systems were anchored in the use of metals, both precious and base ones, and are generally considered to be metallist systems. Under this conception, money is a (preferred) commodity operating as a generally accepted and efficient means of exchange/payment, with its value (price) determined by supply and demand factors. As such, money could only have arisen spontaneously from the need to exchange goods, originated within what many call — in a rather anachronical manner — the "private sector".

In some respects, this is basically the explanation already presented by Aristotle in his writings, namely the *Nicomachean Ethics* and *Politics*, dating back to 350-330 BCE. It is precisely in Aristotle's writings that one may find one of the earliest discussions about the nature and functions of money (Schaps, 2004). To Aristotle, money was also a standard of value and a unit of account used to set the relative values of other assets. Finally, money is a store of value, i.e., it has the ability of holding its purchasing power over time, allowing its use in future transactions without significant loss of value.

Yet money was not an element one could find in nature: quite the opposite. Aristotle believed that money was a product of society, born out of social convention, and that it was in the power of men to change its value and render it worthless (Aristotle, trans. 2004, p. 90). This amounts to say the value of things is not in themselves: it is not a property intrinsic to things, but rather a quality bestowed on things by humans.

Such views recall an alternative conception on money: the so-called nominalism. According to this conception, the nominal value of money is essentially determined by the authorities exerting power over a given territory, and not by the eventual intrinsic or market value (if any) of the material embodying money. In the case of metal currencies, the market value of the constituent metals could not be ignored, at the risk of serious economic predicament, but currencies were understood as a state instrument on which they were entitled to exert almost discretionary power. The success of such monies ultimately rests upon the ability of a sovereign authority (i.e., the state) to exert its powers and impose a value set by law.

From this point of view, money is a representation of value, a widely recognised token that entails a claim on goods and services. It is also a token representing simultaneously a liability of its issuer (debt) and an asset of its holder (credit), so the issuer, as with state monies or private IOUs, assumes the commitment of taking it back and redeeming it for something else when presented with. This is the common ground of the so-called state theories and credit theories of money, which find significant backing in anthropological and historical research (Graeber, 2011). In contrast to metallism, it becomes clear that the nominalist conception of money is genetically open or even prone to the creation of intangible forms of money.

MONEY IN ANCIENT MESOPOTAMIA

As with other technological innovations, the origins of money are most likely polycentric, with two cultural areas at the heart of this historical process: Mesopotamia and China. Regarding the first, there is plenty of documentary evidence dating as back as the end of the 4th millennium BCE.

The ancient Neolithic economies of Mesopotamia revolved around agriculture and seem to have operated mainly on the basis of credit. The use of credit arose from the seasonal nature of production, essentially due to the time lapse between sowing and crop periods. The seed consigned for sowing would be later repaid in grain or silver plus interest. Palaces and temples were the largest landowners, supported important handicraft activities, namely weaving and metallurgy, and were the centres of political, economic and religious power. Additionally, they promoted trade with foreign countries, as most of Mesopotamian territories lacked basic raw-materials like metals and timber.

In this context, crops, handicraft production and silver were all part of a complex system of redistribution and settlement of debts, loans, wages and other obligations which had both palaces and temples at its core. Such a system required the existence of an administrative structure responsible for planning and managing revenue and expenditure. Considering their importance in domestic and foreign transactions, grain and silver emerged as the preferred commodities and units of account for administrative purposes and had a fixed exchange rate. Dates and wool were other means of payment available in the ancient palace and temple economies, but unlike silver their monetary role was mainly domestic (Hudson, 2020; Van De Mieroop, 1997).

The continuous acceptance of grain and silver in the settlement of obligations to the palaces and temples stimulated the widespread use of these commodities in the economy as general-purpose forms of money. The definition of these commodities as standards of value was associated with the refinement standardised systems of weights and measures, stemming from the bureaucratic need to register, count and weigh the different resources and ensure their efficient allocation throughout the year (Hudson, 2020).

This was especially true for silver, which presented obvious advantages when compared to grain, other foodstuffs and perishable products. Silver was durable, divisible without any loss of value, portable, and easily measured and stored. Additionally, silver linked domestic and foreign economies across the ancient Middle East and by the 2nd millennium BCE it had already become a shared standard of value, a monetary instrument and a financial tool in a vast geographical area encompassing Greece, present-day Turkey, Egypt, Syria and Mesopotamia (Van De Mieroop, 2014; Schaps, 2004, pp. 34-56).

Despite the role and functions perform by silver, neither the Mesopotamian city states nor the later kingdoms and empires apparently felt the need to convert silver into standardised and state-controlled monetary objects, i.e., into coinage. Silver served perfectly as money in the form of raw silver and broken pieces of jewellery. A large share of the silver stocks was captured by palaces and temples, either immobilised as treasure, luxury goods and religious offers, or periodically flowed back to these institutions as revenue from taxes and rents. In light of the ancient Mesopotamian laws, a critical aspect in the payment systems was the protection of the system of weights and measures against fraud.

METAL CURRENCIES AND STATE MONEY IN THE WEST

The emergence of state currencies was one the greatest events in the history of money. This evolutionary step took place in Lydia, China (once again) and apparently also in India, between the 7th and 5th centuries BCE. If in the case of Northern India, the researchers discuss the possibility of western influences (Cribb, 2003; Bopearachchi, 2017), the case of China represents a totally independent breakthrough.

The available evidence suggests that Lydia took the lead in this process, but instead of silver, the Lydian state chose electrum, a locally abundant alloy made of gold and silver. The first issues may have used a natural metallic combination of the two metals. However, recent studies suggest that the issues were struck using an artificial alloy from a very early stage. Now the major difference regarding metal used in the form of ingots, chunks of metal or broken pieces of jewellery was the issue of small pieces of metal in standardised weights combined with the imposition of a mark or symbol of authority that also served as a mark of quality and genuineness. In a certain sense, that mark gave a recognised value to a specific weight of metal (Kroll, 2012; De Callataÿ, 2013).

What drove the Lydian state to use coins instead of the former ingots, with no distinctive marks whatsoever, remains unknown. One of the possible explanations suggests that these high-value pieces of metal were used to reward services and pay soldiers (De Callataÿ, 2013). By the middle of the 6th century, under Croesus, Lydia started making separate issues of gold and silver, a decision that might have been triggered by public distrust in the value of electrum coins: the alloy was naturally variable and some researchers suggest the king was even manipulating its composition.

Whatever the reason, coinage proved to be a very successful innovation, as the Greek city states of Ionia absorbed coinage and its use gradually spread to the city states of insular and mainland Greece. While Ionia continued the tradition of issues in electrum for some time, most of the Greek city states preferred silver. By the end of the 3rd century BCE, Greek-style currencies were being issued by dozens of states, from the Iberian Peninsula to Central Asia, and Rome was becoming a monetary power to seriously take into account.

Coinage represented an improved use of precious metals in the economy, reducing the transaction costs resulting from weighing and testing each piece at each transaction. Within the jurisdiction of the issuer, legal tender coins could circulate by tale amongst common users, and only merchants, money-changers, and state officials would keep checking their weight, fineness and genuineness on a regular basis. City states, republics and kingdoms held the full monopoly of coinage, which comprised the rights of producing, issuing and changing the value and legal tender status of any coins circulating in their jurisdiction. Central political authorities were thus the guardians of public faith and trust in the goodness of legal currencies, persecuting and severely punishing those who tampered with coins and violated what had become a firmly entrenched sovereign right.

Above all, the monopoly over monetary rights made coinage a sizeable source of revenue (seigniorage), as well as an exceptional instrument of state financing, especially in times of war and emergency, which were not infrequent. Military expenditures often proved to be disruptive to state finances and to the monetary systems, and governments felt compelled to overuse or abuse their monetary rights to the point of breaking public trust in state currencies.

One of the extreme examples of coin debasement took place in Athens in the last years of the Peloponnesian War, in 406/405 BCE (Giovannini, 1975; Kroll, 1976). Cut off from its silver mines and facing an imminent exhaustion of financial resources, the city government resorted to a highly debased coin issue made of bronze tetradrachms covered with a thin layer of silver, instead of the fine silver tetradrachms traditionally issued by the city and widely accepted throughout the Greek world and Eastern Mediterranean markets.

The intrinsic value of the new tetradrachms was only a small fraction of its nominal value, making this emergency issue an evident example of a truly fiduciary currency. Not because it was willingly accepted as good currency, but because their users certainly expected the city government to later recall this bad currency. To many, trust was probably the best (if not the only) available alternative. This is an extreme example of the way emergency and financially demanding conditions could push governments and rulers to rapidly loosen or even abandon metallism.

THE LIMITS OF METALLISM IN THE GREEK AND ROMAN WORLDS

By the time Athens had its first experience with fiduciary coinage, the use of bronze token coins was already expanding across the Greek world. The increased use of coinage, probably combined with the effect of periodical inflation, even if mild in the long-run, promoted the introduction of fractional bronze coinage more adapted to common everyday transactions and payments in urban contexts. The Greek cities of Sicily (Akragas, Segesta and Himera) were pioneering this process, the beginning of which can be dated back to the middle of the 5th century BCE (Fischer-Bossert, 2012). In fact, the monetary use of weighed bronze was a well-established tradition in Sicily and Central Italy.

In the Greek and Roman worlds, bronze token coins differed from full-bodied coins in that they no longer respected the standard ratios of bronze in relation to gold and especially to silver. Such coins were obviously overvalued and could be theoretically exchanged for silver coins at a profit. But in practical terms exchanging bronze for silver could involve paying fees or even a substantial discount. The controlled output and circulation of bronze coins favoured the enforcement and acceptance of this currency, and sharply reduced the potential profitability of counterfeiting. Counterfeiting would be even less attractive given the limits to convertibility mentioned above. On the other hand, overvaluing coined bronze ensured the retention of petty coinage in the jurisdiction of the issuer and contributed to maintaining an adequate money supply at the lower levels of monetary circulation (Bransbourg, 2011).

Either token or not, bronze coinage supplied the monetary economies throughout the Mediterranean area with sets of low-denominations that composed the new basis of a multi-tiered currency system adapted to both small and large transactions. In a certain sense, bronze issues contributed to make money accessible to larger sectors of the population, despite the persistence of large geographical asymmetries in the monetization process. From the Hellenistic period until early Roman Imperial times, bronze coinage appears most frequently as a concern of civic authorities, be it the Greek city states of the Roman East or the Iberian municipalities under Roman rule, where one even finds civic issues using lead (Burnett, Amandry & Ripollès, 1992, pp. 13-25).

Highly monetised economies were already in place in regions of Roman Italy and Ptolemaic Egypt (which had a closed currency system) by the 2nd century BCE, boosted by the development of market economies, increased economic interregional integration and the growth of large territorial states with considerable financing needs satisfied via coin issuing, taxation and also through the economy of war (booty, war indemnities, tributes, confiscations and ransoms), which promoted huge transfers and redistributions of wealth including sizeable amounts of bullion and coinage (Temin, 2012; Howgego, 1992).

Roman military and political expansion eventually brought under the same rule all the regions around the Mediterranean by the 2nd half of the 1st century BCE, but there was no effort from Roman authorities to impose the Roman monetary system, based on the fine silver denarius, to the whole empire. Whereas the western part of the empire was gradually deprived of its minting concessions from Augustus rule onwards (there was a concentration process underway), the eastern Greek territories had deep-rooted monetary and self-governing traditions, and they were permitted to keep their autonomous local issues. Monetary integration was thus limited and relatively late within the empire, despite the existence of an overarching political structure.

The growth of monetary and market economies, with the intensification of coin use and its wider reach, increased the availability of capital, improved its liquidity and created new business opportunities for those having access to significant amounts of currency, either domestic or foreign. A trustworthy network of money and credit specialists came into being. Especially relevant were money professionals and other businessmen engaging in money-lending activities, namely money-changers, assayers, bankers and pawnbrokers, as well as merchants and tax-farmers; at least in Rome, the political elites also engaged in money-lending and trade activities and represented a large share of the available capital (Andreau, 1999). Dealing with coins was indeed a business requiring specialised knowledge and expertise. Depending on the scale of the business, it would involve the ability to recognise the designs of dozens of coin denominations (mainly gold and silver ones) and their slight variations; checking the size, weight and fineness of coins; knowing their nominal and bullion values, their position in the money market (supply and demand), or their legal tender status and exchange ratios.

Nevertheless, it apparently took a long time until money and financial markets and their professionals could really pose a threat to state control over the monetary stock. State intervention was decisive in tackling the debt and liquidity crisis that periodically affected Roman society. The government was committed to upholding the so-called *fides publica*, "public faith" or "public trust", and this included providing stable currencies and ensuring the normality of payments (Andreau, 1999, pp. 100-111).

But from 64 AD to 195 AD the silver content of Roman denarius, which had been minted with fine silver since about 211 BCE, fell steadily until it reached 50%, without due adjustment in the exchange ratios within the system. The overexpansion of military expenditure was the main drive behind the debasement of silver coinage: the state was clearly financing its budgetary deficits at the expense of the quality of currency and monetary stability. Putting it in other terms, the Roman state was increasingly monetizing its debt, transferring it to society and economy at large through ever-increasing issues of coin.

In 215, Caracalla introduced the antoninianus (or radiate), a coin having about the same silver content as the old denarius but worth 2.5 times more. As a result, general distrust in the new coins broke out and the state felt it hard to enforce the official exchange ratio against the denarius. After the large-scale production of the denarius was discontinued, in 238, the antoninianus rapidly deteriorated in terms of weight and fineness until the late 260s. At the bottom of the slope, the denomination had fallen below half of its primitive weight, with a silver content of only 2.5% (Bland, 2012; Elliott, 2020, pp. 81-82). Dire political and economic conditions (civil strife, invasions, secessions, shortage of precious metals) pushed the collapse of the monetary system and severely damaged public confidence in state currency.

The reactions to such monetary abuse and loss of credibility included widespread distrust on currency, initial rejection of overvalued issues, hoarding of issues with higher intrinsic value and the rise of counterfeiting. Moreover, troubles in the supply and distribution of cash caused episodes of shortage and spurred the appearance of local imitations in peripheral areas of the empire, especially in the Western areas. In contexts of chronic shortage of cash, or undersupply, counterfeiting or low-denomination coins may have even performed a useful function by expanding the money supply (Campo, 2010).

The evolution roughly outlined above shows how the Roman Empire gradually drifted towards a mixed monetary system until the end of the 3rd century AD, combining full-bodied coins (gold aurei) with token issues (silver denarii) and later with truly fiduciary issues (billon radiates) that became the vast majority of the money supply in quantitative terms.

METAL-CURRENCIES AND STATE MONEY IN CHINA

As previously mentioned, China was one of the cradles of metal currencies and state money, along with Lydia and Greece, in the West, and ancient India. It is possibly that cowries were actually used as money since the 2nd half of the 1st millennium BCE (Thierry, 1997, pp. 39-43; Von Glahn, 1996, pp. 23-25), even though some authors argue that they were only a token of value and social distinction within ritualised gift exchanges (Kakinuma, 2014).

Be it as it may, the fact was that the state was once again the main driving force behind the appearance of metal currencies from the 7th or 6th century BCE onwards. However, in contrast with West Eurasia, preference went not for precious metals or alloys, but for cast bronze. Furthermore, the first Chinese "coins" were not reduced versions of ingots, but took the form of miniaturised implements, namely spades and knifes. Round coins with a central hole appeared later, as well as imitations of cowries (Kakinuma, 2014; Thierry, 1997). There were clear regional preferences for determined types of bronze currency, as they were characteristic of different regions displaying only limited overlapping. In general terms, the production of spades, knifes and other bronze currencies occurred in a fragmented and competitive political environment, and was apparently open to private parties, although under government regulation and standardization (Kakinuma, 2014).

Bronze currencies became a shared standard of value and means of payment within complex monetary systems comprising commodities that performed monetary functions: gold, grain, hemp and silk. These commodities were less general means of payment and had no fixed exchange ratios regarding bronze currencies, but they were all complementary with bronze. As warfare amongst several states competing for political hegemony grew endemic, the financing needs of the states increased sharply, and the only way the expand the limited supply of available monetary and reward instruments was the intensification of bronze currencies under state control, in accordance with strict standards. The Qin eventually unified China in 221 BCE and paved the way for monetary unification under its own coins, the bronze *banliang*.

Such a rich monetary experience meant that Chinese statesmen and officials had plenty of opportunities to reflect upon the nature and functions of money and particularly of state-issued metal currencies. Apparently, the dominant underlying conception of money was much closer to nominalism than to metallism, as it becomes apparent not only from the selection of bronze as a standard monetary alloy, but also from the fact that the weights inside a specific currency tended to show considerable variation. Bronze currencies were essentially fiduciary currencies, accepted in the settlement of private and state obligations by tale, and enforced by law (Thierry, 2001).

The *Guanzi*, an ancient compilation of political, economic and philosophical texts from the 5th-2th centuries BCE, contains a surprising amount of thought on monetary economics. The origins of money were placed in the salvific and mythical action of the ancient kings. Created by the state for the benefit of the population, money was deemed a state monopoly. For this reason, the state was entitled with the right to determine the purchasing power of the different forms of money and to regulate the level of prices through law and state expenditure, according to the theory of the "light and heavy" (*qing zhong*), a kind of quantity theory of money that focused on the interplay between the prices of commodities and money (Von Glahn, 1996, pp. 28-33).

Metallist theories were not unfamiliar to Chinese economic thinking and had they share in the monetary policies of the empire since Antiquity. However, it is the deep influence of the nominalist and state theories of money that explains why China took the lead in the development of what are the first successful paper currencies in world history.

PAPER CURRENCIES AND FIAT MONEY IN CHINA

Indeed, China was at the cutting-edge of the "technology of money" and other areas of scientific knowledge and technological development (Robinson, 2004). Some early and limited experiences with paper money or notes representing currency are documented in the 9th century, when the Tang and Song governments started granting special credit facilities to the long-distance merchants with whom they maintained regular trade. Those merchants could deposit their cash, precious metals or silk in the capital treasury and obtain in exchange promissory notes (the *feiqian* and *bianqian*) payable at the provincial treasuries (Von Glahn, 2005). The advantage of this particular arrangement was mutual. On one hand, the central government obtained a kind of zero-interest short-term loan, immediately increasing its liquidity and anticipating revenue from the provincial administration. Chronic problems with the coin supply made this solution even more appealing. On the other hand, merchants avoided the inconvenience and potential risk of transporting bulky sums of low-denomination coins across hundreds of miles.

By the late 10th century, the merchants of Sichuan also developed their own private notes (*jiaozi*) in reaction to a severe coin shortage (this was an endemic problem in China for centuries). The notes were convertible into hard currency (subject to a fee), precious metals and silk and circulated as currency amongst the restricted trust network of local merchants, partially offsetting the lack of liquidity caused by the currency crisis. Litigation around the *jiaozi* forced government intervention. The issue and circulation of the new paper currency was then regulated, standardised and restricted to a selected group of merchants. Yet, the provincial government set no cap to issuance, which floated according to seasonal liquidity needs of interregional trade. Under the combined effect of counterfeiting, bankruptcies and resulting litigation, confidence in the *jiaozi* faltered. The reply of the government was to order the suspension of the notes, already depreciated, and offer a centralised trust solution to the paper currency system. From 1023 onwards, the government called the issues upon itself, setting an overall issuance cap and expiration terms for the new notes. The feedback of the market was encouraging, as the new currency soon began to be traded at a premium (Von Glahn, 2005).

The convertible notes issued by the government coexisted with other state papers issued by the imperial administration, namely promissory notes and vouchers exchangeable into monopolised commodities (salt and tea). Attempts to replace the *jiaozi* for these papers raised doubts about the ability of the provincial government in Sichuan to guarantee their convertibility in the 1080s, and as demand fell, pushed down by changes in the tea market, the *jiaozi* were subject to discounting. In the beginning of the 12th century, the issues of *jiaozi* skyrocketed, turning the notes into an almost fiat currency, soon removed from circulation and replaced for a new paper currency in 1107 (*qianyin*). The step to fiat money was actually close, as within a few years the Sichuan government declared the *qianyin* unredeemable. From there on, the value of notes rested solely on the commitment of the government to accept them in the payment of taxes and other obligations, thus becoming a kind of function of government credibility. As the market reaction showed, that credibility had been severely damaged.

For most of the 12th century, paper money had a troubled existence in China. The Song government was unable to contain the enemy armies of the Jurchen Jin, who took Kaifeng, the Song capital, and submitted Northern China. Printing money was an expeditious way of financing urging war expenses, and so did the Song government in ever-increasing amounts. The government paper money was traded at a considerable discount in the market (over 50%) and could no longer earn the confidence of the market. But the imperial government was in no position to relinquish that virtually unlimited source of financing. Other convertible paper currencies followed, but the trend was clearly towards unredeemable issues and truly worthless fiat currencies, imposed by the state.

In the last decades of the 13th century, the Yuan government took extreme measures to enforce the use of their paper currency, the *zhongtong chao*. In 1282, the use of gold and silver was banned from trade and the notes ceased to be convertible into silver. Other inconvertible notes followed, equally unable to restore trust in state paper currency in the long-run, as the imperial government kept creating money virtually out of nothing, actively contributing to high inflation. In reaction to the reckless monetary policy of the imperial government, the Chinese economy gradually shifted to a silver standard (Von Glahn, 1996, pp. 56-70; Von Glahn, 2005).

The Ming dynasty, which took over China in 1368, was unable to reverse the demise of state paper currency. First launched in 1375, the Ming treasury notes (*Da Ming baochao*) were inconvertible from the onset. At the same time, the mints barely operated, injecting in the economy only small amounts of coins that rapidly disappeared from circulation; coin counterfeiting soared to new heights, stimulated by the rising price of copper and chronic coin shortage. The depreciation of paper money was intense (over 75% in 1390), and the government even resorted to bans on the use of coins and silver in transactions, but to no avail. By 1425, the Ming notes were traded at less than 2% of their nominal value. The state had no reasonable option but to submit to the power of economy, eventually abandoning the paper money issues for centuries (Von Glahn, 1996, pp. 70-82).

The monetary experiences of the Roman Empire and China alike show the obvious: when monetary economies reach a certain scale and level of complexity, it becomes virtually impossible for the state to manipulate the money supply without causing significant damage to the overall economy and seriously hindering stability, predictability and public trust.

BILLS OF EXCHANGE AND BANK MONEY IN EUROPE

Between the 12th and 14th centuries, Europe experienced an unprecedented period of commercial and economic growth, linked with demographic expansion, urbanization, the expansion of international trade and the improvement of monetary and financial instruments, private and public alike (Lopez, 1976; Spufford, 1988, pp. 109-263). Among the financial and monetary innovations characterizing this period were the bill of exchange, bank money, the development of cashless payment systems and the securitization of public debt. All of these innovations took place in the merchant republics of North Italy, ushered in by the activity of merchants, money-changers and bankers. Most of them stemmed from private initiative. Except for public debt, which ended up being converted into perpetuities, all the others heavily relied on the principle of convertibility. Gold and silver coins were still the most real and liquid form of money, but credit remained of paramount importance in long-distance trade: in this context, most sales were in fact sales on credit.

The bill of exchange was born in the 13th century from a notarised exchange contract commonly used in the Italian trade conducted in the context of the Champagne fairs, which had turned into a commercial interface between Northern Europe and the Mediterranean economies (De Roover, 1953). Differently from the exchanged contract, the bill of exchange was an informal arrangement. Being a private IOU, the bill of exchange required strong trust between the parties involved. The exchange operation typically involved different currencies, times and locations and became a vital instrument of payment (settlement), remittance and credit alike, reducing transaction costs, streamlining cash flows and enhancing liquidity. As a result, restrictions on the export of currencies and bullion could be successfully overcome, and the risks of long transportations by sea or land avoided (Kohn, 2020; Denzel, 2014). This was an important piece of the system of cashless payments that was under development; the soundest contributions to it would come from the banking sector.

The growth of international trade and the prominence of Italian merchants and commercial companies resulted in the organization of international networks of branches and agencies settled in the main European business centres. Such networks, built on trust, reputation and creditworthiness, provided the infrastructure on which the bill of exchange could operate, contributing to the progressive integration of commodity, exchange and financial markets across the continent, with Venice and Bruges as two of their major hubs. In its full-fledged form, the exchange operation could take four parties: the deliverer, who bought the bill and thus provided the money; the taker, who sold the bill; the payee, who received the bill from the deliverer; and at last, the payer, who paid the bill to the payee at maturity date. All this implied the previous existence of debt/credit relations between the deliverer and the payee, on the one hand, and between the taker and the payer, on the other hand (Kohn, 2020; Mueller, 1997, pp. 288-303).

The full potential of the bill of exchange was only explored in the 16th century, once endorsement became a standard practice commonly accepted in the financial and money market of Antwerp, the focal point of European economy until at least the middle of the century. Endorsement, associated with the practice of discounting commercial paper, made the bills a fully transferable and negotiable instrument, thus creating what may be considered the first European form of paper money. The bills could now be traded a number of times until they reach maturity and their payment could be conveniently anticipated through discounting in case of need (De Roover, 1953, pp. 83-146; Denzel, 2014; Kohn, 2020). They became private money, at the juncture of units of account, credit and state currencies. Only the bills issued by trustworthy, well-known merchants and companies would earn general acceptance in the markets, and this meant that besides money, the networks circulated increasing amounts of valuable information about the financial position of the intervenient parties. One must remember that defaults and failures were not infrequent. In this context, trust tended to be highly decentralised and unevenly distributed, always adjusting to the evolution of the various components integrating the system (merchants, banks, companies, states, etc.).

In the 16th century, the development of large international exchange markets around the fairs of Lyons, Antwerp, Medina del Campo and other pivotal cities gave rise to another intangible and private money, an abstract unit of account used by merchant bankers for exchange purposes that provided a common link between all relevant territorial units of account: the so-called "exchange money".

Bank money (also called "scriptural money") made its appearance in the same century that witnessed the invention of the bill of exchange, as a by-product of the banking business and the credit facilities provided to clients. Genoa, Florence and especially Venice, probably the best studied case, stood at the cutting edge of this evolution. Bank money was intangible, a stable money unit used for accounting purposes, free from the complexities created by changes in the legal value and legal tender status of coins, and from the inconveniences of accounting deposits and loans in different monetary units and denominations. All assets and liabilities held by the bank could be converted into a convenient unit of account (Lane & Mueller, 1987, pp. 61-64).

In late 13th century Venice, beyond regular banking activities such as taking deposits and granting loans, the Venetian banks offered services that contributed to the development of a cashless payment system. Businessmen having current accounts at the bank could settle their debts by ordering the transfer of funds to the current account of the creditor, without moving any cash. Some clients also benefited from the facility of overdrawing their current accounts. Using these facilities, merchants could easily settle their contracts and obligations by bank transfer, and even craftsmen could receive payment in bank money. By the 1320s, the cashless payment system was fully operational, with the banks at its core performing a crucial clearing function. Thus, in trade cities, banks turned into privileged financial intermediaries, aggregating a large share of public trust (Mueller, 1997, pp. 3-32; Denzel, 2014; Kohn, 2020).

The extension of credit and bank services enhanced the liquidity of the system and freed capital for investment in profitable business opportunities, from commercial ventures to speculation on exchange, bullion and staple commodities. This was possible because banks adopted a system of fractional banking in which only a small part of the deposits and other liabilities were actually covered by reserves in cash, as the amount of cashless payments expanded. However, reducing tied-up capital exposed the Venetian banks to temporary shortages of liquidity related seasonal fluctuations in the money market and trade cycles. The low level of reserves, combined with acute money shortages, wars, famines, as well as panics that ended up in bank runs, could force banks into insolvency or bankruptcy. As matter of fact, bank failures were not infrequent in the 14th and 15th centuries, despite continuous regulation and state supervision (Mueller, 1997). Afterall, trust was as precious as fragile.

One of the most successful cases of bank money is to be found in the Bank of Amsterdam experience, a public exchange bank established in 1609 to protect the money market from currency devaluations and the bad quality of circulating specie. As the bank became a major international clearing centre, holding the near privilege of settling bills of exchange in the Amsterdam, its bank money — the bank guilder, backed by gold and silver coin of good quality — was eventually converted into a trusted fiat medium in exchange in the 1680s, after various reforms limited the convertibility of deposits and further discouraged withdrawals (Van Nieuwkerk, 2009; Quinn & Roberds, 2014).

EUROPEAN PAPER MONEY: THE EMERGENCE AND SPREAD OF BANKNOTES

Despite the refinement of financial markets and credit facilities, it took four centuries before European banks developed their first convertible paper currencies. The first experiment came with the Bank of Stockholm in 1661, more than two centuries after the Ming government abandoned the issue of Treasury notes and finally capitulated to commodity money.

The Bank of Stockholm was established in 1656 as a private exchange and loan bank after a project present by Johann Palmstruch, the son of a rich merchant from the Low Countries. The new bank, under state protection, was intended to respond to usury, facilitate trade and keep the purchasing power of money. Unlike other exchange banks, the Bank of Stockholm did not convert deposits into its own bank money, but kept separate accounts and records of the copper and silver deposits it accepted, which it had to redeem on demand in the same money. The demand for credit rapidly outstripped the cash reserves held by the bank. Loans were granted on a variety of securities, from gold and silverware, to real estate and commodities. In some cases, personal assurances would suffice.

Excessive concession of credit exposed the bank to the risk of sudden liquidity crisis. Monetary reform in 1660 increased the market value of the old copper plate deposited at the bank and soon caused a bank run. Short of liquidity and unable to recover outstanding loans, in 1661 the bank resorted to what was supposed to be a short-term solution: the issue of credit notes acknowledging the right of the bearer to a certain amount of silver or copper money at the counters of the bank (Wetterberg, 2009, pp. 37-38). The notes were a state-guaranteed promise of payment that could be transferred to third-parties without endorsement and became valid in the payment of taxes to the crown. Furthermore, they served as a convenient means of payment in the face of the bulky copper plates that circulated as legal tender but were rather suited to serve as a store of value. Copper plate money had been minted since 1644 and the largest denomination, worth 10 daler silver-money, weighted about 20 kg (Tingström, 1986, pp. 17-21).

The experiment of convertible banknotes proved to be a success, and from 1663 on the concession of credit accelerated, now based on the issue of notes with absolutely no backing (fiduciary money). The crown, chartered companies, political elites and nobility were the largest recipients of this unrestrained credit policy. Withdrawal demands of large sums put the bank in a difficult situation, unable to convert the notes. As distrust spread, the value of notes in the market declined and speculation grew. After sustaining considerable losses, the bank was forced into liquidation by the Swedish Parliament in 1664. In the process of redemption, the value of banknotes recovered, but the experiment was deemed a failure and enthusiasm about paper money slumbered.

In France, the complex financial scheme set up by John Law between 1716 and 1720 was behind another centralised and state-sponsored experience of banknote issuing that radically envisioned the replacement of all silver and gold specie in circulation. The ascension and demise of banknotes in France was as fast as spectacular.

In the preceding years, the Crown had issued interest-bearing bills (the *billets de monnoie*) that originally represented amounts of coin delivered to the mint for recoinage, but that were never reimbursed. The bills were granted limited legal tender status in 1706 and circulated as paper money for some years, subject to discount, before being converted into other forms of debt and also seigniorage credits (Lafaurie, 1981, pp. 62-63).

Law's experience began with the Banque Générale, founded in 1716 as a private bank under the protection of the regent of France. The banknotes it initially issued were denominated and convertible into different types of silver coin, an option devised to protect its bearers from debasements and other monetary manipulations, and were accepted in the payment of taxes. Following its nationalization in 1718, the institution (renamed Banque Royale) eventually switched to banknotes denominated in money of account, no longer guaranteeing the claim to a fixed metallic equivalent (Velde, 2020; Murphy, 1997, pp. 154-162). It must be noted that the bank acted as banker of the state and was part of a larger monetary and financial scheme that within a few years came to include exclusive trading rights over the Louisiana and the monopoly over tobacco, slave trade, Canadian furs and all Eastern trade conducted by France. To these rights, managed by a company, Law later added the collection of all royal taxes, a lease on the royal mints and finally the management of French national debt (Velde, 2020).

In this context, a series of decisions were enacted in order to encourage the use of banknotes in the economy at large and to remove silver and gold from circulation. The state offered a 5% premium to tax payments made in banknotes, determined that all private debts could be settled in banknotes and reduced ceilings above which payments in paper money or gold were mandatory. Additionally, monetary reforms reduced the purchasing power of specie, thus increasing the relative value of banknotes against gold and silver coin (Murphy, 1997). At the end of this process, banknotes had become legal tender in the settlement of all kinds of debt. The monetary system was actively evolving into a paper standard made of pure fiat money.

Ultimately, the overexpansion of banknote issues, combined with steep financial speculation, lead the whole system to collapse. In fact, Law was lending money in the form of banknotes to buy stock of the company, which monopolised French overseas trade and tax-collection, in an attempt to keep their prices high. The price of the shares was guaranteed and this further expanded the potential money supply. When Law tried to limit this liability by gradually reducing the nominal value of shares and banknotes, the price of shares started falling, and fears about the ability of the bank to honour its commitments spread. Within days, crowds of banknote holders were desperately trying to convert them back into specie. Trust had been lost and the way to restore it was to return to the old commodity money system (Murphy, 1997; Velde, 2020).

These were just two of the most relevant paper money experiences in Europe during the 17th and 18th centuries. Paper monies linked to governments and private banks or companies were put in circulation in an increasing number of countries, from Northern to Southern Europe, including the British colonies in North America. That was the case of the Massachusetts colony in 1690, when a failed military operation against Quebec forced the government to issue bills to the troops promising to pay them in specie of commodities at a later time, as soon as the situation of Treasury allowed it (Goldberg, 2009). In Spain and Portugal, as well as in revolutionary France, paper money issues went hand in hand with the need to fund public debt, but invariably faced growing distrust and eventually became discredited, once the promise of later redemption failed to be fulfilled or rumours about the incapacity of the issuer to uphold convertibility spread. Wars, urgent financing needs, increasing public debt and currency shortages were common factors underlying such experiences. After all the political and economic turmoil caused by the French Revolution and Napoleonic Wars, the banks, either private or state-run, emerged as the main trusted issuers of convertible paper money in Europe.

FROM THE GOLD STANDARD TO THE TRIUMPH OF FIAT MONEY

The gold standard was probably the first worldwide monetary and financial response to the problem of confidence in money and repeated state abuse of monetary prerogatives. This overarching monetary structure was built on the trustworthiness and creditworthiness of Great Britain, the centre of the system, and other core countries, namely France, Germany and the United States of America.

The gold standard greatly expanded as an international regime in the second half of the 19th century, reaching its heights between 1880 and 1914. Adhesion to the regime typically implied the commitment of governments to a basic set of conditions and rules: the domestic monetary units were defined in terms of a fixed quantity of gold and the different currencies of the system became interlinked by fixed mint parities; private parties could demand the conversion of gold into coin at the legal fixed price with no limits; Treasury notes and banknotes issued central banks, as well as demand deposits, should be fully convertible into gold; and gold should be allowed to flow freely between economies, with no exchange controls. The practical arrangement of the regime varied from country to country, as rules were essentially implicit and their violation was not infrequent, even in the core countries (Officer, 2020).

The suspension of convertibility was one of the solutions to temporary or structural imbalances: this was the case of Portugal, which formally remained in standard despite abandoning the convertibility of the central banknotes in 1891 (Valério, 2007). In reality, the gold standard was far more beneficial to the core economies, which in reality controlled the system, than to peripheral economies, which often suffered the burden of real adjustment to the imbalances of the system. Nevertheless, while it succeeded, the gold standard did provide a stable monetary architecture that reduced transaction costs and fostered free trade, the free movement of capital and therefore international economic and financial integration. Trust in monetary authorities and governments strongly committed with gold convertibility, balanced budgets and limited monetarization of debt, amongst other aspects, actually allowed the quantity of gold in circulation to decrease, as the amount of credit instruments and other transferable assets convertible into gold increased and the primary use of gold shifted to fulfilling a reserve function. Instead of gold, given the centrality of London in the financial and gold markets, the system came to rely essentially on foreign-exchange, namely sterling (Officer, 2020).

The serious economic and financial disturbances brought by World War I caused the collapse of the gold standard. The convertibility of currencies in gold was then suspended and governments strongly resorted to banknote issuing to finance growing expenditure and debt. Gold coins completely vanished from circulation, replaced by huge amounts of pure fiat money. In the face of necessity, the practical nominalist approach to money rapidly displaced the metallist orthodoxy of the gold standard.

Despite the attempts to reinvent the system, which was actually revived a gold-exchange standard in the interwar period, the transition to pure fiat currencies was steadily on the move. Inflationary and hyperinflationary processes during and in the aftermath of the war, partially related to the overexpansion of money supply through banknote issuing, gradually drove gold coins out of circulation and accelerated the expulsion of all precious metals from domestic monetary systems, replaced by base metals and alloys, circulating alongside paper. In Germany, a country hit hard by hyperinflation, the banknotes issued in ever-increasing quantities were truly fiat money, without any kind of backing, and money, either physical or in the form of demand deposits, was losing its purchasing power every day. Distrust in the monetary authorities and lack of confidence in money was complete, but still there was no real alternative to the use of the available monetary instruments; barter could only provide a very limited alternative

At the lowest level of the monetary supply, the rising price of base metals heavily impacted the supply of fractional coinage. Between 1914 and 1923, countries like France, Germany and Portugal experienced severe shortages of coinage and the explosion of local emergency notes, vouchers, metal tokens and other forms of IOUs issued by municipalities, banks, companies, shops, charity works and other public and private entities, sometimes unlawfully and having no backing whatsoever (Orléan, 2008; Gadoury & Élie, 1990; Almeida, 1982).

In the context of economic crisis, convertibility to gold, even if indirectly, had become a source of instability and a liability to the system, exposed to panics and speculative attacks. By 1933, as the consequences of the Great Depression unfolded, convertibility had been abandoned by all the great economies, with only short-lived agreements before the outbreak of World War II.

The Bretton-Woods system, created in 1944, was the last international monetary agreement to rely on gold. Just as with the classic gold standard, it was the importance of gold in the reserves of the dominant country, now the United States of America, that determined its role in the new system. In fact, the United States held at the time almost three-quarters of the world official stocks of gold and was responsible for more than one-third of international trade. The central currency was now the US dollar, which was directly convertible into gold at the fixed price of $35 per ounce; all other currencies were pegged to the dollar and were thus indirectly convertible into gold (Kugler & Straumann, 2020, pp. 667-668). To holders of US dollars in the United States, this convertibility commitment meant nothing: common citizens could not convert the notes they possessed into gold if they desired to do so.

However, problems of liquidity, credibility and adjustment accrued to the system, as the available reserves were insufficient to support the growth of international trade and finance, the deficit in the US balance of payments was raising concerns about the stability of the dollar, and international imbalances could not be properly offset. Despite the introduction of several equilibrium mechanisms (special drawing rights on the IMF, gold pool, swap deals), the system deteriorated with the adoption of an expansionist monetary and fiscal policy by the US government from 1965 onwards, with inflationary consequences extensive to other countries. Confidence in the system eventually faltered, as France left the gold pool and devalued its currency, following the sterling devaluation. The sharp decrease of US liquid reserves and a run on the dollar forced the government to suspend the convertibility of the currency in 1971. Within a few years and after some speculative attacks to some currencies, the system of fixed exchange rates also collapsed, bringing an end to the whole Bretton Woods arrangement (Kugler & Strauman, 2020, pp. 675-683).

At this point, the transition to pure fiat money was complete. Banknotes were intrinsically worthless and coins virtually so, with only marginal intrinsic value. But they were only the small and visible tip of the money supply iceberg, especially in economically developed countries with a long-lasting and sophisticated banking networks providing services not only to trade and business, but also to citizens. This was the case of Great Britain and the United States of America, where there had been a variety of instruments (especially checks) allowing the holders of demand deposits to remit or transfer their money to other bank accounts without it ever taking any physical form (Quinn & Roberds, 2008). Thus, a large share of the money supply was increasingly becoming intangible, reduced to information registered in central and commercial bank records. The advent of electronic and digital technologies, ATMs, debit cards and the extension of banking services to the overall population further deepened the path to the dematerialisation of money. In the process, monetary authorities, central banks and the banking system, rather than governments, had become the primary trusted intermediaries (and creators) of virtually all forms of money.

It seems forceful to conclude that digital money and cryptocurrencies appear as a logical conclusion to a centuries-old process of money evolution, as money becomes more abstract but no less important, as it expands its ability to incorporate and transform value. Actually, that is what money is since the beginning: a social technology of value.

BLOCKCHAIN, CRYPTOCURRENCIES AND FIAT MONEY

Blockchain and cryptocurrencies developed after the severe crisis of trust in banks and governments that ensued the international financial crisis of 2008, the crisis of sovereign debts in Europe, bank bailouts and their spillover effects across the world. The feeling that public trust had been misplaced and betrayed, because the traditional guarantors and intermediaries of the system had misused and abused the powers they were entrusted with, led Satoshi Nakamoto to propose a radical approach to part of the problem: cut out the potentially untrustworthy middlemen and replace trust by reliance in a decentralised and cooperative system of electronic payments cryptographically empowered and based in an immutable and distributed chain of records (blockchain) open to everyone (Nakamoto, 2008).

The risks and dangers arising from trusting are theoretically eliminated by software codes, cryptography and embedded governance mechanisms, including limits to the money supply. Additionally, both the validation and integrity of the information no longer rest upon unscrutinised central authorities, which could manipulate accounts without being noticed, but upon the consensus (majority) of a peer-to-peer network of participants. Therefore, blockchain, cryptography and distributed ledgers provided the ground for the emergence of cryptocurrencies (also called "virtual currencies"), an alternative to centralised fiat currencies issued under the authority of states and to the intervention of financial intermediaries. As such, cryptocurrency systems have the power to make secure transactions faster and cheaper. By their very design, they are also resistant to censorship and governmental interference and preserve the relative anonymity of their users, qualities that may be highly detrimental to society when it comes to fighting criminal activities such as money laundering, tax evasion, drug trafficking and terrorism (Werbach, 2018), but of paramount importance in non-democratic regimes and economies crippled by problems such as chronic corruption and hyperinflations.

Despite the intents of its founders, neither bitcoin nor any other cryptocurrencies can survive without trust. Blockchain technology does help to solve many of the traditional problems generated by the need to trust, replacing most of it with confidence. But as the DAO incident with Ethereum showed, there are no perfect systems. The systems are always subject to problems and flaws that might expose their users to manipulation and fraud. Ultimately, the credibility of the system relies on the trustworthiness of its participants, above all, of its developers and validators. The asymmetries of power of these participants are evident (Werbach, 2018).

From a certain point of view, one can look at cryptocurrencies as an attempt to democratise the control of money by turning that power over the community. Nevertheless, from where does the value of cryptocurrencies come from? From the trust or reliance that his users put in the goodness of the system in itself or the benefits they expect the system to create? From the input of sovereign fiat currencies that users pour into the system in order to have access to units of cryptocurrency? Or from the expectation of making a profit by selling cryptocurrency later at a higher price, as in the biggest fool theory? (Wray, 2015, pp. 138-139). The answers diverge.

The nature of cryptocurrencies is a controverted issue. In contrast to many state-approaches and conventional views, the authors consider that cryptocurrencies do share with fiat currencies a series of attributes and essential functions that support the idea that they should be considered at least a limited form of money with a tremendous potential of growth in the context of burgeoning digital economies. Cryptocurrencies are actually used and accepted as a means of payment in both domestic and international private transactions, although the number of businesses accepting payments in cryptocurrency worldwide is still very restricted and unevenly distributed. They are also well adapted to operate as a unit of account, providing a reasonably convenient way of expressing the prices of all kinds of goods and services. Currently, bitcoin cryptocurrency is divisible into its one-hundredth-millionth part or 0.00000001, but the protocol could be easily changed to increase or reduce its divisibility if consensus is reached. Yet, the limited acceptance of cryptocurrencies represents a heavy impediment to their use as effective units of account and consequently as a real standard of value. Moreover, transaction fees may be low, but they become significant in the case of micropayments (Stroukal, 2018; Gerba & Rubio, 2019).

Given its digital and decentralised nature, cryptocurrencies are highly portable, as they can be easily moved across borders without any restrictions, durable, as they have no deterioration risks associated, and easily storable at low cost. Finally, cryptocurrencies are also fungible, liquid and relatively scarce (Stroukal, 2018; Gerba & Rubio, 2019). The inelastic supply of some cryptocurrencies, as in the case of bitcoin (capped at 21 million units), causes its price to rise as demand increases, but it is also one reason price is so volatile. Furthermore, volatility is one of the major handicaps of cryptocurrencies in the battle to be accepted as universal currencies. For that reason, and despite their general appreciation over time, cryptocurrencies are not reliable means of payment and a store of value. Cryptocurrency holders are exposed to the risks of a sharp depreciation in the value of their holdings.

Volatility, limited acceptance and lack of scale are obvious disadvantages of cryptocurrencies compared to sovereign fiat currencies, further aggravated by the fact that cryptocurrencies are monetary instruments not recognised — or even bluntly disavowed — by monetary authorities and states. Cryptocurrencies still have no legally recognised power to discharge debts as legal tender currencies do, and therefore are not accepted in the payment of state taxes, fees, fines or other kinds of legal obligations, considered by many economists the main drive behind money. Moreover, cryptocurrencies are not liabilities of the issuer, and there is no underlying guarantee system, no commitment to redeem them at a fixed nominal value (Wray, 2015, pp. 138-157). As the history suggests, the continued surge of cryptocurrencies will eventually come to an end, and it is a matter of time until a crash happens. When that happens, the absence of guarantee mechanisms may result in dramatic losses for common cryptocurrency holders.

At the moment, even though cryptocurrencies do perform functions commonly ascribed to money and display typical monetary attributes, they apparently fail to respond to some of the basic expectations and beliefs on which confidence in money (and trust in monetary authorities and governments) seem to rest, namely that money will be accepted as a legal means of payment in the settlement private and public obligations, and that the value of money (i.e. its purchasing power) will remain fairly constant over time (Lascaux, 2012). Both expectations are crucial when it comes to stability and predictability. Private cryptocurrencies may not be able to assert themselves as international currencies, but monetary authorities are already learning the lessons and incorporating both blockchain technologies into their own digital currencies (Gerba & Rubio, 2019). One thing seems certain: neither fiat currencies nor cryptocurrencies can dispose of trust.

CONCLUSION

As previously argued, trust is essentially a relational (interpersonal) phenomenon that requires the willingness to be vulnerable to others and the trustor's confident, positive expectations towards the trustee. Hence, the risk of being deceived or betrayed is intrinsic to the trusting attitude. If that risk is absent, there is no room for trust, precisely what Satoshi Nakamoto and his successors were proposing after the disruptive effects of the international financial and economic crisis of 2008.

According to Harari (2014), "money is the most universal and the most efficient system of mutual trust ever devised" (p. 201). The historical evidence strongly suggests that trust performed a pivotal role in the success and continuous sophistication of the "technology of money," even though the use of many hard currencies, at least on the lower level of the monetary systems, often seemed to be base on reliance, habit or need. Extreme cases show that it was even possible to keep using distrusted currencies in the face of political coercion, endemic shortages, hyperinflation, or significant counterfeiting. However, such currencies were unable to gain widespread acceptance and were eventually doomed to fail.

The most successful historical currencies were state or state-backed currencies based on the existence of solid trust towards issuers, i.e., the willingness to accept currency trusting that its issuer would at least endeavor to uphold its value. This typically implied the issuer's commitment to accept its own currency at its full nominal value in settlement of obligations, to maintain its convertibility, or to redeem it if discontinued, depending on the type of currency at stake. Ultimately, the issuer's commitment to currency holders involves creating guarantee systems to be executed in case of collapse.

From a strictly formal point of view, trust in money or any specific currency is just a convenient metaphor. At the bottom of the issue, what people are actually trusting in (assuming that trust is there) is always other people, either directly or indirectly. In the case of sovereign fiat currencies, this includes a trusted network involving different intervenient parties at different levels of the monetary and payments system, from states, monetary authorities, and commercial banks to local businesses and ordinary citizens, i.e., end-users, intermediaries, issuers and guarantors.

As for cryptocurrencies, trust in third-party intermediaries is being replaced by software codes and cryptography, but that is just part of the problem of trust. Moreover, blockchain creates conditions for a decentralized and more robust form of trust. With cryptocurrencies, power is being transferred from political and monetary authorities to the system's developers and validators, who are vested with the power of maintaining its integrity, security, and reliability (and it is not irrelevant to ask where they are based). Developers probably stand at the apex of this structure, as they can change the code and cause forks, which present a challenge to the community's cohesion. The stronger the trust, the larger the acceptance of such forks. Furthermore, as flaws are detected and problems emerge (including fraudulent attacks), all cryptocurrency systems need governance mechanisms and some degree of flexibility that inevitably lay beyond their embedded codes and protocols. Regulation and guarantee systems implementation will contribute to enhancing trust amongst cryptocurrency users (Werbach 2018; De Filippi, Mannan & Reijers, 2020).

Cryptocurrencies have made a decisive contribution to expose the true nature of modern money: "a trusted form of information that conveys value" (Werbach, 2018, p. 96). Cryptocurrencies do possess key attributes shared with sovereign fiat currencies, but they are still too volatile, unstable, and unsatisfactorily regulated, as well as subject to an inherent conflict between its crypto asset (speculative) and money functions. The exponential growth of the digital economy and similar growth on the Internet of value, coupled with the increased tokenization of assets (as royalties, equity, claims on services, cryptocurrencies, or real estate), will undoubtedly contribute to expanding private cryptocurrencies soon. It is impossible to say whether cryptocurrencies will succeed against state or central bank digital currencies, but their contribution to developing more efficient payment systems and a new world of value cannot be denied.

REFERENCES

Almeida, M. (1982). *Catálogo geral de cédulas de Portugal / Low emergency paper Money of Portugal.* Sociedade Portuguesa de Numismática.

Aristotle. (2004). *Nicomachean Ethics* (R. Crisp, Trans.). Cambridge University Press. doi:10.1017/CBO9781139600514

Bencsik, A., Jakubik, M., & Juhasz, T. (2020). The Economic Consequences of Trust and Distrust in Knowledge-Intensive Organizations. *Journal of Competitiveness*, *12*(3), 28–46. doi:10.7441/joc.2020.03.02

Bland, R. (2012). From Gordian III to the Gallic Empire (AD 238-274). In W Metcalf (Ed.), *The Oxford Handbook of Greek and Roman Coinage* (pp. 514-537). Oxford University Press. https:// doi:10.1093/oxfordhb/9780195305746.013.0029

Bopearachchi, O. (2017). Achaemenids and Mauryas: Emergence of coins and plastic art in India. In A. Patel & T. Daryaee (Eds.), *India and Iran in the Longue Durée* (pp. 15–47). UCI Indian Centre for Persian Studies.

Bransbourg, G. (2011). *Fides et pecunia numerate.* Chartalism and metallism in the Roman World. Part 1: The Republic. *American Journal of Numismatics*, *2*(23), 87–152.

Burnett, A., Amandry, M., & Ripollès, P. P. (1992). Roman Provincial Coinage (vol. 1). British Museum Press / Bibliothèque nationale de France.

Campo, M. (2010). Producción i circulació de moneda falsa a la Península Ibèrica (s. IV aC – I dC). In M. Campo (Ed.), *Falsificació i manipulació de la moneda. XIV Curs d'Història monetària d'Hispània* (pp. 23–39). MNAC – Gabinet Numismatic de Catalunya.

CoinDesk. (n.d.). *Bitcoin.* Retrieved January 22, 2021, from https://www.coindesk.com/price/bitcoin

Cribb, J. (2003). The origins of the Indian coinage tradition. *South Asian Studies*, *19*(1), 1–19. doi:10.1080/02666030.2003.9628617

De Callataÿ, F. (2013). White gold: An enigmatic start to Greek coinage. *American Numismatic Society Magazine*, *12*(2), 7–17.

De Filippi, P., Mannan, M., & Reijers, W. (2020). Blockchain as a confidence machine: The problem of trust & challenges of governance. *Technology in Society*, *62*, 1–24. doi:10.1016/j.techsoc.2020.101284

De Roover, R. (1953). *L'Évolution de la lettre de change XIVe-XVIIIe siècles.* Librairie Armand Colin.

Denzel, M. A. (2014). Monetary and financial innovations in Flanders, Antwerp, London and Hamburg: fifteenth to eighteenth century. In P. Bernholz & R. Vaubel (Eds.), Explaining monetary and financial innovation: a historical analysis (pp. 252-282). Springer. doi:10.1007/978-3-319-06109-2_10

Elliott, C. E. (2020). The role of money in the economies of Ancient Greece and Rome. In S. Battilossi, Y. Cassis & K. Yago (Eds.), Handbook of the History of Money and Currency (pp. 67-86). Springer. doi:10.1007/978-981-13-0596-2_46

Erikson, E. H. (1982). *The life cycle completed.* W. W. Norton & Company.

Fukuyama, F. (1995). *Trust: The social virtues and the creation of prosperity*. Free Press.

Fulmer, C. A., & Gelfand, M. J. (2012). At what level (and in whom) we trust: Trust across multiple organizational levels. *Journal of Management, 38*(4), 1167–1230. doi:10.1177/0149206312439327

Gadoury, V., & Élie, R. (1990). *Monnaies de nécessité françaises, 1789-1990*. Éditions Victor Gadoury.

Gerba, E., & Rubio, M. (2019). *Virtual money: how much do cryptocurrencies alter the fundamental functions of money?* (PE 642.360). European Parliament. https://www.europarl.europa.eu/cmsdata/190132/PE%20642.360%20LSE%20final%20publication-original.pdf

Giovannini, A. (1975). Athenian currency in the late fifth and early fourth century B.C. *Greek, Roman and Byzantine Studies, 16*(2), 185–195.

Goldberg, D. (2009). The Massachusetts paper money of 1690. *The Journal of Economic History, 69*(4), 1092–1106. doi:10.1017/S0022050709001399

Goldberg, S. C. (2020). Trust and reliance. In J. Simon (Ed.), *The Routledge handbook of trust and philosophy* (pp. 97–108). Routledge. doi:10.4324/9781315542294-8

Graeber, D. (2011). *Debt: the first 5,000 years*. Melville House Printing.

Harari, Y. N. (2014). *Sapiens: a brief history of mankind* (Y. N. Harari, J. Purcell, & H. Watzman, Trans.). Vintage Books.

Howgego, C. (1992). The supply and use of money in the Roman World 200 B.C. to A.D. 300. *Journal of Roman Studies, 82*, 1–31. doi:10.2307/301282

Hudson, M. (2020). Origins of Money and Interest: Palatial Credit, Not Barter. In S. Battilossi, Y. Cassis & K. Yago (Eds.), Handbook of the History of Money and Currency (pp. 45-65). Springer. doi:10.1007/978-981-13-0596-2_1

Kakinuma, Y. (2014). The emergence and spread of coins in China from the Spring and Autumn Period to the Warring States Period. In P. Bernholz & R. Vaubel (Eds.), *Explaining monetary and financial innovation: a historical analysis* (pp. 79–126). Springer. doi:10.1007/978-3-319-06109-2_5

Kohn, M. (2020). Money, trade, and payments in Preindustrial Europe. In S. Battilossi, Y. Cassis & K. Yago (Eds.), Handbook of the History of Money and Currency (pp. 223-244). Springer. doi:10.1007/978-981-13-0596-2_15

Kroll, J. (1976). Aristophanes' *ponera chalkia*: A reply. *Greek, Roman and Byzantine Studies, 17*(4), 329–341.

Kroll, J. (2012). The monetary background of early coinage. In W. Metcalf (Ed.), *The Oxford Handbook of Greek and Roman Coinage* (pp. 33–42). Oxford University Press., doi:10.1093/oxfordhb/9780195305746.013.0003

Kugler, P., & Straumann, T. (2020). International monetary regimes: the Bretton Woods system. In S. Battilossi, Y. Cassis & K. Yago (Eds.), Handbook of the History of Money and Currency (pp. 665-685). Springer. doi:10.1007/978-981-13-0596-2_25

Lafaurie, J. (1981). *Les assignats et les papiers-monnaies émis par l'État au XVIIIe siècle*. Le Leopard d'Or.

Lane, F. C., & Mueller, R. C. (1987). Coins and moneys of account. In F. C. Lane & R. C. Mueller (Eds.) Money and banking in medieval Renaissance Venice (Vol. 1). The John Hopkins University Press.

Langfred, C. W. (2004). Too much of a good thing? Negative effects of high trust and individual autonomy in self-managing teams. *Academy of Management Journal, 47*(3), 385–399. doi:10.5465/20159588

Lascaux, A. (2014). Money, trust and hierarchies: Understanding the foundations for placing confidence in complex economic institutions. *Journal of Economic Issues, 46*(1), 75–100. doi:10.2753/JEI0021-3624460103

Lewicki, R. J., McAllister, D. J., & Bies, R. J. (1998). Trust and distrust: New relationships and realities. *Academy of Management Review, 23*(3), 438–458. doi:10.5465/amr.1998.926620

Lopez, R. S. (1976). *The commercial revolution of the Middle Ages*. Cambridge University Press.

Lowry, P. B., Schuetzler, R., Giboney, J. S., & Gregory, T. (2015). Is trust always better than distrust? The potential value of distrust in newer virtual teams engaged in short-term decision-making. *Group Decision and Negotiation, 24*(4), 723–752. doi:10.100710726-014-9410-x

Luhmann, N. (1988). Familiarity, confidence, trust: Problems and alternatives. In D. Gambetta (Ed.), *Trust: Making and breaking cooperative relations* (pp. 94–107). Basil Blackwell.

Mangus, S. M., Jones, E., Folse, J. A. G., & Sridhar, S. (2020). The interplay between business and personal trust on relationship performance in conditions of market turbulence. *Journal of the Academy of Marketing Science, 48*(6), 1138–1155. doi:10.100711747-020-00722-6

Mayer, R. C., Davis, J. H., & Schoorman, F. D. (1995). An integrative model of organizational trust. *Academy of Management Review, 20*(3), 709–734. doi:10.5465/amr.1995.9508080335

McLeod, C. (2020). Trust. In E. N. Zalta (Ed.), *Stanford Encyclopedia of Philosophy*. Retrieved March 1, 2021, from https://plato.stanford.edu/archives/fall2020/entries/trust/

Mueller, R. C. (1997). The Venetian money market: Banks, panics, and the public debt, 1200-1500. In F. C. Lane & R. C. Mueller (Eds.), Money and banking in medieval Renaissance Venice (Vol. 2). The John Hopkins University Press.

Murphy, A. E. (1997). *John Law: economic theorist and policy-maker*. Clarendon Press. doi:10.1093/019828649X.001.0001

Nakamoto, S. (2008). *Bitcoin: A peer-to-peer electronic cash system* [White paper]. https://bitcoin.org/bitcoin.pdf

Officer, L. H. (2020). International monetary regimes: the gold standard. In S. Battilossi, Y. Cassis & K. Yago (Ed.), Handbook of the History of Money and Currency (pp. 599-631). Springer. doi:10.1007/978-981-13-0596-2_23

Orléan, A. (2008). Crise de la souveraineté et crise de la monnaie: l'hyperinflation allemande des années 1920. In B. Théret (Ed.), La monnaie dévoilée par ses crises, vol. 2, Crises monétaires en Russie et en Allemagne au XXe siècle. Éditions de l'EHESS.

Peters, S., & Bilton, D. (2018). 'Right-Touch' trust: Thoughts on trust in healthcare. In R. H. Searle, A. I. Nienaber, & S. B. Sitkin (Eds.), *The Routledge companion to trust*. Routledge.

Quinn, S., & Roberds, W. (2008). The evolution of the check as a means of payment: A historical survey. *Economic Review (Kansas City, Mo.)*, *93*(4), 1–28.

Quinn, S., & Roberds, W. (2014). The Bank of Amsterdam through the lens of monetary competition. In P. Bernholz & R. Vaubel (Eds.), *Explaining monetary and financial innovation: a historical analysis* (pp. 283–300). Springer. doi:10.1007/978-3-319-06109-2_11

Robinson, K. G. (Ed.). (2004). General conclusions and reflections. In J. Needham, Science and civilisation in China (vol. 7.2). Cambridge University Press.

Schaps, D. M. (2004). *The invention of coinage and the monetization of Ancient Greece*. The University of Michigan Press. doi:10.3998/mpub.17760

Schoorman, F. D., Mayer, R. C., & Davis, J. H. (2007). An integrative model of organizational trust: Past, present, and future. *Academy of Management Review*, *32*(2), 344–354. doi:10.5465/amr.2007.24348410

Spufford, P. (1988). *Money and its use in medieval Europe*. Cambridge University Press. doi:10.1017/CBO9780511583544

Stroukal, D. (2018). Can bitcoin become money? Its money functions and the regression theorem. *International Journal of Business and Management*, *6*(1), 36–53. doi:10.20472/BM.2018.6.1.004

Tapscott, A., & Tapscott, D. (2007). *How blockchain is changing finance* [White paper]. Harvard business review. https://hbr.org/2017/03/how-blockchain-is-changing-finance

Temin, P. (2013). *The Roman market economy*. Princeton University Press.

Thagard, P. (2019). *Mind-society: From brains to social sciences and professions*. Oxford University Press. doi:10.1093/oso/9780190678722.001.0001

Thierry, F. (1997). Monnaies chinoises, vol. I – L'Antiquité préimpériale. Bibliothèque nationale de France.

Thierry, F. (2001). La fiduciarité idéale à l'épreuve des couts de production: Quelques éléments sur la contradiction fondamentale de la monnaie en Chine. *Revue Numismatique*, *6*(157), 131–152. doi:10.3406/numi.2001.2323

Tingström, B. (1986). *Plate money: the world's largest currency*. Royal Coin Cabinet.

Valério, N. (2007). From the first Portuguese bank to the Bank of Portugal's role as central bank. In N. Valério (Ed.), *History of the Portuguese banking system* (Vol. 1). Banco de Portugal.

Van De Mieroop, M. (1997). *The ancient Mesopotamian city*. Clarendon Press.

Van De Mieroop, M. (2014). Silver as a financial tool in ancient Egypt and Mesopotamia. In P. Bernholz & R. Vaubel (Eds.), *Explaining monetary and financial innovation: a historical analysis* (pp. 17–29). Springer. doi:10.1007/978-3-319-06109-2_2

Van Nieuwkerk, M. (2009). How a city bank became a world-famous bank. In M. van Nieuwkerk (Ed.), *The Bank of Amsterdam: on the origins of central banking* (pp. 12–27). De Nederlandsche Bank / Sonsbeek Publishers.

Von Glahn, R. (1996). *Fountain of fortune: money and monetary policy in China, 1000-1700*. University of California Press. doi:10.1525/9780520917453

Von Glahn, R. (2005). The origins of paper money in China. In W. N. Goetzmann & K. G. Rouwenhorst (Eds.), *The origins of value: financial innovations that created modern capital markets* (pp. 65–89). Oxford University Press.

Werbach, K. (2018). *The blockchain and the new architecture of trust*. The MIT Press. doi:10.7551/mitpress/11449.001.0001

Wetterberg, G. (2009). *Money and power: From Stockholms Banco 1656 to Sveriges Riksbank today*. Sveriges Riksbank.

Wray, L. R. (2015). *Modern money theory: a primer on macroeconomics for sovereign monetary systems* (2nd ed.). Palgrave Macmillan. doi:10.1057/9781137539922

Chapter 3

Blockchanging Money:
Reengineering the Free World Incentive System

Dario de Oliveira Rodrigues
https://orcid.org/0000-0002-2817-5115
Instituto Politécnico de Santarém, Portugal

ABSTRACT

Blockchain technology is changing the world incentive system, making programmable money. This kind of money is only fruitful and democratically livable in a transparent political environment. Otherwise, instead of unleashing innovation and collective action with the market's visible hand of qualified money, the new internet of value will deliver a digital money with the same algorithmic fate that social media met on the previous internet. The latter allows digitizing users' data and has been used to manipulate consumers and public opinion (possibly in the last two U.S. Presidential elections). Similarly, the former will let states and corporatocracy cross-reference social media and digital money's data, hurting privacy even more. As blockchains disseminate, having the crucial economic advantage of reducing transaction costs, only free-market competition between private and public blockchains guarantee transparency and democracy. Blockchain technology is the real McCoy, and decentralizing digital money is the free world's best shot, especially in the new normal triggered by COVID-19.

INTRODUCTION

"Technology comes in packages, big and small." (Kranzsberg, 1986) Kranzberg's Third Law

This chapter's main objective is to show both auspicious and worrisome implications of *Blockchain Technology* (BT), which has recently empowered money as the newest type of economic media (Beller, 2020) aired on the *Internet of Value* (Twesige, 2015). Several central banks are making efforts to develop their digital currencies (Náñez Alonso et al., 2021), and it will be discussed how to deal with the *blockchain* kind of money. It is thought that digital money's implications will be crucial to society in a

DOI: 10.4018/978-1-7998-7363-1.ch003

post-pandemic new normal (Berwick, 2020) that requires a watchful consideration of "how institutions are designed and formed, and how the balance between institutions' control and the public's freedom is negotiated in society" (Tam, 2021, p.9).

As stated by Ebadi et al. (2020), "The idea of a secure digital currency that is not managed by a central authority has been an interesting field of research for decades. Bitcoin showed this ideal is reachable" (p. 54).

Whatever consumers may say, in the end, they want quality before anything else. [...] To keep in pace with this growing trend, initiatives flourish to help increase transparency and traceability. [...] More than just a buzzword, a blockchain is an opened ledger of every transaction between the stakeholders. The records are permanent and verifiable, and are not managed by a central authority. (Tonin et al., 2018, p. 3)

Following a rationale shared by economists like Keynes and Friedman but going against the conventional belief about *money* and not following the orthodox theory of most economic books, one can draw a line between one-dimensional centralized, traditional money and multi-dimensional programmable tokens. Not complying with rulers' perspective (see *Seigniorage* in Key Terms and Definitions), BT allows decentralizing money globally in a structured and secure way for the first time in history (Nakamoto, 2008). To understand such a paradigm shift is convenient to begin investigating what *money* is.

Although we usually assume a sharp line of distinction between what is money and what is not, and the law generally tries to make such a distinction so far as the causal effects of monetary events are concerned, there is no such clear difference. What we find is instead a continuum in which objects of various degrees of liquidity, or with values which can fluctuate independently of each other, shade into each other in the degree to which they function as money" (Hayek 1990, p. 56)

BT's predictable diffusion makes it possible to envision a "political transformation [that] requires the possibility of a redesign of the protocols of money" (Beller, 2020, p. 217), diversifying humans incentive systems and assuring freedom of choice on the *Internet of Money* (Peters & Panayi, 2016; Antonopoulos, 2017; Pocher, 2019; Srivastava et al., 2021).

It should be mentioned the author's liberal perspective. The investigation method was based on qualitative research, and the methodology chosen was the literature review, which is adequate to overview several thematic areas on a given topic. Among the literature review methods available, the most used for business studies are systematic review, semi-systematic review, and integrative review (Snyder, 2019). Considering the need to carry out a synthesis conducive to envision the economic and *crypto-economic* implications of BT, the author chose the integrative literature review, which is indicated to frame a study from new perspectives, especially when it comes to research themes and topics little explored (Torraco, 2005). As far as it was possible to observe, the author concludes there are few studies regarding specifically the economic impact of cryptocurrencies and other *crypto assets*.

This chapter is organized as follows. It begins demystifying money's nature and checking if cryptocurrency has the necessary properties to redesign money's protocols. It will be shown that these protocols are changing, and it is still pretty much unsure that it will be for the best. After providing a background regarding BT and observing some critical elements of the blockchain ecosystem, digital money's competitive advantages will be presented. It will be argued that *blockchain money* should not remain solely a creature of the state (Reiners, 2020). It is thought that besides changing society's fundamental ethical dilemmas (see the same book, Chapter 1 - *Blockchanging Trust: Ethical Metamorphosis in Business & Healthcare*), BT will make-or-break democracy (see Chapter 4 - *Blockchanging Politics: Opening a Trustworthy But Hazardous Reforming Era*), offering a civilizational opportunity to nurture community ecosystems by equipping multidimensional financial incentives systems with *qualified money* (Helbing, 2014). A liberal scenario of decentralized markets will be introduced where a new breed of socio-financial incentives will be the *economic media hyperlink* to Friedrich Hayek's premonitory vision of private currencies backed by free competition (Hayek, 1976).

BACKGROUND

The Essence of Money

According to economic books, money fulfills three core functions, performing as (i) a medium of exchange, intermediating trade by paying for goods and services; (ii) a reserve of value, maintaining its value to be reliable spent later; (iii) a unit of account, measuring value and setting the price of goods, services, assets, and liabilities (Monroe, 1923; Ingham, 2013; Mattke et al., 2020).

Supposedly, trading without using a medium of exchange would always demand business parties' compatible desires since barter always requires coincidental interests. However, as will be seen below, this presumed inevitability is truly a misconception, which is crucial to correct in the dawn of the *blockchain era*.

It is thought that is useful drawing a parallel between digital money and social media, the two modern types of *economic media* (Beller, 2020). Social media comes from a long time ago. As stated by Hurlburt & Voas (2011), "our walls are just more likely to be on Facebook than deep inside caves" (p. 11). In a certain sense, cave painting constituted prehistoric *posts*, and cave walls of human ancestors were the social media *murals* possible to edit and program with the technology then available (Safko, 2010). Therefore, for thousands of years, an economic *value-of-use* (see Key Terms and Definitions) is being created and signalled by attention and reputation raised in social media. Firstly, through physical and handcrafted work, then industrialized, and finally digitalized, an increasing network effect enhanced this economic media (Beller, 2020).

Money is the main economic media, and while "likes and retweets are a form of "voting" but are not optimal [because] there is no scarcity of likes and therefore no real value beyond signaling" (Martinelli, 2017, p. 4), digital money is a new breed of valuable economic media.

Several authors trace money's path from ancient times (Szabo, 2002; Zelmanovitz, 2011; Martin, 2013; Lannoye, 2020). As in the social media case, it may be useful to observe this economic media's past. In the article "Banking on Stone Money: Ancient Antecedents to Bitcoin," published in the field of economic anthropology, Fitzpatrick & McKeon (2019) compare the *stone money* system of the small islands of Yap, in Micronesia, which has been studied for many decades (Furness, 1910; de Beauclair, 1963, 1971; Friedman, 1991; Fitzpatrick, 2004), with the modern financial sector given similarities between such *stone money* and cryptocurrencies. As stated by Fitzpatrick & McKeon (2020), "stone money was a conceptual precursor to Nakamoto's Bitcoin white paper, which introduced a modern invention to solve similar societal problems." (p. 13).

Yap Islands' *stone money* consisted of stone discs, many with several tons, called *fei* or *rai* (the name *rai* was used in the northern part of Yap, and *fei* in the southern part). This *stone money* was not easy to transport, and it certainly would not have been a smart choice to move around as a medium of exchange (Martin, 2013).

Regardless of transactions and money transfers that took place, the physical transportation of *fei* from one owner's home to another was infrequent, as the debts incurred were typically only offset with the expectation of further exchanges later on. Albeit the character of *stone money* was strictly symbolic, when it was associated with the Yap's natives' *oral ledger*, either the *stone money'* value and changes in its ownership could be tracked, and trade went fine on the Yap Islands. As stated by Furness (1910), "after concluding a bargain which involves the price of a "fei" too large to be conveniently moved [some of these "coins" weighed several tons], its new owner is quite content to accept the bare acknowledgment of ownership and without so much as a mark to indicate the exchange, the coin remains undisturbed on the former owner's premises." (p. 96.).

Yap's *stone money* may seem just anecdotal, but prominent economists like John Maynard Keynes and Milton Friedman thought it would be more than that. These two brilliant minds recognized that Yap's monetary system could hold an essential and universal lesson that defied conventional money theory. Keynes would state the following about what was written, in 1910, by the American anthropologist, William Henry Furness III, in a book describing his travels to Borneo and the Yap Islands (located where are today the Federated States of Micronesia):

[Furness' book] has brought us into contact with a people whose ideas on currency are probably more truly philosophical than those of any other country. Modern practice in regard to gold reserves has a good deal to learn from the more logical practices of the island of Yap. (Keynes, 1915, p. 281)

As it was referred, Keynes was not the only worthy of twentieth-century economics to exalt Yap's inhabitants for their clear understanding of the nature of money (Martin, 2013). Also, Friedman (1991) praised the people of the Yap Islands' discernment, saying that they have escaped the conventional obsession with money-merchandise and recognized that money is not a commodity but a system of credit and clearing. So, the basic assumption that money has evolved primarily as a medium of exchange (the intuitive idea that money emerged out of barter) must be questioned. Pointing out that Keynes and Friedman reverberated Yap's money, Martin (2013) referred that "to win the praise of one of the two greatest monetary economists of the twentieth century may be regarded as chance; to win the praise of both deserves attention…" (p. 14).

This same author also stated that "seek as they might, not a single researcher was able to find a society, historical or contemporary, that regularly conducted its trade by barter." (p. 14). As told by the American scholar George Dalton, in 1982, "Barter, in the strict sense of moneyless market exchange, has never been a quantitatively important or dominant mode of transaction in any past or present economic system about which we have hard information" (p. 183).

Also, the Cambridge anthropologist Caroline Humphrey concludes that "no example of a barter economy, pure and simple, has ever been described, let alone the emergence from it of money; all available ethnography suggests that there has never been such a thing" (Humphrey, 1985).

If one villager needed a pig for a feast, he may be able to obtain it from another villager for four clay pots, or a different villager for ten pairs of shoes. Constantly making mental calculations to determine the best value for a pig, or whatever else you are trying to acquire, is time consuming, thus, money is "born." The problem with this story is that it is simply not true. In reality, these villagers know one another, and rather than exchange ten pairs of shoes for one pig, the villager who provides the pig simply takes note of the contribution and that his fellow villager owes him something of comparable value. This is the same thing as credit, and the archaeological record reveals that credit systems of this sort preceded the invention of coinage by thousands of years. (Reiners, 2020, p.2)

Hence, it is considered appropriate to ask the following question: if the *stone money* from the Yap Islands were not a medium of exchange, how did it work well as being money for so many years? What is the secret so that the physical movement, from person to person, of the specific thing considered to be the money has proved irrelevant? The answer is that money itself is not a specific thing or object with intrinsic value, but rather it is an underlying system of credit and clearing accounts that these objects help represent and keep in track. The stone disks were just tokens portraying how the entire accounting record was kept in place at any given moment. Yap's oral ledger was the real money, *i.e.*, the credit accounts' system and their clearing that currency represents (Martin, 2013).

Thinking of money as a *thing* or commodity whose *intrinsic value* constitutes the incentive to exchange goods and services by such a thing (currency) could be intuitive when coins were minted in precious metals or money was backed by gold. However, this is no longer the case, and today should be easier to understand that fiduciary currencies or *fiat money* (see Key Terms and Definitions) are just symbols or tokens. Additionally, since the last century, most currencies exist in an electronic version, obviously being intangible and without *intrinsic* value, and the physical version of these coins is a minority (Prinzs, 1999). Moreover, some authors think that *fiat currencies* soon will cease to have a physical format (Quian, 2019; Bindseil, 2019).

A dollar, whether under a Gold Standard or not, is something that would be intimately familiar to the faceless bureaucrats of the International Bureau of Weights and Measures: it is a unit of measurement—an arbitrary increment on an abstract scale. So, like a metre or a kilogram, a dollar itself doesn't refer to any physical thing at all—even if the length or mass or value of some particular physical thing has been agreed on as its standard. (Martin, 2013, p. 51)

As Keynes and Friedman soon understood, Yap's economic and financial worldview considered *stone money* as tokens of an underlying credit relationship, being the former nothing more than a way of representing the latter. The sound money was the oral ledger.

The weighty argument provided by the heavy *stone-money* of the Yap Islands, praised by no less weighty figures of the economic thought, perhaps will be able to shake out the idea that *intrinsic value* has to exist and go from hand in hand to make money work as a portable medium of exchange. Even after the gold-standard, the *intrinsic value* false belief helped keep the prerogative of currency-issuing in sovereign hands. However, the source of trust created by blockchain technology (BT) dismantles such wrong allegation with mathematical precision.

The idea of a technology for recording and transferring monetary obligations from one person to another, dispensing central coordination, may appear to be subversive and dangerous to some. After all, the invention of coins in the Kingdom of Lydia, located in what is now the western part of Turkey, nearly three thousand years ago (Weatherford, 2009), ushered in the conversion of traditional social obligations into financial relationships, a giant step in individual emancipation, challenging the previously undisputed authority of a centralized economy and a historical immutable social hierarchy. However, this enfranchisement process is by no means complete. Today, societies face the historical inevitability (because BT is not neutral) of taking another giant monetary step, and one should be keen this new step would be given towards freedom, for there is a considerable risk of following the opposite direction which entails the risk of a complete loss of privacy, and subsequently the demise of democratic regimes.

Understanding cryptocurrency requires letting go of the notion of money as an incentive system made up of things with intrinsic value. Practicing barter requires an available credit and clearing system, a language with which people can negotiate without intermediaries. In this sense, BT allowed creating a global ledger or *hyperledger* of digital tokens. These tokens are recognized as money; likewise, the natives' *oral ledger* and *stone money* were hundreds of years ago in the Yap Islands. A decentralized money system made it possible to offset obligations without reference to a central authority in both cases. As stated by Fitzpatrick & McKeon (2020), there are striking similarities between bitcoin and the Yap Islands' *stone money*:

The principles by which Blockchains—in oral and digital forms—operate and how Yapese stone money (rai) can be considered analogous to modern cryptocurrencies along several dimensions. In many ways, the process through which these monetary units are created, transacted, and recorded is similar, demonstrating that the concept behind Bitcoin and the underlying blockchain technology have their roots in the ancient past. (Fitzpatrick & McKeon, 2020, p. 13)

Therefore, Yap's *stone money* shows how a small island society crafted an effective system for monitoring asset ownership and trade. In a very similar way, albeit using a digital *hyperledger* instead of an *oral ledger*, information about money' ownership is managed collectively with cryptocurrency, even without their owners physically possess any medium of exchange. Hence, both systems ensure financial transparency and security with no central bank.

Long before the Internet and BT protocols were created, the protocol of money (6th century BC) allowed people to start negotiating with each other something essential to individual freedom: *the offsetting of obligations without reference to a centralized authority* (Martin, 2013). This decentralized negotiability was responsible for the pioneering idea of an objective and lifelong economic space, and probably then the *market* concept was born.

For markets to work, a shared concept of value given by a standardized unit is needed. For the market's sake, it does not matter if there is or not a preconceived collective idea about the value for a product or a service since that value's determination is, itself, the essential market's task. What is required then is just a shared idea on how to measure the market's value. Without such a common language, trade is not possible.

The costliness of information is the key to the cost of transacting, part of the transaction costs in any deal is associated with the gathering of information about the best opportunities for trade. (...) So, a unit of exchange was introduced in order to make transactions easier among barterers by lowering their transaction costs in acquiring information about the relative prices among their respective goods and services. (Zelmanovitz, 2011, p. 76)

Therefore, *money* and *market* are inseparable concepts, in the absence of which ancient people used to depend on a central authority to receive directives on how to act. These two concepts brought the powerful and emancipatory notion of a new political-economic reality: due to money, traditional social obligations started to be valued on a universal scale and became transferable between individuals.

The great fear associated with violating rules of conduct has always been that the result would be anarchy. This fear is why conserving social order may be at odds with innovation, ambition, entrepreneurship, and social mobility. Hence, the introduction of money into society was undoubtedly disruptive, daring to combine political stability with social mobility:

Money made its miraculous promise to combine apparent opposites on the personal level as well. It catered to two fundamental aspects of human psychology: the desire for freedom and the desire for stability. The ethics of the traditional society had sacrificed the former on the altar of the latter. The new world of monetary society promised both. Money's claim that its new way of organising society would not end in disaster, but would combine the power of social mobility and personal freedom with that of social stability and economic security (Martin, 2013, p.62)

No wonder that the notion of *hyperledger* as a *distributed ledger* replicated on a network of computers that is able to decentralize trust due to a common cryptographic language, will find resistance coming from those who do not want to give up of central power. Understanding that money is an accounting system and that tokens are merely symbolic and not mandatorily made of specific *things* with intrinsic value is crucial to grasp into cryptocurrencies' nature and realize how digital money's intangibility is not by no means a limitation. On the contrary, such intangibility can be a considerable advantage given the desirable characteristics of money (see the next sections).

Distributed Ledger Technologies (DLT), such as BT, are digital versions of Yap Islands' oral ledger (Fitzpatrick & McKeon, 2020). It was that same kind of trust that Yap Islands' natives used as money during centuries, a *distributed trust* that was really the essence of their money. Although natives' network was not digital, Yap's money was based on a trustable collective memory, *i.e.*, on the tribal knowledge about the property whereabouts of the conspicuous *stone-money*. Some of the stones were marked upon after transactions, but most changed hands verbally without being moved around. The truth is that Yap Islands' monetary system relied above all upon an oral ledger.

In the Pacific Islands, as in many other societies, "money" developed from locally available, but comparatively rare resources that were assigned value and exchanged, primarily for foodstuffs and other goods. Some common examples of money in the Pacific include thorny oysters (Spondylus sp.) and pearl shells (Pinctada sp.) [...] It is important to note that in none of these or other cases in the Pacific did the exchange of shells or other resources evolve into what would strictly be defined as a currency. (...) only in the case of Yapese stone money did an exchange valuable have its ownership recorded orally in a social ledger that allowed possession of an object to be tracked and henceforth "titled" to an individual or group. (Fitzpatrick & McKeon, 2020, p. 5).

Thus, the *stone money* shows that the widespread belief in money's intrinsic value indispensableness is historically false. Nevertheless, several authors are convinced that "Bitcoin has no fundamental value and that sooner or later the market will recognize this fact." (Andolfatto & Spewak, 2019, p.1). Although such causality notion can be intuitive and shared enough (Sanz Bas, 2020), it was soon denied in the Yap Islands where during centuries *stone money* worked just fine (Fitzpatrick & McKeon, 2020) despite being nothing more than bulky rocks with no intrinsic value.

Finally, another essential lesson about cryptocurrencies can be learned by looking at Yap Islands' *stone money*. It is known that several authors do not consider cryptocurrencies as being real currencies (Mittal, 2012; Grant, 2014; Lo, 2017; Passinsky, 2021; Brummer & Yadav, 2018), mainly due to their high volatility, which is usually attributed to the fact that the states and the central banks do not backed them. For example, Andolfatto & Spewak (2019) state that "the price dynamic of an unbacked asset is likely to be highly volatile" (p. 2). However, disproving this belief, it is observed that it was exclusively the difficulty of producing the *stone money* of the Yap Islands that backed its value, and this money has worked for centuries even though its acceptance was exclusively dependent on perceived rarity. The truth is that any authority or other third party never backed the *stone money* of the Yap Islands.

As mentioned by Fitzpatrick & Diveley (2004) about the Yap Islands *stone-money* production process, "This would have required months of planning, extensive labor, and significant energy to complete the process" (p. 133). Later, Fitzpatrick would recognize that the same production difficulty characterizes cryptocurrencies like Bitcoin, with such a guarantee of value working similarly. In his words, "the same [costly production process] could be said of today's digital blockchains, which need tremendous computing power to create and verify new cryptocurrency units along with other ancillary considerations (mathematical and computer programming expertise)" (Fitzpatrick & McKeon, 2020, p. 9). The production difficulty underlying the bitcoin creation process was explained in the first white paper that introduced Bitcoin to the world, where one can read that "the steady addition of a constant amount of new coins is analogous to gold miners expending resources to add gold to circulation. In our case, it is CPU time and electricity that is expended." (Nakamoto, 2008, p. 5)

The Bitcoin protocol limits inflation, and these limits are visible to all market participants. Analogously, supply of new rai [(the stone-money of the Yap Islands)] was also constrained. The constraints were not imposed by a digital protocol but rather by physical means since limestone was not present on Yap. Creating new supply required a trip over open ocean to neighboring Palau and the exertion of manual labor. Additionally, Palauans controlled access to suitable limestone deposits, and a discussion or negotiation was required for new production, further limiting new supply. In a sense, this process is similar to other monetary stores of value throughout history in which there was a constrained stream of supply. (Fitzpatrick & McKeon, 2020, p. 8)

There is little doubt that it was the constraints and difficulties in issuing the Yap Islands 'stone money, prominent determinants of the respective rarity, that were at the origin of the respective perceived value: "[the stone-money] were transported around jagged coral rock islands, through labyrinths of reefs, and over an ocean filled with often unpredictable winds, currents, and swells. (Fitzpatrick, 2004a, p. 23).

It becomes clear that both ancient and modern forms of consensus-based ledgers require immense power to operate. The Yapese version relied on human power to construct boats; sail to Palau; negotiate with Palauan clans or chiefs for access to limestone; carve the rai; construct stone docks, platforms, and other architectural features to facilitate manufacture and movement of stone within and outside of the quarries; and then return home with their [heavy] cargo using some type of watercraft (Fitzpatrick & McKeon, 2020, p. 9).

Therefore, it is necessary to demystify the belief that money will inevitably have to be backed up by the state or any other entity. Although the persistence of such an idea may be convenient for coin issuers, given the income resulting from *seigniorage costs* (see Key Terms and Definitions), it does not seem to be true, nor in the pre-industrial age at the isolated Yap Islands, nor in the digital age at the global village where everyone lives. Although a seal granted by third parties may be a sufficient condition to classify money as so, it is not anymore, a necessary one. Furthermore, in the *blockchain era*, as it will be seen below, in addition to being unnecessary, this wrong belief can be dangerous for democracy and freedom (see Chapter 4).

Private Money

From what was exposed in the previous section, trust on the correct accounts 'memory (oral or digital) is the basis of money, i.e., *trust* on the more or less distributed ledger that ensures such right balances. In *fiat money* trust is ensured by the issuing entity's credibility, which mainly depends on states' ability to collect taxes. This prerogative is the most significant guarantee of confidence underlying the currencies of sovereign states, and therefore "every such country declares at least one type of fiat money to be legal tender for taxes (and contractual debts)." (Goldberg, 2012, p. 23), as well as a way to ensure that state currencies will always be needed. As stated by Goldberg (2012), "Given that the government collects taxes in any case, it can easily promote any money by merely insisting on accepting only that money. (P. 27).

In the 70s, Friedrich Hayek, winner of the Nobel Prize for Economics (1974), for his work on the monetary theory of the trade cycle (Boettke & Prychitko, 2011), proposed what it would be like to replace confidence in the currency issuer (*e.g.*, the state) by confidence in the currencies' competition process itself. In his view, the market share dispute for competitive currencies supremacy will result in the *mutual supervision* of private currency issuers themselves (Hayek, 1976). According to Hayek, this would be enough for that the "gold standard would re-emerge as a result of the competitive process" (Garrison & Kirzner, 1989).

Hayek considered that an intrinsic guarantee of quality would emanate from the competitive struggle among the various private currencies, which is the case of cryptocurrencies "since they have emerged from a private initiative, not from a state" (Sanz Bas, 2020, p. 19). With more than 5000 private cryptocurrencies competing in the market (Fousekis & Grigoriadis, 2021), it is thought that Hayek's words about private money should be taken into due account. Besides competition, further considerations about private money's confidence should include the fact that cryptocurrencies are issued accordingly to algorithmic rules and advanced encryption techniques. For example, Bitcoin's algorithm defines a maximum number of units which is slightly less than 21 million and can never be exceeded (Nakamoto, 2008).

Thus, one can consider that trust in the issuer is now advantageously replaced by trust in cryptographic math operating in a distributed way. As it will be seen, there are good reasons to anticipate that such *distributed trust* (Bellini et al, 2020) will support an epic shift in money creation prerogatives, which can lead to unprecedented financial democratization (decentralized scenario) or to the end of consumer privacy (centralized scenario). As stated by Birch (2020), "Digital currency is a political issue as much as a technological issue." (p. 10) and it is thought that such a change in the foundation of money will have paramount importance to society's development.

Programmable Money

Programmable money comes in different types. For instance, Central Bank Digital Currency (CBDC) is defined by some authors as "a digital representation of a sovereign currency issued by and as a liability of a jurisdiction's central bank or other monetary authority" (Kiff et al., 2020, p. 9). However, it is thought that CBDC is much more than that, and one should emphasize that such centralized digital money should require "a traceable, transferable and divisible digital currency system that protects user's privacy while enabling the retrieval of user's identity in case of suspicious transactions, e.g., suspicion of fraud or money laundering activities" (Barki & Gouget, 2021).

CBDC is not the only programmable money let alone the first. Cryptocurrencies are tradable peer-to-peer (P2P), eliminating the constraints associated with centralization and intermediation, taking advantage of the positive network effects of a structured decentralization. Thus, they can benefit from the cross-pollination, creativity, and intelligence of civil society, including, of course, all qualified programmers in different ecosystems and communities of interest on a planetary scale.

Cryptocurrency is a virtual currency that is used as an alternative currency that the currency is produced and traded through a cryptographic process. The most of the cryptocurrency is decentralized in computer-based networks and is based on peer-to-peer technology and open source cryptography that does not depend on central authorities such as central banks or other administrative institutions. (Adiyatma & Maharani, 2020, p. 71)

It is judged that non-programmable money is outdated and has to go. "Denmark, for example, has adopted legislation that calls for a cashless economy within five years" (Turi, 2020). Nevertheless, the departure of traditional money can both be good or bad news. As it will be seen, even though there is a severe risk of dealing with new centralized money that compromises privacy and freedom, society also has the chance to create a much better version of money. As stated by Helbing (2014):

Currently, money is a scalar, i.e., the simplest mathematical quantity one can think of. It is neither multidimensional nor does it have a memory. But mathematics offers a much richer spectrum of concepts to define exchange processes, such as vectors, i.e., multidimensional quantities, and network graphs. In fact, money comes from somewhere and goes somewhere else. Who transfers money to whom defines a network of money flows. Therefore, money should be represented by network quantities. And money should be multidimensional to allow other things to happen apart from the eternal ups and downs. (p. 3)

Money that comes from somewhere and goes somewhere else is not fungible because it is traceable and has an identity. In fact, "fungibility and anonymity are effectively synonymous" (Berg, 2020, p. 11). So, defending privacy rights in a blockchain world requires balancing transparency and anonymity, and one can agree with Helbing (2014) when he says that money should be multi-dimensional and have a memory for creating the right balance between transparency and anonymity. In his words, "Such money could earn reputation and, with this, additional value!" (p. 3). Therefore, it can be supposed that non-fungibility will allow money's programmable reputation to contribute to an ethical monetary system's faithful balance.

Central banks basically only can print more money and change the interest rate, as banks control the custodian game and governments control banks (Ammous, 2018). However, this is not enough because more control variables are needed, like in any ecosystem.

This problem [of few control variables] is actually well-known from control theory. (…) It is also instructive to compare this with ecosystems. The plant and animal life in a place will not just be determined by a single control variable such as the amount of water, but also by the temperature, humidity, and various kinds of nutrients such as oxygen, nitrogen, phosphor, etc. Our bodies, too, require many kinds of vitamins and nutrients to be healthy. So, why should our economic system be different? Why shouldn't a healthy financial system need several kinds of money? (Helbing, 2014, p. 7)

Since programmable money is here to stay, it is advisable to examine how society reached this point-of-no-return. Once gone digital, money will never go back to a one-dimensional mindless form again, and this is why present stakes are high in the author's perspective.

The two modern economic media, *social media* and *digital money* (Beller, 2020) can be affected by Internet protocols. The 2020 United States Presidential Election dramatic events have shown a pungent example of how disruptive social media and data centralization can be. Social networks are selling the influence that they indeed have over their users on the *Internet of Information*, and it is considered that Washington D.C. riots were largely induced by algorithms "that are telling lies" (O'Neill, 2017. p .7), exacerbating opinions and polarizing society to better segment users and feed rapacious business models.

If the dramatic and violent attempts to take over the Capitol building in Washington DC in January 2021 amount to a historically significant or crucial 'event', much of the subsequent attempts at analysis, explanation, and public debate have focused heavily on the role and influence of the contemporary media system, social media in particular. Fingers were quickly and consistently pointed at social media platforms, such as Twitter and Facebook (…) were widely blamed for "polarising political opinion, normalising extremism and mobilising violent protest (Thornhill, 2021).

It is thought that things can even worse. The Internet of Value (Twesige, 2015) globally distributes the next level of trust, the distributed trust created by BT, which can be a good thing or damaging privacy even harder than has happened so far on the Internet.

It is thought that Blockchain Technology is a game changer that allows the emergence of an Internet of Value by making the digital integration of two very different levels of confidence a reality. The first level is necessary to deal with information and to share its value, but it is not enough to deal with transactions which demand a second level of trust. (De Oliveira Rodrigues, 2021, p. 46)

This time there is a severe risk that the main economic media will serve the political agenda with a never seen granularity, turning corporate or state-sponsored digital currencies into powerful instruments to conditioning citizens' political opinions.

China was the first country to launch a CBDC, the *Digital Yuan*. It is not unreasonable to notice that this is a nation with "normative power and global governance reform aspirations" (Breslin, 2021). One should notice that this digital currency is a second programmable economic media whose semiotic value can be cross-referenced with the first one: social media (*e.g.*, WeChat). Such data matching is now being done in China. Thus, it is thought that Digital Yuan can be simultaneously a currency and an influential political vector, coming from a high-tech central bank sponsored by the most potent authoritarian regime worldwide. Of course, this is not good news when decentralization of finance and cryptocurrencies' free competition is highly recommended to preserve freedom and democracy (Antonopoulos, 2017; Harrison, 2018; Jain, 2020).

Observers have criticised China's social credit scoring system. Called "Sesame Credit," it's billed as mostly a credit score, but it may also function as a way of keeping tabs on an individual's political opinions [(for instance on the WeChat social network)], and for that matter as a way of nudging people towards compliance. (O'Neill, 2017)

Blockchain technology (BT) represents a historical milestone and a crucial crossroads to humankind. BT's *hyperledger* has a social structuring role digital emulation of the *oral ledger* who backed the Yap Islands' natives' stone money for centuries, whose confidence is now digitally extended to the *global village*. Once again, *the medium is the message*, and artifacts as media will affect society by their characteristics or content (McLuhan & McLuhan, 1994). Digitally orchestrated this time, if data centralization prevails, dark times for freedom of thought may be repeated:

In the Soviet communist bloc, and other sectors where state-controlled broadcasting prevailed, systems of broadcasting were intended to reproduce the dominant national culture or state ideology, while serving as instruments of social integration and conformity. (Kellner & Durham, 2001, p. xix)

On the contrary, a very different political-economic history will be written in the following years if decentralization prevails. Thanks to BT, the decentralized requirements underlying the uncensored and non-corruptible transactions on the Yap Islands can now be globally fulfilled over the Internet. A *hyperledger* based on *distributed trust* has just arrived in the Internet's *global village* (McLuhan & Powers, 1989), whose inhabitants can now speak to each other a dealing language, and not just a chat one.

The unusual monetary granularity, provided by the blockchain protocol, together with the seamless integration of the production factors *labor* and *capital* in the same unit of value, which is a cryptocurrency, is paving the way for incorporating in money other values besides *trade value* (Helbing, 2014), a fact that is thought to constitute a notable landmark in the evolution of money itself (Antonopoulos, 2016).

Programmable money allows a much more fine-grained control of a monetary system: token supply can be capped or non-capped leading to deflationary or inflationary currency; tokens can be destroyed ("burnt") and removed from the supply; demurrage, expiration, and many more characteristics can be made inherent properties of a token. However, as these possibilities did not exist before, it is hard to predict the potential of large-scale, bottom-up, open cryptocurrency systems, that are democratically governed and accessible to anyone. (Dapp, 2019)

Programmable money should cause considerable disruption at the political-economic level (Eikmanns, 2019). If threats to privacy and freedom are overcome, it is believed that digital money will create a myriad of opportunities for innovation that can be seized by civil society.

Digital currencies are more competitive than traditional ones, allowing individuals and organizations, including *decentralized autonomous organizations* (DAOs), to make self-executing contracts or *smart contracts* (see next section and Key Terms and Definitions), decisively reducing transaction costs and streamlining transactions by diminishing uncertainty and increasing confidence in business.

In 1937, Ronald Coase (Economics Nobel Prize, 1991), in a remarkable statement, said that companies are formed to reduce transaction costs (Coase, 1937). Today, it is known that business competitiveness is determined by the ability to do so, and this is precisely what cryptocurrency and *smart contracts* are expected to deliver. Thus, probably these new monetary and contractual instruments will become the preferred way for making deals and bindings agreements considering their decisive advantages, namely:

- Efficiency: they are fast and low cost.
- Trust: they are safe and accurate.

Blockchain adoption will increase the scale of economic activity coordinated through *distributed trust*, and *smart contracts* will create what can be considered a more polycentric economic order (Aligica & Tarko, 2012), further away from the single thought regimes, and governments coordination and oriented in a market perspective. As referred by Aligica and Tarco (2012), "[the market] should be seen as a polycentric system involving a web of many agents that constantly adjust their behavior to the decisions made by others. [In turn,] socialism implies the transformation of the system into a monocentric one." (p. 238). Therefore, the *crypto-economy* is oriented towards the diversity of thought of economic agents and probably will "unfold as a process of disintermediation and dehierarchicalisation." (Berg, 2018, p. 9).

As mentioned above, the acceptance or liquidity of Yap Islands money was never due to the intrinsic value or portability of such stones, which were, in fact, giant and heavy. Nevertheless, such *stone money* worked well for centuries as a medium of exchange, thanks to Yap's oral ledger ability to register the collective memory of natives' financial movements. Of course, an *oral ledger* has little scalability, and such a monetary system could only function (providing sufficient liquidity to their users) in a limited geographical scope, as was the case of such then isolated Pacific Ocean islands. Thus, as time went by and after some entangled adventures regarding the English crown's difficulties to tax the Yap's natives (Furness, 1910), the stone money was naturally replaced by more available money. Therefore, the Yap Islands' official money (nowadays is the dollar) success never had anything to do with a supposed intrinsic value but with factors that increased its liquidity or "salability."

It is important to note that media of exchange do not become money because of their direct utility (consumption) but rather because of their salability (liquidity). Many goods served as money until they were demonetized because a new more salable and less costly (to transact) money emerged. (Thagapsov & Kozlovskiy, 2020).

Like most economists, businessmen, and academics, David Yermack, in his article "Is Bitcoin a Real Currency? An Economic Appraisal." referred to "currency functions as a medium of exchange, a store of value, and a unit of account" (2015). These functions determine the functional currency requisites. As stated by Harrison (2018), "while some scholars still maintain that cryptocurrency does not qualify for this categorization, when analyzed in depth, cryptocurrency does satisfy each of these criteria and can therefore be classified as a currency." (p. 1-2)

Money has six attributes: *durability, portability, fungibility, scarcity, divisibility, and recognizability* (Vassiliadis et al., 2017). Cryptocurrency has them all, as shown by pioneer Bitcoin (Thagapsov & Kozlovskiy, 2020).

Today it is conceded that bitcoin possesses the characteristics of money (durability, portability, fungibility, scarcity, divisibility and recognizability) based on the properties of mathematics rather than relying on physical properties (like gold and silver) or trust in central authorities (like fiat currencies) (Vassiliadis, 2017, p. 3)

Indeed, Bitcoin shows outstanding performances regarding several attributes of money, such as *durability* (bits can last forever, which is reassuring), *portability* (data has no weight or physical volume, which is convenient), and *scarcity* (bitcoin units are programmed to be less in number than 21 million, which give it immunity to inflation).

Considering the *divisibility* attribute: each bitcoin unit is programmed to be divisible in one hundred million sub-units called *satoshis* (Bjercke & Finlow-Bates, 2020, p. 1). It is thought that cryptocurrencies that allow straightforward transactions on the Internet-of-Things (IoT), will be a marketing must. The "servitization of consumption" (Wilczak, 2018, p. 298) will rely on *self-servuction interactions* (De Oliveira Rodrigues, 2021, p. 49), which are a digital type of self-service where *prosumers* (see Key Terms and Definitions) participate in the *servuction process* (Eiglier & Langeard, 1987) by giving intellectual inputs which can be integrated into atomized transactions thanks to BT. Hence, cryptocurrencies' micropayment features will eventually be highly marketable. Using products *as-a-service* instead of owning them, consumers' behavior will form a *pay as you go* and *pay only for what you use* consumption pattern (Perera et al., 2014). These patterns should translate into consumers' preference for highly fragmented cryptocurrencies tailored to make micropayments on the IoT (Tennant, 2017), as is the case of the IOTA cryptocurrency (www.iota.org).

Crypto will form the foundation of a new micro-subscription economy, with our wallets constantly feeding a vast and shifting array of goods and services and media.[...] You'll top off a wallet and fractions of a cent will flow out of it over time to watch various videos or play games or rent an app. The payments will be so small that you won't really pay attention to them, until you login to your dashboard to see what you spent. (Jeffries, 2021)

As for Bitcoin's *recognizability* attribute, it seems to be a work in progress. Companies, entrepreneurs, and public figures like Elon Musk and Mark Cuban accept *crypto payments* for their products and services, namely Bitcoin and other cryptocurrencies. In May 2021, Elon Musk showed his preference for Dogecoin. "Launched in December 2015, Dogecoin started as a joke" (Ghaiti, 2021) but was later accepted to buy goods as valuable as luxury real estate (McIntosh, 2021; Jha, 2021; Mack, 2021). Thus, it is not too risky to say that cryptocurrencies will enter the financial mainstream, perhaps sooner than expected, if there is no political repression, which is not sure, of course. After all, as mentioned above, "Digital currency is a political issue as much as a technological issue." (Birch, 2020, p. 10).

Finally, regarding *fungibility*, two supposed paradoxical aspects must be considered. On the one hand, BT allows avoiding cryptocurrencies' *double-spending* (Nakamoto, 2008). On the other hand, unlike conventional currencies, different cryptocurrency units may look equal but, after all, be unique. For example, each traded bitcoin unit or sub-unit carries the history of its previous transactions and has its own identity (Möser et al., 2014). Thus, Bitcoin and many other cryptocurrencies are not fungible because they are traceable, which can be an advantage in fighting crime.

The cryptocurrency Bitcoin is an example of a pseudo anonymous currency, where encrypted accounts can theoretically be traced back to their successive owners while remaining anonymous for everyday practical purposes. Value can thus be held and exchanged in cryptocurrencies without public disclosure of personal identity (Dierksmeier & Seele, 2018, p. 2).

The fact that digital currencies are programmable allows to assign them with specific properties, which can be translated into an unusual convenience and granularity, hopefully serving to catalyze innovation and encourage entrepreneurship. Despite its increased convenience in terms of liquidity and privacy, which are reminiscent of anonymous living cash characteristics, some authors think that bitcoin features will give rise to fraud and crimes over the Internet, such as money laundering and tax evasion (Kethineni & Cao, 2020).

However, unlike traditional cash, cryptocurrencies are not all the same, and their traceability facilitates the criminal investigation. Nothing can be altered or deleted from a blockchain, as the records inserted in it are immutable (Nakamoto, 2008). It is crucial to understand this reality because the alternative to cryptocurrencies is centralized digital money, programmed in closed source code. Misrepresenting Bitcoin with the antithetic and surreptitious ideas of insecurity and opacity is gaining strength by feeding itself on people's fears, which can be good for the *status quo* but very dangerous for freedom and democracy.

Our freedom of choice in a competitive society rests on the fact that, if one person refuses to satisfy our wishes, we can turn to another. But if we face a monopolist we are at his absolute mercy. And an authority directing the whole economic system of the country would be the most powerful monopolist conceivable... it would have complete power to decide what we are to be given and on what terms. It would not only decide what commodities and services were to be available and in what quantities; it would be able to direct their distributions between persons to any degree it liked. (Hayek, 1944)

Bitcoins are not alike. Each transaction is a descendant of a unique transaction history, which is readily available in the public block chain. Therefore, markets participants can, in principle, scrutinize the history and become selective in which transactions they accept; or, with more granularity, how much they value it (Möser et al., 2014)

Bitcoin is based on a *public-permissionless* blockchain (see Chapter 4), which means that any technically savvy person or entity can verify how its protocol is encoded and securely access its transaction features by using private cryptographic keys. Thus, Bitcoin transactions can be openly carried out, safely and reliably, directly between individuals, without the intervention of banks or other intermediaries, which has been happening since 2009 with Bitcoin price climbing considerably, although showing high volatility (Jain, 2020).

Bitcoin's non-inflationary protocol makes it immune to hyperinflation (Nakamoto, 2008). Friedrich Hayek argued that states will always have tremendous difficulty maintaining *fiat* currencies' purchasing power in the long run. Therefore, it is not difficult to imagine what he would think about nowadays risks of uncontrolled inflation since the Federal Reserve's printing orders for dollars, in 2021, have an increase of more than 35% to the year 2020, from 7.6 billion notes to 9.6 billion notes. (Federal Reserve System, 2020).

Adding up to the seigniorage costs inconvenience (Buiter, 2007), Hayek revealed his disbelief regarding the ability of governments to control inflation due to the continued temptation to manipulate the currency to please interest groups or achieve political-economic objectives (Hayek, 1976). His thought on the matter is evident, as quoted by Ametrano (2016): "I do not think it an exaggeration to say that history is largely a history of inflation, and usually of inflations engineered by governments and for the gain of governments." (p. 7)

Seigniorage refers historically, in a world with commodity money, to the difference between the face value of a coin and its costs of production and mintage. In fiat money economies, the difference between the face value of a currency note and its marginal printing cost are almost equal to the face value of the note – marginal printing costs are effectively zero. Printing fiat money is therefore a highly profitable activity – one that has been jealously regulated and often monopolized by the state (Buiter, 2007)

During the XX century, and particularly after World War II, the international community grew from a few dozens to over 200 independent territories and countries, most of which started printing their own money. The incredible growth of central banking and the extensive use of fiat money resulted in many terrible episodes of high inflation and outright hyperinflation. (…) We sometimes forget that central banking, as we know it today, is, in fact, largely an invention of the past hundred years or so, even though a few central banks can trace their ancestry back to the early nineteenth century or before. It is a sobering fact that the prominence of central banks in this century has coincided with a general tendency towards more inflation, not less. (Cordeiro, 2003, p. 110)

Ultimately there is a finite number of Bitcoins that can ever exist. Avoiding inflation through an algorithmic limitation established by consensus between thousands of people is something new in the political and financial world, and, in these times of *fiat money*, it eventually constitutes one of the reasons behind Bitcoin´s value appreciation.

Hyperinflations have never occurred when a commodity served as money or when paper money was convertible into a commodity. The curse of hyperinflation has only reared its ugly head when the supply of money had no natural constraints and was governed by a discretionary paper money standard. (Hanke & Kwok, 2009, p. 353)

I would say, we cannot take it for granted that the current financial system will still work in 10 or 20 years from now. Most industrial states have debts of the order of 100 to 200 percent of the gross domestic product (GDP), sometimes even a multiple of this. Controlled inflation has been considered to be a recipe to reduce these debts. The trick can work, if applied by a single country or just a few ones. However, if the USA, Europe, Japan, and further countries are all trying to reduce their debts in such a way at the same time, this may trigger an inflationary spiral that can get out of hand. (Helbing, 2014, p. 5)

A fundamental aspect of cryptocurrencies is the nature of the mechanism that controls its offer, namely the automatic, transparent, and rigorous process of applying the algorithms that regulate each cryptocurrency's existing quantity. This aspect constitutes a precious asset, obviating the need to trust the issuing entity (that is why the expression "trustless" is used to suggest the lack of need for third-party verification). Thus, even though cryptocurrency has no *intrinsic value* in the tangible and conventional sense of the term, it can be recognized, in a pragmatic way, that the referred mathematical trust can be understood as a valuable attribute of them. The only relevant intrinsic value is that of trust, in this case, that of *distributed trust*.

One should remember the Yap Islands' people discernment, who decentralized its financial system, recognizing and proving, during centuries, that money is not something with intrinsic value but a system of credit and clearing. The algorithm responsible for trusting such a system did not have the BT's mathematical accuracy, which relied on the collective tribal memory and the good word of the Yap's natives. Nowadays, thanks to BT, credit and clearing systems can be globally decentralized. Not only can digital money be programmed to be immune to inflation (let alone hyperinflation), as it is also possible to mint digital tokens and cryptocurrencies as multidimensional incentives that integrate both *labor* and *capital* in their toolbox. Hopefully, it will be possible to use the conspicuous market *visible hand* acknowledging sustainable innovation and ethical entrepreneurship to induce collective action, as seen in the following sections.

Tokens, Smart Contracts, and Decentralized Autonomous Organizations

Blockchain Technology (BT) allows the creation of cryptocurrencies and other digital tokens.

Just as some protocols or languages are communication standards on the Internet (*e.g.*, HTTP) and other protocols are standards for formatting digital content (*e.g.*, JPEG), the blockchain protocol allows the creation of transaction standards to store and deal with data safely.

Unlike most of the Internet's data, which are mere copies (the "copy-paste" digital function replicates data with a neglectable marginal cost), blockchain encrypted data keep its originality. Therefore, such data can be directly traded on the Internet rather than merely shared. This feature can be a reality today because BT's encryption method guarantees data authenticity, immutability, and confidentiality (Nakamoto, 2008). Thus, it has become doable to use the Internet to store and transfer digital assets without third party intervention.

A token is not a financial asset but rather a digital good (Shin et al., 2019). There are multiple token formats (Lipusch et al., 2019). For instance, the Swiss Financial Market Supervisory Authority (FINMA) established the following token classes:

Payment tokens (synonymous with cryptocurrencies) are tokens which are intended to be used, now or in the future, as a means of payment for acquiring goods or services or as a means of money or value transfer. Cryptocurrencies give rise to no claims on their issuer. Utility tokens are tokens which are intended to provide access digitally to an application or service by means of a blockchain-based infrastructure. Asset tokens represent assets such as a debt or equity claim on the issuer. Asset tokens promise, for example, a share in future company earnings or future capital flows. In terms of their economic function, therefore, these tokens are analogous to equities, bonds or derivatives. Tokens which enable physical assets to be traded on the blockchain also fall into this category. (Mueller et al., 2018, p. 16)

FINMA points out that the individual token classifications are not mutually exclusive and that hybrid tokens are possible, which leads to legal uncertainty in practice.

It is essential to understand that digital tokens only exist conceptually as entries in a ledger, the blockchain *hyperledger*. In other words, an individual has a *token* because he or she has a key that allows the creation of a new entry in the ledger, reassigning ownership of that token to another person. Thus, having a certain amount of tokens is not having them stored on a computer but knowing the keys that reassign ownership of that same number of tokens (Lewis, 2015).

Some several standards or protocols determine programming logic for tokenizing digital assets. For example, the ERC-20 standard, created in 2014 (Buterin, 2014), makes it possible to ensure that tokens are fungible. The Merriam-Webster dictionary defines fungible as "of such a kind or nature that one specimen or part may be used in place of another specimen or equal part in the satisfaction of an obligation; or capable of mutual substitution." In other words, the ERC-20 standard guarantees that tokens have properties that make them equal one to another in terms of their type and value, thus making them replaceable (the same number of tokens of a given type) will always have the same value. As stated by Perez (2018), "a token is "a unit of value (...) a specific amount [or number] of digital resources which you control and can reassign control of to someone else".

There is also a standard to endow tokens with properties that allow representing non-fungible assets. These are the Non-Fungible Tokens (NFTs), which are one of a kind, like a signature, and can be used to represent *virtual memorabilia*, which are virtual objects that can be made unique by "a class of tokens introduced in late 2017 with the ERC-721 standard" (Regner et al., 2019, p. 4). This standardization is a way to turn originals (*e.g.*, paintings) into collectibles, capturing the art of the moment by catching past events to owning them in marketable formats. So, tokens can represent a wide range of digitalized assets and play many essential roles in *crypto-economics* (see Key Terms and Definitions). Its market value "depends on the value of the underlying assets and services they represent [and] can be transferred easily among users or traded for other cryptocurrencies such as Bitcoin and Ether" (Chen, 2018, p. 569).

Besides empowering digital currencies, blockchain technology has given innovators the capability of creating digital tokens to represent scarce assets, potentially reshaping the landscape of entrepreneurship and innovation. Blockchain tokens may democratize entrepreneurship by giving entrepreneurs new ways to raise funds and engage stakeholders, and innovation by giving innovators a new way to develop, deploy, and diffuse decentralized applications. BT and tokens have sparked a new wave of innovation, which may start to revolutionize entrepreneurship and innovation. (Chen, 2018, p. 567)

Tokens have the particularity of performing both the functions they are programmed to and being a financing platform to quantify the participants' commitment to new projects. Such fund-raising operations are called Internet Coin Offering (ICO). Besides being a global crowdfunding financial instrument, ICOs are a new way of engaging early stakeholders in building an ecosystem (Massey et al., 2017). Therefore, tokens "reshape the landscape of entrepreneurship [and] allow innovators to build developer communities." (Chen, 2018, p. 573). It is undisputed that cryptocurrencies and other tokens represent a different breed of value (a programmable one) and, as stated by Mueller et al. (2018), "tokens are qualified for decentralized, open-sourced and community-based projects, which do not need a centralized issuer" (p. 17). As stated by Muzzy (2018), "as all tokens of a particular blockchain are created equal, multiple transactions can occur rapidly and instantly without the participants worrying if the tokens all store the same value." It is this mathematical certainty that makes tokens the critical element to set self-executing contracts. Without the tokens, the so-called *smart contracts* would not be possible. The expression *smart contract* was invented in the 1990s by Nick Szabo, a US lawyer, and computer scientist. He defined *smart contract* as "a set of promises, specified in digital form, including protocols within which the parties perform on other promises" (Szabo, 1997). Smart contracts enforce the computer code they have been programmed for (Jaccard, 2018).

Figure 1. Using "smart contracts" to make efficient and trustable deals.

TRANSACTION DEALS IN THE PRE-BLOCKCHAIN ERA

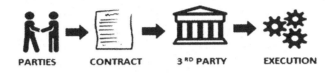

PARTIES   CONTRACT   3ᴿᴰ PARTY   EXECUTION

TRANSACTION DEALS IN THE POST-BLOCKCHAIN ERA

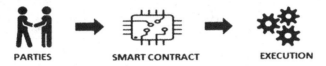

PARTIES   SMART CONTRACT   EXECUTION

As stated by Dwyer (2017), "If Bitcoin tries to obviate central institutions for the management of money, the smart contract works to obviate the institution of law, [because] much of the work required to implement, observe, verify and enforce contracts between parties might be delegated to cryptographic protocols." (p. 15) (see Figure 1).

The first and most popular blockchain protocol that supports a *Turing complete* scripting languages is Ethereum (Buterin, 2014). A blockchain is characterized as *Turing complete* if it can perform any computation. Ethereum, which is a *public-permissionless* blockchain, uses a language that is "Turing complete" (Wood, 2014), allowing any user to create and deploy programs on its shared global infrastructure Today, a vibrant community has evolved, running many pieces of software code (*smart contracts*) on the Ethereum blockchain (Regner et al., 2019, p. 3).

Smart contracts are event-driven computer programs running on the public ledger. [They] can handle and transfer assets of considerable value. (…) Specifically, smart contracts are some scripts or codes that are deployed in blockchain. Once the predefined conditions are activated, the scripts on the contract content could be executed without the help of an external trusted authority. The entire process is automated, and the executed transactions are recorded in the public ledge for auditing (Liu et al., 2018, p. 2).

According to the consensus mechanism established in a *smart contract*, prescribed programming codes are executed *on-chain*, *i.e.*, the correspondent transactions occur on a blockchain whenever such smart contract's mathematical conditions are met:

[Smart-contracts] implement forward-chaining operational semantics for Condition-Action rules where changing conditions trigger update actions, like IF/THEN/ELSE (derivative reasoning), IF/DO (production rules), ON/DO (trigger rules), ON/IF/DO (Event-Condition-Action or ECA) or a variation of ON/IF/DO and IF/THEN (Knowledge Representation). (Kruijff & Weigand, 2018, p. 152)

The accuracy and security of *smart-contracts* depend on external data (*off-chain*), which acts as inputs that change the *hyperledger* by executing blockchain state transitions (*on-chain*). These data feeds are provided by the so-called *validation oracles* (Xu et al., 2016). Thus, oracle systems constitute a link between blockchain's data and external data resources (see Figure 2).

Figure 2. Oracles: bridging blockchains and the outside world

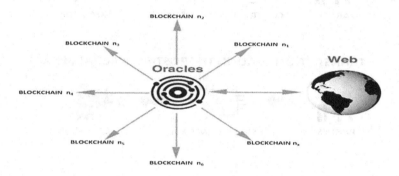

As stated by Heiss et al. (2019), "oracles are middleware systems situated at the edge of the blockchain that intermediate between smart contracts and external systems." (p. 497). *Oracles* provide *smart contracts* with external information. They serve as bridges between blockchains and the outside world. As stated by Beniiche (2020), "the data transmitted by oracles come in many forms, *e.g.*, information, the successful completion of a payment, [digital asset prices, exchange rates, real-time flight information] or the temperature measured by a sensor." (p. 606).

Smart contracts are executed in code that no party controls or can shut down (Nakamura et al., 2020), opening a whole new range of possibilities for defining and engaging stakeholders around innovative projects and building decentralized applications to create value. The ecosystems thus created are called *decentralized autonomous organizations* (DAO), a new kind of electronic communities (see figure 3) that smart contracts cast together (Norta, 2016). As stated by Wang et al. (2019), DAOs are organizations whose management rules are typically encoded on blockchain in the form of smart contracts and can autonomously operate without centralized control or third-party intervention.

A DAO is nothing more than a series of smart contracts to which all participants choose to refer, locking some of their resources and letting the code enforce the rules they have collectively formulated. These organizations can be programmed to spend common funds, modify their own algorithms (i.e., intervention patterns), claim rights, activate machines and devices, enhance/restrict the abilities of some members' accounts, let in/kick out some members; the input would be the fulfillment of some pre-set conditions, probably with the aid of IoT applications. [...] In a DAOs, law is replaced with digital contractual relations [...] any action that is reducible to algorithmic relations (if x happens, then y happens) regarding registered data can be organized with no third parties, as a matter of principle. (Martinelli, 2017, pp. 3, 5).

Through polls carried out with their tokens, the DAO's constituents can trigger update actions and automatically configure management acts, carrying out events such as hiring staff, making payments, or adjudicating a work, among many other possibilities. One should note that these actions also reach the physical world, being able to trigger actions as mundane as locking or unlocking a door depending on whether a property's rent is paid or not, as well as connecting equipment or preventing a vehicle from starting its march if its driver delays the payment of the respective lease (Reisenwitz, 2014).

The Internet of Things (IoT) will lead people to live surrounded by intelligent digital artifacts (Lindley et al., 2019), and it is believed that BT's cost reduction will be decisive for optimizing transactions related to the data that will be collected and issued by such ubiquitous artifacts. Hence, it is thought that most of the data will be processed on blockchain networks. After all, these networks have the tremendous competitive advantage of sharing information and allowing straighforward trade with low transaction costs and without intermediaries. Enabled by BT, DAOs can run themselves alone under the control of code rules and business decisions, determining their execution regardless of human involvement. (see Figure 3).

Figure 3. Decentralized autonomous organizations
(Adapted from [Yablonskaya, 2018]).

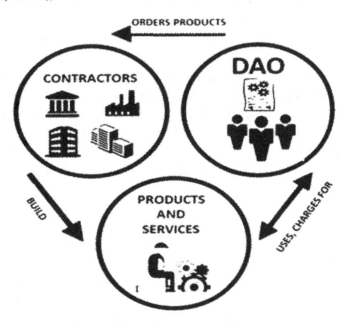

To have a clear explanation of DAOs, see the same book in Chapter 5 - *The Real Blockchain Game Changer: Protocols and DAOs for Coordinating Work to Provide Goods and Services.*

BLOCKCHAIN ECONOMIC IMPLICATIONS

Crypto-Economy: Upgrading Collective Action

Crypto-economics can be defined as "the optimization of incentive design to evoke social behavior in a decentralized token-based economy" (Hülsemann & Tumasjan, 2019, p. 4). It is thought it is about emancipation, decentralization, and collective action. Thanks to blockchain technology (BT), personal data and private digital assets will hopefully be dealt with together only when that conjoint operation proved to be advantageous for the individual. Everyone will never lose their *crypto identity*, always retaining its privacy and data ownership privileges (see Chapter 1).

Institutional economics predicts that the adoption of blockchain technology will increase economic activity coordinated through markets and reduce demand for hierarchic organisation, including firms and government. Many sectors of the economy will be disrupted by this growth of markets and networks, with new types of market forms emerging, such as data markets, and more direct P2P exchanges for newly "tokenised" assets and services. (Berg et al., 2018, p. 8)

BT will have profound economic repercussions. However, it is thought that only free competition between private and public cryptocurrencies will conveniently stimulate innovation, aligning individual entrepreneurship with collective interests. Such diversity is fundamental, augmenting the motivational range of monetary incentives and eventually making consumer behavior contribute to community ecosystems' sustainability (Dapp, 2019).

One of the major problems of the current economic system is that it causes systemic sustainability failures called *externalities*. According to Padfield (2019), *externalities* are "a manifestation of a failure to assign property rights, then, when feasible and under certain conditions, assigning property rights would allow for efficient trading." (p. 291). Due to BT's civilizational impact on privacy and ownership trade-offs, *crypto-economics* brings the possibility of representing and dealing with *externalities* in the market. This *financial chimera* is technically feasible because, on the one hand, it has become possible to create monetary systems accessible to anyone on the Internet and, on the other, *digital tokens* are programmable and can be endowed with special features to accomplish specific goals like optimizing the supply chains:

The solution to the problem of minimizing negative externalities within the framework of the current model of the economic system is associated with the creation of a mechanism for recording externalities and a mechanism for stimulating economic entities to minimize the negative external effects produced by their activities and maximize positive external effects. Tokenization on the supply chain platform creates the possibility of forming this mechanism. The system of tokenizing the externalities includes: (a) the formulation of the target behaviour of economic agents, (b) the creation of a supply chain platform that provides token issuance, (c) the determination of the exchange rate of tokens by economic agents for economic incentives (tax breaks, grants, investments, etc.), (d) an assessment of the effectiveness of economic agents in reducing negative externalities and increasing positive externalities. (Safiullin et al., 2020, p. 1)

It also can be financially interesting for individuals and communities to design incentive systems focused on externalities, namely, to encourage production and consumption behaviors beneficial to community ecosystems and discourage harmful ones. On the other hand, as Helbing (2014) states, "a considerable fraction of people care about ethics and fair products [and] financial investors are getting interested in ethical investments, as they tend to be more sustainable." (p.12).

Some of the tension between ethical and pragmatic business considerations becomes aggravated by the fact that humanity's primary incentive system is limited to a fungible one-dimensional type of money, whose market value rests alone on the undifferentiated prerogative of being exchanged for scarce goods.

The current system of frictionless convertible currencies reduces the number of money-related control variables effectively to one. (…) this one dimensionality is the cause of the recurrent bubbles and crashes in the financial system for thousands of years. But now we can create new, complementary forms of money that enable a better self-organization of our economy. (Helbing, 2014, p. 1)

A one-dimensional incentive system is very limited in its options, as the legendary Midas King of Greek mythology felt when cursed to turning everything he touched into gold. By reducing value to just one dimension, the money someone wins is always equal to the money someone loses, which leads to a *zero-sum game* (Fisher et al., 1991). However, in the *blockchain* era, it does not have to be like that. Incentive systems composed of cryptocurrencies and "purpose-driven token that produces a common good as a side product - a positive externality" (Fritsch et al., 2021) may incorporate other value dimensions than the single *value-of-exchange* monotonously exhibited by the non-programmable traditional money, as is the case of reputational value. It is thought that digital currencies will enrich the monetary system thanks to a savvy combination of value propositions relating to *capital* and *labor*, two production factors that can be integrated into the same unit of value once registered on a DLT, creating diversity enough to bring about multidimensional reputational *trade-value* and *win-win* business situations (Fisher et al., 1991).

Reputation changes the transaction from a single-stage zero-sum game into a repeated positive-sum game. The value that is created in the transaction is that the reputation of both parties is improved in a harmonious profit-able transaction for the long-term. (Calcaterra & Kaal, 2021)

Hence, it is thought that BT paves the way to engineer *smart monetary systems* that may contribute to foster collective action leading to more sustainable human development. Therefore, in the *blockchain* era, a *crypto Midas King* could make an even more valuable wish without regrets, as he would not be cursed with a one-dimensional *golden touch* but blessed with untouchable cryptographic money protocols.

Several ways of integrating reputation and community values into financial incentive systems will be looked at in the following sections in a conceptual and prospective approach. The exploratory idea is seeking out a brighter future overcoming the limitations of one-dimensional money, which invites more speculation than production (French, 2009), impoverishing humanity's motivational spectrum.

Tailoring Monetary Policies

Cryptocurrencies and other digital currencies can increase the granularity of monetary policies and also sharpen political power. They are actionable through *smart contracts* programmed to exert precise effects, for example, depending on the time elapsed until the respective use, the economic sector, or the interest rate. Thus, they can reach specific sectors on any stipulated dates and with discretionary loan rates adapted to many market vicissitudes. Due to blockchain technology (BT), these and other conditions will always be met with mathematical certainty.

It is believed that many governments will try to sponsor and launch digital currencies. After all, the money supply will no longer need to be aggregated, and digital currencies will allow the allocation of financial assets with *ballistic precision*, giving a new meaning to the very expression *monetary policy*. For example, central banks will set interest rates depending on the sector, the transaction date, and market fluctuations. Of course, that all of these conditions can be optimized insofar as "all digital currencies can be programmed" (Kiff et al., 2020, p. 10).

In a free market system, centralized and decentralized digital currencies will be able to compete. In another scenario, cryptocurrencies will not compete freely in the market, nor public blockchains with free and unconditional access for law-abiding citizens will thrive. Eventually, only the state and corporatocracy will issue digital currencies and private blockchains will dominate. In this case, digital money can lead to a *new normal* (Tam, 2021) where the *post-covid-19* and *blockchain* realities will come together for an even stronger centralization of political-economic power, increasing the risk of people losing their privacy and even their freedom. This scenario is already confirmed in China, where at least some consumer behavior traits are already carried out according to citizens' social ranking (Troshchinskiy, 2021). Thus, it is believed that digital currencies will make it possible to refine the control over citizens, and some authoritarian states and powerful companies maybe will use digital money as an exportable *app* to extend their influence (see Chapter 4).

Even in the so-called free world, it is believed that public digital currencies, sponsored by states such as the USA and Japan, or economic blocs such as Europe, will make it possible to create absolute obligations and specifically targeted monetary policies, rather than recommendations. Thus, it is considered that the states will be able to implement monetary policies with granular effects that were never seen before.

Regarding community ecosystems, one agrees with Dapp (2019) when he refers that "one of the core problems is that today's economic system is creating systemic market failures in the form of so-called market externalities." (p. 156). As mentioned above, *externalities* are the side effects of a decision for those who do not participate in it (Dahlman, 1979), which can be negative or positive. The idea is to "expose such priced externalities to new (dis)incentive systems (*i.e.,* markets) [extending] the economic system itself by systematically including externalities and making them tradable on markets" (Dapp, 2019, p. 157). This author considers that BT enables a new governance paradigm, "which would motivate people to act more sustainably while remaining decentralized, self-organizing, multi-layered, and circular." (p.157).

On the other hand, in what is considered an irreversible process pushed by the pandemic crisis, more and more online services are being consumed with an increasing number of devices connected to the *electronic cloud*. It is believed that this new reality will contribute to making digital currencies and cryptocurrencies more convenient than traditional money. Due to their extreme divisibility and the fact that they can be incorporated into *smart contracts*, such digital tokens may be the preferable way for people and machines to manage the countless number of transactions and micro-transactions that will have to be dealt with in the IoT.

It is thought that the foreseeable development of IoT will be facilitated by new sensory capabilities, which will allow measuring many physical phenomena representing the above-mentioned economic externalities. The also referred to *oracles* will be used to introduce those measurements into blockchains using suitable tokens. Also, it will be possible to encumber or relieve token transactions according to smart contracts' rules using artificial intelligence (AI). Hopefully, a free-market scenario will allow private initiatives to continuously launch innovative cryptocurrencies to contribute to more sustainable human development, as seen in the following sections

Tokenization, Innovation and Entrepreneurship

The creation of tokens is called *tokenization*. In addition to financing projects, it allows to design multifaceted incentive systems. Hopefully, such incentives will ethically reconcile individual profit with collective action favoring the communitys' ecosystems.

Tokenization refers to the issuance of smart contracts tokens, conventionally (but not necessarily) through the ritualized event of an Initial Coin Offering (ICO), which allows access to the existing or prospective value generated by a specific asset – such as gold, computing power, storage, even artworks, and, more generally, an alluring value proposition for a decentralized ecosystem. (Lotti, 2019, p. 287)

Tokens are digitally programmed, allowing financial and economic attributes to be integrated into seamless value propositions that can fit community ecosystems' goals. It is thought that token's properties will contribute decisively to redefining societies' value creation in the *blockchain era*.

[Tokens] introduce differences in kind in the ways in which value generation and distribution are expressed and accounted for in digital environments. [Tokenization] opens up new ways to reimagine and reprogram financial and social relations, and gesture toward new opportunities and challenges for a practice of digital design focused on the ideation and realization of cryptoeconomic systems. (Lotti, 2019, p. 287)

To understand the blockchain economic and the new financial reality, one should know that digital tokens, including cryptocurrencies, are more resourceful than traditional money. Tokens can be thought of as digital financial instruments capable of triggering events in both the digital and physical world. Digital money's features may seem like magic to some but are just technology. While traditional currencies can only trigger automatic actions in a few cases (for example, a physical coin can trigger a self-service vending machine or release a shopping cart in a supermarket), digital tokens can be designed to aggregate and deliver *value-of-exchange* and *value-of-use* (see Key Terms and Definitions). It is thought that market competition will distinguish the most creative and innovative digital tokens, which will be scrutinized by fulfilling people's needs in decentralized markets for which they have been designed. Hopefully, these tokens' value propositions will be appropriate for a more sustainable human development. After all, not being necessarily fungible, tokens do have a memory. They are traceable, so they have an identity. Unlike his analogic predecessor, digital money can carry a reputation (of being done good or bad deeds), potentially affecting its value in every transaction.

In addition to serving as a bargaining chip, digital tokens can have a functional or utilitarian dimension, hopefully corresponding to community members' expectations. In other words, they can represent community benefits, hitherto financially unattainable, allowing quantifying positive externalities like recycling, education, cooperation, community service, and negative externalities like pollution, pathological contagions, and waste of food or energy and deforestation. The idea is to sum or discount cryptocurrency's transactions with those externalities' values, encouraging behaviors that contribute to ecosystems' sustainability and discouraging the harmful ones. One should note that these externalities can be related to production or consumption and be positive or negative. For example, pollution from a factory is a negative production externality. In the same way, the Washington DC riots (2020 US Presidential Elections) can be understood as a negative externality derived from pernicious digital platforms' business model, which was denounced by whistle-blowers (Beever et al., 2019) (see Chapter 1). In turn, considering consumption, traffic congestion and passive smoking are two examples of negative externalities. As positive externalities, at the production level, one can refer, for example, R&D synergies and recycling. In terms of consumption, it can be mentioned the protective effect that a particular vaccinated individual offers to others, especially in his or her community, and the added utility that some private appliances provide even to third parties not involved in its acquisition. For example, when an individual installs a collaborative application on his smartphone, anyone with whom he is interconnected also can use this functionality. Hence, in all these examples there are externalities, triggered either by production or consumption, that can be encouraged or discouraged. Hopefully, next generations will use *smart contracts* and *ethical tokens* to act proactively in many economic situations.

Therefore, digital tokens allow programming new incentive and reward systems. This monetary approach can expand financial capital accounting to capture social and environmental capital (Bakarich et al., 2020). In a free market, the most valued tokens can help community members guide collective action pragmatically. In the bottom-line, tokens' market capitalization will represent the total value of specific assets or rights featured as a whole in such communities' ecosystems.

It is essential not to confuse collective action with collectivism. Digital tokens can have specific uses, acting as individual incentives even if programmed from a community perspective. This feature of digital money is critical to let individuals pursue their interests and seek personal profits, which is natural and human. The good social news is that when transacting digital tokens whose value can be indexed to factors linked to human development and communities' sustainable progress, individual behavior impacts collective action positively. Also, the concept of personal profit needs to be expanded to quantify the individual reputation.

Using programmable tokens in incentive systems enables the creation of metrics akin to reputation. For example, maintaining a consistently above-average balance of "CO2 coins" would indicate that an individual has made a credible effort to keep his/her ecological footprint low (if the user decides to make this information public). Several externality measurements combined would gradually form a rich user profile with some degree of reliability and accuracy. Under the control of the user, such profiles could be used for job interviews, political campaigns, insurance policies, etc. (Dapp, 2019, 164)

One can think that performing all these features may seem difficult or even impossible due to their complexity. However, it is essential to consider the vertiginous evolution of information technologies like *Big Data* and *Artificial Intelligence*. Berg et al. (2018) stated that "in the near future personal artificially intelligent machine agents will be able to conduct exchanges with a matrix of liquid digital assets (such as [tokens and] cryptocurrencies)" (p. 4).

Hybrid blockchains of the *public-permissioned* type (see Chapter 1) already offer agility, transparency, and speed (when operating the consensus-building mechanism), while simultaneously favor stakeholders' reputation visibility. These rewards can be translated into individual incentives helping each person to climb Maslow's Pyramid, satisfying a well-established hierarchy of psychologic human needs (social affiliation, self-esteem, and self-realization) (Maslow, 1943). Moreover, it is considered that a myriad of decentralized applications (dApps) probably will make this whole reputational process seamless and user-friendly.

Although crypto-economics (see Key Terms and Definitions) is still poorly understood, the new programmable money can encourage building circular economies (Narayan, 2020), aligning individuals with collective interests and favoring ecosystems thanks to a network effect (Metcalfe & Metcalfe, 2013).

It is thought that a healthy tokenized economy should stimulate the circulation of tokens within an ecosystem (Dapp, 2019). For example, in a given dental ecosystem, if the circulation of tokens only results from purchases done by users/patients and sales done by providers/dentists on currency and tokens' exchange platforms, those tokens' life cycles will be too short. In this case, the exchange platform will be the only way for users to acquire the tokens necessary to pay for dental service and for the providers to exchange the tokens received from their customers. In other words, tokens will practically do not circulate among the members of such a system, just entering and exiting the system before and shortly after each transaction. Therefore, this system is not an ecosystem, as the respective tokens representing community members' symbiotic interests do not flow inside the system. In such a dental system, the tokens' value is one-dimensional, maximized at transaction moments, and *individually* captured just at the exchange events, like traditional money does, reducing all value to a single tradable dimension.

For instance, in the dental ecosystem called Dentacoin there are several ways for members to earn tokens, for example, using the *Dentacare App* or writing comments on the platform itself using *Dentavox* and *Trusted Reviews* platforms (Salah et al., 2019).

The platform will reward patients in the form of Dentacoins tokens (DCN) for participating. The program will ultimately help users save money by using DCN to pay for their dental treatment or to purchase dental products. In the long run, it envisions that dentists could potentially consider DCN as a financial investment. For example, they could use it to remunerate employees or to pay suppliers with no middlemen and no high international transaction costs. This direct connection between producers and dentists will ultimately allow dentists to provide lower prices to patients. (Fang, 2021, p. 4)

Therefore, for the cryptocurrencies of a given ecosystem to work, their tokens must circulate and be sufficiently moved for various reasons and in several directions. Thus, buyers and sellers of products and services must spend and earn tokens within the ecosystem, namely by interacting and transacting with each other (Dapp, 2019).

The competitive power of networks should not be underestimated (Metcalfe & Metcalfe, 2013), and *decentralized autonomous organizations* (DAO) will probably create more value to society than traditional organizations. In a scenario of political freedom, *blockchain* technologies will digitally extend network effects to both *economic media*, leading communities to use *social media* and *digital money* for, respectively, sharing information and transacting value. Hence, transactions will be increasingly done in a decentralized way rather than relying on the intermediation provided by hierarchically structured companies. Thus, the DAOs may be the source of a new breed of products and services entirely committed to a community-based marketing perspective (see the same book, Chapter 5 - *The Real Blockchain Game Changer: Protocols and DAOs for Coordinating Work to Provide Goods and Services*). In this scenario, the commercially programmed obsolescence of products and services and other unethical corporate quests for unilateral gains according to blind monetization schemes may have their days numbered for the sake of a more fair and sustainable society.

Cryptocurrencies and other digital tokens may represent an entirely new way of guiding society contributing to the algorithmic institution of community-based capitalism. This political-financial chimera may be possible to achieve by letting individual economic behavior align itself with *the visible hand of the market* endorsed by civil society and ethical entrepreneurship, only possible to attain once the premises of collaborative and sustainable development are tokenized. In this case, individual financial incentives may be synergetic with the public interest due to multidimensional tokens that are very different from the unidimensional traditional money. Therefore, it is thought that free competition between such tokens is essential to encourage innovation, entrepreneurship, and value creation, simultaneously avoiding the privacy risks due to data centralization inherent to Central Bank Digital Currency (CBDC).

SOLUTIONS AND RECOMMENDATIONS

The first recommendation is that states themselves use cryptocurrencies to diversify their financial reserves strategically. Not only to set up a new range of intervention in the money markets but also to have a hedging instrument (see Key Terms and Definitions), given the risk of global crises and the possibility of a conflict escalation (Ghabri et al., 2020; Mamun et al., 2020). Nowadays, the world can change quickly. Berwick (2020) stated, "tectonic changes in health care mirror similar ones in societies overall," and who could have imagined billions of people willingly sheltering in place or social distancing barely 2 two months after almost no one knew those terms?" (p. 2126). Moreover, several studies indicate the convenience of doing hedging using Bitcoin to emulating gold's traditional role.

Evidence supporting the particularity of Bitcoin in the cryptocurrency market as a valuable asset in terms of providing a shelter to political risk, which is in line with previous studies (Aysan et al., 2019). (…) finding nicely complements previous studies arguing that Bitcoin is a hedge against geopolitical risk. (Bouriey al., p. 9)

Bitcoin could provide the sought-after diversification benefits during turbulent times. A similar result is obtained for gold, confirming its well-recognized status as a haven when a crisis happens. Furthermore, we find a low extreme correlation between bitcoin and gold, which implies that both assets can be used together in times of turbulence in financial markets to protect equity positions. Such evidence indicates that bitcoin can be considered as the new digital gold. (Gkillas & Longin, 2018, p.1)

It is thought that cryptocurrencies must belong to the people and be for the people. The only way to do it is by not prohibiting or coarcting each law-abiding citizen from using personal secret keys. Especially when living *new normal* (Tam, 2021) times of fear and crisis, it is considered imperative to keep this in mind. Such cryptographic private keys will always open the door of free-will and democracy, even if someone tries to close it. Of course, they also guarantee cryptocurrencies' free competition. It is thought that individual private cryptographic keys are a pre-requisite of democracy and the only way to deal with the severe risks of losing privacy and freedom. These risks are associated with data centralization harvested from economic media human interactions, firstly social (social media) and now also financial (digital currencies). Private cryptographic keys, decentralized markets, and decentralized applications are considered as essential to prevent bad actors like authoritarian states from using the new multidimensionality of money as a panopticon to control citizens and consumer behavior.

With those new CBDCs, countries will have full surveillance right in your pocket at all times at all times. Every transaction you ever make. Everywhere you ever go. All of it tied to your identity and history and geolocation data. A decade after that you won't file your taxes, they'll get yanked out automatically every time you buy a second-hand toaster at a garage sale. If there's a mistake, you'll call to fight it or have an accountant try to get you a refund while the government takes a free loan from you for a year.

The money won't even pass from central banks to private banking institutions, it will go right into your pocket and those panopticoins will know everything you ever did from cradle to grave. (Jeffries, 2021)

It is though that due to BT it is crucial to liberate human society wit to face present and future challenges. Cryptocurrencies are necessary due to their duality: they have a private genesis, and they are public in their open, transparent, and decentralized market philosophy, making it possible to stimulate an ethical and conscious' entrepreneurship, giving rise to money's programming protocols defined according to society's expectations. So, cryptocurrency probably will attend less to concealed political-economic interests than traditional money.

Giving the floor to civil society will stimulate the talent and shrewdness necessary to design and develop digital currencies particularly useful in communities with shared interests, exploring how individual gains can be correlated with collective successes. This symbiosis can become an essential feature of future monetary systems. It may seem strange to some that any person or group of people now have the opportunity to create a currency, mainly due to the common belief that governments should exercise control over monetary policy and that each country should structure and control its monetary units. However, already the Nobel in Economics Friedrich Hayek had strongly criticized such state control prerogative (Hayek, 1976) even before money becomes a programmable economic media too much dangerous to be centralized.

Objectively, a new prerogative of creating private cryptocurrencies was introduced by blockchain technology (BT). This technology will not be *uninvented*, nor will Internet go back to the time when money was not yet programmable, and more and more people will realize that the Internet is becoming to have several bank features (*e.g.*, Bitcoin). It is thought that such evolution will not be reversed unless democracy, the free-market, and freedom will be reversed as well. However, it would be naive not to realistically consider this worse scenario. It is thought that, unfortunately, from the perspective of democratic development of societies, there is a considerable possibility of repeating in the *Internet of Value*, the same situation verified in the former *Internet of Information*.

Current money issuers will probably try to emulate content publishers' past efforts to protect their business models. These models were quickly made obsolete right in the first phase of the Internet and replaced by others whose algorithms centralize user data with impressive financial results (e.g., Facebook), and lobbying to ban content from being shared on the Internet did little good incumbent publishers. In fact, such prohibitions currently benefit the new digital oligopolies that have been formed to replace the previous players obliterating all competition (Galloway 2017; Ducci, 2020). The same kind of data centralization can now hit digital currencies, and a new digital social contract is of utmost need:

When undertaken in tandem with comprehensive privacy reforms and the institution of transparency into collecting and using personal information, a robust new competition policy regime will necessarily redistribute the allocation of power between the industry, the government, and the individual. (...) What is most of all necessary in this new age of technology is the formulation of a new "digital social contract" that conclusively recognizes the individual's rights. (Gohsh, 2019, p. 11)

It is thought that, again, prohibitions will not work as intended and will turn against the incumbents, probably inviting the appearance of new voracious players whose character, this time, probably will be as economical as political. In the new Internet made possible by BT, the vanishing gap between political and economic power can be closed for good by digitally encompassing the second and most essential economic media: money itself. It is believed that this is a particularly threatful scenario for democracy (see Chapter 4).

The two modern economic media reached the Internet, *social media*, and *digital currencies* (Beller, 2020). It is thought that the quality of financial incentives attributed to the different routes to share information (using social media) and to transact value (using digital tokens) will dictate the next political-economic paradigm: *collective action* or *collectivism*. The way it will go, of course, will depend on politics. In this author's opinion, in order that freedom and democracy can prevail, digital decentralization should not be by any means constrained. It is thought that the unrestricted use of private cryptographic keys and decentralized applications by law-abiding citizens is a fundamental requisite of democracy in the new blockchain digital era.

As they constitute a new kind of non-replicable data, digital tokens can be programmed to be exchanged only for specific data in particular circumstances. In other words, depending on how and when individuals exchange data with each other (encompassing assets, rights, and functionalities), a token's deal may result, simultaneously, in individual gains and collective benefits (Noyen et al., 2014). In decentralized ecosystems (see *DAOs* in the previous section), according to the smart contract's specifications, tokens may reward merit and encourage productive work and positive externalities, *i.e.,* behaviors with social value and favorable impact on human ecosystems (*e.g.,* recycling). In turn, while also fulfilling ethical principles and social purposes, other tokens can be programmed to limit or penalize the production/consumption of goods and services burdened with negative externalities, *i.e.,* harmful productive/consumptive behaviors, with an unfavorable impact on ecosystems (*e.g.,* pollution).

Contrary to today's economic system, agents will use a variety of currencies that represent classes or types of externalities. People do not use one single currency, but many: each currency represents a type of externality and acts as a signal on the market for externalities. These signals will make preferences and priorities in the demand and supply of externalities to a greater extent visible than in today's markets. Besides, agents will be able to participate by trading the different currencies/externalities actively. (Dapp, 2019, p. 162)

Cryptocurrencies and other digital tokens come with built-in memory, as they leave a *digital footprint* of previous transactions. Digital currencies allow tracking its previous whereabouts and applying a *reputation-dependent conversion factor* in the successive financial transactions. Hence, a multidimensional incentive system will result from differentiating tokens and cryptocurrencies. As stated by Helbing (2014), "possible qualifiers could be, how the money was earned, its origin or destination location, the reputation of the product bought [(*e.g.,* is it a recycled product, or a polluting one?)], or the reputation of the producer or seller [(*e.g.,* is it a vegan entrepreneur selling eco-friendly farming products?)].

It should be people and communities to decide about *crypto rewards* relevance transparently, encouraging ethical behavior. As such, the range of choice in terms of cryptocurrencies and digital tokens should not be limited politically. The author thinks this is a way to withdraw money from politics and vice-versa, avoiding promiscuity between the public and private sectors and keeping privacy safe to preserve freedom and democracy. As stated by Berg (2018), alluring to Bitcoin's inventor, "Capitalism after Satoshi will be flatter, more distributed, and less regulated" (p. 12), which is thought to be the formula of letting digital currencies contribute to a sustainable development of society.

From the author's perspective, in nowadays political-economic crossroads, the best hope for humanity is to use the most recent and powerful cryptographic techniques to creatively foster cryptocurrencies and other applications that use *crypto assets* as a multidimensional incentives system. Hopefully, this will drive the free world through the *new normal* post-pandemic times (Berwick, 2020; Tam, 2021) to a new era of transparency, collaborative innovation, and ethical entrepreneurship, benefiting community's ecosystems and sustainable development.

LIMITATIONS AND FUTURE RESEARCH DIRECTIONS

Bitcoin and other cryptocurrencies are not considered as eligible to be real money by many authors (Mittal, 2012; Grant, 2014; Lo, 2017; Passinsky, 2021; Brummer & Yadav, 2018). Cryptocurrencies' lack of *intrinsic value* and *volatility* are argued as being strong reasons against such classification preventing their acceptance in the market. For example, Sanz Bas (2020), refers that "many experts and analysts believe that cryptocurrencies are not currently money, but rather digital assets", and just a few years ago the European Central Bank (ECB 2015, 23-24) seemed to be sure about such limitation as recently referred by this same author:

Indeed, certainly in the case of Bitcoin, (…), virtual currencies have a limited function as a medium of exchange because they have a very low level of acceptance among the public. In addition, the high volatility of their exchange rates to currencies – and therefore in terms of most goods and services – renders virtual currency useless as a store of value even for short-time purposes, let alone for the purpose of being a longer-term savings instrument. Finally, both the low level of acceptance and the high volatility of their exchange rates and thus purchasing power make them unsuitable as a unit of account. Therefore, although it cannot be excluded that more stable virtual currencies will emerge and be used by a much wider group of users, [cryptocurrencies] such as Bitcoin cannot be regarded as full forms of money at the moment. (Sanz Bas, 2020, p. 18)

However, the acceptance of digital currencies has been growing significantly, as proved by the market price of Bitcoin and other cryptocurrencies. It was so even during the pandemic crisis. As referred by Kurihara (2021), "COVID-19 has promoted risk-on attitudes in financial markets, so Bitcoin prices have gone up" (p. 50). As these lines are being written, more and more businesses and public figures (*e.g.,* Elon Musk) accept cryptocurrencies and tweet about them. As time goes by, one can observe the "significant impact that social media activity of influential and well-known individuals can have on cryptocurrencies" (Ante, 2021, p.1).

Therefore, Bitcoin's *lack of intrinsic value* and *high volatility* does not explain its irregular but overall growing level of acceptance in the market, and it is thought that the best explanation relies on the new type of trust that underlies it, which can be called *distributed trust*. Although very recent, taking into account the history of human trust (see Chapter 1), distributed trust should consolidate as the public opinion catch the thought leadership and gets to know how trustable its mathematical nature is. Therefore, the current volatility of Bitcoin and other cryptocurrencies is coherent with what is considered a concise definition of money given by Niall Ferguson: *money is trust inscribed and portable power* (Ferguson, 2008, pp. 30, 22). Considering that these two prerogatives are undoubtful advantages of cryptocurrencies, it is thought that this nuclear definition of money will endure in the digital realm.

Besides its financial implications, the *intrinsic value* of the new *distributed trust* created by blockchain technology (BT) also justifies the new level of disintermediation that probably will take place in the coming years globally due to *smart contracts*. As noted by Chambers (2019), "Blockchain isn't just a new technology, it is a political disrupter that takes away the state's monopoly on money. Try as they might, governments won't be able to legislate it away." (p. 13).

Governments may cripple this innovation. They'll want all kinds of tracking and compliance and know your customer/anti-money laundering rules built for old-world finance but there won't be anybody home. There won't be a big compliance department because there won't be a bank, just a lot of open source code running on micro-nodes in the cloud and the fog, doing atomic swaps and matching lenders and borrowers without any people in the mix at all. (Jeffries, 2021)

It can be argued that this independence from third parties establishes new causal relationships for the acceptance of Bitcoin and other cryptocurrencies. Such acceptance, measured by the market price, may depend on the difficulty or cost involved in producing a currency based on distributed trust, whether this trust is spoken over oral ledgers or digitally encrypted on blockchains. Both in the case of Yap Islands's stone money and Bitcoin, it was and still is the cost or difficulty of coinage that establishes a perceived value linked to scarcity.

As stated by Hayes (2017), "[once analyzed] the causes of relative value formation among cryptocurrencies, it was found that relative differences in costs of production on the margin are the main determinants. [...] Cost of production drives value." (p.1319)

[To determine the causal direction between the two variables], a Granger causality test was run on price and aggregate hashpower. The results strongly indicate that causality runs one-way from mining effort to price and not the other way. [...] Hypothesis H1 is supported in that the coefficient is positive as expected a priori (prices increase as computational power increases), and the t-statistic indicates that it is highly statistically significant that computational power influences price. (Hayes, 2017, pp. 1312, 1313)

The more aggregate computational power employed in mining for a cryptocurrency, the higher the value. (...) First, the more mining power there is, the more acceptance for that 'coin' can be inferred – since mining also serves to verify transactions, the amount of mining power in use is a proxy for overall use and acceptance of that altcoin. A cryptocurrency with no acceptance or usage will have neither value nor computational power directed at it. Second, a rational miner, motivated by profit, would only seek to employ mining resources to a profitable pursuit. Therefore, if the marginal cost of mining exceeded the marginal product of mining, that miner would redeploy his resources elsewhere, removing the computational power from the network of that altcoin and into another. (Hayes, 2017, p. 1312)

The causal relationship between the cost of production and market acceptance also invalidates another argument against Bitcoin, namely the allegedly excessive energy consumption necessary to carry out the Proof-of-Work (PoW) mechanism required to establish consensus, which demands considerable computing effort. As stated by Sedlmeir (2020), "participation in the mining process is only profitable as long as the expected revenue from mining is higher than the associated costs [(e.g., electricity)] (p. 601). Thus, considering that production costs are driving cryptocurrency acceptance, as confirmed above, energy costs will only be paramount if Bitcoin reveals itself successful. However, in this case, energy consumption will be avoided at other significant levels, so this issue must be considered in a broader perspective. For example, "by enabling the digitization of supply-chain processes, blockchain can substantially reduce the amount of paperwork and transport, including air-freight (Jensen et al., 2019). Furthermore, as was also mentioned above, cryptocurrencies can be used to nurture communitarian ecosystems' and manage sustainability through collective action, which ecological effects probably will surpass many times Bitcoin's energetic consumption.

Considering what is thought to be an actual limitation of cryptocurrencies, one should look at the difficulty related to the handling and care required from its users, who have to deal with secret cryptographic keys to store and transact them. As stated by Moniruzzaman et al. (2020), "the software (wallets) used to access any cryptocurrency suffer from serious usability issues, in particular for general users." (p. 642). On the other hand, keychains are different from coin purses, involving other levels of care and attention. Otherwise, individuals will eventually lose or forget their private keys, which, by definition, constitutes an irreversible and irremediable error. Furthermore, the "possession of these alphanumeric codes is not risk-free for their owners since cases of robbery and fraud have been detected." (Sans Bas, 2020, p. 17). Thus, it is thought that more research is needed to create decentralized applications and the right set of usability guidelines to set secure, user-friendly cryptocurrency wallets.

On the other hand, it can be seen in the literature that the demand for Bitcoin and other cryptocurrencies is highly speculative. According to Sanz Bas (2020), "Proof of this is the high number of inactive Bitcoin accounts" (p. 20). However, it is difficult to agree that inactive accounts provide speculation. To hold Bitcoin can mean saving (setting money aside). After all, investing can be a long-term process, as it seems to be the case with Bitcoin (DeMartino, 2018). Inactive accounts do not suggest putting money at risk with the hope of earning a high return in a short period, as it happens in the case of day trading, and such guessing intention obviously cannot be extrapolated from Bitcoin accounts' inactiveness. Meaningfully, "true Bitcoiners use the term 'HODL' to describe holding on to their Bitcoin rather than selling to fiat" (Knittel & Wash, 2019, p. 4). As stated by Drutarovska (2015), "speculation can be defined as the activity of guessing the possible answer to a question without having enough information to be certain" (p. 345)", and the high number of inactive Bitcoin accounts can mean that many of Bitcoin holders will be confident in the value of Bitcoin in the long run. Now, this eventual certainty is objectively dependent on the mathematical rigor underlying the proper functioning of the respective cryptographic protocol. Of course, society at large still does not trust BT's merit, not in the same way, ignoring the contours of this technology which is still very recent and relatively immature. Thus, the high volatility recorded in the cryptocurrency markets must be viewed with relative ease, because there is an entirely new type of trust in society, called "distributed trust" (Bellini et al. 2020). Several authors have reported this contingence for years, warning that the volatility in question may be only circumstantial, like Brito et al. (2014), who mentioned that "Bitcoin may not be inherently volatile, however. So, its volatility is likely attributable to the fact that it is a new currency, still in the process of discovering its stable price." (p. 156).

It should also be noticed that to conducting business deals with *crypto assets*, a more consolidated legal framework is needed. "Business dislikes uncertainty and invests more when the rules of the game are set" (Bate, 2017), and perhaps due to BT's newness, legal uncertainty is a limitation that has been plaguing the *crypto assets* world. That said, it is judged that finding a clear set of legislative solutions will be just a matter of time, either for better or worse, depending on political will and the clairvoyance of public opinion.

Finally, it is believed that the perspective of making direct and operative transactions between individuals is a sufficiently robust political-economic drive to motivate the overcoming of technical limitations. It is thought that, sooner or later, BT will have a significant ethical, political, and financial-economic impact. Such an implication indicates that BT and digital currencies should urgently deserve further investigation.

CONCLUSION

Humankind arrived at a historic milestone that is also a critical political-economic crossroads. The Internet allowed to put the information in people's hands, at least in theory. Nowadays, the blockchain protocol allows Internet users to do the same with other economic media: *money*. Money is essentially a system to offset financial obligations, a trustable ledger. Blockchain technology created a new distributed trust, emulating digital ledgers to forge secure hyperledgers. Hence, money is now in people's hands. Again, at least in theory. However, sometimes from theory to practice, it goes a big difference, as shown by the centralization that occurred with the first economic media on the Internet, *social media*. With *digital money*, another economic media arrives on the Internet bringing back the hope of decentralization and openness, although Covid-19 triggered a worrying *new normal* (Tam, 2021).

TThe blockchain protocol empowers digital money with a never seen functional granularity, allowing the integration of labor and capital (the two main factors of production) in the same unit of account. Hopefully, such multidimensionality will pave the way to creating cryptocurrencies with innovative value propositions aligning individual economic incentives and social goals. Cryptocurrencies are programmable. They are *apps*, which can be decentralized and represent new *qualified money*. Besides having *trade-value*, the single attribute of traditional money, such *apps* also can represent *use-value*. *Tokens* and other *crypto assets* allow the automated execution of *smart contracts*, streamlining transactions, reducing transaction costs, and diminishing business uncertainty. As a result, cryptocurrencies can be more competitive than traditional currencies.

It is thought that free competition between cryptocurrencies will decentralize value creation, stimulate innovation, and avoid political risks inherent to data centralization. If every law-abiding citizen has the inalienable right to use cryptographic private keys, there will be a massive explosion of decentralized apps, the *big bang* of the digital money *multiverse* (whether or not such universe is called a *bubble*). Private keys are a democracy's safe conduct in the *blockchain era*. They represent the right to own and protect personal data when dealing with economic media, assuring privacy, free-market competition, and eventually free will.

Suppose the *post-pandemic new normal* (Tam, 2021) brings along with its closure premissas the prohibition of private cryptographic keys. In that case, it will be possible to watch the globalization of a political-economic scenario prepared by totalitarian regimes, where consumption patterns will be based on citizen's social ranking and monitored on social networks (*e.g.,* WeChat). Then, *social media* and *digital currency* (*e.g.,* Digital Yuan) data will be centralized and cross-referenced, which is not good news as the free competition among cryptocurrencies is considered to be a requirement of democracy. Unlike traditional money, digital currencies and other *crypto assets* can be programmed to exert very granular effects. For instance, these effects can be as auspiciosos as continuously setting interest rates accordingly to niche market fluctuations or as worrisome as clearing consumer payments correspondingly to individual political profiles monitored and cross-referenced in social networks and other applications.

Nevertheless, if freedom prevails, cryptocurrencies will represent an entirely new democratic way of guiding *collective action*, which has nothing to do with collectivism. Such a political-economic accomplishment, paradoxical in the pre-blockchain era, can be now achieved by symbolizing or monetizing the premises of sustainable development, creating a multidimensional community incentive system to unleash civil society's free initiative. Then, the digital money will be qualified to foster innovation and ethical entrepreneurship.

Hopefully, the digital opportunity to design money will be taken for ethical and sustainability reasons, decentralizing the collective memory to build hyperledgers of disintermediating trust. Following the opposite path will centralize people's data even further, probably reinforcing authoritarian regimes and corporatocracy, seizing privacy, freedom, and democracy.

REFERENCES

Adiyatma, S. E., & Maharani, D. F. (2020). Cryptocurrency's Control in the Misuse of Money Laundering Acts as an Effort to Maintain the Resilience and Security of the State. *Lex Scientia Law Review*, *4*(1), 70–82. doi:10.15294/lesrev.v4i1.38257

Akhtar, Z. (2019, November). From Blockchain to Hashgraph: Distributed Ledger Technologies in the Wild. In *2019 International Conference on Electrical, Electronics and Computer Engineering (UPCON)* (pp. 1-6). IEEE. 10.1109/UPCON47278.2019.8980029

Al Mamun, M., Uddin, G. S., Suleman, M. T., & Kang, S. H. (2020). Geopolitical risk, uncertainty and Bitcoin investment. *Physica A*, *540*, 123107. doi:10.1016/j.physa.2019.123107

Aligica, P. D., & Tarko, V. (2012). Polycentricity: From Polanyi to Ostrom, and beyond. *Governance: An International Journal of Policy, Administration and Institutions*, *25*(2), 237–262. doi:10.1111/j.1468-0491.2011.01550.x

AmetranoF. M. (2016). Hayek money: The cryptocurrency price stability solution. *Available at* SSRN 2425270.

Ammous, S. (2018). *The bitcoin standard: the decentralized alternative to central banking*. John Wiley & Sons.

Andolfatto, D., & Spewak, A. (2019). Whither the price of bitcoin? *Economic Synopses*, (1), 1–2.

AnteL. (2021). How Elon Musk's Twitter Activity Moves Cryptocurrency Markets. *Available at* SSRN 3778844.

Antonopoulos, A. M. (2016). *The Internet of Money* (Vol. 1). Merkle Bloom LLC.

Antonopoulos, A. M. (2017). *The Internet of Money: Volume Two*. Merkle Bloom LLC.

Aysan, A. F., Demir, E., Gozgor, G., & Lau, C. K. M. (2019). Effects of the geopolitical risks on Bitcoin returns and volatility. *Research in International Business and Finance*, *47*, 511–518. doi:10.1016/j.ribaf.2018.09.011

Baird, L. (2016). *The swirlds hashgraph consensus algorithm: Fair, fast, byzantine fault tolerance*. Swirlds Tech Reports SWIRLDS-TR-2016-01, Tech. Rep.

Baird, L., Harmon, M., & Madsen, P. (2018). *Hedera: A governing council & public hashgraph network. The trust layer of the internet, whitepaper,* 1, 1-97.

Bakarich, K. M., Castonguay, J. J., & O'Brien, P. E. (2020). The Use of Blockchains to Enhance Sustainability Reporting and Assurance. *Accounting Perspectives, 19*(4), 389–412. doi:10.1111/1911-3838.12241

Bate, R. (2017). *India's dodgy pharmacy. AEI Paper & Studies.* COVB.

Beever, J., McDaniel, R., & Stanlick, N. A. (2019). *Understanding Digital Ethics: Cases and Contexts.* Routledge. doi:10.4324/9781315282138

Beller, J. (2020). Economic Media: Crypto and the Myth of Total Liquidity. *Australian Humanities Review, 66,* 215–225.

Bellini, E., Iraqi, Y., & Damiani, E. (2020). Blockchain-based distributed trust and reputation management systems: A survey. *IEEE Access: Practical Innovations, Open Solutions, 8,* 21127–21151. doi:10.1109/ACCESS.2020.2969820

Beniiche, A. (2020). *A study of blockchain oracles.* arXiv preprint arXiv:2004.07140.

Berg, A. (2020). The Identity, Fungibility and Anonymity of Money. *Economic Papers: A Journal of Applied Economics and Policy, 39*(2), 104-117.

Berg, C., Davidson, S., & Potts, J. (2018). *Beyond money crypto currencies.pdf.* Scribd. https://www.scribd.com/document/426669100/Beyond-money-crypto-currencies-pdf

Bernabe, J. B., Canovas, J. L., Hernandez-Ramos, J. L., Moreno, R. T., & Skarmeta, A. (2019). Privacy-preserving solutions for Blockchain: Review and challenges. *IEEE Access: Practical Innovations, Open Solutions, 7,* 164908–164940. doi:10.1109/ACCESS.2019.2950872

Berwick, D. M. (2020). Choices for the "new normal". *Journal of the American Medical Association, 323*(21), 2125–2126. doi:10.1001/jama.2020.6949 PMID:32364589

Bindseil, U. (2019). Central Bank Digital Currency: Financial System Implications and Control. *International Journal of Political Economy, 48*(4), 303–335. doi:10.1080/08911916.2019.1693160

Birch, D. (2020). *Digital Currency Revolution.* Centre for the Study.

Bjercke, B., & Finlow-Bates, K. (2020). *Decoupling Bitcoins from Their Transaction History Using the Coinbase Transaction.* Academic Press.

Boettke, P. J., & Prychitko, D. (2011). 1985: A defining year in the history of modern Austrian economics. *The Review of Austrian Economics, 24*(2), 129–139. doi:10.100711138-011-0142-8

Bouri, E., Gupta, R., & Vo, X. V. (2020). Jumps in Geopolitical Risk and the Cryptocurrency Market: The Singularity of Bitcoin. *Defence and Peace Economics,* 1–12. doi:10.1080/10242694.2020.1848285

Breen, M. (2018, May 2). *An Introduction to district0x: A Network of Decentralized Communities.* CryptoSlate. https://cryptoslate.com/district0x/

Breslin, S. (2021). *China Risen?: Studying Chinese Global Power.* Policy Press. doi:10.2307/j.ctv1gm00k4

Brinks, V. (2019). 'And Since I Knew About the Possibilities There…': The Role of Open Creative Labs in User Innovation Processes. *Tijdschrift voor Economische en Sociale Geografie, 110*(4), 381–394. doi:10.1111/tesg.12353

Brito, J., Shadab, H., & Castillo, A. (2014). Bitcoin financial regulation: Securities, derivatives, prediction markets, and gambling. *Colum. Sci. & Tech. L. Rev., 16*, 144. doi:10.2139srn.2423461

Brummer, C., & Yadav, Y. (2018). Fintech and the innovation trilemma. *Geological Journal, 107*, 235.

Buiter, W. H. (2007). *Seigniorage* (No. w12919). National Bureau of Economic Research.

Busygina, I., Filippov, M., & Taukebaeva, E. (2018). To decentralize or to continue on the centralization track: The cases of authoritarian regimes in Russia and Kazakhstan. *Journal of Eurasian Studies, 9*(1), 61-71.

Buterin, V. (2014). *A next-generation smart contract and decentralized application platform.* Retrieved from http://buyxpr.com/build/pdfs/EthereumWhitePaper.pdf

Buyle, R., Taelman, R., Mostaert, K., Joris, G., Mannens, E., Verborgh, R., & Berners-Lee, T. (2019). *Streamlining governmental processes by putting citizens in control of their personal data.* Academic Press.

Calcaterra, C., & Kaal, W. A. (2021). The Importance of Reputation for the Evolution of Decentralization. In *Decentralization-Technology's Impact On Organizational And Societal Structure.* DeGruyter Publishers.

Cawthorn, D. M., Kennaugh, A., & Ferreira, S. M. (2020). The future of sustainability in the context of COVID-19. *Ambio,* 1–10. PMID:33289053

Chambers, C. (2019). Money+ markets: Blockchain isn't just a new technology, it is a political disrupter that takes away the state's monopoly on money. try as they might, governments won't be able to legislate it away. *Engineering & Technology, 14*(7/8), 13–13.

Chen, J. (2017). Can online social networks foster young adults' civic engagement? *Telematics and Informatics, 34*(5), 487–497. doi:10.1016/j.tele.2016.09.013

Chen, Y. (2018). Blockchain tokens and the potential democratization of entrepreneurship and innovation. *Business Horizons, 61*(4), 567–575. doi:10.1016/j.bushor.2018.03.006

Choi, M. K., Yeun, C. Y., & Seong, P. H. (2020). A Novel Monitoring System for the Data Integrity of Reactor Protection System Using Blockchain Technology. *IEEE Access: Practical Innovations, Open Solutions, 8*, 118732–118740. doi:10.1109/ACCESS.2020.3005134

Coase, R. H. (1991). *The nature of the firm (1937). The Nature of the Firm.* Origins, Evolution, and Development.

Cointelegraph. (2018, February 13). *What is DAO and how it works.* https://cointelegraph.com/ethereum-for-beginners/what-is-dao

Cordeiro, J. L. (2003). Different Monetary Systems: Costs and Benefits to Whom? *Revista Venezolana de Análisis de Coyuntura, 9*(1), 107–140.

Dahlman, C. J. (1979). The problem of externality. *The Journal of Law & Economics*, *22*(1), 141–162.

Dalton, G. (1982). Barter. *Journal of Economic Issues*, *16*(1), 181–190.

Dapp, M. M. (2019). Toward a Sustainable Circular Economy Powered by Community-Based Incentive Systems. In *Business Transformation through Blockchain* (pp. 153–181). Palgrave Macmillan. doi:10.1007/978-3-319-99058-3_6

Darlington III, J. K. (2014). *The future of Bitcoin: mapping the global adoption of world's largest cryptocurrency through benefit analysis*. Academic Press.

De Beauclair, I. (1963). The Stone Money of Yap Island. *Bulletin of the Institute of Ethnology, Academia Sinica*, *16*, 147–160.

De Beauclair, I. (1971). Studies on Botel Tobago, and Yap. In *Asian Folklore and Social Life Monographs, edited by Lou Tsu-k'uang* (pp. 183–203). Orient Cultural Service.

De Oliveira Rodrigues, D. (2021). Marketing-Mix Metamorphosis and New Trusted Business Practices. In *Competitive Drivers for Improving Future Business Performance* (pp. 46–66). IGI Global. doi:10.4018/978-1-7998-1843-4.ch004

DeMartino, I. (2018). *The Bitcoin Guidebook: How to Obtain, Invest, and Spend the World's First Decentralized Cryptocurrency*. Simon and Schuster.

Dierksmeier, C., & Seele, P. (2018). Cryptocurrencies and business ethics. *Journal of Business Ethics*, *152*(1), 1–14. doi:10.100710551-016-3298-0 PMID:30930508

District0x. (2020). *An Introduction To Decentralization. District0x Education Portal*. https://education.district0x.io/general-topics/what-is-decentralization/introduction/

Dixon, C. (2018). *Why Decentralization Matters*. https://medium.com/s/story/why-decentralization-matters-5e3f79f7638e

Drutarovska, J. (2015). The Linkage between Speculation and Derivatives' Trading Society. Academic Press.

Ducci, F. (2020). *Natural Monopolies in Digital Platform Markets*. Cambridge University Press. doi:10.1017/9781108867528

Dumas, J. G., Jimenez-Garcès, S., & Şoiman, F. (2021, March). Blockchain technology and crypto-assets market analysis: vulnerabilities and risk assessment. The 12th International Multi-Conference on Complexity, Informatics and Cybernetics: IMCIC 2021.

Dush, L. (2015). When writing becomes content. *College Composition and Communication*, 173–196.

Dwyer, R. (2017). *Code! = Law: Explorations of the Blockchain as a Mode of Algorithmic Governance*. Retrieved March 23, 2021, from https://www.academia.edu/34734732/Code_Law_Explorations_of_the_Blockchain_as_a_Mode_of_Algorithmic_Governance

Ebadi, E., Yajam, H., & Akhaee, M. (2020, September). Improvements on Easypaysy: The Bitcoin's Layer-2 Accounts Protocol. In *2020 17th International ISC Conference on Information Security and Cryptology (ISCISC)* (pp. 54-59). IEEE.

Ebner, N. (2017). Negotiation is changing. *J. Disp. Resol., 99*.

Eiglier, P., & Langeard, E. (1987). *La servuction: stratégie et managment*. Ediscience.

Eikmanns, B. C. (2018). *Blockchain: Proposition of a new and sustainable macroeconomic system*. Frankfurt School, Blockchain Center.

Emmer, T. (2020, June). *Virtual Hearing - Inclusive Banking During a Pandemic: Using FedAccounts and Digital Tools to Improve Delivery of Stimulus Payments*. US House Committee on Financial Services. https://financialservices.house.gov/calendar/eventsingle.aspx?EventID=406617

Ethereum. (2020). *Home*. https://ethereum.org/en/

Faber, B., Michelet, G. C., Weidmann, N., Mukkamala, R. R., & Vatrapu, R. (2019, January). BPDIMS: a blockchain-based personal data and identity management system. In *Proceedings of the 52nd Hawaii International Conference on System Sciences*. 10.24251/HICSS.2019.821

Fang, H. S. A. (2021). *Commercially Successful Blockchain Healthcare Projects: A Scoping Review*. Blockchain in Healthcare Today.

Federal Reserve System. (2020, October 6). *Federal Reserve Board - Currency Print Orders*. https://www.federalreserve.gov/paymentsystems/coin_currency_orders.htm

Feldstein, S. (2019). The road to digital unfreedom: How artificial intelligence is reshaping repression. *Journal of Democracy, 30*(1), 40–52. doi:10.1353/jod.2019.0003

Fenwick, M., & Vermeulen, E. P. (2019). Technology and corporate governance: Blockchain, crypto, and artificial intelligence. *Tex. J. Bus. L., 48*, 1.

Ferguson, N. (2008). *The ascent of money: A financial history of the world*. Penguin.

Fisher, R., Ury, W., & Patton, B. (1991). Getting to yes: Negotiating agreement without giving in (No. 158.5). FIS. CIMMYT.

Fitzpatrick, S. (2004a). Banking on Stone Money. For the Yapese of Micronesia, a disk of sculpted limestone could buy just about anything. *Archaeology*, 19–23. https://www.researchgate.net/profile/Scott-Fitzpatrick/publication/255687068_Banking_on_Stone_Money/links/0c9605202df58df571000000/Banking-on-Stone-Money.pdf

Fitzpatrick, S. M., & Diveley, B. (2004). Interisland exchange in Micronesia: a case of monumental proportions. *Voyages of discovery: The archaeology of islands*, 129-146.

Fitzpatrick, S. M., & Diveley, B. D. (2004). Interisland Exchange in Micronesia: A Case of Monumental Proportions. In S. M. Fitzpatrick (Ed.), *Voyages of Discovery: The Archaeology of Islands* (pp. 129–146). Praeger.

Fitzpatrick, S. M., & McKeon, S. (2020). Banking on Stone Money: Ancient Antecedents to Bitcoin. *Economic Anthropology*, 7(1), 7–21. doi:10.1002ea2.12154

Fousekis, P., & Grigoriadis, V. (2021). Directional predictability between returns and volume in cryptocurrencies markets. *Studies in Economics and Finance, ahead-of-print*(ahead-of-print). Advance online publication. doi:10.1108/SEF-08-2020-0318

French, D. E. (2009). *Early speculative bubbles and increases in the supply of money*. Ludwig von Mises Institute.

Friedman, M. (1991). *The Island of Stone Money*. Hoover Institution, Stanford University.

Fritsch, F., Emmett, J., Friedman, E., Kranjc, R., Manski, S. G., Zargham, M., & Bauwens, M. (2021). Challenges and Approaches to Scaling the Global Commons. *Frontiers in Blockchain*, 4, 9. doi:10.3389/fbloc.2021.578721

Furness, W. H. III. (1910). *The Island of Stone Money, Uap of the Carolines*. J. B. Lippincott.

Galloway, S. (2017). *The four: the hidden DNA of Amazon, Apple, Facebook and Google*. Random House.

Garrison, R. W., & Kirzner, I. M. (1989). Friedrich August von Hayek. In *The Invisible Hand* (pp. 119–130). Palgrave Macmillan. doi:10.1007/978-1-349-20313-0_14

Ghabri, Y., Guesmi, K., & Zantour, A. (2020). Bitcoin and liquidity risk diversification. *Finance Research Letters*, 101679.

Ghaiti, K. (2021). *The Volatility of Bitcoin, Bitcoin Cash, Litecoin, Dogecoin and Ethereum* (Doctoral dissertation). Université d'Ottawa/University of Ottawa.

Ghosh, D. (2019). *A New Digital Social Contract to Encourage Internet Competition*. Antitrust Chronicle.

GkillasK.LonginF. (2018). Is Bitcoin the new digital gold? Evidence from extreme price movements in financial markets. SSRN. Available at https://papers.ssrn.com/sol3/papers.cfm doi:10.2139srn.3245571

Goldberg, D. (2012). The tax-foundation theory of fiat money. *Economic Theory*, 50(2), 489–497. doi:10.100700199-010-0564-8

Grant, J. M. (2014). *Is Bitcoin Money? Implications for Bitcoin derivatives regulation and security interest treatment of bitcoins under article 9 of the uniform commercial code*. Implications for Bitcoin Derivatives Regulation and Security Interest Treatment of Bitcoins Under Article 9.

Gurguc, Z., & Knottenbelt, W. (2018). *Cryptocurrencies: overcoming barriers to trust and adoption*. eToro.

Harrison, M. (2018). *Decentralizing the International Monetary System: An Assessment of Regulatory Structures for Cryptocurrencies in the Age of Digital Finance*. Academic Press.

Hasselgren, A., Kralevska, K., Gligoroski, D., Pedersen, S. A., & Faxvaag, A. (2020). Blockchain healthcare and health sciences—A scoping review. *International Journal of Medical Informatics*, 134, 104040. doi:10.1016/j.ijmedinf.2019.104040 PMID:31865055

Hassine, M. B., Kmimech, M., Hellani, H., & Sliman, L. (2020, September). Toward a Mixed Tangle-Blockchain Architecture. In *Knowledge Innovation Through Intelligent Software Methodologies, Tools and Techniques: Proceedings of the 19th International Conference on New Trends in Intelligent Software Methodologies, Tools and Techniques (SoMeT_20)* (Vol. 327, p. 221). IOS Press.

Hayek, F. (1944). The road to serfdom. London. *George Routledge & Sons*, *67*, 84.

Hayek, F. (1976). *Denationalization of money*. Institute of Economic Affairs.

Hayek, F. (1990), Denationalisation of Money-The Argument Refined. An Analysis of the Theory and Practice of Concurrent Currencies (3rd ed.). Academic Press.

Hayes, A. S. (2017). Cryptocurrency value formation: An empirical study leading to a cost of production model for valuing bitcoin. *Telematics and Informatics*, *34*(7), 1308–1321. doi:10.1016/j.tele.2016.05.005

Heiss, J., Eberhardt, J., & Tai, S. (2019, July). From oracles to trustworthy data on-chaining systems. In *2019 IEEE International Conference on Blockchain (Blockchain)* (pp. 496-503). IEEE. 10.1109/Blockchain.2019.00075

HelbingD. (2014). *Qualified money-a better financial system for the future*. Available at SSRN 2526022 doi:10.2139srn.2526022

Hopkins, J. C., III, Prasad, B., Jameson, H. R., & Rangan, G. (2019). *U.S. Patent No. 10,521,780*. Washington, DC: U.S. Patent and Trademark Office.

Hoxtell, W., & Nonhoff, D. (2019). *Internet Governance: Past, Present and Future*. Konrad Adenauer Stiftung. https://www.gppi.net/media/Internet-Governance-Past-Present-and-Future.pdf

Hülsemann, P., & Tumasjan, A. (2019). *Walk this Way!* Incentive Structures of Different Token Designs for Blockchain-Based Applications.

Humphrey, C. (1985). Barter and Economic Disintegration. *Man*, *20*(1), 48–72. doi:10.2307/2802221

Hurlburt, G. F., & Voas, J. (2011). Storytelling: From cave art to digital media. *IT Professional*, *13*(5), 4–7. doi:10.1109/MITP.2011.87

Ingham, G. (2013). *The nature of money*. John Wiley & Sons.

Insights, L. (2020, June 12). *Congressman argues for permissionless digital dollar to demonstrate U.S. values*. Ledger Insights - Enterprise Blockchain. https://www.ledgerinsights.com/digital-dollar-congress-permissionless/

JaccardG. (2018). Smart contracts and the role of law. Available at SSRN 3099885. doi:10.2139srn.3099885

JainD. (2020). The Economics of Cryptocurrencies-Why Does It Work? Available at SSRN 3644159.

Jeffries, D. (2021, May 21). *Dan Jeffries: It's 2031. This Is the World That Crypto Created*. Retrieved May 22, 2021, from https://www.coindesk.com/its-2031-this-is-the-world-that-crypto-created

Jha, P. (2021, May 14). *Guaranty Escrow to Accept Dogecoin Payment For Real Estate Purchases*. Retrieved May 14, 2021, from https://coingape.com/guaranty-escrow-to-accept-dogecoin-payment-for-real-estate-purchases/amp/

Kellner, D. M., & Durham, M. G. (2001). Adventures in media and cultural studies: Introducing the keyworks. *Media and cultural studies: Keyworks*, 1-29.

Kethineni, S., & Cao, Y. (2020). The rise in popularity of cryptocurrency and associated criminal activity. *International Criminal Justice Review*, *30*(3), 325–344. doi:10.1177/1057567719827051

Keynes, J. M. (1915). The Island of Stone Money. *Economic Journal (London)*, *25*(98), 281–283. doi:10.2307/2222196

Khare, R. (2003). *Extending the REpresentational State Transfer REST Architectural Style for Decentralized Systems* (Doctoral dissertation). University of California, Irvine.

Khare, R., & Taylor, R. N. (2004, May). Extending the representational state transfer (rest) architectural style for decentralized systems. In *Proceedings. 26th International Conference on Software Engineering* (pp. 428-437). IEEE.

KiffJ.AlwazirJ.DavidovicS.FariasA.KhanA.KhiaonarongT.ZhouP. (2020). A survey of research on retail central bank digital currency. Available at SSRN 3639760.

Kim, S. (2020). *Fractional Ownership*. Democratization and Bubble Formation - The Impact of Blockchain Enabled Asset Tokenization.

Kirillova, E., Bogdan, V. V., Filippov, P., Tkachev, V., & Zulfugarzade, T. (2020). The Main Features of Blockchain Technologies Classification. *COMPUSOFT: An International Journal of Advanced Computer Technology*, *9*(10), 3900–3905.

Knittel, M. L., & Wash, R. (2019, May). How "True Bitcoiners" work on reddit to maintain bitcoin. In *Extended Abstracts of the 2019 CHI Conference on Human Factors in Computing Systems* (pp. 1-6). ACM.

Kranzberg, M. (1986). Technology and History:" Kranzberg's Laws. *Technology and Culture*, *27*(3), 544–560. doi:10.2307/3105385

Kruijff, J. T., & Weigand, H. (2018, February). An introduction to Commitment Based Smart Contracts using ReactionRuleML. In VMBO (pp. 149-157). Academic Press.

Kurihara, Y. (2021). *Has the Price of Bitcoin changed during COVID-19?* Academic Press.

Lamport, L., Shostak, R., & Pease, M. (2019). The Byzantine generals problem. In Concurrency: The Works of Leslie Lamport (pp. 203-226). Academic Press.

Lan, R., Upadhyaya, G., Tse, S., & Zamani, M. (2021). *Horizon: A Gas-Efficient, Trustless Bridge for Cross-Chain Transactions.* arXiv preprint arXiv:2101.06000.

Lannoye, V. (2020). *The History of Money for Understanding Economics.* Vincent Lannoye.

Leach, M., MacGregor, H., Scoones, I., & Wilkinson, A. (2020). Post-pandemic transformations: How and why COVID-19 requires us to rethink development. *World Development*, *138*, 105233. doi:10.1016/j.worlddev.2020.105233 PMID:33100478

Lewis, A. (2015). *A gentle introduction to digital tokens.* https://bitsonblocks.net/2015/09/28/a-gentle-introduction-to-digital-tokens/

Li, G. (2008). *Economic sense of Metcalfe's Law*. Academic Press.

Lindley, J., Coulton, P., Akmal, H. A., Hay, D., Van Kleek, M., Cannizzaro, S., & Binns, R. (2019). *The Little Book of*. Academic Press.

Liu, J., Li, X., Ye, L., Zhang, H., Du, X., & Guizani, M. (2018, December). BPDS: A blockchain based privacy-preserving data sharing for electronic medical records. In *2018 IEEE Global Communications Conference (GLOBECOM)* (pp. 1-6). IEEE. 10.1109/GLOCOM.2018.8647713

LoY. C. (2017). Blockchain and bitcoin: technological breakthrough or the latest tulip price bubble? Available at SSRN 3198530. doi:10.2139srn.3198530

Lopez, P. G., Montresor, A., & Datta, A. (2019, July). Please, do not decentralize the Internet with (permissionless) blockchains! In *2019 IEEE 39th International Conference on Distributed Computing Systems (ICDCS)* (pp. 1901-1911). IEEE.

Lotti, L. (2019). The Art of Tokenization: Blockchain Affordances and the Invention of Future Milieus. *Media Theory*, *3*(1), 287–320.

Lu, Y., & Pan, J. (2020). Capturing Clicks: How the Chinese Government Uses Clickbait to Compete for Visibility. *Political Communication*, 1–32. doi:10.1080/10584609.2020.1765914

Mack, C. A. (2011). Fifty years of Moore's law. *IEEE Transactions on Semiconductor Manufacturing*, *24*(2), 202–207. doi:10.1109/TSM.2010.2096437

Mack, E. (2021, May 14). *Wow, much value: Dogecoin seals New England real estate deal*. Retrieved May 14, 2021, from https://www.cnet.com/google-amp/news/wow-much-value-dogecoin-seals-new-england-real-estate-deal/

Mamun, M. A., Bhuiyan, A. I., & Manzar, M. D. (2020). The first COVID-19 infanticide-suicide case: Financial crisis and fear of COVID-19 infection are the causative factors. *Asian Journal of Psychiatry*, *54*, 102365. doi:10.1016/j.ajp.2020.102365 PMID:33271687

Manovich, L. (2002). *The Language of New Media*. MIT.

Manovich, L. (2013). *Software Takes Command*. Bloomsbury Academic.

Martin, F. (2013). *The Unauthorised Biography*. Random House.

Martinelli, E. (2017). *The Politics of Bitcoin*. http://www.brunoleonimedia.it/public/Mises2018/Papers/Mises2018-Paper_Martinelli.pdf

Maslow, A. H. (1943). A theory of human motivation. *Psychological Review*, *50*(4), 370–396. doi:10.1037/h0054346

Massey, R., Dalal, D., & Dakshinamoorthy, A. (2017). *Initial coin offering: A new paradigm*. Deloitte. Available at https:// www2.deloitte.com/content/dam/Deloitte/us/Documents/ process-and-operations/us-cons-new-paradigm.pdf

Mattke, J., Maier, C., & Reis, L. (2020, June). Is cryptocurrency money? Three empirical studies analyzing medium of exchange, store of value and unit of account. In *Proceedings of the 2020 on Computers and People Research Conference* (pp. 26-35). 10.1145/3378539.3393859

McIntosh, R. (2021, May 12). *While Tesla Decides on Dogecoin, FNTX Users Can Buy Condos with DOGE*. Retrieved May 13, 2021, from https://www.financemagnates.com/cryptocurrency/news/while-tesla-decides-on-dogecoin-fntx-users-can-buy-condos-with-doge/?tg=1620799861

McLuhan, M., & McLuhan, M. A. (1994). *Understanding media: The extensions of man*. MIT Press.

McLuhan, M., & Powers, B. R. (1989). *The Global Village: Transformations in World, Life and Media in the 21st Century*. Oxford University Press.

Mertes, T. (2002). Wall Street. *Amass, 12*(2), 80.

Metcalfe, B. (2013). Metcalfe's law after 40 years of Ethernet. *IEEE Computer, 46*(12), 26–31. doi:10.1109/MC.2013.374

Mittal, S. (2012). *Is bitcoin money? bitcoin and alternate theories of money*. Bitcoin and Alternate Theories of Money.

Mollick, E. (2006). Establishing Moore's law. *IEEE Annals of the History of Computing, 28*(3), 62–75. doi:10.1109/MAHC.2006.45

Moniruzzaman, M., Chowdhury, F., & Ferdous, M. S. (2020, February). Examining Usability Issues in Blockchain-Based Cryptocurrency Wallets. In *International Conference on Cyber Security and Computer Science* (pp. 631-643). Springer. 10.1007/978-3-030-52856-0_50

Monroe, A. (1923). *Monetary Theory before Adam Smith* (Vol. 25). Harvard University Press. doi:10.4159/harvard.9780674183438

Möser, M., Böhme, R., & Breuker, D. (2014, March). Towards risk scoring of Bitcoin transactions. In *International Conference on Financial Cryptography and Data Security* (pp. 16-32). Springer.

Mouial-Bassilana, E., Restrepo, D., & Colombani, L. (2018). Le déséquilibre significatif dans les contrats commerciaux: nouvel outil de lutte contre les GAFA. *Actualité juridique. Contrat, 471*.

Mueller, L., Glarner, A., Linder, T., Meyer, S. D., Furrer, A., Gschwend, C., & Henschel, P. (2018). *Conceptual Framework for Legal and Risk Assessment of Crypto Tokens*. Academic Press.

Muzzy, E. (2018, October 9). *CryptoKitties Isn't About the Cats - Everett Muzzy*. Retrieved April 27, 2021, from https://medium.com/@everett.muzzy/cryptokitties-isnt-about-the-cats-aef47bcde92d

Nakamoto, S. (2008). *A peer-to-peer electronic cash system*. Bitcoin. https://bitcoin.org/bitcoin.pdf

Nakamura, Y., Zhang, Y., Sasabe, M., & Kasahara, S. (2020). Exploiting smart contracts for capability-based access control in the Internet of Things. *Sensors (Basel), 20*(6), 1793. doi:10.339020061793 PMID:32213888

Náñez Alonso, S. L., Jorge-Vazquez, J., & Reier Forradellas, R. F. (2021). Central Banks Digital Currency: Detection of Optimal Countries for the Implementation of a CBDC and the Implication for Payment Industry Open Innovation. *Journal of Open Innovation*, 7(1), 72. doi:10.3390/joitmc7010072

Naudet, L. B. (2021). *Regard sur les conséquences des mutations organiques de la monnaie dans la manifestation des conflits armés depuis l'éclatement du système de Bretton-Woods*. Academic Press.

Norta, A. (2016, November). Designing a smart-contract application layer for transacting decentralized autonomous organizations. In *International Conference on Advances in Computing and Data Sciences* (pp. 595-604). Springer.

Noyen, K., Volland, D., Wörner, D., & Fleisch, E. (2014). *When money learns to fly: Towards sensing as a service application using bitcoin*. arXiv preprint arXiv:1409.5841

O'Neil, C. (2017). How can we stop algorithms telling lies? *The Guardian*, 7-16.

Overview, D. A. O. (2020). *A List of Ethereum's Top DAOs and DAO Structures*. DeFi Rate. https://defirate.com/daos/

Paik, H. Y., Xu, X., Bandara, H. D., Lee, S. U., & Lo, S. K. (2019). Analysis of data management in blockchain-based systems: From architecture to governance. *IEEE Access: Practical Innovations, Open Solutions*, 7, 186091–186107. doi:10.1109/ACCESS.2019.2961404

Passinsky, A. (2021). Should Bitcoin Be Classified as Money? *Journal of Social Ontology*.

Pasuthip, P., & Yang, S. (2020). *Central Bank Digital Currency: Promises and Risks*. Academic Press.

Perera, C., Zaslavsky, A., Christen, P., & Georgakopoulos, D. (2014). Sensing as a service model for smart cities supported by internet of things. *Transactions on Emerging Telecommunications Technologies*, 25(1), 81–93. doi:10.1002/ett.2704

Perez, S. (2018, June 20). *Does a Blockchain Need a Token? The Startup*. Retrieved February 20, 2021, from https://medium.com/swlh/does-a-blockchain-need-a-token-66c894d566fb

Peters, G. W., & Panayi, E. (2016). Understanding modern banking ledgers through blockchain technologies: Future of transaction processing and smart contracts on the internet of money. In *Banking beyond banks and money* (pp. 239–278). Springer. doi:10.1007/978-3-319-42448-4_13

Pocher, N. (2019). The Internet of Money between Anonymity and Publicity: Legal Challenges of Distributed Ledger Technologies in the Crypto Financial Landscape. In *JURIX*. Doctoral Consortium.

Prinz, A. (1999). Money in the real and the virtual world: E-money, c-money and the demand for cb-money. *NETNOMICS: Economic Research and Electronic Networking*, 1(1), 11–35. doi:10.1023/A:1011441519577

Qian, Y. (2019). Central Bank Digital Currency: optimization of the currency system and its issuance design. *China Economic Journal, 12*(1), 1-15.

Qiang, X. (2019). The road to digital unfreedom: President xi's surveillance state. *Journal of Democracy*, 30(1), 53–67. doi:10.1353/jod.2019.0004

Rajapashe, M., Adnan, M., Dissanayaka, A., Guneratne, D., & Abeywardena, K. (2020). Multi-Format Document Verification System. *American Scientific Research Journal for Engineering, Technology, and Sciences, 74*(2), 48–60.

Regner, F., Urbach, N., & Schweizer, A. (2019). *NFTs in Practice–Non-Fungible Tokens as Core Component of a Blockchain-based Event Ticketing Application.* Academic Press.

ReinersL. (2020). *Cryptocurrency and the State: An Unholy Alliance.* Available at SSRN 3682724.

Reisenwitz, C. (2014). Smart contracts promise for the Poor. *Bitcoin Mag.* https://bitcoinmagazine.com/articles/smart-propertys-promise-poor-1390852097/

Rooney, D., & Chavan, M. (2017). Globalization/internationalization. The International Encyclopedia of Organizational Communication, 1-15.

Sadowski, J. (2020). *Too smart: How digital capitalism is extracting data, controlling our lives, and taking over the world.* MIT Press. doi:10.7551/mitpress/12240.001.0001

Safiullin, M., Savelichev, M., Elshin, L., & Moiseev, V. (2020). *Increasing stability of economy through supply chain management and the circular economy.* Electronic archive of the Kazan Federal University. https://dspace.kpfu.ru/xmlui/handle/net/163214

Safko, L. (2010). *The social media bible: tactics, tools, and strategies for business success.* John Wiley & Sons.

Salah, K., Alfalasi, A., & Alfalasi, M. (2019, April). A Blockchain-based System for Online Consumer Reviews. In *IEEE INFOCOM 2019-IEEE Conference on Computer Communications Workshops (INFOCOM WKSHPS)* (pp. 853-858). IEEE. 10.1109/INFCOMW.2019.8845186

Sanz Bas, D. (2020). Hayek and the cryptocurrency revolution. *Iberian Journal of the History of Economic Thought, 7*(1), 15–28. doi:10.5209/ijhe.69403

Schaller, R. R. (1997). Moore's law: Past, present and future. *IEEE Spectrum, 34*(6), 52–59. doi:10.1109/6.591665

Scott-Briggs, A. (2018, January 12). *Introduction to Decentralized Autonomous Organization.* TechBullion. https://techbullion.com/introduction-decentralized-autonomous-organization/

Sharma, P., Jindal, R., & Borah, M. D. (2020). Blockchain technology for cloud storage: A systematic literature review. *ACM Computing Surveys, 53*(4), 1–32. doi:10.1145/3403954

Shirky, C. (2008). *Here comes everybody: The power of organizing without organizations.* Penguin.

SMA. (2018, November). *FLIPHODL.* https://www.fliphodl.com/social-media-alternatives-series-ep-1-what-you-need-to-know/

Sosnovik, V., & Goga, O. (2021). *Understanding the Complexity of Detecting Political Ads.* arXiv preprint arXiv:2103.00822.

Srivastava, A., Jain, P., Hazela, B., Asthana, P., & Rizvi, S. W. A. (2021). Application of Fog Computing, Internet of Things, and Blockchain Technology in Healthcare Industry. In *Fog Computing for Healthcare 4.0 Environments* (pp. 563–591). Springer. doi:10.1007/978-3-030-46197-3_22

Starr, R. M. (1989). The structure of exchange in barter and monetary economies. In *General Equilibrium Models of Monetary Economies* (pp. 129–143). Academic Press. doi:10.1016/B978-0-12-663970-4.50014-1

Sunyaev, A. (2020). Distributed ledger technology. In *Internet Computing* (pp. 265–299). Springer. doi:10.1007/978-3-030-34957-8_9

Swan, M. (2015). *Blockchain: Blueprint for a new economy*. O'Reilly Media, Inc.

Szabo, N. (1997). Formalizing and Securing Relationships on Public Networks. *First Monday*, *2*(9). Advance online publication. doi:10.5210/fm.v2i9.548

Szabo, N. (2002). *The Origins of Money (No. 0211005)*. University Library of Munich.

Tam, K. P., Leung, A. K., & Khan, S. (2021). The new normal of social psychology in the face of the COVID-19 pandemic: Insights and advice from leaders in the field. *Asian Journal of Social Psychology*, *24*(1), 8–9. doi:10.1111/ajsp.12468 PMID:33821135

Tapscott, D., & Euchner, J. (2019). Blockchain and the Internet of Value: An Interview with Don Tapscott Don Tapscott talks with Jim Euchner about blockchain, the Internet of value, and the next Internet revolution. *Research Technology Management*, *62*(1), 12–19. doi:10.1080/08956308.2019.1541711

Tapscott, D., & Tapscott, A. (2016). *Blockchain revolution: how the technology behind bitcoin is changing money, business, and the world*. Penguin.

Tennant, L. (2017). *Improving the Anonymity of the IOTA Cryptocurrency*. Academic Press.

Thagapsov, A., & Kozlovskiy, M. (2020). Bitcoin as Money. *Economic Analysis*.

Thornhill, J. (2021) The tech platforms are not entirely to blame for Washington unrest: knee-jerk reactions in the wake of the storming of Capitol Hill could have unintended consequences. *Financial Times*. Available at: https://www.ft.com/content/ef64b160-5f01-404a-bb39-d013fde808ca

Tonin, P., Gosselet, N., Halle, E., & Henrion, M. (2018). Ideal oil and protein crops–what are users ideotypes, from the farmer to the consumer? *OCL*, *25*(6), D605. doi:10.1051/ocl/2018060

Troshchinskiy, P. V. (2021, February). Main Directions of Digitalization in China. In *International Scientific and Practical Conference "Russia 2020-a new reality: economy and society" (ISPCR 2020)* (pp. 451-454). Atlantis Press.

Turi, A. N. (2020). Currency Under the Web 3.0 Economy. In Technologies for Modern Digital Entrepreneurship (pp. 155-186). Apress.

Twesige, R. (2015). *A simple explanation of Bitcoin and Block Chain technology*. Academic Press.

Urgo, A. K., Lestan, M., & Khoriaty, A. (2017, September 17). *A cooperative of decentralized marketplaces and communities*. Powered by Ethereum, Aragon, and IPFS. District0x. https://district0x.io/docs/district0x-whitepaper.pdf

Vassiliadis, S., Papadopoulos, P., Rangoussi, M., Konieczny, T., & Gralewski, J. (2017). Bitcoin value analysis based on cross-correlations. *Journal of Internet Banking and Commerce, 22*(S7), 1.

Veblen, T. (1899). Mr. Cummings's Strictures on The Theory of the Leisure Class. *Journal of Political Economy, 8*(1), 106–117. doi:10.1086/250640

Veitas, V., & Weinbaum, D. (2017). Living cognitive society: A 'digital'world of views. *Technological Forecasting and Social Change, 114*, 16–26. doi:10.1016/j.techfore.2016.05.002

Vergne, J. P. (2020). Decentralized vs. Distributed Organization: A Framework for the Future of Blockchain and Machine Learning and for Avoiding Digital Platform Dystopia. *Distributed Organization: A Framework for the Future of Blockchain and Machine Learning and for Avoiding Digital Platform Dystopia.*

Wang, S., Ding, W., Li, J., Yuan, Y., Ouyang, L., & Wang, F. Y. (2019). Decentralized autonomous organizations: Concept, model, and applications. *IEEE Transactions on Computational Social Systems, 6*(5), 870–878. doi:10.1109/TCSS.2019.2938190

Weatherford, J. (2009). *The history of money*. Currency.

Weber, M. (1958). *The Protestant Ethic and The Spirit of Capitalism*. Charles Scribner's Sons.

Wilczak, A. (2018). Between Consumerism and Deconsumption – Attitudes of Young People as a Challenge for Marketers. *Economic and Social Development: Book of Proceedings*, 297-305.

Wood, G. (2014). Ethereum: A secure decentralised generalised transaction ledger. *Ethereum Project Yellow Paper, 151*(2014), 1-32.

Xu, X., Pautasso, C., Zhu, L., Gramoli, V., Ponomarev, A., Tran, A. B., & Chen, S. (2016, April). The blockchain as a software connector. In *2016 13th Working IEEE/IFIP Conference on Software Architecture (WICSA)* (pp. 182-191). IEEE. 10.1109/WICSA.2016.21

Yablonskaya, T. (2018, October 18). *Ethereum-Based Organization The DAO Launches and Raises Millions Worth of... Coinspeaker*. https://www.coinspeaker.com/dao-new-breath-of-blockchain-ethereum/

Young, S. (2018). Changing governance models by applying blockchain computing. *Catholic University Journal of Law and Technology, 26*(2), 87–128.

Zaprutin, D. G., Nikiporets-Takigawa, G., Goncharov, V. V., Sekerin, V. D., & Gorokhova, A. E. (2020). Legal Practice in the Blockchain Era. *Revista Gênero e Interdisciplinaridade, 1*(1).

Zelmanovitz, L. (2011). Money: Origin and essence. *Criterio Libre, 9*(14), 65–90. doi:10.18041/1900-0642/criteriolibre.2011v9n14.1232

Zhang, X. Z., Liu, J. J., & Xu, Z. W. (2015). Tencent and Facebook data validate Metcalfe's law. *Journal of Computer Science and Technology, 30*(2), 246–251. doi:10.100711390-015-1518-1

Zheng, Z., Xie, S., Dai, H. N., Chen, X., & Wang, H. (2018). Blockchain challenges and opportunities: A survey. *International Journal of Web and Grid Services, 14*(4), 352–375. doi:10.1504/IJWGS.2018.095647

KEY TERMS AND DEFINITIONS

Crypto-Economics: Is the combination of cryptographic proofs of past events and economic incentives to encourage future events inside a blockchain system. On the cryptography side, components used centre mainly around consensus algorithms, digital signatures, and hash functions, plus more recently, zero-knowledge proofs, multi-party computation and homomorphic encryption. On the economy side, things are more complex and an active area of research involving game theory, mechanism design, and network economics.

Decentralized Autonomous Organization (DAO): A new decentralized business model (open source) for organizing both commercial and non-profit endeavours.

Fiat Money: Is the government-issued currency that is not backed by a physical commodity, such as gold or silver, but rather by the government that issued it. Its value is derived from the demand-supply relation and the stability of the issuing entity (government) rather than by the worth of a commodity backing it (commodity money). Most modern paper currencies are *fiat currencies*, including the U.S. dollar, the euro, and other major global currencies.

Hedging: A hedge is an investment that is made with the intention of reducing the risk of adverse price movements in an asset. Normally, a hedge consists of taking an offsetting or opposite position in a related security.

Peer-to-Peer (P2P) Network: A group of computers that are linked together with equal permissions and responsibilities for processing data. Each connected machine has the same rights as its "peers" and can be used for the same purposes.

Prosumer: A proactive consumer that voluntarily and when stimulated to do so, participates in the design, creation or improvement of products and services.

Seignoriage: Seigniorage is the difference between the face value of money, and the cost to produce it. The economic cost of producing a currency within a given economy or country is lower than the actual exchange value, which generally accrues to governments who mint the money.

Self-Servuction: The process of production of a service carried out in a strategic partnership and close collaboration with the prosumers.

Smart Contracts: Software programs that code business arrangements and that execute themselves automatically under pre-determined circumstances which are also coded.

Token: An object (either in hardware or software) which represents the right to perform some operation. Traditional currencies are physical "tokens" and cryptocurrencies are virtual tokens.

Value-of-Exchange: The trade value that justify transacting something, for instance in the blockchain stage of the Internet (Internet of Value or Internet of Money).

Value-of-Use: The utility value that justify sharing something, for instance in the pre-blockchain stage of the Internet (Internet of Information).

Chapter 4
Blockchanging Politics:
Opening a Trustworthy but Hazardous Reforming Era

Dario de Oliveira Rodrigues

https://orcid.org/0000-0002-2817-5115

Instituto Politécnico de Santarém, Portugal

Pedro Santana Lopes

GlobalLawyers, Portugal

ABSTRACT

There has been a fundamental change in the genesis of political-economic trust, with the arrival of a decentralized but structured way to reach consensuses and automatically implementing decisions through self-executable contracts. Blockchain technology (BT) is a distributed, consensus-based, and secure way for individuals to make enforceable censorship-resistant quantifiable agreements. Every vote is a transaction, and BT is paving the way for decentralizing politics, defending privacy, and streamlining voting procedures. It has the potential to provide much more granular governance that hopefully will preserve freedom and defend democracy. However, especially in an embarrassing post-COVID-19 world, BT's centralization can, instead, pave the way for citizens' control, turning cryptographic protocols into an authoritarian digital corset tightened by some to menace the privacy and freedom of many.

INTRODUCTION

"Invention is the mother of necessity." (Kranzberg, 1986) Kranzberg's Second Law

To change the world is the dream of some. Blockchain Technology (BT) empowers humankind with the potential to fulfill that dream or make it a nightmare. In this chapter it will be discussed why BT can make-or-break democracy in a "post-Covid uncertain future" (Leach et al., 2020, p.1), being uncertain who will benefit the most now that confidence is embedded on the Internet "through a distributed consensus protocol" (Faber et al., 2020, p. 6857).

DOI: 10.4018/978-1-7998-7363-1.ch004

A permanent record of all transactions is set in "cryptographic stone" on the ledger, which means no one can rewrite or deny history. In other words, it is impossible to cheat with blockchain because everything is in the open to those involved and authorized to see. Risk is minimized in a system in which governance is truly shared. I can't think of a better definition of trust. (Dwyer, 2017, p. 12)

As argued by Young (2018), BT's *distributed-trust* makes it possible to dream about a political transformation that includes a never seen democratic authenticity where granular decisions will be made by citizens holding governments directly accountable thanks to decentralized blockchain-based transactions and a "smart social contract" (Young, 2018, p. 61).

Blockchain technology has the potential to reshape the organizational landscape, rendering traditional, hierarchical ways of organizing obsolete. Its distributed nature enables organizing in nonhierarchical ways. [...] nonhierarchical ways of organizing the structures needed to build new social contracts [(smart social contracts)] for sustainability and further shape the transition to a sustainable development. (Faber & Hadders, 2016, p. 17)

It is thought that BT can be used to enhance or disrupt democracy, and this chapter highlights what is believed to be a historic opportunity to guarantee political transparency to build trust. Such trust has never been as necessary as today to preserve privacy and freedom aiming for a digital responsive democracy that leads to a sustainable and fair society.

The authors approached BT's political implications from a liberal democratic perspective. They opted for an investigation method based on qualitative research. The research methodology chosen was the literature review, which is considered adequate to overview several thematic areas on a given topic. Among the literature review, the most used for business studies are systematic review, semi-systematic review, and integrative review (Snyder, 2019). Considering the need to carry out a synthesis of social sciences knowledge, which is required to make the intended political-economic analysis, the authors used an integrative literature review, which is indicated to frame a study from new perspectives, especially when it comes to research themes and topics little explored (Torraco, 2005). As far as the authors were able to observe, this lack of research still characterizes the study of BT's political implications.

This chapter is organized as follows: BT and decentralization will be considered first before discussing why the Internet is entering a new stage to change society again, this time with an even more significant political-economic impact. The opposite effects of using two very different digital currencies will illustrate how BT can serve two contrasting political regimes. After discussing such political implications, strategic solutions will be recommended advocating BT's resourceful use to face a challenging *new normal* (Berwick, 2020) where *post-Covid-19* physical reality and *blockchain* digital reality will inevitably merge, creating a new political era whose outlines are still open.

BACKGROUND

Blockchain: A Civilizational Milestone

It is thought that blockchain's political best novelty is the prompt execution of people's will. Intermediaries usually establish trust, but they can also break it (which is not an exception in politics). The authors consider that the new guarantee of trust provided by Blockchain Technology (BT) represents an inflection point in human development. As everybody can rely on the blockchain-based distributed trust (Bellini et al., 2020, p.1127), thanks to the auditability of the blockchain protocol (Zheng, 2018), even strangers can now blindly trust each other. Hence, individuals do not need to walk alone anymore depending on institutional third parties to establish reliable political-economic ties between themselves. Hopefully, BT will help remove the considerable agency costs due to many tempting but empty promises sometimes used by politicians, which, at least in democratic regimes, are supposed to be honest intermediaries.

It is argued that digital technologies offer "particular benefits to authoritarian and illiberal regimes" (Feldstein, 2019, p.42). Indeed, information is an instrument of power (Heitman & User, 2018), and new digital technologies combined with centralized data can make life too easy for governments that eventually want to control and manipulate their citizens. However, BT's decentralizing properties make this digital technology ambivalent, being that "theoretical and empirical studies have identified that decentralization is strongly associated with democracy" (Busygina et al., 2018, p. 61). As stated by Sir Tim Berners-Lee, the creator of the *World Wide Web*, "blockchain is a way for different parties that do not know each other to reach an agreement without the need for a referee or a trusted third party" (Buyle et al. 2019, p.2). According to Alcazar (2017), "concisely stated, blockchain is a technology that stores data in a way that makes it incorruptible, doing so via its integrated data ledgers [*hyperledger*)]." (p. 91).

Digital systems develop faster than analogic ones, and systems distributed over a network appear to be more competitive. Gordon Moore, a founder, and CEO of Intel (Mack, 2011), accurately predicted in 1965 that "the speed of computers, as measured by the number of transistors that can be placed on a single chip, will double every year or two" (Mollick, 2006, p. 62). In the '80s, Robert Metcalfe, the inventor of Ethernet (the connection architecture for local area networks - LAN- most used globally), referred that a network's value is proportional to the square of its size. This statement was later named Metcalfe's "law" (Metcalfe, 2013).

Several decades after these statements were made, it turns out that, in the case of the two most prominent social networks in the world, Facebook and WeChat (Chen, 2017), data fit Metcalfe's "law" quite well, and significantly their costs are inversely proportional to the square of network size (Zhang et al., 2015). So, it seems to be true that digital networks' competitive advantage can be inferred from their size (the number of network nodes).

The cost of the computing and communication used to create connectivity is halved every two years according to the Moore's Law. Combining Moore's and Metcalfe's Laws together, the number of users at which a network's value exceeds its cost halves every two years. In the same time, the value of connectivity has been going up. (Li, 2008, p. 23)

In the last years, information and communication technologies (ICT) have diminished social media sharing costs. However, that reduction had no parallel in terms of *transaction costs*: "The Internet vastly improved the flow of data within and between organizations, but the effect on how we do business has been more limited. The Internet was designed to move information - not value - from person to person "(Tapscott & Tapscott, 2017).

However, the Internet changed. In the *blockchain era*, the *Internet of Information* is replaced by the *Internet of Value*, and regarding transaction costs (Coase, 1993), some authors consider that a much more significant reduction is expected (Davidson et al., 2018; Berg et al., 2019).

Such a critical cost reduction anticipates the economic success and the pervasiveness of this technological innovation, which justifies introducing the expression *Information and Transaction Technologies* (ITT) herein proposed by the authors. It is thought that this new designation attends to both economic media shared and transacted on today's Internet, respectively, social media and digital tokens.

As stated by Jain (2020), "digitization pushed verification prices for various types of transactions close to zero [and] Blockchain technology completes this method by providing free verification." (p. 5). According to Chen (2018), "blockchain technology is one of the most revolutionary general-purpose technologies, and it may have far-reaching implications for entrepreneurship and innovation" (p. 573).

Blockchain technology allows the creation of platforms where the exchange and provision of digital assets does not have need/rely on an intermediary. On these platforms, trust in a platform operator is replaced by trust in the underlying incentives, code, and consensus rules. This is possible because blockchain technology decreases the cost of networking. (…) In the case of blockchain, by reducing the market power of intermediaries, the technology conjointly permits platforms to work with lower barriers to entry and innovation. (Jain, 2020, p. 5,6).

As published in the "The Economist" cover page, BT is a powerful "trust machine" (2015) based on cryptography and mathematical certainty, making it possible to carry out secure transactions even in the absence of intermediaries. As it will be seen, BT's transaction features encompass electoral tokens ("cryptovotes"), which can be a game-changer in politics.

The fascination with the blockchain derives from the fact that it establishes the truth of an event without recourse to a trusted third party in an adversarial environment where no-one can be trusted. The truth of an event, i.e., the creation and/or transfer of tokens, is established by means of "distributed consensus," i.e. the confirmation by a majority of nodes in a decentralized network that a given block has [been validated]. Consequently, the blockchain itself is "trustless" because it creates and confirms a certain state of affairs and replaces the need to trust third parties with the ability to trust the technology itself. (Mik, 2017, p. 7)

A Blockchain is just a database that works as a distributed ledger, verifying and validating sequential blocks containing transaction data. This ledger replication is called a *hyperledger*.

There are different types of blockchains configured in two main dimensions. According to Dumas et al. (2021), those are the *permission dimension* (which sets limitations concerning the user's right to write and amend the ledger) and the private dimension (which sets limitations concerning the users' right to access and submit data into the ledger). These dimensions are represented in the axis of Table 1.

Most transactions carried out by citizens throughout their lives involve third parties on whom it is impossible to place complete trust. It is believed that such transactions will tend to be carried out on blockchain networks, which involve lower transaction costs than traditional solutions.

Landermore (2012) defines *democracy* as "a procedure for collective choice decisions" (p. 10), and the authors consider that, in the *Blockchain Era*, it will not be possible to live in a democracy without the kind of transparency achieved by *public blockchains*. An exhaustive explanation of blockchain technicalities goes beyond this chapter's scope, but it is politically essential to understand *public blockchains* and *private blockchains*. There are also two types of *public blockchains,* which are *public-permissionless* blockchain and *public-permissioned* blockchains. The other types of blockchains are privately or state-owned, resulting in user's data centralization, with the consequent loss of privacy. Although *private blockchains* have usefulness (plenty of use cases already exist, and many others will arise), they should not resume the alternatives that must be available in a blockchain democracy since "contractual terms can be manifested in a computer code, what is not generally prohibited based on the *freedom of contract* principle." (Savelyev, 2017, p. 10).

Table 1. Blockchain types

Editability	Openness		
	Public (open access: all can read/join)	**Private** (restricted access)	
Permissionless (free validation rights)	Public-Permissionless Blockchain (reading & mining rights)	Hybrid Blockchains: Private-Permissionless (publicly mineable only)	
Permissioned (restricted validation rights)	Hybrid Blockchains: Public-Permissioned (publicly readable only)	Consortium Blockchains	Private Blockchains

Source: Authors' work.

Personal rights on the Internet can be guaranteed by using private cryptographic keys to access *public blockchains*, while transactions carried out on *private blockchains* stay dependent on third parties. In other words, some blockchains decentralize power, and others do the opposite.

Some ideas and critical elements about decentralization will be seen in the following section, whose understanding is considered fundamental before addressing BT's political-economic implications, blockchain governance issues, and the authors' solutions and recommendations.

Decentralization

In the *blockchain era*, *decentralization* should be understood "as a property similar to redundancy and no single point of control" (Vergne, 2020, pp. 3,4). To investigate the decentralizing potential of Block-chain Technology (BT) applied to communities' ecosystems, one should start to see the role that *tokens*, *smart contracts*, and *decentralized autonomous organizations* (DAO) will likely play perhaps sooner than expected. Some of these concepts are not of intuitive or easy apprehension to *non-digitally born* mindsets (as is the authors' case), but one should give it a try because they are fundamental pieces to understand the reasons behind the predictable expansion of the blockchain universe.

DAOs are one of the most notorious results of the new type of structured digital decentralization made possible by BT. According to several authors (Zwitter & Hazenberg, 2020); Dwyer, 2017; Young, 2018, 2018a), although DAOs having started to strictly care about the creation of economic value, they may extend to public administration and the direction of the state. BT's structured decentralization may lead to the third sector's emancipation and the self-organization of civil society in ways that have not been thought possible until recently (see Figure 1).

In this sense, Dwyer (2017) points that "a key aspect of the DAO is that it takes traditional aspects of governance that were previously enacted by the state and implements these through software-defined processes with an underlying liberal free-market ideology." (p. 14)

Figure 1. Rules flows in centralized and decentralized networks.
(Adapted from [Fliphodl, 2018])

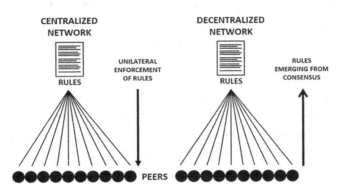

As self-sufficient social structures, DAOs can make and implement decisions. Despite not being hierarchical, they can generate consensus among their constituents about managing socio-economic resources (see the same book, Chapter 5 – *The Real Blockchain Game Changer: Protocols and DAOs for Coordinating Work to Provide Goods and Services*).

With the concept of decentralized autonomous organizations (DAOs), blockchain technology can not only cure all sorts of blown-up bureaucratic structures, by coordinating people, resources, and processes in more transparent and efficient ways. It will even allow one to build a new form of socio-ecological, liberal, efficient and democratic kind of capitalism. This will consider externalities of everyone's activities on their environment and others by combining blockchain technology with the Internet of Things, creating a socio-ecological finance system. In such a way, it is possible to boost a sustainable circular and sharing economy, with a variety of incentives, i.e. new socio-economic feedbacks. (van den Hoven et al., 2019, p. 166)

It is thought that in a free-market system and once technically optimized, DAOs will be unstoppable infrastructures. Relying on *smart contracts* to trigger a *collective action* that can be encouraged by tokens' transactions, DAOs can manage resources in a decentralized way. Such decentralization of value is possible due to the tokens' programmability accomplished by BT.

Tokens are objects or symbols that represent and quantify physical or digital assets. Thanks to *smart contracts*, tokens can be programmed to perform precise functions. They can integrate *social capital* and *social work* to manage consensus among DAOs' users. Thus, besides being valuable to trade, tokens can also perform concrete tasks to reach specific objectives and accomplish certain missions. Hence, hopefully, tokens can be used as individual incentives to manage communities' sustainability through collective action.

In turn, *smart contracts* allow to move, lock or unlock digital tokens (*e.g.*, cryptocurrencies) in a decentralized way through the Internet, which is only possible thanks to Blockchain Technology (BT). For example, smart contracts developed on the Ethereum blockchain make it possible to go beyond mere monetary transactions, adding rules and logic to transactions. This new feature is the great novelty and evolution of the blockchain protocol paving the way to a digital decentralization spreading from the strictly monetary sphere to the economic, social, and political sphere, eventually in this order.

While Blockchain was born with Bitcoin, its applications have gone far beyond Bitcoin or digital currency. Many people believe that blockchain could revolutionize many fields, such as finance, accounting, management, and law leading to three generations of blockchains, namely, Blockchain 1.0 for digital currency, Blockchain 2.0 for digital finance, and Blockchain 3.0 for digital society (Zhao et al., 2016)

Whenever it is financed with the required tokens to comply with its clauses, a smart contract will self-execute like and when stipulated. For instance, considering political elections, a smart contract can link the electoral choices (results = x votes) with quantifiable commitments made by the winning party (budgets = y dollars/euros/bitcoins). Such a smart contract may be triggered to transfer funds automatically, on specific dates, to adjudicate public services or finance any mensurable electoral proposal (y = f (x)). Such sequences of aggregated automatisms are possible because each vote is a single token's transaction.

It is thought that a substantial reduction in transaction costs (*e.g.*, agency costs) is achievable probable in the next few years due to falling costs of trust mediation, which should have a profound political-economic impact. The auto-enforceable code under a blockchain and smart contracts can substitute the middlemen and lower bureaucracy (Shermin, 2017), diminishing transaction costs and allowing a more efficient economic organization and better governance (Davidson et al., 2016).

The political way to generate trust is very compelling. It is the key to the state's power, the "Leviathan" of Thomas Hobbes (Gibbons, 2001), giving rise to the ability to collect taxes and other dividends. However, BT introduced a new kind of trust, built and distributed in a decentralized way (powerful even among strangers), coming from everywhere through the Internet instead of centrally issued as before, which one can think makes sense:

Everything is in the edge: not only the humans that use the services, but also the activities that put them in contact in the first place. Control must be at the edge, because both the information needed to take decisions and the effects that the decisions may have are located there (Lopez et al. 2019, p. 1909).

The migration from centralized to decentralized organizations characterizes the evolution of complex systems (Kauffman, 1993). It occurs in several domains, such as the spontaneous institution of the order in free markets (Hayek, 1976), in computer systems (open-source and peer-to-peer networks), communication systems (digital social media), and political systems (democracy). All these systems show an evolution towards decentralization, which is also natural in politics because, over time, centralization is vulnerable to exploitation in the form of inflation, corruption, and rent-seeking. The authors agree with Kim & Lee (2011), who stated that "the centralization of government is the fundamental source of corruption" (p. 523). On the contrary, the costs of decentralization fall over time, often due to technological progress and computers, as in blockchain (Davidson et al., 2016).

The lesson is that when you compare centralized and decentralized systems you need to consider them dynamically, as processes, instead of statically, as rigid products. Centralized systems often start out fully baked, but only get better at the rate at which employees at the sponsoring company improve them. Decentralized systems start out half-baked but, under the right conditions, grow exponentially as they attract new contributors. (Dixon, 2018)

However, even though decentralized systems are more competitive due to their low transaction costs, governments (*i.e.*, politicians and bureaucrats) have themselves rents to protect, which is easier to do with a monopoly over governance. It is thought that in the *post-Covid-19 new normal* (Berwick, 2020), such monopolies, unfortunately, can be more than a politicians' megalomaniac dream. Hence, threats for *blockchain governance* acceptance can be expected to rise in proportion to the politicians' rents at risk (Lessig 2015, Hendrickson et al. 2015).

Entrepreneur-driven technological competition is often met with political response (…) So we should expect that while centralized ledgers may not always be able to compete on cost, they can still compete through co-option of force, through enacting legislation or regulation to artificially drive up the cost of decentralized technologies—including by rendering them illegal (Davidson et al., 2016, p. 4).

Therefore, even in democratic regimes, the path of decentralization is not open, which puts democracy and freedom at risk, given the digitally enhanced political power of centralized data. As stated by Kranzberg (1986), "technology is neither good nor bad, nor is it neutral." (p. 545), and it is thought that BT will in no way be neutral or innocuous to society. Thus, it is convenient to look at the concept of decentralization and understand BT's political implications to make sufficiently informed choices in the light of a challenging global technological framework.

According to Khare (2003), *centralized* means "drawn toward a center or brought under the control of a central authority" (p. 20), and *decentralized* means "withdrawn from a center or place of concentration; especially having power or function dispersed from a central to local authorities" (p.27). In this last case, the control is not vertically exerted directly anymore but instead emerges organically through the collaboration and aggregation of peers.

[In a] decentralized database multiple databases are distributed over a network (…) with no central authority managing the database. (…) [BT] is a system of recording information in a way that makes it difficult or impossible to change (…) hundreds and thousands of computers working together so they can verify data by reaching a "consensus". The consensus illustrates that the uploaded data is valid. (Rajapashe, 2020, p. 50)

Baran (1964) differentiated networks based on the number of nodes that needed to fail to break down communications, ranging from a single node in centralized networks to a few in decentralized networks and a majority in distributed networks. (Vergne, 2020, p. 5)

In a distributed network, data is replicated across multiple storage devices (nodes) with equal rights (see Figure 2). Resources like data storage or processing power are spread among peers and network nodes to accomplish a particular job or task, for instance, increasing processing power or creating a global ledger (*hyperledger*). In turn, a decentralized system can also be geographically distributed, but it will always rely upon the control of the node operators (*e.g.*, Bitcoin). Therefore, building a decentralized system is all about distributing trust locations across all participants of the system.

Decentralized systems provide the benefit of being distributed and authority agnostic [(censorship resistant)]. On the contrary, a distributed system might span geographical boundaries but [still be] owned and controlled by a single entity (with the advent of cloud computing this is a very common scenario). Trust in such a system is still centralized (District0x, 2020)

Figure 2. Baran's typology of communication networks
(Adapted from [Baran, 1964])

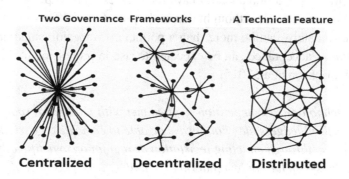

Two Governance Frameworks   A Technical Feature

Centralized   Decentralized   Distributed

Cloud storage services like Dropbox, Box or Google Drive are definitely centralized: these companies control how the information flows on their respective client-server architecture. However, their networks most probably have a distributed component in order to provide a sufficiently fast and secure service around the world. (SMA, 2018)

Components of a decentralized system operate on local information to accomplish goals rather than under the influence of a central ordering (see Figure 1). In turn, when it refers to distribution is all about communication and messaging. A distributed system computation is shared across components that communicate and coordinate their actions by sending messages. In other words, the components interact to achieve a common goal.

Therefore, these are two very different concepts. While distributed network designs configure a technical feature, a (de)centralized network sets a *governance framework* (see Figure 2).

Having observed valuable introductory concepts about blockchain and decentralization is time to move on to BT's political-economic implications, starting by distinguishing two very different types of digital currencies to envision their profound impact on society.

POLITICAL-ECONOMIC IMPLICATIONS OF BLOCKCHAIN TECHNOLOGY

Cryptocurrencies Impact: The Good, the Bad, and the Ugly

For better or worse, digital currencies are here to stay for political and economic reasons. Programmability is a decisive competitive advantage, bringing with it the possibility of stipulating the features of each currency on a case-by-case basis. Such a profound change should lead society to think twice about what is really at stake. However, unfortunately, blockchain's theme is not readily acknowledged by ordinary people, especially when the pandemic crisis is a severe problem enough to fill people's minds and keep them concerned.

Considering both economic media, digital money, and social media (Beller, 2020), the authors think that the most significant matter that people have to deal with is protecting privacy. The privacy lost on social media should not also happen on the primary economic media because consequences to society will probably worsen. A story of The Economist (2017) was titled "The world's most valuable resource is no longer oil, but data," and as argued by Lopez (2020), "if data is like oil, then the owner is the first one who drills [...] This is what is precisely happening now on the Internet, where data brokers and tech companies benefit from personal data drilled from users. "(p. 3).

The reality is that there is a wide range of technologies (hardware, software, biological) that can help companies or governments to drill our data without our permission. Accessing, trading, or making money using our personal data without our consent is unethical, and basically a theft of our privacy rights. Governments should protect individuals of abuses to their privacy by third parties. But either they are weak in front of big multinational companies or authoritarian states themselves are interested in this information (Lopez, 2020, p.3)

Such a loss of privacy is not a good thing, but a latent move against citizens can be even worse: after drilling the oil of peoples' social data, corporatocracy and authoritarian states can mine the gold of peoples' money data, supremely crowning their financial and political power. Unfortunately, funding such a mission will not be hard with centralized digital currencies in those hands.

Perhaps the most extraordinary impact of digital money, which is programmable and thus entirely different from current electronic money, will result from its pioneering capacity to diversify human incentives systems (see the same book, Chapter 3 - *Blockchanging Money: Reengineering the Free World Incentive System*). Obviously, such programming should be done ethically and wisely. If this will not be the case, digital money's features can be gloomy. Hence, programmable money can be *good*, *bad*, or *ugly*, according to the elected (hopefully not dictated) policies. Great opportunities come with significant risks, which is the case with blockchain technology (BT), especially when combined with artificial intelligence (AI) and Big Data. Blockchains and trusted data will reinforce the ability of computers to learn, rationalize, and take actions to achieve specific goals (Rath, 2019). However, it is up to politicians to set the right goals.

As stated by Fenwick & Vermeulen (2019), "one reason to believe that the economic, cultural and social impact of *new* digital technologies will be much greater than we have experienced before is that new technologies increasingly *amplify* each other" (p. 13). Numerical data is programmable and infinitely variable. As such, digital media is always "subject to algorithmic manipulation" (Dush, 2015; Manovich, 2002, 2013: O'Neill, 2017). Thus, *algorithmic manipulation* can now affect not just one but two economic media. Social media manipulation has been happening with notorius ethical repercussions: monetizing techniques adopted by ubiquitous digital platforms (*e.g.*, Facebook) which "puts the expressive (attentional, cognitive, affective) power of people to work [while] platform owners reap the spoils and externalize the costs [(*e.g.*, the Washington riots)]." (Beller, 2020, p. 216):

The values we project and create in media factories are abstracted by means of new sets of metrics (of which 'like' is only the most primitive), and, in the processes of monetisation are converted and collapsed into the value-form priced by the code of money. They are, in short, liquidated and placed on the market. After being sold to attention brokers, this value, realised as money, flows upwards to platform owners. (Beller, 2020, p. 216)

In a *post-Covid-19* world, programmable money will probably defeat traditional money due to allowing an inexorable reduction of *transaction costs* (Coase, 1937). It is thought that in a financial scenario of digital money ubiquitously, defending democracy requires "decoding the protocols of money already operating today in semiotic media to make it possible for users to redesign them more in accord with their interests." (Beller, 2020, p. 216).

Money's good old days probably will be gone. Perhaps soon one will say that traditional money was bad enough coming from "a speculative financial system with a life of its own" (Mertes, 2002), or something even worse will be spoken if the inflation reach levels such where "it can quickly become an ugly beast" (Darlington III, 2014, p. 7). State-sponsored digital currencies are coming, and private cryptocurrencies are entering the financial mainstream. The authors agree with Dumas et al. (2021), who stated that cryptocurrencies "[not being backed by any government], could serve well, especially during moments of turmoil, when countries with vulnerable economy might consider crypto assets an interesting tool, less exposed to monetary risks (*e.g.*, hyperinflation, an issue affecting the national currencies)" (p. 16). One way or the other, digital currencies are coming. As referred to by Naudet (2021), "in this conception, [of cryptocurrency,] we could realistically consider the emergence of a resolutely reliable and egalitarian international monetary system, at the origin of a consecration of social peace by the energetic mutation of the currency." (p. 7).

It should be noticed that the first strategic choice when evaluating a future digital currency should consider two opposite political scenarios:

1. Centralization - resulting from a prohibition or severe constraint (*e.g.*, fiscal) of all cryptocurrencies except those based on *private blockchains* (*state-sponsored, fully private*, or *consortia* blockchains);
2. Decentralization – resulting from free use of private cryptographic keys by any law-abiding citizen to operate cryptocurrencies on *public blockchains* (*public-permissionless,* or in a somehow minor degree *public-permissioned* blockchains).

According to several authors (Antonopoulos, 2016, 2017; Tapscott, 2016, 2017; Young, 2018; Lopez et al., 2019), programmable money should not be "captured by the state," staying available to be freely used and traded on open networks, where each citizen can use *private keys* to move it around without constraints in and out their communities. Hence, it is thought that *private and state-sponsored digital currencies must freely compete in decentralized markets.*

Also, regarding the desirable nature of digital money, one should notice Congressman Tom Emmer' words in the US Congress, outlining his vision of a *digital dollar* open to all:

It is American values like freedom, privacy, openness and permissionless entrepreneurship that have led [the USA] to dominate global commerce and innovation. We should have the courage of our convictions to build these values into a digital dollar and not to emulate systems like China's new digital yuan, which is closed, centralized, surveilled and permissioned so that access can be denied and payments blocked by those in power. (…) The same rules that apply to physical cash should apply to the digital dollar. While this may not go far enough for some, the only way to go farther would be to create a permissioned closed and surveilled system like China. (…) Technologies like this can empower individuals and make their governments more accountable directly to them. We can't cede this power to the government at the expense of the individual. (Ledger Insights, 2020)

This speech made clear that the USA (and implicitly also the rest of the free world) must follow an open model to create *good* digital currencies to stimulate innovation and entrepreneurship. Choosing a closed model would originate a *bad* centralized digital dollar that can be engineered to feed certain powers and eventually become *ugly* enough to obliterate the US founding fathers' checks and balances system in *the land of the free* (Blaustein, 1987). The authors could not agree more with this Congressman's words.

It is judged that centralized opaque versions of state-sponsored digital currencies can induce citizens' submission to non-auditable political power, allowing governments to monitor consumption, raising the bar of state surveillance and citizens' control. Therefore, digital currencies are a challenging type of money that can increase the government's control over citizens who are also consumers. It is thought that voters understand the long-lasting need to withdraw the money from politics, but, unfortunately, it is doubtful that the urgent need to separate politics from digital money can be timely and sufficiently understood given the population's lack of knowledge about BT. Moreover, people's attention is being disputed by sanitarian and economic concerns. Thus, this chapter aims to contribute to filling that gap.

The pioneering example of such global threat to privacy and freedom is the so-called *Digital Yuan*, China's central bank digital currency - the Digital Currency / Electronic Payment (DCEP) which marked "the first launch by a major economy of a sovereign digital currency [technically enabling] the merger of the monetary and payment systems." (Didenko et al., 2020).

Digital Yuan's network access is controlled, and all transactions are subject to central validation. The use of this digital currency requires the consent of the network's master keys holder because such keys are hidden in an opaque computer code. In other words, the computer system administrator (in this case, an authoritarian political regime) can discretionarily prevent payments made by any individual, thus being able to condition each user's consumption behavior, perhaps not only in China when Digital Yuan becomes global. As stated by Slawotsky (2020), "a blockchain powered digital Yuan — the currency of the world's second biggest economy (already digitalized to a far greater extent than the United States) might serve as an intriguing pathway towards a Chinese alternative to the USD. "(p. 39). According to Hoxtell & Nonhoff (2019), "authoritarian states are not only restricting the flow of information within their own countries and using the Internet as a tool to repress their citizens, but they are also exporting this model of Internet governance to other countries" (p .13).

The Internet is now "a global ledger" (Tapscott & Euchner, 2019), which empowers those who have the right keys to use it freely. It should be emphasized that the owner of the master keys of a centralized digital network also controls the respective data flows, being able to validate or change all network's transactions. Thus, privacy and private property depend on each individual ability to protect his data by using secure cryptographic keys. Only the possession of those digital secret keys will guarantee citizens' rights to privacy, private property, and even free will. Thus, in the authors' perspective, all law-abiding citizens should have the right to use private cryptographic keys. Moreover, it is thought that this is the most crucial safe conduct of every democratic system in the *blockchain era*.

As the story goes, when people are afraid and feel insecure, as in the face of the pandemic crisis of COVID-19, they are predisposed to compromise in matters of freedom to achieve the desired security. This *syndrome*, of an anxious nature, can lead people to accept restrictive measures that would otherwise be unlikely to see the light of day. Moreover, these measures are not just a reality in undemocratic countries with authoritarian regimes.

In China, the outbreak has strengthened and advanced a pre-existing authoritarian project that relied on emerging technologies and data to implement Xi Jinping's "prevention and control" doctrine with respect to Chinese society. But similar tools have been employed by democracies, including several that have become international models for their successful handling of the public health crisis introduced by the coronavirus (Greitens, 2020, p. 18).

As stated by Degeling et al. (2020), "many individuals are likely to accept limits on personal autonomy in pursuit of population health benefits at times when members of the public are being told to prepare for a major health emergency" (p. 7), and there are concerns about privacy risks due to pandemics, including mass surveillance in a *post-Covid-19* world (Wang, 2021). Information means power, and having too much data about citizens' lives can be tempting for some governments. Much personal information is being collected (*e.g.,* in apps and social networks), aimed at favoring governments and companies. Henceforth, due to digital currencies' properties, regimes may go even further, compromising people's privacy and ruining democracy.

Digital Yuan is quite different from *Bitcoin*. The latter is based on an open-sourced public blockchain, and no single entity can shut it down or even change its network protocols. Every user has its private secret keys, and changing blockchain's governance protocol requires most of its members' consensus (Nakamoto, 2008). On the contrary, the former is a digital currency native from a state-sponsored *permissioned blockchain* with its access requisites stipulated at a central level by the political regime (Buckley et al., 2021). The same happens with the Chinese social network WeChat, a platform whose use has become an authentic lifestyle for the Chinese citizens. Indeed, the Chinese government has emphasized WeChat, which began as a messaging app like WhatsApp, but was later described as a *super-app* (Chen et al. 2018).

WeChat users can send free messages with text, image, video, and/or audio to individual contacts and groups of contacts. However, WeChat functionality vastly exceeds interpersonal communication because it integrates internal apps that enable users to conduct a wide array of activities—make mobile payments, hail taxis, order food, book hotels, give to charity, play games—from within the WeChat app environment. This integration of utilities creates new gratifications that may increase the "stickiness" of WeChat and increase time spent on WeChat. (Lu & Pan, 2020, p.12)

Despite the usual secrecy that prevails in China, there are reports that BT has been tested on WeChat social networks (Iwamoto, 2021). As mentioned above, this technology allows registering and executing peer-to-peer (P2P) transactions with units representing value (tokens), and the WeChat network accounts for *social value* and *financial value*. Furthermore, it is possible to convert everyday personal experiences into computable transaction rules by indexing those values. The criteria followed to balance individual accounts, increasing or decreasing the social capital displayed by each individual in the WeChat network, will be established by the Chinese regime. Later on, Digital Yuan may function as *ration coupons*, aligning (or suppressing) individual rights to make payments according to each one's *social credit*.

Bitcoin and Digital Yuan clearly define the boundaries of digital currencies' political and economic role. Unlike traditional money, digital currencies work not only as exchange units but also as utility units, storing a political-economic value that stems from their specific features. Bitcoin was openly programmed to be an autonomous reserve of value due to its limited supply (Nakamoto, 2008), while Digital Yuan programming is not known nor auditable. Hopefully, other cryptocurrencies, instead of being economically used as *digital gold* (Bitcoin) or serve as a political instrument (Digital Yuan), will be used as "qualified money" (Helbing, 2014) to diversify financial incentives. The new multidimensionality of money is globally possible by dealing in hyper ledgers with units of value that cryptographically merge *labor* and *capital*. For the first time in history, these two productive factors can be integrated into the same unit of value, allowing to deal with value in a richer way (see Chapter 3).

"We are inventing a type of trust that can grease the wheels of business and facilitate person-to-person relationships [and DAOs] in the age of distributed networks and collaborative marketplaces." (Ebner, 2017, p. 132).

Given that there are different ways of building a blockchain-based society, we must avoid to fall into the trap of a totalitarian post-privacy world, in which people might be restricted—and unnecessarily restrained in unfolding their knowledge, ideas, and talents. If we want to see a world with a level playing field for everyone, we need to insist on responsible blockchain innovations and on using distributed ledger mechanisms for the greater good, rather than allowing them to be usurped and harnessed by a very limited group of people for private interests. (van den Hoven et al., 2019, p. 166)

If freedom prevails, which needs to be proactively guaranteed in the face of a *new normal* (Berwick, 2020) triggered by the confluence of the pandemic crisis and the *blockchain paradigm*, programmable money will not be centralized and used as a corset to control citizens. On the contrary, it will be used to promote collective action, which is very different from collectivism. One should not ignore the harsh reality of central state planning experienced in the 20th century behind eastern Europe's "iron curtain" (Applebaum, 2012) and be aware of BT's disruptive *dark side* of centralization. It is believed that it is crucial to enlighten citizens about the upsurge risks of totalitarianism, from the left and the right, given that technologies such as AI or BT can change the world quickly. Suppose there is room to preserve democracy and freedom. In that case, digital currencies may serve *to expand the pie before dividing it*, taking advantage of the new multidimensionality of money to induce a *collective action* based on individual merit and creativity, innovation, and ethical entrepreneurship focused on a sustainable human development.

Blockchanging Governance

Governance can be defined as the process whereby power is exercised, decisions are made, citizens or stakeholders are given a voice, and account is rendered on important issues (Plumptre, 2006). Blockchain Technology (BT) can be used to perform such processes. Although BT started with the purpose of ensuring bitcoin transactions (blockchain 1.0), it now is used to act proactively in rendering many other accounts, securing and verifying diverse assets and contracts (blockchain 2.0 and 3.0) (Xu et al., 2019).

The notion of *power* is linked to the notion of *hierarchy*, but decentralized networks are changing this notion. The Internet is the Information Age's decisive technology (Castells, 2014), and BT has empowered the Internet even more. As in any hierarchical system, the governance of a network is a prerogative of those who rule. However, the same does not happen in a completely decentralized system, as is the case of *public-permissionless blockchains*, which rely only on open code and public scrutiny. Hence, BT creates a new *distributed trust* whose impact on citizens' behavior will be framed only by the cryptographic rules chosen and political rules allowing or forbidden accessing different blockchains.

Open-source code guarantees transparency and auditing, which is essential to build citizens' trust and grant free access to blockchain networks. On the contrary, closed source-code and centralized protocols can restrain access on an individual basis, obviously limiting citizen's choices. These are two substantially different processes of letting transactions be carried out on blockchains. While the latter requires trust in specific persons or organizations, *i.e.*, trust on *private blockchains* (either privately, governmental, or consortium owned), the former is censorship-resistant, depending only on trusting a large community-based consensus (*public-permissionless* blockchains) or, alternatively, a consensus emerging of a smaller group of *delegated witnesses* trusted by such communities (*public-permissioned* blockchains).

All these protocols to reach a consensus about what should be trusted entails unavoidable trade-offs. According to Qin & Gervais (2018), the *scaling trilemma* dictates that blockchains can have at most two of the following three properties: *decentralization, scalability,* and *security.* This scaling trilemma is the reason why *hybrid blockchains* try to combine the best of three worlds, aiming for *security* pursuing the right trade-offs between the *scalability* advantage of *private-permissioned* blockchains and the *decentralization* feature of *public-permissionless* blockchains, which does not arise without a considerable burden:

In a permissionless blockchain, all the transactions and blocks are broadcast, verified and recorded among all participants in a decentralized peer-to-peer network. This process ensures that the whole system is immutable, stable and resistant as long as more than half of the computing resources remain honest. Honest majority is required for an appropriate security property, which however is very costly on the scalability side as all participants need to be informed and to implicitly agree [to reach the consensus]. (Qin & Gervais, 2018, pp. 3, 4)

Hopefully, BT will evolve and adapt to overcoming technical limitations and complying with regulations that will be flexible enough to satisfy the transaction needs of the so-called free world. However, powerful interests can mislead BT's public perception disproportionally connoting Bitcoin with negative factors, such as excessive energy consumption and criminality (see the LIMITATIONS AND FUTURE RESEARCH section). Thus, the lousy reputation can harm the credibility of all BT's applications, eventually diverting blockchain's evolution to protect the status quo. In other words, it can happen the same that happens every time a technological innovation reveals itself as a threat to someone's business (Antonopoulos, 2017). Nevertheless, it is considered that a decentralized approach might provide the most reliable alternative to deal with political and financial affairs, especially at times of institutional distrust. As stated by Atzori (2015), "while the State bases its action on coercion, the blockchain can provide governance services in a more efficient and decentralized way, without having to rely on force. This approach allows a more horizontal and distributed diffusion of authority, in which the source of legitimacy are the individuals themselves." (p. 7)

The collective relationship between individuals and the State can be fully or partially automated by "a series of instant atomic interactions [...] Instead of a hierarchical structure managed by a set of humans interacting in person...via the legal system, a decentralized organization involves a set of humans interacting with each other according to a protocol specified in code, and enforced on the blockchain. (Buterin, 2014)

As it goes in Estonia for almost a decade, governments can benefit from BT by instituting digital transparency and secure open access to information, a fact that should be especially appreciated in an area so sensitive to voters' eyes as healthcare.

Estonia is at the forefront, securing more than one million citizens' records in a [blockchain].

The system has proven that interoperability is an achievable goal and demonstrated that the ability to analyze data has helped the government become aware of and more easily track health epidemics. (Vazirani et al. 2020, p. 3)

This Baltic republic is an excellent example of how transparency and openness can benefit a country and improve citizens' lives (Adeodato & Pournouri, 2020). One should remark that such *openness* may not always be followed in the physical world (*e.g.*, for security reasons), but in the digital world, it can make sense, as in the case of the successful Estonian e-residency program (e-resident.gov.ee) (Blue, 2020).

BT allows storing proofs of data's authenticity for reference instead of the data itself (Nakamoto, 2008), guaranteeing privacy and convenience. This feature presents the best of two worlds and can be called a "win-win situation" (Fisher et al., 2011), benefiting all players of the blockchain-based identity management ecosystem (Kuperberg, 2019). For instance, opting for decentralized identity management solutions will increase people´s access to online services, contributing to protecting citizens' privacy and solving many unbanked and identityless people's problems (Keweel et al., 2017). More than two billion people with no bank account but with a mobile phone (Ardo & Zamani, 2019) can benefit from low-cost BT solutions to prove their identities and immediately start accessing financial services to make micro-transfers or small remittances of currency (cryptocurrency).

On the other hand, new decentralized media apps (*dapps*) will provide censorship-resistant access to the entire spectrum of information and opinions expressed by social media users. This kind of information can release citizens from the biased content available in today´s social networks, which is managed by machine learning algorithms that feed predatory business models (O'Neill, 2017). The same goes for the biggest state-controlled social network (WeChat) which contents are also being managed by machine learning algorithms, this time to feed an authoritarian regime (Lu & Pan, 2020).

In the *blockchain era*, to expose democracy worldwide to *virulent* ideologies, it is enough to prohibit people from achieving the *group immunity* conferred by private cryptographic keys (*the masks*) and open-sourced code programming (*the vaccines*). Without digital decentralization and transparency, privacy and freedom will not be *immunized against* malignant software *backdoors* (see Key Terms and Definitions) eventually hosted in non-auditable close-sourced programming codes of *private blockchains*. Moreover, both economic media (digital money and social media) will be ideal propagation vectors for *enforcing ideological memes* and *tailoring money rules* cleverly dictated by statistical bias algorithms "that are telling lies" (O'Neill, 2017. p.7).

A Trustworthy Digital Democracy

Electronic Voting

Democracy needs reliable data and citizens' privacy to function effectively. Thus, transparency is a fundamental element of democracy. For instance, without the secret vote, there can be no freedom of choice or independent decisions. If constructive criticism can be stopped by the fear of reprisals and witnesses' anonymity is not guaranteed, fight corruption and organized crime cannot be properly enduring, compromising the rule of law (Helbing, 2014). On the other hand, transparency promotes accountability, which may induce ethical and responsible behavior. Thus, there is an urgent need to find an ethically recommended balance between privacy and transparency (see the same book, Chapter 1 - *Blockchanging Trust: Ethical Metamorphosis in Business & Healthcare*).

A *digital democracy* requires electronic voting (e-voting), and it is thought that e-voting systems must be decentralized. By considering a vote as a transaction, citizens can vote on the blockchain (Barnes et al., 2016). The same process can be used for rapid voting on relevant issues and not just voting for officials (Young, 2018). According to Atzori (2015), "democracy can become more effective through the direct participation of citizens in the decision-making process [and] blockchain technology can implement new models of participation" (p. 9).

Once technical issues have been solved (Specter et al., 2020; Waldron, 2019), whose description would go beyond the scope of this book, Blockchain Technology (BT) eventually will allow coding the electoral decision process directly in *smart contracts*, using open, transparent, and auditable code-source to make the electoral system verifiable and incorruptible. For this reason, it is considered that the electoral process will eventually be reformed by using BT. After all, the same mathematical precision that made Bitcoin's hyperledger secure, tamper-proofing its accounts for more than ten years now, also can be used to certify and audit electronic voting systems. As stated by Wright & De Filippi (2015), "[BT offers] a distributed, irreversible and encrypted public paper trail that can be easily audited."

The technology already exists to have a voting system on the blockchain. "With the cost of voting drastically reduced, politicians hampered by scandal, corruption, or incompetence could easily be removed from their offices, making governance more efficient and decreasing the impact of politicians who have lost the confidence of their constituency. (Young, 2018, p. 9)

E-voting is among the key public sectors that can be disrupted by blockchain technology. The idea in blockchain-enabled e-voting (BEV) is simple. To use a digital-currency analogy, BEV issues each voter a "wallet" containing a user credential. Each voter gets a single "coin" representing one opportunity to vote. Casting a vote transfers the voter's coin to a candidate's wallet. A voter can spend his or her coin only once. However, voters can change their vote before a preset deadline. (Kshetri, 2018, p. 95)

Robust voting systems, either traditional or digital, should satisfy obligatory requirements. Barański et al. (2020) reviewed several of such conditions mentioned in the literature (Qadah, 2005; Schneier, 2007; Ayed, 2017; Hjálmarsson et al., 2018; Sadia et al., 2019; Vo-Cao-Thuy et al., 2019) and proposed the following seven mandatory conditions for having a secure and effective e-voting system:

- *Immutability*: No one can change the vote after it was made.
- *Verifiability*: Everyone should be able to verify if his or her vote has been counted correctly.
- *Scalability*: The system should be able to handle large-scale elections, both in terms of votes per second and voting costs.
- *Authorization*: Only authorized voters can vote, and no one can vote more than once.
- *Privacy*: Relation between voter and his vote must be kept in secret. Each voter must be sure about his vote privacy.
- *Coercion resistance*: It should be illegal to sell or exchange votes.
- *Fairness*: No partial results are available until the end of the election.

An extended review of the literature showed that another condition must be added (Takabatake et al., 2016, p. 127):

- *Completeness*: The administrator always accepts an eligible voter, and all valid votes are counted correctly.

Heiberg et al. (2020) consider that "the search for a better balance is on-going" (p. 95), identifying several threat actors that can compromise an *Internet Voting System*: (i) Civil hacktivist seeking publicity; (ii) Single candidate trying to get more votes; (iii) Political party trying to increase the number of seats; (iv) Organization aiming at influencing policy decisions, and (v) Foreign state-level actor trying to gain more control over the country.

Thus, considering so many restrictive conditions of effectiveness, and the possible attack angles, assembling a secure and effective e-voting system seems to be a complex issue. As stated by Çabuk et al. (2020), "security term includes integrity, verifiability, and non-repudiation of votes; authentication and singularity of voter accounts; immutability and trackability of all the records." (p. 132). However, despite these and other requirements, this author adds that "using blockchain mechanisms that support smart contracts (or similar), such as Ethereum, can be a good fit since it would natively support distributed applications on the chain." (p. 132).

The blockchain technology offers a decentralized storage and computation mechanism for e-voting systems, where the voting records are transparent to all the voters and independent observers. (…) It offers a system, in which everyone can trust. This trust is not just about the perception, but rather the mathematical, analytical, and logical means of security, provided by the blockchain technology. (Çabuk et al. 2020, p. 132)

However, "privacy and confidentiality of votes is rather an implementation-dependent, and it is possible to find the relation between a voter and his / her vote, by digging into the chain" (Çabuk et al. 2020, p. 132), being that BT still presents vulnerabilities. These are not good news when a solution with total robustness in all parameters is desired. Therefore, the various electronic voting systems using BT (Benítez-Martínez et al., 2021; Dhinakaran, et al., 2021: Yang et al., 2020) should be viewed with moderate optimism. Some of these systems propose to increase the granularity of public scrutiny even in times of pandemic (Wattegama, et al., 2021), including using remote validation of votes with biometric parameters (Priyadharshini et al., 2021).

Given the complexity and the degree of demand for entirely satisfactory electronic voting solutions, it will be practically mandatory to give up something to obtain the desired convenience. Thus, trade-offs will become necessary. As stated by Çabuk et al. (2020), "any voting protocol suite is a complex set of mechanisms balancing between conflicting requirements. Improving one component may decrease the overall security level of the whole system. Thus (...) a holistic study of the whole suite needs to be conducted. (p. 132). The same rationale is patent in the following quotation of the political philanthropist Bradley Tusk, a Voatz backer speaking to the Harvard Business Review:

It's not that the cybersecurity people are bad people per se. I think it's that they are solving for one situation, and I am solving for another. They want zero technology risk in any way, shape, or form [...] But in my view, then you can't resolve the issues on guns, on climate, on immigration, because the middle 70% doesn't participate in primaries [...] I am solving for the problem of turnout. (Specter et al, 2020, p. 14)

The authors' opinion on BT-based electronic voting systems coincides with that expressed by Waldron (2019), which states that "it is a useful tool, but it is not a solution that address all of the concerns (...) solution not bad but rather incomplete "(p. 4). Simply put, a blockchain is an authenticity tool, not a privacy tool (MX Technologies Inc., 2016). Even so, despite understanding the existing reservations, one should be pragmatic when factors such as the abstention rate and democratic representativeness of national elections are at stake. As such, giving up electronic voting is not a solution.

These are turbulent times, and the pace is one of accelerated change. The future will no longer be a reissue of the past, requiring the capacity for innovation under penalty of obtaining diminishing returns (Hamel, 2000) that can culminate in a resounding civilizational failure. Thus, future elections must include not only "the middle 70%" above mentioned by Tusk (Specter et al, 2020, p. 14), but also the younger voters, the *generation y*, or *millennials*, which *grown-up digital* unlike their parents (the *baby boomers*) and are a tech-savvy group of users instead of mere viewers (Tapscott, 1997; Almeida, 2017).

Weighing the respective pros and cons, the authors consider that electronic voting is highly recommended, and BT's systems are in the pole position to win the challenging race to find a bulletproof system. Meanwhile, Voatz, a BT-based system, was used with its results officially approved in the 2020 US Presidential Elections, although contested by some and including fights in courts (this was the first time people cast votes via smartphone in a Presidental Election). Nevertheless, BT-based electronic voting systems should be improved and eventually combined with other technologies (e.g., homomorphic cryptography) to deal with privacy issues. Still, it can be said that BT is an auspicious solution for using electronic voting systems over the Internet.

Algorithmic Governance

Any dream of making the world better must include political transparency and digital openness as fundamental requisites for protecting democracy and freedom in the *blockchain era*. Otherwise, powerful computing resources, eventually including state-sponsored digital currencies, will put at the mercy of powerful interests, not only personal data, as happening so far in social media, but also citizen's consumption prerogatives. One can think this is wrong, as the government must be scrutinized and conditioned by the citizens, not the other way around. The menace of such an unethical future state-of-affairs is one of the main reasons digital decentralization is considered crucial to keeping the free world on a democratic path.

If people do not preserve the dignity of their data and do not defend privacy, every citizen will be subject to the power of digital centralization. The states and other third parties will take control of even the slightest detail of everyone's life. This level of control is not only possible but highly probable, as partially shown on the *pre-blockchain* version of the Internet (see Chapter 1).

The research about *algorithmic governance* has been mentioned the risks of *datafication* (see Key Terms and Definitions) and mass surveillance. Monitoring entire populations and citizens' profiling create ample opportunities for social sorting, discrimination, state oppression, and manipulating consumers and citizens (Gandy, 2010; Lyon, 2014). However, in the cryptographic *blockchain era*, the digital tools go both ways, also letting citizens protect themselves. Hence, *algorithmic governance* highlights that digital technologies can produce social ordering in a specific way (Katzenbach & Ulbricht, 2019). In the new *Internet of Value*, debauching privacy can easily include consumer behavior monitoring and restraint because the prerogatives of digital currencies can be automated according to each payer political profile. Nevertheless, the authors hope that in the so-called free world things could happen transparently and democratically.

The inherent consensus-seeking, scalability, and decentralization make blockchain computing the next step in evolution for public governance. Controlling a government's institutions by connecting them to a blockchain system will create greater oversight of the government and will prevent government actors from acting beyond their mandate. (...) When attached to government property, blockchain computing allows for potentially unlimited checks and balances on a government. (Young 2018, pp. 33,34)

BT's auditability and irreversibility can give a decisive contribution to governments' accountability. As stated by Young (2018a), "the future regulatory structure that can be built with blockchain technology has been called "*Lex Cryptographia*" (...) This, like *lex mercatoria*, is executed outside the government control, and independent from the state" (p. 15). "Centralization refers to the degree to which authority and decision-making is concentrated at the top" (Matseshe et al., p. 383), and it is known that for many centuries and still today " "decision power is concentrated at the top of the hierarchy" (Alexandru, 2018, p. 9). However, in the new *Internet of Value* (Tapscott & Euchner, 2019), blockchain computing allows "the decision-making process of a decentralized organization [to be] encoded directly into source code [to] distribute authority throughout without the need for any trusted centralized party" (Wright & De Filippi, 2015).

Several government initiatives are underway (Clavin et al., 2020; Amend et al., 2021). Such pioneering efforts demonstrate that BT foreshadows a new level in governance and human development models. As referred in Atzori (2015), "decentralization through the blockchain technology represents a "natural progression of humanity"(Andreas Antonopoulos, 2014) and a "natural efficiency process "(Swan 2015, p. 31)" (p. 11).

Thanks to smart contracts, the integrity, and fairness of government commitments can directly migrate from the winning party's political proposals, and be precisely executed, with no scope for unattended electoral promises or tricky subjective interpretations. As referred by Young (2018), "In addition to being an ideal tool for scaling democracy, blockchains are also an ideal tool for ensuring a party does not act outside of its mandate because parties cannot act outside of the encoded powers granted to them" (p. 66). This same author proposed a *social smart contract* and two kinds of *blockchain governmental tokens*, which are presented in Table 2, to be used by individuals in their relationship both with the government and is fellow citizens:

Table 2. "Blockchain governmental tokens"

GovernmentCoins (Credits Given to the Government)	CitizenCoins (Credits Given to the Citizens)
It provides power within or over the government	It provides access to the government institutions
When a government's blockchain is established, each citizen would vote and do all the things its government ID empowers him to do. The citizens would exercise oversight into the Government's blockchain, see every transaction, and verify that the source-code has not changed.	When a citizens' blockchain is established, citizens would receive a unique cryptographic token as an ID that would identify them to take advantage of government-distributed benefits, enabling each citizen to work (vote) within the government system, and also with other citizens.

Source: Adapted from Young (2018), and Barnes et al. (2016).

As stated by Young (2018), "the code of the Smart Social Contract will determine what abilities the holder of each GovernmentCoin has." (p. 28).

When voters elect someone to a leadership or a bureaucratic role, that person's GovernmentCoin will receive greater privileges, and then have access to the government infrastructure (computers, vehicles, intelligence, military) assigned to the function to which they were elected. This way something for which the individual is responsible [or voted for] can be tracked to the exact individual. Additionally, an individual could be prevented from acting ultra vires, [(see Key Terms and Definitions)] because the government's checks and balances are built into the system. (Young, 2018)

The proposed new type of blockchain-based governance may determine mayors and government officials' direct election. As each vote is a transaction, citizens can command algorithms on the blockchain, treating the political affairs like business deals, which can be called "algorithm governance" (Dwyer, 2017).

Through smart contracts, it is possible to stipulate the scope of political scrutiny, determining the transactions of GovernmentCoins and their practical consequences. In turn, CitizenCoins can manage the entire relationship between the citizen and the state, guaranteeing access to public services and directly influencing everything open to voting. The CitizenCoins can even encourage collective action, which is very different from collectivism as seen below.

Liberal democracy is often associated with an ethical model where consensus results from reason and rational debate between peers (Habermas & Rehg, 1997). This deliberative model, which "claims that collective public deliberation is the definitive democratic experience" (Gabardi, 2001), was replaced by another one, advocated by the neo-liberal policy initiated in the middle of the last century (Schumpeter, 1942). According to neoliberals, consensus should not result from the debate between equals, morally based on a common good's notion, which is always debatable, but instead on the aggregation of individual preferences and interests. This aggregative model of democracy, assuming an economic subject motivated by self-interest, considers that political institutions' organization must result from a sum of individual preferences and interests (Cunningham, 2010).

If these two modes of governmentality, one imagining a mode of politics arising from free reasoning among equals and the other a politics of consensus founded on self-interest are in competition in liberal governmentality, algorithmic governmentality is the total succession of this aggregative model of democracy. It does away with claims towards a rational, discursive public sphere in favour of a bland social unanimity. It replaces politics with economics (Dwyer, 2017, p. 5)

It is thought that a new evidence-based policy is mandatory, where words cannot be broken, and deeds cannot be lacking. In a time of uncertainty and few reliable indicators, it is believed that authenticity, transparency, and mathematical certainty are necessary political assets.

Both liberal and algorithmic approaches make use of quantitative techniques. Numericity was and still is seen as a kind of disinterested politics, where techniques of calculation are understood to be less biased or politically motivated than the excesses of rhetoric or theoretical disputes. [...] Here, liberal knowledge provides a historic precedent for viewing numbers as self-evident, for the universal belief that the numbers don't lie. (Dwyer, 2019)

In the following section, the authors will present solutions and political recommendations to place BT's "truth machine" (Economist, 2015) at the service of liberal democracy.

SOLUTIONS AND RECOMMENDATIONS

Fulfilling electoral promises is one of the most ethical commandments of democracy. It is thought that Blockchain Technology (BT) can translate political party programs into immutable computer protocols, scrutinized, and validated on blockchain networks. Thus, BT can bring a new era of confidence in translating political promises into deeds.

In the *blockchain era*, data's legitimacy and transactions' authenticity can be verified in a decentralized way through consensuses, which may be automatically established among citizens instead of relying on third parties' validation mechanisms. BT's political implications will emphasize the need for a much more often voters' involvement in public policies and decisions that concern them, congregating the younger generations presently dismissed from the public cause. Thus, the authors think it will be convenient to adopt transparent proximity mechanisms to guarantee citizens' participation through open, collaborative platforms.

It is understood that the power to control citizens' lives must reside on the periphery of traditional centers of power, i.e., with the citizens themselves, because that is where is the information needed to make decisions and the effects that result from these same decisions (Lopez, 2019). Thus, it is believed that the decentralization of entities and services will promote social justice and transparency through equal opportunities while increasing government accountability and citizen's autonomy by using private keys in controlling their own personal and procedural data.

The blockchain protocol should also change the paradigm of trust in justice (Zaprutin et al., 2020), democratizing access and guaranteeing equality. It is not possible, for example, *losing* documents or lawsuits issued and registered through a *blockchain protocol*. This censorship resistance is because blockchain documents are replicated in a vast as-needed computer network, becoming immutable and practically incorruptible, unlike what happens with documents issued by centralized systems. Thus, the authors think that adopting the blockchain protocol will undoubtedly reform areas where the issue of corruption is more sensitive and harmful to society, as is the case with politics and justice (Aarvik, 2020).

A new digital reality triggered by BT and synergistically pushed by two other powerful technologies, Artificial Intelligence and Big Data, increases the effectiveness of information systems opening business possibilities that all can enjoy in a decentralized free market scenario.

The new-fangled Business world requires better treatment of enormous information and better use with more knowledge incorporated in all business processes. Fundamentally, block chain is apprehensive with keeping correct records, verification, and implementation while AI helps in conducting assessment, examining, and coming to conclusion of certain patterns and datasets, eventually engendering selfdirected interaction. [...] Artificial Intelligence and Block Chain needs sharing of data. The decentralized approach of database focuses the significance of data sharing among various clients on a meticulous network. In the same way, AI depends very much on Big Data, exclusively, for data distribution. Including more provisions of data analysis, the future trends prediction and assessments of machines are measured more correctly, and the algorithms developed are more consistent. (Rath, 2019, p. 1031)

It is judged that these new possibilities can be used by the third sector to reinforce its political, economic importance. Hence, civil society must be allowed to be responsible for its future, believing that the private sector's role will be key to innovate and create decentralized markets using DAOs (see Key Terms and Definitions), which may benefit from a substantial reduction of *transaction costs* and tax burden. The authors consider that it will be very difficult or even impossible to continue to raise taxes on wealth creation in the new digital paradigm and keep democracy on track. Given the new horizons opened by technological advances in information systems (Sadowski, 2020), it is thought that such a fiscal ambition makes no sense, and further insistence on taxation would bring the shadow of the totalitarian regimes where market laws are suppressed. Unfortunately, the non-democratic path of authoritarianism cannot be excluded, especially in the light of the crisis triggered by the SARS-CoV-2 virus (Cawthorn et al., 2020), and considering digital surveillance and citizens' control procedures that are being tested in the East (Qiang, 2019).

In the authors' opinion, well-known political options aimed at centralization and ideological uniformization, historically positioned against democracy and freedom, may postpone or even make lose the historical opportunity of using BT to benefit humankind. Hopefully, free world democracies will show enough resilience to adapt to the double edge sword of digital pragmatism. For the first time in human history, it is possible to distinguish collectivism from collective action (Tapscot, 2016). While collectivism implies state planning and coercive central control, collective action is based on the freedom of choice, with the *public-blockchain protocols* ensuring access to transacting freely and ensuring data's ownership (Nakamoto, 2008). Digital money can quantify public and individual benefits simultaneously since digital tokens and cryptocurrencies may have a *multidimensional value*, which is not the case with traditional money. Cryptocurrencies and other digital tokens should be programmed to integrate *labor* and *capital* into single units of account creatively (see Chapter 3). This *financial socio-economic chimera* is strategically recommended in the *blockchain era*. Hopefully, it will constitute a political choice to benefit both individuals and their community ecosystems, promoting unity between community members but respecting individual differences without falling into the old trap of collectivistic single-minded ideologies.

The *blockchain protocol* allows individuals to organize their transactions without traditional organizations, creating decentralized and secure digital infrastructures to produce wealth (see Chapters 4 and 5). It is highly recommended that everyone has free access to *public-blockchain* networks openly promoted by governments, businesses, and civil society. This openness is the generic solution proposed by the authors to democratize and disintermediate transactions, pursuing a transparent reform of the state in the *blockchain era*.

LIMITATIONS AND FUTURE RESEARCH DIRECTIONS

Bitcoin is the most visible face of Blockchain Technology (BT). As stated by Rath (2019), "Bitcoin popularized Blockchain Technology" (p. 1033). Two limitations pointed out to Bitcoin are (i) its volatility allegedly due to its lack of intrinsic value (as stated by Alan Greenspan, referring himself to Bitcoin, "It's a bubble. It has to have intrinsic value." (Ametrano, 2016, p. 11), and (ii) the high energy consumption required to carry out the Proof-of-Work (PoW) mechanism used to establish blockchain network consensus, which demands considerable computing effort. Regarding specifically the first of these two criticisms, the argument of Bitcoin's excessive volatility due to lacking intrinsic value, the authors recommend reading in the same book the homonymous section on Chapter 3, where it is presented a scientifically positive correlation between cryptocurrencies production costs and their respective prices. Considering the argument of Bitcoin's excessive energy consumption, although further research to increase BT's efficiency is recommended, it seems evident that, as observed by Hayes (2017), "a cryptocurrency with no acceptance or usage will have neither value nor computational power directed at it "(p. 1312). Thus, low price will mean low production costs, and it is judged as a paradox arguing about Bitcoin's unacceptance due to excessive volatility and lack of intrinsic value and, simultaneously, fearing that it provokes an excessive energy consumption.

The decision to mine for bitcoin comes down to its profitability given its relative cost of production (...) a rational agent would not undertake production of bitcoins if they incurred a real ongoing loss in doing so. Bitcoin mining employs computational effort which requires the consumption of electricity to function, which must be paid for. This computational effort is directed at mining bitcoin, in competition with many other miners who presumably are also motivated by profit, on average. (Hayes, 2017, p. 1315)

Production costs drive cryptocurrency acceptance, and energy costs will only be paramount if Bitcoin reveals itself successful (Hayes, 2017), but in this case energy consumption will be avoided at other significant levels, so this issue must be considered in a broader perspective. For example, according to Sedlmeir et al. (2020), "by enabling the digitization of supply-chain processes, blockchain can substantially reduce the amount of paperwork and transport, including air-freight (Jensen et al. 2019), or allow for more targeted recalls, leveraging many opportunities to reduce carbon emissions" (p. 607).

As stated by Sedlmeir et al. (2020) about the energetic waste argument, "this perception inevitably raises concerns about the further adoption of blockchain technology, a fact that inhibits rapid uptake of what is widely considered to be a ground-breaking and disruptive innovation." (p. 599). One can agree about the political impact of such criticism considering that sustainability is a central issue on many agendas. Nevertheless, it is judged that this critique should be rejected for several reasons. In the first place, "participation in the mining process is only profitable as long as the expected revenue from mining is higher than the associated costs [(*e.g.*, electricity)] (Sedlmeir, 2020, p. 601). In the second place, although being true that the redundant ledger's replication over the Bitcoin network nodes increases energy consumption, especially compared to other conventional solutions that are not redundant and less secure (involving centralized databases and single servers), it is also true that trust has a price, and it turns out that the increased security, provided by BT, also avoids energy consumption at other important levels, so the issue of energy consumption must be considered in a broader perspective. For instance, cryptocurrencies may contribute to managing communitarian ecosystems through collective action (Dapp, 2019), which potential ecological effects will probably surpass Bitcoin's energetic consumption globally, eventually resulting in a better entropy balance (Leonard & Treiblmaier, 2019), especially considering renewable energy:

As electric power systems around the world rely more heavily on intermittent renewable energy, distributed energy resources, and sophisticated digital technologies, the industry will need to cope with rising complexity. Blockchain technology has the potential to help manage that complexity. (...) blockchain can be used to underpin a vast, distributed network that records transactions swiftly, immutably, and transparently. Now, substantial investment is flowing toward ventures that apply blockchain technology to the electric power sector. (Livingstone et al., 2018, p. 19)

The authors think it is essential to overview the environmental impact of cryptocurrencies considering other factors relevant for sustainability, such as the gold mining industry. As argued by McCook (2018), some critics have labelled Bitcoin as an environmental disaster. However, it has been demonstrated that Bitcoin is dramatically less harmful to the environment than the gold mining industry (p. 28). The energy consumption of the banking system is even greater.

The Bitcoin network consumes an estimated ~113.89 TWh/yr in total. (…) The gold industry utilizes roughly 240.61 TWh/yr. (…) With the publicly available information that we could find, we estimate the banking system uses 263.72 TWh of energy each year. Deriving a comprehensive number for this sector's energy consumption would require individual banks to self-report. (…) To have an honest conversation about Bitcoin's energy use, a comparison to the most analogous incumbents—the gold industry and the banking system—is appropriate. (Rybarczyk et al., 2021, pp. 4-13)

Finally, there are alternatives to BT's consensus mechanisms besides Proof-of-Work (PoW).

Huge energy consumption is by no means necessary for the creation of a block from a technical perspective and alternative ways for finding consensus are currently being discussed in various communities (e.g., proof of stake, proof of burn, proof of elapsed time, Byzantine fault tolerance and variations thereof, Federated Byzantine agreement) (Leonard & Treiblmaier, 2019, p. 202)

Among these alternatives, the second most consensus mechanism is the so-called Proof-of-Stake (PoS), a planned future improvement of Ethereum which involves much less energy consumption than Bitcoin's PoW (Alfieri, 2019).

Furthermore, new cryptographic protocols are being discovered, some of them presenting already greater energy efficiency, solving scalability issues and maintaining or even increasing the level of decentralization, as seems to be is the case of Holochain, an open-source framework for developing microservices (and micropayments) that run *peer-to-peer* applications entirely on end-user devices without central servers (Holochain, 2020). As stated by Zaman et al. (2021), "in contrast to blockchain, holochain liberates the communicating agents from any form of centralized control by running the applications (hApps) entirely at the user side." (p. 14).

Another criticism made to BT is that cryptocurrencies serve, above all, to illegal purposes, facilitating criminal activities such as *money laundering*, tax evasion, terrorism, among others. As stated by Turner et al. (2020), "illicit bitcoin transactions could take the form of money laundering, terrorism financing or the movement of proceeds from other crimes such as ransomware attacks." (p. 53). However, this criticism is based on a misconception because the very design of a blockchain implies immutable records tracking the history of transactions. This feature improves traceability and facilitates the detection of eventual police cases. Nothing can be deleted from a blockchain, as the records inserted in it are immutable (Nakamoto, 2008).

Unlike fungible traditional currencies, the different units of the same cryptocurrency may be distinguished between themselves. They are made unique because each one of them carries the digital history of its prior transactions. If compared to physical money, *pseudo-anonymous* cryptocurrencies are more traceable (Antonopoulos, 2017). This traceability is a feature of Bitcoin, which does not oblige its users to register or reveal their real-world identity explicitly, although the patterns of user's behavior might themselves be identifying (Nath, 2020).

Ultimately, the literature shows that there is no lack of available data on the Bitcoin blockchain. By providing open data this allows the community to flag certain behavior or orientation of Bitcoin addresses and transactions. (...) The emergence of machine learning and its application to graphs is providing a powerful analysis capability for disrupting Bitcoin related criminal activity. (Turner et al., 2020, p. 63)

Meanwhile, the so-called privacy coins such as Monero and Zcash use complex cryptography to hide special anonymity features, and it seems reasonable to admit a need for some regulation in this regard. Nevertheless, anonymity still has essential roles to play, and digital money's programmability can be used in such regulatory efforts. For instance, Helbing (2014) pointed out that building in the anonymous cryptocurrency's protocol an obligation to spend it quickly (by programming a devaluation timeline) can be a market solution to benefit traceability and still keeping some degree of freedom:

Most of us don't want anybody to know, which toys someone buys in a sex shop. For such and many better reasons, we still need sufficient amounts of cash besides traceable electronic money, even though it should lose its value quickly enough to make traceable transactions sufficiently attractive. (p. 14)

It is advisable not to confuse the tree with the forest by labeling all cryptocurrencies equally. Cryptocurrencies should be classified by authorities, and ethically rated by communities according to the benefits and inconveniences determined by the computer programs that designed them (see Chapter 3). To facilitate such an assessment is another reason why open-source code is highly recommended in a blockchain. The privacy cryptocurrencies case shows the importance of researching how to optimize the trade-off between privacy and security.

Electronic voting is another area where undoubtedly more research is needed, as mentioned above. A general-purpose electronic voting system is a complex problem. Both privacy (votes have to be anonymous to prevent coercion) and public verifiability are required (otherwise, the provider of the e-voting solution, or someone who managed to compromise it, can change the votes), and trade-offs are unavoidable (Wüst & Gervais, 2018). Unlike Young (2018), the authors are unsure if there is yet a "robust voting system" (p. 9) on a blockchain. Observing the current state of electronic voting in "the most digital country in the world" (Butt et al., 2020), this is not precisely so. As referred to by Heiberg et al. (2020), "the Estonian Internet voting scheme does not provide full end-to-end verifiability" (p. 95), relying heavily on the electronic identity infrastructure, which can be problematic as these same authors "consider the user's personal computing environment to be the weakest point in the e-ID ecosystem." (p. 84)

The most serious implication of this threat is an attacker submitting a vote using a compromised e-ID environment without the voter noticing. This is a problem both in the scenario when the attacker changes the originally submitted vote by re-voting, and also when the voter did not intend to vote at all (which is her legal right in Estonia). (Heiberg et al, 2020, p. 20)

Thus, more research is needed on electronic voting systems, because fraud risks are very high and because democratic representativeness is very much at stake due to abstentionism.

Finally, one should keep in mind that BT goes, perhaps decisively, against the *status quo* and the interest of powerful intermediaries, which will certainly try to resist change. Although no one can de-invent BT, nor the Internet will go back to its previous stage, some will probably try to halt or delay the thrive of *public-permissionless* blockchains. Surprisingly enough, BT makes it possible for civil society to use digital prerogatives usually only used by large organizations. Thus, BT may change power dynamics in politics and economy favoring the third sector.

The authors think that few things in politics and the economy will remain the same in the *blockchain era*, and it is thought that more research into BT is required to educate politicians and citizens better to protect privacy, freedom, and democracy.

CONCLUSION

Networked organizations and distributed systems are unbeatable. For decades, the Internet has allowed sharing of information between people. Due to Blockchain Technology (BT), transactions can also be carried out directly from one person to another without intermediaries. In the *Blockchain Era*, the Internet will be more impactful to society because transacting is even more vital to humankind than sharing. BT was firstly used to execute secure financial transactions *peer-to-peer* (*e.g.*, Bitcoin), but with *smart contracts*, it is possible to automate other transaction agreements, which are being done, including those of a political nature.

There is a natural evolution from centralized to decentralized organizations, in the markets, in computer governance, in digital communication, and in the political system itself (democracy). Nevertheless, the political path of decentralization will not be easy to follow. Dealing only with private and opaque blockchains can be a dangerous option to democracy, and such closed alleys must be avoided. Instead, citizens must enter the brighter avenue recently opened by public and transparent blockchains. Otherwise, people can lose freedom, that is, lose practically everything. The authors think that the *open & decentralized vs. closed & centralized* dichotomy will become the most prominent political dispute of the 21st century. Anywhere freedom triumphs, citizens will be allowed to use *public and transparent open access blockchains*, whose transactions can be executed and verified by everyone. If law-abiding citizens can use *private cryptographic keys*, to freely transact in *public blockchains,* there will be freedom of choice among many *easy-to-use decentralized applications* (*dApps*), which is the case of *cryptocurrencies*.

Not only state-sponsored digital currencies but many private cryptocurrencies should be free to compete in the market. In this scenario, a paradigm of transparency will probably emerge. Thus, *private cryptographic keys* are a pre-requisite of democracy and the only way to deal with the severe risks of losing privacy and freedom in the *Blockchain Era*. People will have more power over information, reinforcing individual autonomy and government officials' accountability. Of course, crimes and police cases will continue to be increasingly sophisticated, as has been the case since the beginning. However, supposing public blockchains' transparency can thrive, the criminal investigation will be strengthened by combining powerful technologies (*e.g.*, Big Data and Artificial Intelligence) to a great extent, thanks to the immutable and auditable character of transactions once registered in a blockchain. However, ICTT availability (see Key Terms and Definitions) demands full transparency, under penalty of losing freedom and democracy, because once that centralization and closed-source computing dominate the Internet, the state and corporatocracy will cross-reference both *economic media* (social media and digital currencies). This is not considered a very auspicious thing because data extracted from digital money users becomes a database with semiotic value (see Chapter 1), and if each digital coin can have a different cryptographic *color*, some governments can be tempted to *paint* them according to each consumer's political vests. In this scenario, such *colored money* will condition consumer behavior and citizens' freedom. So, instead of being confronted with police cases, citizens would be harassed by the policing of all cases. Such a level of citizens' control is typical in authoritarian states. For instance, in China, the state is sponsoring both the social network "WeChat" and Digital Yuan, eventually combining data handy for the regime. As for the rest of the world, it is known that worse news travels quickly.

Hopefully, political choices will protect democracy and freedom. Then, the *Internet of Value* will serve human ingenuity to foster innovation and entrepreneurship, letting the free world take advantage of the *Blockchain Era*, surpassing any political pitfalls created by the status quo.

REFERENCES

R3. (2020a, September 16). *How "public-permissioned" blockchains are not an oxymoron.* https://www.r3.com/blog/how-public-permissioned-blockchains-are-not-an-oxymoron-2/

R3. (2020b, October 30). *Should we already be using blockchain as a voting system for elections?* Corda. https://www.corda.net/blog/should-we-already-be-using-blockchain-as-a-voting-system-for-elections/

Aarvik, P. (2020). *Blockchain as an anti-corruption tool. Case examples and introduction.* Academic Press.

Adeodato, R., & Pournouri, S. (2020). Secure Implementation of E-Governance: A Case Study About Estonia. In *Cyber Defence in the Age of AI, Smart Societies and Augmented Humanity* (pp. 397–429). Springer. doi:10.1007/978-3-030-35746-7_18

Ahluwalia, S., Mahto, R. V., & Guerrero, M. (2020). Blockchain technology and startup financing: A transaction cost economics perspective. *Technological Forecasting and Social Change, 151,* 119854. doi:10.1016/j.techfore.2019.119854

Alexandru, I. (2018). *Comparative administrative law issues regarding central and local government.* Societatea de Stiinte Juridice si Administrative.

Alfieri, E. (2019). *Cryptocurrencies and market efficiency. Business administration.* Université Grenoble Alpes.

Almeida, R. J. F. D. (2017). *Generation Y: an analysis of millennials' skills, perceptions, values and expectations against the promise (s) of the Gen-Y City project* (Doctoral dissertation). Universidade de Coimbra.

Amend, J., Kaiser, J., Uhlig, L., Urbach, N., & Völter, F. (2021). *What Do We Really Need? A Systematic Literature Review of the Requirements for Blockchain-based E-government Services.* Academic Press.

AmetranoF. M. (2016). *Hayek money: The cryptocurrency price stability solution.* Available at SSRN 2425270.

Antonopoulos, A. M. (2016). *The internet of money* (Vol. 1). Merkle Bloom LLC.

Antonopoulos Andreas, M. (2017). *The Internet of Money: Volume Two.* Merkle Bloom LLC.

Applebaum, A. (2012). Iron curtain: the crushing of Eastern Europe 1944-56. Penguin UK.

Ardo, A. A., & Zamani, E. D. (2019, April). Mobile phone for financial inclusiveness and empowerment: a case study of anchor borrowers programme. In *Proceedings of 2019 UK Academy for Information Systems International Conference*. AIS.

AtzoriM. (2015). Blockchain technology and decentralized governance: Is the state still necessary? Available at SSRN 2709713. doi:10.2139srn.2709713

Ayed, A. B. (2017). A conceptual secure blockchain-based electronic voting system. *Int. J. Netw. Secur. Its Appl.*, *9*, 1–9.

Baran, P. (1964). On distributed communications networks. *IEEE Transactions on Communications Systems*, *12*(1), 1–9. doi:10.1109/TCOM.1964.1088883

Barański, S., Szymański, J., Sobecki, A., Gil, D., & Mora, H. (2020). Practical I-Voting on Stellar Blockchain. *Applied Sciences (Basel, Switzerland)*, *10*(21), 7606. doi:10.3390/app10217606

Barnes, A., Brake, C., & Perry, T. (2016). *Digital Voting with the use of Blockchain Technology*. Team Plymouth Pioneers – Plymouth University.

Baudier, P., Kondrateva, G., Ammi, C., & Seulliet, E. (2021). Peace engineering: The contribution of blockchain systems to the e-voting process. *Technological Forecasting and Social Change*, *162*, 120397. doi:10.1016/j.techfore.2020.120397 PMID:33071364

Beller, J. (2020). Economic Media: Crypto and the Myth of Total Liquidity. *Australian Humanities Review*, *66*, 215–225.

Bellini, E., Iraqi, Y., & Damiani, E. (2020). Blockchain-based distributed trust and reputation management systems: A survey. *IEEE Access: Practical Innovations, Open Solutions*, *8*, 21127–21151. doi:10.1109/ACCESS.2020.2969820

Benhabib, S. (1997). Between Facts and Norms: Contributions to a Discourse Theory of Law and Democracy. *The American Political Science Review*, *91*(3), 725–726. doi:10.2307/2952099

Beniiche, A. (2020). *A study of blockchain oracles*. arXiv preprint arXiv:2004.07140.

Benítez-Martínez, F. L., Hurtado-Torres, M. V., & Romero-Frías, E. (2021). A neural blockchain for a tokenizable e-Participation model. *Neurocomputing*, *423*, 703–712. doi:10.1016/j.neucom.2020.03.116

Berg, C., Davidson, S., & Potts, J. (2019). Blockchain technology as economic infrastructure: Revisiting the electronic markets hypothesis. *Frontiers in Blockchain*, *2*, 22. doi:10.3389/fbloc.2019.00022

Bernabe, J. B., Canovas, J. L., Hernandez-Ramos, J. L., Moreno, R. T., & Skarmeta, A. (2019). Privacy-preserving solutions for Blockchain: Review and challenges. *IEEE Access: Practical Innovations, Open Solutions*, *7*, 164908–164940. doi:10.1109/ACCESS.2019.2950872

Berwick, D. M. (2020). Choices for the "new normal". *Journal of the American Medical Association*, *323*(21), 2125–2126. doi:10.1001/jama.2020.6949 PMID:32364589

Blaustein, A. P. (1987). Our Most Important Export: The Influence of the United States Constitution Abroad. *Conn. J. Int'l L.*, *3*, 15.

Blue, A. (2020). Evaluating Estonian E-residency as a tool of soft power. *Place Branding and Public Diplomacy*, 1–9. doi:10.105741254-020-00182-3

Brinks, V. (2019). 'And Since I Knew About the Possibilities There…': The Role of Open Creative Labs in User Innovation Processes. *Tijdschrift voor Economische en Sociale Geografie, 110*(4), 381–394. doi:10.1111/tesg.12353

Buckley, R. P., Arner, D. W., Zetzsche, D. A., Didenko, A. N., & Van Romburg, L. J. (2021). Sovereign digital currencies: Reshaping the design of money and payments systems. *Journal of Payments Strategy & Systems, 15*(1), 7–22.

Busygina, I., Filippov, M., & Taukebaeva, E. (2018). To decentralize or to continue on the centralization track: The cases of authoritarian regimes in Russia and Kazakhstan. *Journal of Eurasian Studies, 9*(1), 61-71.

Buterin, V. (2014). DAOs, DACs, DAs and more: An incomplete terminology guide. *Ethereum Blog, 6*, 2014.

Butt, S. A., Pappel, I., & Õunapuu, E. (2020, November). Potential for Increasing the ICT Adaption and Identifying Technology Readiness in the Silver Economy: Case of Estonia. In *International Conference on Electronic Governance and Open Society: Challenges in Eurasia* (pp. 139-155). Springer.

Buyle, R., Taelman, R., Mostaert, K., Joris, G., Mannens, E., Verborgh, R., & Berners-Lee, T. (2019). *Streamlining governmental processes by putting citizens in control of their personal data*. Academic Press.

Çabuk, U. C., Adiguzel, E., & Karaarslan, E. (2020). *A survey on feasibility and suitability of blockchain techniques for the e-voting systems*. arXiv preprint arXiv:2002.07175.

Castells, M. (2014). The impact of the internet on society: A global perspective. *Change, 19*, 127–148.

Cawthorn, D. M., Kennaugh, A., & Ferreira, S. M. (2020). The future of sustainability in the context of COVID-19. *Ambio*, 1–10. PMID:33289053

Chamola, V., Hassija, V., Gupta, V., & Guizani, M. (2020). A comprehensive review of the COVID-19 pandemic and the role of IoT, drones, AI, blockchain, and 5G in managing its impact. *IEEE Access: Practical Innovations, Open Solutions, 8*, 90225–90265. doi:10.1109/ACCESS.2020.2992341

Chen, J. (2017). Can online social networks foster young adults' civic engagement? *Telematics and Informatics, 34*(5), 487–497. doi:10.1016/j.tele.2016.09.013

Chen, Y. (2018). Blockchain tokens and the potential democratization of entrepreneurship and innovation. *Business Horizons, 61*(4), 567–575. doi:10.1016/j.bushor.2018.03.006

Chen, Y., Mao, Z., & Qiu, J. L. (2018). *Super-Sticky Design and Everyday Cultures', Super-Sticky Wechat and Chinese Society*. Emerald Publishing Limited. doi:10.1108/9781787430914

Choi, M. K., Yeun, C. Y., & Seong, P. H. (2020). A Novel Monitoring System for the Data Integrity of Reactor Protection System Using Blockchain Technology. *IEEE Access: Practical Innovations, Open Solutions, 8*, 118732–118740. doi:10.1109/ACCESS.2020.3005134

Clavin, J., Duan, S., Zhang, H., Janeja, V. P., Joshi, K. P., Yesha, Y., Erickson, L. C., & Li, J. D. (2020). Blockchains for Government: Use Cases and Challenges. *Digital Government: Research and Practice*, *1*(3), 1–21. doi:10.1145/3427097

Coase, R. H. (1991). *The nature of the firm (1937). The Nature of the Firm.* Origins, Evolution, and Development.

Conway, D., & Garimella, K. (2020). Enhancing Trust in Business Ecosystems With Blockchain Technology. *IEEE Engineering Management Review*, *48*(1), 24–30. doi:10.1109/EMR.2020.2970387

Cunningham, S. (2010). Joseph A. Schumpeter, Capitalism, socialism, and democracy. *International Journal of Cultural Policy*, *16*(1), 20–22. doi:10.1080/10286630902807278

Dalton, G. (1982). Barter. *Journal of Economic Issues*, *16*(1), 181–190. doi:10.1080/00213624.1982.11503968

Dapp, M. M. (2019). Toward a Sustainable Circular Economy Powered by Community-Based Incentive Systems. In *Business Transformation through Blockchain* (pp. 153–181). Palgrave Macmillan. doi:10.1007/978-3-319-99058-3_6

Darlington III, J. K. (2014). *The future of Bitcoin: mapping the global adoption of world's largest cryptocurrency through benefit analysis.* Academic Press.

DavidsonS.De FilippiP.PottsJ. (2016). *Economics of blockchain.* Available at SSRN 2744751.

Davidson, S., De Filippi, P., & Potts, J. (2018). Blockchains and the economic institutions of capitalism. *Journal of Institutional Economics*, *14*(4), 639–658. doi:10.1017/S1744137417000200

De Beauclair, I. (1963). The Stone Money of Yap Island. *Bulletin of the Institute of Ethnology, Academia Sinica*, *16*, 147–160.

De Beauclair, I. (1971). Studies on Botel Tobago, and Yap. In *Asian Folklore and Social Life Monographs, edited by Lou Tsu-k'uang* (pp. 183–203). Orient Cultural Service.

Degeling, C., Chen, G., Gilbert, G. L., Brookes, V., Thai, T., Wilson, A., & Johnson, J. (2020). Changes in public preferences for technologically enhanced surveillance following the COVID-19 pandemic: A discrete choice experiment. *BMJ Open*, *10*(11), e041592. doi:10.1136/bmjopen-2020-041592 PMID:33208337

Dhinakaran, K., Raj, P. B. H., & Vinod, D. (2021). A Secure Electronic Voting System Using Blockchain Technology. In *Proceedings of the Second International Conference on Information Management and Machine Intelligence* (pp. 307-313). Springer. 10.1007/978-981-15-9689-6_34

Didenko, A. N., Zetzsche, D. A., Arner, D. W., & Buckley, R. P. (2020). *After Libra, Digital Yuan and COVID-19: Central Bank Digital Currencies and the New World of Money and Payment Systems.* Academic Press.

District0x. (2020). *An Introduction To Decentralization.* District0x Education Portal. https://education.district0x.io/general-topics/what-is-decentralization/introduction/

Dixon, C. (2018). *Why Decentralization Matters.* https://medium.com/s/story/why-decentralization-matters-5e3f79f7638e

Dumas, J. G., Jimenez-Garcès, S., & Șoiman, F. (2021, March). Blockchain technology and crypto-assets market analysis: vulnerabilities and risk assessment. The 12th International Multi-Conference on Complexity, Informatics and Cybernetics: IMCIC 2021.

Dush, L. (2015). When writing becomes content. *College Composition and Communication*, 173–196.

Dwyer, R. (2017). *Code! = Law: Explorations of the Blockchain as a Mode of Algorithmic Governance.* Retrieved from https://www.academia.edu/34734732/Code_Law_Explorations_of_the_Blockchain_as_a_Mode_of_Algo rithmic_Governance

Dzieduszycka-Suinat, S., Murray, J., Kiniry, J., Zimmerman, D., Wagner, D., Robinson, P., Foltzer, A., & Morina, S. (2015). *The Future of Voting End-to-End – Verifiable Internet Voting. Specification and Feasibility Assessment Study.* U.S. Vote Foundation. https://usvotefoundation-drupal.s3.amazonaws.com/prod/E2EVIV_full_report.pdf

Ebner, N. (2017). Negotiation is changing. *J. Disp. Resol., 99*.

Eikmanns, B. C. (2018). *Blockchain: Proposition of a new and sustainable macroeconomic system.* Frankfurt School, Blockchain Center.

Faber, B., Michelet, G. C., Weidmann, N., Mukkamala, R. R., & Vatrapu, R. (2019, January). BPDIMS: a blockchain-based personal data and identity management system. *Proceedings of the 52nd Hawaii International Conference on System Sciences.* 10.24251/HICSS.2019.821

Faber, N. R., & Hadders, H. (2016, June). Towards a blockchain enabled social contract for sustainability, Creating a fair and just operating system for humanity. In *Proceedings of the First International Conference on New Business Models, Toulouse, France* (pp. 16-17). Academic Press.

Feldstein, S. (2019). The road to digital unfreedom: How artificial intelligence is reshaping repression. *Journal of Democracy, 30*(1), 40–52. doi:10.1353/jod.2019.0003

Fenwick, M., & Vermeulen, E. P. (2019). Technology and corporate governance: Blockchain, crypto, and artificial intelligence. *Tex. J. Bus. L., 48*, 1.

Fisher, R., Ury, W. L., & Patton, B. (2011). *Getting to yes: Negotiating agreement without giving in.* Penguin.

Fitzpatrick, S. M., & Diveley, B. D. (2004). Interisland Exchange in Micronesia: A Case of Monumental Proportions. In S. M. Fitzpatrick (Ed.), *Voyages of Discovery: The Archaeology of Islands* (pp. 129–146). Praeger.

Fitzpatrick, S. M., & McKeon, S. (2020). Banking on Stone Money: Ancient Antecedents to Bitcoin. *Economic Anthropology, 7*(1), 7–21. doi:10.1002ea2.12154

Fliphodl, F. (2018, November 22). *Social Media Alternatives Series, EP. 1: What You NEED to Know.* Fliphodl. https://www.fliphodl.com/social-media-alternatives-series-ep-1-what-you-need-to-know/

Friedman, M. (1991). *The Island of Stone Money.* Hoover Institution, Stanford University.

Furness, W. H. (1910). *The Island of Stone Money, Uap of the Carolines.* J. B. Lippincott.

Gabardi, W. (2001). Contemporary models of democracy. *Polity*, *33*(4), 547–568. doi:10.2307/3235516

Gandy, O. H. Jr. (2010). Engaging rational discrimination: Exploring reasons for placing regulatory constraints on decision support systems. *Ethics and Information Technology*, *12*(1), 29–42. doi:10.100710676-009-9198-6

Gibbons, R. (2001). Trust in social structures: Hobbes and Coase meet repeated games. *Trust in Society*, *2*, 332-353.

Greitens, S. C. (2020). Surveillance, Security, & Democracy in a Post-COVID World. *International Organization*, *74*(S1), E169–E190. doi:10.1017/S0020818320000417

Gurguc, Z., & Knottenbelt, W. (2018). *Cryptocurrencies: overcoming barriers to trust and adoption*. eToro.

Habermas, J., & Rehg, W. (1997). *Contributions to a discourse theory of law and democracy*. Polity Press.

Hamel, G. (2000). *Leading the revolution*. Harvard Business School Press.

Haneem, F., Bakar, H. A., Kama, N., Mat, N. Z. N., Ghazali, R., & Mahmood, Y. (2020). *Recent Progress of Blockchain Initiatives in Government*. Academic Press.

Harari. (2020). *The world after coronavirus*. https://www.ft.com/content/19d90308-6858-11ea-a3c9-1fe6fedcca75

Harrison, M. (2018). *Decentralizing the International Monetary System: An Assessment of Regulatory Structures for Cryptocurrencies in the Age of Digital Finance*. Academic Press.

Hasselgren, A., Kralevska, K., Gligoroski, D., Pedersen, S. A., & Faxvaag, A. (2020). Blockchain in healthcare and health sciences—A scoping review. *International Journal of Medical Informatics*, *134*, 104040. doi:10.1016/j.ijmedinf.2019.104040 PMID:31865055

Hayek, F. A. (1976). *Denationalisation of money*. Ludwig von Mises Institute.

Heiberg, S., Krips, K., & Willemson, J. (2020). Planning the next steps for Estonian Internet voting. *E-Vote-ID*, *2020*, 82.

Heiss, J., Eberhardt, J., & Tai, S. (2019, July). From oracles to trustworthy data on-chaining systems. In *2019 IEEE International Conference on Blockchain (Blockchain)* (pp. 496-503). IEEE. 10.1109/Blockchain.2019.00075

HelbingD. (2014). *Qualified money-a better financial system for the future*. Available at SSRN 2526022 doi:10.2139srn.2526022

HendricksonJ.HoganT.LutherW. (2015). The political economy of bitcoin. SSRN.

Hjálmarsson, F. Þ., Hreiðarsson, G. K., Hamdaqa, M., & Hjálmt'ysson, G. (2018). Blockchain-based e-voting system. *Proceedings of the 2018 IEEE 11th International Conference on Cloud Computing (CLOUD)*, 983–986. 10.1109/CLOUD.2018.00151

Holochain.org. (2020). *What is Holochain?* https://developer.holochain.org/docs/what-is-holochain/

Hoxtell, W., & Nonhoff, D. (2019). *Internet Governance: Past, Present and Future*. Konrad Adenauer Stiftung. https://www.gppi.net/media/Internet-Governance-Past-Present-and-Future.pdf

Humphrey, C. (1985). Barter and Economic Disintegration. *Man, 20*(1), 48–72. doi:10.2307/2802221

Ingham, G. (2013). *The nature of money*. John Wiley & Sons.

Insights, L. (2020, June 12). *Congressman argues for permissionless digital dollar to demonstrate U.S. values*. Ledger Insights - Enterprise Blockchain. https://www.ledgerinsights.com/digital-dollar-congress-permissionless/

Iwamoto, K. (2021, February 15). *China's New Year digital yuan tests hasten Asia e-currency race*. Nikkei Asia. https://asia.nikkei.com/Spotlight/Asia-Insight/China-s-New-Year-digital-yuan-tests-hasten-Asia-e-currency-race

JaccardG. (2018). Smart contracts and the role of law. Available at SSRN 3099885. doi:10.2139srn.3099885

JainD. (2020). The Economics of Cryptocurrencies-Why Does It Work? Available at SSRN 3644159.

Jensen, T., Hedman, J., & Henningsson, S. (2019). How tradelens delivers business value with blockchain technology. *MIS Quarterly Executive, 18*(4), 221–243. doi:10.17705/2msqe.00018

Katzenbach, C., & Ulbricht, L. (2019). Algorithmic Governance. *Internet Policy Review, 8*(4), 1–18. doi:10.14763/2019.4.1424

Kauffman, S. A. (1993). *The origins of order: Self-organization and selection in evolution*. Oxford University Press.

Kewell, B., Adams, R., & Parry, G. (2017). Blockchain for good? *Strategic Change, 26*(5), 429–437. doi:10.1002/jsc.2143

Keynes, J. M. (1915). The Island of Stone Money. *Economic Journal (London), 25*(98), 281–283.

Khare, R. (2003). *Extending the REpresentational State Transfer REST Architectural Style for Decentralized Systems* (Doctoral dissertation). University of California, Irvine.

Khare, R., & Taylor, R. N. (2004, May). Extending the representational state transfer (rest) architectural style for decentralized systems. In *Proceedings. 26th International Conference on Software Engineering* (pp. 428-437). IEEE.

Khezr, S., Moniruzzaman, M., Yassine, A., & Benlamri, R. (2019). Blockchain technology in healthcare: A comprehensive review and directions for future research. *Applied Sciences (Basel, Switzerland), 9*(9), 1736. doi:10.3390/app9091736

Kim, S. (2020). *Fractional Ownership*. Democratization and Bubble Formation - The Impact of Blockchain Enabled Asset Tokenization.

Kim, Y. S., & Lee, J. W. (2011). Corruption and Government Roles: Causes, Economic Effects, and Scope. *Korea and the World Economy, 12*(3), 513–553.

Kranzberg, M. (1986). Technology and History:" Kranzberg's Laws. *Technology and Culture, 27*(3), 544–560. doi:10.2307/3105385

Kshetri, N., & Voas, J. (2018). Blockchain-enabled e-voting. *IEEE Software*, *35*(4), 95–99. doi:10.1109/MS.2018.2801546

Kuperberg, M. (2019). Blockchain-based identity management: A survey from the enterprise and ecosystem perspective. *IEEE Transactions on Engineering Management*, *67*(4), 1008–1027. doi:10.1109/TEM.2019.2926471

Landemore, H. (2012). *Democratic reason: Politics, collective intelligence, and the rule of the many*. Princeton University Press.

Lannoye, V. (2020). *The History of Money for Understanding Economics*. Vincent Lannoye.

Leach, M., MacGregor, H., Scoones, I., & Wilkinson, A. (2020). Post-pandemic transformations: How and why COVID-19 requires us to rethink development. *World Development*, *138*, 105233. doi:10.1016/j.worlddev.2020.105233 PMID:33100478

Leonard, D., & Treiblmaier, H. (2019). Can cryptocurrencies help to pave the way to a more sustainable economy? Questioning the economic growth paradigm. In *Business transformation through Blockchain* (pp. 183–205). Palgrave Macmillan. doi:10.1007/978-3-319-99058-3_7

Lessig, L. (2015). *De ja vu all over again*. Talk given at Sydney Blockchain workshop.

Lewis, A. (2015). *A Gentle Introduction to Digital Tokens*. Bits on Blocks. https://bitsonblocks.net/2015/09/28/a-gentle-introduction-to-digital-tokens

Li, G. (2008). *Economic sense of Metcalfe's Law*. Academic Press.

Liu, J., Li, X., Ye, L., Zhang, H., Du, X., & Guizani, M. (2018, December). BPDS: A blockchain based privacy-preserving data sharing for electronic medical records. In *2018 IEEE Global Communications Conference (GLOBECOM)* (pp. 1-6). IEEE. 10.1109/GLOCOM.2018.8647713

Livingston, D., Sivaram, V., Freeman, M., & Fiege, M. (2018). *Applying blockchain technology to electric power systems*. Academic Press.

Lopes, J., Pereira, J. L., & Varajão, J. (2019). *Blockchain based E-voting system: a proposal*. Academic Press.

Lopez, P. G., Montresor, A., & Datta, A. (2019, July). Please, do not decentralize the Internet with (permissionless) blockchains! In *2019 IEEE 39th International Conference on Distributed Computing Systems (ICDCS)* (pp. 1901-1911). IEEE.

Lotti, L. (2019). The Art of Tokenization: Blockchain Affordances and the Invention of Future Milieus. *Media Theory*, *3*(1), 287–320.

Lu, Y., & Pan, J. (2020). Capturing Clicks: How the Chinese Government Uses Clickbait to Compete for Visibility. *Political Communication*, 1–32.

Lyon, D. (2014). Surveillance, Snowden, and Big Data: Capacities, consequences, critique. *Big Data & Society*, *1*(2). Advance online publication. doi:10.1177/2053951714541861

Mack, C. A. (2011). Fifty years of Moore's law. *IEEE Transactions on Semiconductor Manufacturing*, *24*(2), 202–207. doi:10.1109/TSM.2010.2096437

Manovich, L. (2002). *The Language of New Media*. MIT Print.

Manovich, L. (2013). *Software Takes Command*. Bloomsbury Academic Print.

Massey, R., Dalal, D., & Dakshinamoorthy, A. (2017). *Initial coin offering: A new paradigm*. Deloitte. Available at https:// www2.deloitte.com/content/dam/Deloitte/us/Documents/ process-and-operations/ us-cons-new-paradigm.pdf

Matseshe, L. K., Arasa, R., & Yohannes, T. H. (2017). *The Moderating Effect Of Decision-Maker On The Relationship Between Strategy And Organizational Structure*. Academic Press.

Mattke, J., Maier, C., & Reis, L. (2020, June). Is cryptocurrency money? Three empirical studies analyzing medium of exchange, store of value and unit of account. In *Proceedings of the 2020 on Computers and People Research Conference* (pp. 26-35). 10.1145/3378539.3393859

Mertes, T. (2002). Wall Street. *Amass*, *12*(2), 80.

Metcalfe, B. (2013). Metcalfe's law after 40 years of Ethernet. *IEEE Computer*, *46*(12), 26–31. doi:10.1109/ MC.2013.374

Mik, E. (2017). Smart contracts: Terminology, technical limitations and real world complexity. *Law, Innovation and Technology*, *9*(2), 269–300. doi:10.1080/17579961.2017.1378468

Mollick, E. (2006). Establishing Moore's law. *IEEE Annals of the History of Computing*, *28*(3), 62–75. doi:10.1109/MAHC.2006.45

Monroe, A. E. (1923). *Monetary Theory before Adam Smith* (Vol. 25). Harvard University Press. doi:10.4159/harvard.9780674183438

Möser, M., Böhme, R., & Breuker, D. (2014, March). Towards risk scoring of Bitcoin transactions. In *International Conference on Financial Cryptography and Data Security* (pp. 16-32). Springer.

Mouial-Bassilana, E., Restrepo, D., & Colombani, L. (2018). Le déséquilibre significatif dans les contrats commerciaux: nouvel outil de lutte contre les GAFA. *Actualité juridique. Contrat, 471.*

Mueller, L., Glarner, A., Linder, T., Meyer, S. D., Furrer, A., Gschwend, C., & Henschel, P. (2018). *Conceptual Framework for Legal and Risk Assessment of Crypto Tokens*. Academic Press.

MX Technologies Inc. (2016). *Checks, Balances, and Bitcoin: The Genius of the Blockchain*. Retrieved from https://www.mx.com/moneysummit/checks-balances-and-bitcoin-the-genius-of-the-blockchain/

Nakamoto, S. (2008). *A peer-to-peer electronic cash system*. Bitcoin. https://bitcoin.org/bitcoin.pdf

NathG. V. (2020). *Cryptocurrency and Privacy-An Introduction to the Interface*. Available at SSRN 3658459. doi:10.2139srn.3658459

Naudet, L. B. (2021). *Regard sur les conséquences des mutations organiques de la monnaie dans la manifestation des conflits armés depuis l'éclatement du système de Bretton-Woods*. Academic Press.

Norta, A. (2016, November). Designing a smart-contract application layer for transacting decentralized autonomous organizations. In *International Conference on Advances in Computing and Data Sciences* (pp. 595-604). Springer.

Noyen, K., Volland, D., Wörner, D., & Fleisch, E. (2014). *When money learns to fly: Towards sensing as a service applications using bitcoin.* arXiv preprint arXiv:1409.5841

O'Neil, C. (2017). How can we stop algorithms telling lies? *The Guardian*, 7-16.

Pasuthip, P., & Yang, S. (2020). *Central Bank Digital Currency: Promises and Risks.*

Peters, G. W., & Panayi, E. (2016). Understanding modern banking ledgers through blockchain technologies: Future of transaction processing and smart contracts on the internet of money. In *Banking beyond banks and money* (pp. 239–278). Springer. doi:10.1007/978-3-319-42448-4_13

Plumptre, T. (2006). *"How Good is our Board?" How Board Evaluations Can.* Policy.

Pocher, N. (2019). The Internet of Money between Anonymity and Publicity: Legal Challenges of Distributed Ledger Technologies in the Crypto Financial Landscape. In *JURIX*. Doctoral Consortium.

Poovey, M. (1998). *A history of the modern fact: Problems of knowledge in the sciences of wealth and society.* University of Chicago Press. doi:10.7208/chicago/9780226675183.001.0001

Prinz, A. (1999). Money in the real and the virtual world: E-money, c-money and the demand for cb-money. *NETNOMICS: Economic Research and Electronic Networking, 1*(1), 11–35. doi:10.1023/A:1011441519577

Priyadharshini, A., Prasad, M., Raj, R. J. S., & Geetha, S. (2021). An Authenticated E-Voting System Using Biometrics and Blockchain. In *Intelligence in Big Data Technologies—Beyond the Hype* (pp. 535–542). Springer. doi:10.1007/978-981-15-5285-4_53

Qadah, G. Z. (2005). Requirements, design and implementation of an e-voting system. *Proceedings of the IADIS International Conference on Applied Computing*, 405–409.

Qiang, X. (2019). The road to digital unfreedom: President xi's surveillance state. *Journal of Democracy, 30*(1), 53–67. doi:10.1353/jod.2019.0004

Qin, K., & Gervais, A. (2018). *An overview of blockchain scalability, interoperability and sustainability.* Hochschule Luzern Imperial College London Liquidity Network.

Rajapashe, M., Adnan, M., Dissanayaka, A., Guneratne, D., & Abeywardena, K. (2020). Multi-Format Document Verification System. *American Scientific Research Journal for Engineering, Technology, and Sciences, 74*(2), 48–60.

Rath, M. (2019, November). A review of Artificial Intelligence Emerging technologies and challenges in Block Chain Technology. In *2019 International Conference on Smart Systems and Inventive Technology (ICSSIT)* (pp. 1031-1035). IEEE. 10.1109/ICSSIT46314.2019.8987807

Regner, F., Urbach, N., & Schweizer, A. (2019). *NFTs in Practice–Non-Fungible Tokens as Core Component of a Blockchain-based Event Ticketing Application.* Academic Press.

ReinersL. (2020). *Cryptocurrency and the State: An Unholy Alliance.* Available at SSRN 3682724.

Reisenwitz, C. (2014). Smart contracts promise for the Poor. *Bitcoin Mag*. https://bitcoinmagazine.com/articles/smart-propertys-promise-poor-1390852097/

Rooney, D., & Chavan, M. (2017). Globalization/internationalization. The International Encyclopedia of Organizational Communication, 1-15.

Rybarczyk, R., Armstrong, D., & Fabiano, A. (2021, May). *20210513 Galaxy Digital Mining - On Bitcoin Energy Consumption*. Retrieved June 1, 2021, from https://docsend.com/view/adwmdeeyfvqwecj2

Sadia, K., Masuduzzaman, M., Paul, R. K., & Islam, A. (2019). *Blockchain Based Secured E-voting by Using the Assistance of Smart Contract*. arXiv:1910.13635.

Sadowski, J. (2020). *Too smart: How digital capitalism is extracting data, controlling our lives, and taking over the world*. MIT Press. doi:10.7551/mitpress/12240.001.0001

Safko, L. (2010). *The social media bible: tactics, tools, and strategies for business success*. John Wiley & Sons.

Savelyev, A. (2017). Contract law 2.0: 'Smart' contracts as the beginning of the end of classic contract law. *Information & Communications Technology Law*, 26(2), 116–134. doi:10.1080/13600834.2017.1301036

Schaller, R. R. (1997). Moore's law: Past, present and future. *IEEE Spectrum*, 34(6), 52–59. doi:10.1109/6.591665

Schneier, B. (2007). Applied Cryptography: Protocols, Algorithms, and Source Code in C (2nd ed.). John Wiley & Sons, Inc.

Schumpeter, J. A. (1942). *Capitalism, socialism and democracy*. Routledge.

Sedlmeir, J., Buhl, H. U., Fridgen, G., & Keller, R. (2020). The energy consumption of blockchain technology: Beyond myth. *Business & Information Systems Engineering*, 62(6), 599–608. doi:10.100712599-020-00656-x

Sharma, P., Jindal, R., & Borah, M. D. (2020). Blockchain technology for cloud storage: A systematic literature review. *ACM Computing Surveys*, 53(4), 1–32. doi:10.1145/3403954

Shermin, V. (2017). Disrupting governance with blockchains and smart contracts. *Strategic Change*, 26(5), 499–509. doi:10.1002/jsc.2150

Shirky, C. (2008). *Here comes everybody: The power of organizing without organizations*. Penguin.

Slawotsky, J. (2020). US Financial Hegemony: The Digital Yuan and Risks of Dollar De-Weaponization. *Fordham Int'l LJ*, 44, 39.

SMA. (2018, November). *FLIPHODL*. https://www.fliphodl.com/social-media-alternatives-series-ep-1-what-you-need-to-know/

Snyder, H. (2019). Literature review as a research methodology: An overview and guidelines. *Journal of Business Research*, 104, 333–339. doi:10.1016/j.jbusres.2019.07.039

Specter, M. A., Koppel, J., & Weitzner, D. (2020). *The Ballot is Busted Before the Blockchain: A Security Analysis of Voatz, the First Internet Voting Application Used in U.S. Federal Elections*. Available online: https: //www.usenix.org/system/files/sec20-specter.pdf

Srivastava, A., Jain, P., Hazela, B., Asthana, P., & Rizvi, S. W. A. (2021). Application of Fog Computing, Internet of Things, and Blockchain Technology in Healthcare Industry. In *Fog Computing for Healthcare 4.0 Environments* (pp. 563–591). Springer. doi:10.1007/978-3-030-46197-3_22

Starr, R. M. (1989). The structure of exchange in barter and monetary economies. In *General Equilibrium Models of Monetary Economies* (pp. 129–143). Academic Press. doi:10.1016/B978-0-12-663970-4.50014-1

Swan, M. (2015). *Blockchain: Blueprint for a new economy*. O'Reilly Media, Inc.

Szabo, N. (2002). *The Origins of Money (No. 0211005)*. University Library of Munich.

Takabatake, Y., Kotani, D., & Okabe, Y. (2016). An anonymous distributed electronic voting system using Zerocoin. *IEICE Technical Report, 116*(282), 127–131.

Tapscott, D. (1997). *Growing Up Digital: The Rise of the Net Generation*. Harvard Business Press.

Tapscott, D., & Euchner, J. (2019). Blockchain and the Internet of Value: An Interview with Don Tapscott Don Tapscott talks with Jim Euchner about blockchain, the Internet of value, and the next Internet revolution. *Research Technology Management, 62*(1), 12–19. doi:10.1080/08956308.2019.1541711

Tapscott, D., & Tapscott, A. (2016). *Blockchain revolution: how the technology behind bitcoin is changing money, business, and the world*. Penguin.

Thagapsov, A., & Kozlovskiy, M. (2020). Bitcoin as Money. *Economic Analysis*.

Torraco, R. J. (2005). Writing integrative literature reviews: Guidelines and examples. *Human Resource Development Review, 4*(3), 356–367. doi:10.1177/1534484305278283

Turner, A. B., McCombie, S., & Uhlmann, A. J. (2020). Analysis techniques for illicit Bitcoin transactions. *Frontiers of Computer Science, 2*, 53.

Urgo, A. K., Lestan, M., & Khoriaty, A. (2017, September 17). *A cooperative of decentralized marketplaces and communities. Powered by Ethereum, Aragon, and IPFS*. District0x. https://district0x.io/docs/district0x-whitepaper.pdf

van den Hoven, J., Pouwelse, J., Helbing, D., & Klauser, S. (2019). The blockchain age: Awareness, empowerment and coordination. In *Towards digital enlightenment* (pp. 163–166). Springer. doi:10.1007/978-3-319-90869-4_13

Vassiliadis, S., Papadopoulos, P., Rangoussi, M., Konieczny, T., & Gralewski, J. (2017). Bitcoin value analysis based on cross-correlations. *Journal of Internet Banking and Commerce, 22*(S7), 1.

Vazirani, A. A., O'Donoghue, O., Brindley, D., & Meinert, E. (2020). Blockchain vehicles for efficient medical record management. *NPJ Digital Medicine, 3*(1), 1–5. doi:10.103841746-019-0211-0 PMID:31934645

Vergne, J. P. (2020). *Decentralized vs. Distributed Organization: A Framework for the Future of Blockchain and Machine Learning and for Avoiding Digital Platform Dystopia*. Academic Press.

Vo-Cao-Thuy, L., Cao-Minh, K., Dang-Le-Bao, C., & Nguyen, T. A. (2019). Votereum: An Ethereum-Based E-Voting System. *Proceedings of the 2019 IEEE-RIVF International Conference on Computing and Communication Technologies (RIVF)*, 1–6.

Voatz. (2021, February 4). *Voatz Response to Researchers' Flawed Report*. Voatz. https://voatz.com/2020/02/13/voatz-response-to-researchers-flawed-report/

Waldron, C. (2019). *Viability of the Usage of Blockchain Technology in Electronic Voting*. Academic Press.

Wang, J. (2021). *An In-depth Review of Privacy Concerns Raised by the COVID-19 Pandemic*. arXiv preprint arXiv:2101.10868.

Wattegama, D., Silva, P. S., Jayathilake, C. R., Elapatha, K., Abeywardena, K., & Kuruwitaarachchi, N. (2021). *"iSAY": Blockchain-based Intelligent Polling System for Legislative Assistance*. Academic Press.

Weatherford, J. (2009). *The history of money*. Currency.

Wright. De Filippi, Primavera. (2015). Decentralized Blockchain Technology and the Rise of Lex Cryptographia, SSRN 1, 16 (Mar. 20, 2015)

Wüst, K., & Gervais, A. (2018, June). Do you need a blockchain? In *2018 Crypto Valley Conference on Blockchain Technology (CVCBT)* (pp. 45-54). IEEE. 10.1109/CVCBT.2018.00011

Xu, M., Chen, X., & Kou, G. (2019). A systematic review of blockchain. *Financial Innovation*, *5*(1), 1–14. doi:10.118640854-019-0147-z

Xu, X., Pautasso, C., Zhu, L., Gramoli, V., Ponomarev, A., Tran, A. B., & Chen, S. (2016, April). The blockchain as a software connector. In *2016 13th Working IEEE/IFIP Conference on Software Architecture (WICSA)* (pp. 182-191). IEEE. 10.1109/WICSA.2016.21

Yang, X., Yi, X., Nepal, S., Kelarev, A., & Han, F. (2020). Blockchain voting: Publicly verifiable online voting protocol without trusted tallying authorities. *Future Generation Computer Systems*, *112*, 859–874. doi:10.1016/j.future.2020.06.051

Young, S. (2018). Changing governance models by applying blockchain computing. *Catholic University Journal of Law and Technology*, *26*(2), 87–128.

Young, S. (2018a). Enforcing constitutional rights through computer code. *Cath. UJL & Tech*, *26*, 52.

Zaman, S., Khandaker, M. R., Khan, R. T., Tariq, F., & Wong, K. K. (2021). *Thinking Out of the Blocks: Holochain for Distributed Security in IoT Healthcare*. arXiv preprint arXiv:2103.01322.

Zaprutin, D. G., Nikiporets-Takigawa, G., Goncharov, V. V., Sekerin, V. D., & Gorokhova, A. E. (2020). Legal Practice in the Blockchain era. *Revista Gênero e Interdisciplinaridade, 1*(1).

Zelmanovitz, L. (2011). Money: Origin and essence. *Criterio Libre*, *9*(14), 65–90. doi:10.18041/1900-0642/criteriolibre.2011v9n14.1232

Zhang, X. Z., Liu, J. J., & Xu, Z. W. (2015). Tencent and Facebook data validate Metcalfe's law. *Journal of Computer Science and Technology, 30*(2), 246–251. doi:10.100711390-015-1518-1

Zhao, J. L., Fan, S., & Yan, J. (2016). *Overview of business innovations and research opportunities in blockchain and introduction to the special issue.* Academic Press.

Zheng, Z., Xie, S., Dai, H. N., Chen, X., & Wang, H. (2018). Blockchain challenges and opportunities: A survey. *International Journal of Web and Grid Services, 14*(4), 352–375. doi:10.1504/IJWGS.2018.095647

Zwitter, A., & Hazenberg, J. (2020). Decentralized Network Governance: Blockchain Technology and the Future of Regulation. *Frontiers in Blockchain-Blockchain for Good, 3,* 12. doi:10.3389/fbloc.2020.00012

KEY TERMS AND DEFINITIONS

Agency Costs: Are the costs associated with the differences between the intentions of an agent and a principal, where the principal does not have complete control over the situation.

Backdoor: A hidden part of a computer program that may be used to gain access to privileged information like passwords, corrupt or delete data on hard drives, or transfer information within networks without consent.

Consensus: A group decision-making process in which group members develop and agree to support a decision in the best interest of the whole group.

Cryptocurrencies: A digital or virtual currency that is secured by cryptography. It is a special case of a digital token which has its own blockchain.

Datafication: A modern technological tendency to transform different aspects of our life into data that are later transformed into information perceived as a new form of value.

Decentralized Autonomous Organization (DAO): A group of people with no central management that coordinate over the internet around a shared set of rules to achieve a common mission. It relies on a system created by a group of developers to automate decision-making, including assigning voting rights.

E2E-VIV: End-to-End Verifiable Internet.

ICTT: Information, Communication, and Transaction Technologies (an original expression proposed by the authors).

Meme: It is for memory just as the gene is for biology. It is the minimum unit of information that multiplies from brain to brain or between places where information is stored.

Proof of Stake: A type of consensus mechanism used by blockchain networks to achieve distributed consensus. It requires users to stake their tokens to become a validator in the network.

Proof of Work: The pioneer consensus mechanism. A proof of work is a piece of data which was difficult (costly, time-consuming) to produce to satisfy certain requirements. It must be trivial to check whether data satisfies said requirements.

Smart Contract: An auto-executable piece of code implementing arbitrary rules on a computer with distributed consensus (a blockchain), such that when the code is live it cannot be censored or shut down. Smart contracts are analogous to the business logic instantiated in code in businesses and organisations around the world, the difference being that here the code runs on a code that no one party controls or can turn off.

Token: A unit of value secured by cryptography that represents an asset or a specific use. It can be created on top of a blockchain by using smart contracts.

Transaction Costs: The costs incurred in making any economic trade when participating in a market. They are costs that do not accrue to any participant of the transaction.

Ultra Vires: (Latin - "Beyond the Powers") A Latin phrase used in law to describe an act which requires legal authority but is done without it.

Chapter 5
The Real Blockchain Game Changer:
Protocols and DAOs for Coordinating Work to Provide Goods and Services

Mitchell Loureiro

Immunefi, Portugal

Ana Pêgo

Centro de Estudos de Doenças Crónicas (CEDOC), NOVA Medical School, Universidade NOVA de Lisboa, Lisbon, Portugal

Inês Graça Raposo

ISEG Executive Education, Lisbon School of Economics and Management, University of Lisbon, Portugal

ABSTRACT

The single critical output of a blockchain is creating trust where previously impossible. While this feature delivers compelling value for many use cases (bitcoin for money, standards setting and data sharing for permissioned blockchains, audit trails and protection against liability in supply chains), the most novel use case has been something unexpected: the birth of a new type of social structure to provide goods and services. The early examples of this new type of social structure have shown themselves to be incredibly effective at providing those services to their users.

INTRODUCTION

Many historical developments, whether technological or social, were relatively unappreciated in their early days. Their utility is compared against the existing order of things: steam engines against animal-drawn carriages, paper money against gold, and so on. Eventually, their paradigm-shattering nature

DOI: 10.4018/978-1-7998-7363-1.ch005

becomes evident to all, and a rough transition takes place. Blockchain technology seems like it is on the verge of that same transition.

When Bitcoin was first revealed in 2008, its potential was visible to only a tiny group (Nakamoto, 2009). Over the last ten years, Bitcoin slowly gained ground, and in the process, it birthed generalized Blockchain Technology (BT). What was challenging to see in 2008 is now on the edge of clarity: BT is a dramatic technological step into the future because it enables social coordination that would be otherwise impossible (De Filippi, 2016).

The single critical output of a blockchain is trust, upon which social coordination is built, provided that a specific set of rules have been followed (as determined by the consensus algorithm), you can be confident that information in a blockchain is accurate, and you can audit the entire history of additions and changes to that information (Namasudra et al., 2020; Zheng et al., 2018).

While this feature delivers compelling value for many use cases (Bitcoin for money, data sharing for permissioned blockchains, audit trails, and protection against liability in supply chains), the most novel use case was something unforeseen: the birth of a new type of social structure to provide goods and services (Li, 2019). Automated and decentralized protocols were generated within a network that controls transactions, but the individuals do not even need to know or speak to each other, as their trust in the system is on a token-based incentive scheme (Voshmgir, 2020). These social structures are generally called protocols or Decentralized Autonomous Organizations (DAOs) in the blockchain community, and they have a unique advantage over previous social structures (clans, empires, and corporations) in producing wealth. DAOs are the highest form of a smart contract. They are run by rules created by members through a consensus process, which are then written into a set of contracts run through a computer code, thus, enabling the automated management of a distributed organization (Sims, 2020).

Traditional Organizations and DAOs

Until today, only a few major social structures have contributed to the material advancement of humankind. First among them is the family, which grows until it becomes the clan and then the tribe before hitting the limits of its ability to coordinate work. The tribe is based primarily on blood relationships and the trust that comes from looking out for oneself. It fails to effectively coordinate work for those outside the tribe (Greif, 2006; Werbach, 2018).

The second central structure is the state, which lays claim to sovereignty over a place or a group of people. Urbanizing tribes formed states which could coordinate a far greater number of people under their codified laws, caste structures, and unified ideology. Most of written history is the history of states and their competition for power and resources (Biersteker & Weber, 2011).

The third primary structure is the corporation, which aligns a core group of contributing stakeholders (the shareholders) to achieve specific material aims. The shareholders contribute capital, which they use to contract labor to produce some good or service sold for profit to consumers (Maher & Andersson, 2005). The corporation is a relatively recent development, becoming a standard institution only over the last 300 years. The corporation's age begins with the age of exploration (Weber, 1978; Pomeranz, 2001).

The development of each social structure unleashed a torrent of materially creative forces for humankind. The tribe was able to support more sophistication and technological development than a bunch of families could. In turn, the state organized far more labor and specialization of labor than any number of tribes could. Finally, the corporation and multinationals organize labor far more efficiently and at a grander scale than states do (Morgan, 2009).

In particular, the corporation has been a central player over the last 300 years, for it was corporations that drove the industrial revolution and presided over a dramatic expansion in technological development (Pomeranz, 2001). This technological development ultimately created material wealth orders of magnitude larger than all previous human history combined. It was not the state as a social structure that birthed the telegraph, electric generators, or steelworks. Corporations and private industry birthed these technologies and facilitated their spread for profit (Bruland & Mowery, 2004).

The corporation's great advantage is its ability to align capital holders and labor incentives together to create goods and services (Hill, 1977). The corporate structure makes it advantageous for any capital holder to participate in a commercial venture as a shareholder to gain more capital in future cash flows to shareholders. The value of participation is abstracted away from the shareholder's personal history, nationality, and religious affiliation, as all shareholders have shared and agreed upon privileges and responsibilities. These privileges and responsibilities are further secured by limitations of liability, which effectively cap the downside of a venture to the equity's value, making further risk-taking possible. With a corporation, people from anywhere and everywhere can provide capital to pursue a common aim, and this capital provides the generalized incentive for labor to help realize those commercial goals. The corporation has been, up until the rise of blockchain, the most effective way of coordinating labor because it accounts for the interests of capital and labor in a generalized way, which tribes and states cannot do. "Multinationals are essentially market actors; their goals and strategies are driven by issues of market positioning, not by issues of institutional change and redesign" (Morgan, 2009, p. 10).

As a result of the corporation's effectiveness as a social structure, these social-economic architectures have become the leading creators of material wealth in modern society. Today, most of the wealth is owned directly by corporations and indirectly by their shareholders (Transformation, 2010). The clearest example of the predominance of the corporate structure is in the world's largest company, Apple, with a fully diluted valuation of over USD 2.2 trillion at the time of publication, which is more than the GDP of the vast majority of countries around the world (Sergent, 2020).

DAOs are aimed to be the next step of the current traditional top-down organizations (Popova & Butakova, 2019; Voshmgir, 2020). In opposition to the last ones, DAOs do not have a hierarchical structure or entity to enforce decisions, as individuals can be geographically anywhere and independently-run different architecture nodes. This equality vote on the DAOs' decisions, and their transactions are stored on a transparent blockchain-based system. The code upgrade is the only point of centralization of these organizations. By using small contracts, DAOs members are not bound to anything by a formal contract, and their connection to the organization is based on token-based incentives.

These distributed organizations try to avoid situations where people become overly influenced or persuaded by any highly influential member. They try to harness a diversity of perspectives from all the members. Distributed organizations try to embody evolution in their design, similar to the evolutionary process built into our market economy. Distributed organizations work through a process whereby members create a stock of new ideas, decisions, or initiatives. They essentially invest their tokens into those that they believe are the most viable receiving rewards if the initiative is beneficial to the organization (Cryptoswede, 2020).

Blockchain-enabled DAOs have emerged as a new form of collective governance, in which communities may organize themselves, relying on decentralized infrastructure. In this chapter, the reader will be introduced to DAOs and their history. Current examples of DAOs will be reviewed, highlighting their potential for a technological transition and what still needs to be done and improved.

ENTER BITCOIN: THE FIRST DAO

Enter BT, with its progenitor Satoshi Nakamoto, the pseudonymous creator of Bitcoin. Nakamoto aimed to create a censorship-resistant store of value, and ideally, an uncensorable money, meaning an exchange value that cannot be controlled by an authority, as ordinary money. To realize his aim, Nakamoto combined public-key cryptography, elliptic curve cryptography, proof of work, and a host of other cryptographic innovations to create Bitcoin, the first blockchain (Nakamoto, 2009).

The system's technical components made for a censorship-resistant database that anyone could contribute to, audit, and use (Nakamoto, 2009). It created the world's first record of truth, "the trust machine", that could be comprehensively trusted by one's own experience alone, without the need for a trusted third party (Lansiti & Lakhani, 2017). Provided one has the technical skills to audit the code, anyone can download the Bitcoin client, check the code, run it themselves, and verify if Bitcoin exactly does what it says it will do and only that (Arslanian et al., 2019).

However, the technical invention of Bitcoin was only half the innovation. The other innovation, and a more major one, was aligning the incentives of those interested in Bitcoin to drive adoption and use of the nascent currency. Such alignment was achieved to no small extent via the Bitcoin mining scheme. The combination of a temporarily inflationary asset that can only be acquired by performing a specific kind of work (proof of work) and open, transparent nature of the database upon which this asset lives, created the first incentive scheme of this kind, the first DAO (Saiedi et al., 2020). This first example revealed the characteristic properties that make DAOs a unique vehicle for producing material wealth (Hsieh, Vergne, Anderson, Lakhani, & Reitzig, 2018).

Bitcoin was unique (and uniquely successful) because it was the first social structure of its kind to provide the market with something it desperately wanted: a censorship-resistant, transparent store of value (Tomescu & Devadas, 2017). It did so without shareholders, without the use of force, without any legal entity, and without any employees. It did so by aligning the interests of consumers, capital, and labor in the same motion.

Bitcoin provided consumers with a store of value that could not be stolen from them (Yermack, 2015). It provided labor with a standardized protocol for providing that labor and a limitless, yet transparent way to make that provision. It provided the capital with a straightforward path to preserve wealth and benefit from Bitcoin's adoption, which was to buy and hold Bitcoin. Finally, it provided these means so that any of the three parties supplying made the value proposition to the other two parties more compelling. In this way, participation in any part of the Bitcoin ecosystem (consumers seeking to preserve wealth from state confiscation and other forms of censorship, capital seeking capital growth, and labor seeking returns) drove value for the other components.

In this first instance of BT, we have a foretaste of the dramatic, global changes that blockchain could bring. Bitcoin, at the end of the first quarter of 2021, standed at almost $59 million, for a total market capitalization of almost $1 trillion USD, making it by far the largest financial 'institution' in the world financial market (CoinDesk, 2021). All this achieved in less than 13 years since Bitcoin was first revealed, making it the fastest-growing financial asset in world history (Liquid, 2020). Notably, it has achieved this dramatic valuation entirely thanks to its ability to align capital, labor, and consumer interests, so that all three parties are driving its adoption. The power to align these participants in creating material value is the non-obvious, novel use case of blockchains that we are only now starting to see clearly.

Since the emergence of Bitcoin and its identification as a DAO, a few hundred more of these organizations have been created, notably Ethereum and, subsequently, Yearn Finance. (Hsieh et al., 2018).

ETHEREUM AND YEARN FOLLOW

The characteristics of Bitcoin as a social structure are not one-offs; they are not unique to Bitcoin alone. Instead, they are familiar to a host of different cryptocurrency projects, and a number of those projects have been executed in a manner akin to Bitcoin with comparable rates of growth and adoption. First among those is Ethereum, which launched in 2015 and whose market value at the end of the first quarter of 2021 stands at $221 billion USD (CoinMarketCap, 2020a), and Yearn Finance, which launched in 2020 and whose market value stands in the same date at $1.3 billion USD (CoinMarketCap, 2020b). Both projects are decentralized, lack liable legal entities or reporting hierarchies, and both have grown rapidly (Becker, 2020; Wood Gavin, 2014). Ethereum has its blockchain, while Yearn Finance lives on Ethereum's blockchain as a smart contract set (yearn.finance, 2021). As is becoming clear, the characteristics of Bitcoin were not "a flash in the pan"; they were the harbingers of a new social structure for creating material wealth and getting work done.

The authors will detail four examples and take a more in-depth look into the value being created and into the parties that create such value, starting with Bitcoin.

Bitcoin's value creation depends on a host of parties and has dramatically increased in complexity over the years. The central value creators in the Bitcoin network are the miners (SFOX, 2018b; Tuwiner, 2020), the Bitcoin Core developers (SFOX, 2018b), the exchanges and wallets (Edwood, 2020; Volety et al., 2019), and the block explorers (Romano & Schmid, 2017).

There are also many other parties offering a host of technical and financial services, but the above four groups sit at the center of value creation for Bitcoin.

The Bitcoin miners do the crucial work of mining blocks in the Bitcoin network, which they do by executing challenging computation puzzles. Those who mine fastest receive Bitcoin block rewards (Kroll et al., 2013). The mining difficulty increases with the amount of computation in play (measured in hashrate), so the more hash power there is, the harder it gets to earn rewards. This increasing difficulty makes Bitcoin more secure, since any hostile third party must bring more hash power to bear than at least 51% of the miners, which becomes more expensive as the mining difficulty increases (Yang et al., 2019).

The second major group of value creators is the Bitcoin Core developers. Spread worldwide, the Bitcoin Core developers oversee the Bitcoin Core codebase maintenance and add new features as time goes by. They are the primary reason Bitcoin has proven resilient (Cuneta, 2017).

The third major group of value creators is exchanges and wallets. Exchanges provide on-ramps from fiat currencies into Bitcoin and off-ramps from Bitcoin into fiat currencies. These parties help users store their Bitcoin, make Bitcoin liquid, and put Bitcoin to work to purchase goods and services (Edwood, 2020; Volety et al., 2019).

The fourth major group of value creators is the generators and maintainers of block explorers. These parties provide an interface for interacting with the Bitcoin network and auditing on-chain activity. Without them, the utility of the network decreases significantly (Romano & Schmid, 2017).

The Bitcoin network effectively incentivizes these groups to work together and create value in an accessible, censorship-resistant store of value. As they do this well, the consumers purchase more Bitcoin, which further drives cash flow to these parties (Agrawal et al., 2014).

The most crucial factor is the consumers themselves; for the above parties' value creation work to be justifiable, Bitcoin needs to accrue to it early on, which must come from a set of early adopters. Bitcoin supplies these early adopters effortlessly because the creators of most of these services (mining, Bitcoin

Core developers, exchanges and wallets, and block explorers) themselves want censorship-resistant money, and so serve as the early adopters that put the Bitcoin adoption cycle in motion (Agrawal et al., 2014).

When we understand that the infrastructure Bitcoin needed to grow as a censorship-resistant store of value was built by the early consumers of the network itself, the importance of DAOs as a new social structure becomes apparent. These early consumers do not just benefit from the service itself; they also benefit from any adoption of the service following them, by virtue of their owning the value capture instrument of service itself (Bitcoin in the case of the Bitcoin network; Lecarme, 2019).

As such, the alignment between early (and generic) capital to fund a venture, the labor needed to build it, and the consumers that validate and perpetuate the service is clear.

ETHEREUM AS THE WORLD COMPUTER

The second great example of a DAO as a new social structure is Ethereum, the decentralized smart contract blockchain. Started by a small group of Bitcoin early adopters in late 2013 (Buterin, 2013), Ethereum has become the market leader of smart contract blockchains, and its growth was marked by the same properties that catapulted Bitcoin to success.

A smart contract is a piece of code implementing arbitrary rules on a computer with distributed consensus (a blockchain), such that when the code is live, it cannot be censored or shut down (Szabo, 1997). Smart contracts are analogous to the business logic instantiated in code in businesses and organizations worldwide, the difference being that here the code runs on a code that no one party controls or can turn off (Nakamura et al., 2020).

From the start of Ethereum's journey, a core group of consumers looking to use its service gathered around the project. Their support began as private investment contributions and led to a USD 18 million crowd sale, the largest of its kind up to that time. These users became the first parties to build decentralized applications (dApps) on top of the Ethereum network. This movement is most clearly seen in Consensys (https://consensys.net), created by the Ethereum co-founder Joseph Lubin, the first company to begin building dApps en masse. These include Metamask (the dominant browser-based wallet for blockchain applications) and Gitcoin (the most extensive developer grants product in crypto). Once again, we see the early alignment of consumers with the capital and labor necessary to birth the project in the first place (Zheng et al., 2020).

Whereas Bitcoin started entirely grassroots and was limited to no funding whatsoever, Ethereum began its life with a massive capital injection (SFOX, 2018a). It also requires an ecosystem of services around it to produce value for its consumers in the form of a trustworthy platform for smart contracts. In the case of Ethereum, these services are the miners, ethereum core developers, exchanges and wallets, block explorers, and lastly, dapp developers.

These services quickly gathered around Ethereum in the same way that they gathered around Bitcoin, except for Dapp developers (Smith, 2019). For a while, Ethereum could leverage the same communities, resources, and early adopter spirit that Bitcoin had already built, but there was no previously existing community of Dapp developers. Here, Ethereum had to break new ground.

The challenge with creating a Dapp developer community is that demand for Dapps depends on the demand for whatever value individual Dapps provide. To tackle this, the Ethereum community started building applications for things they needed, including data feeds (Santiment, Cindicator), DAO smart contracts (The DAO, Aragon, DAOstack), decentralized exchanges (Bancor, Uniswap), and more. This growth was once again facilitated by the core community itself, which invested its Ether (the native currency of the Ethereum network) into a great many crowd sales for these Dapps, funding them the same way Ethereum was funded.

Eventually, this resulted in thousands of Dapps and billions of dollars of value backing them being birthed on the Ethereum network, which is where we find ourselves today (Faridi, 2020). The same early consumers of Ethereum's value helped create demand for Ethereum's service and captured that value in the form of upside on Ether. Once again, we see the alignment between capital, labor, and consumers in a blockchain-based organization catapulting a new technology to dramatic valuation and adoption.

At the end of the first quarter of 2021, Ethereum's market valuation stands at around $221 billion USD, with a price of almost $2 million USD per Ether (CoinMarketCap, 2020a).

YEARN FINANCE: DECENTRALISED YIELD AGGREGATOR

Whereas the two previous examples are protocols built into a blockchain network, the next example is a custom-built DAO that lives on the Ethereum Network, called Yearn Finance (https://yearn.finance/). Even though Yearn lacks a native blockchain, its operation and the manner of its growth parallels those of Bitcoin and Ethereum (Ivan on Tech, 2020).

Publicly launched in early 2020, Yearn is a decentralized yield aggregator for decentralized financial (DeFi) products. Users deposit funds into a Yearn Finance smart contract called a vault. These vaults then redirect those funds to whichever DeFi product offers the highest annual percentage return via lending those funds out to other parties. Yearn Finance provides value by having the simplest to use, most up to date Annual Performance Report (APR) data, thereby maximizing Yearn users' yield.

Yearn was launched as a product by a single developer, Andre Cronje, and has since moved all operational ownership and responsibilities to a DAO, called Yearn Finance. Since moving to the DAO, the accumulation of funds in Yearn has grown dramatically (from $0 in early January 2020 to approximately $247 million USD as of March 31st, 2021), and the combined market cap of the Yearn governance token (YFI) sits at $1.3 billion USD (CoinMarketCap, 2020b).

Yearn's growth is due to a combination of the open nature of DeFi and its close alignment with its consumers. First and foremost, the creator of Yearn, Andre Cronje, created Yearn just for his use, but when he opened up access to Yearn, he found that all users had similar interests to his own. To further fuel growth and decentralize ownership of Yearn, Andre created the Yearn DAO, governed by holders of a token called YFI, which was distributed entirely to early users of Yearn Finance over nine days.

With Yearn, the alignment with its service consumers is so explicit that its users entirely own the governance token, YFI. This cohesion gives Yearn several substantial advantages over other products in its space. It gets rapid and immediate feedback on its product from its users. Its users provide the labor to build out and drive adoption of new products. It has a limitless pool of labor seeking to build out new services to solve the problems Yearn has in-house.

Again, we see the defining feature of Yearn as a protocol that drove its own growth: the alignment between consumers of a service, the capital necessary to start it, and the labor necessary to provide the service. This collaboration is possible only because of the decentralized and uncensorable nature of the Yearn smart contracts, making it effortless for anyone to get involved in Yearn and contribute to its growth.

API3: A DECENTRALISED DATA FEEDS NETWORK

Whereas the previous three examples provide censorship-resistant money, trustless computation, and a permissionless hedge fund, API3 uses the same economic structure to provide trustworthy data feeds to decentralized applications. Data feeds are defined as mechanisms that provide updated data from data sources to users. They are typically used on websites, apps, or another online tools.

For perspective, modern commerce is dependent on the interaction between a massive number of application programming interfaces (APIs; Thorneycroft, 2020). These APIs provide standardized communication and data structuring, allowing an online storefront to securely communicate with its payment processor, which in turn securely communicates with Know Your Customer (KYC) and fraud detection services (Hyduchack, 2020; Team, 2019).

In the blockchain industry, APIs represent a more difficult challenge. Whereas a standard API - trusted and operated by a company or individual - may satisfy the security needs in a traditional e-commerce context, they do not satisfy decentralized finance's security requirements. A critical attack vector for decentralized financial applications is manipulating data feeds (called 'oracles' in the blockchain industry) for profit. If a data feed misreports key information, this can lead to mispricing by any application depending on that data feed, such as decentralized exchanges, derivatives markets, and insurance protocols (Apis & Benligiray, 2020).

API3 uses a token incentive scheme and DAO to bootstrap a network of trustworthy data feeds. API3 participants can stake their DAO tokens to get access to staking fees. These begin as inflation and are eventually derived from API fees. Afterwards, staking tokens put that stake up as collateral. In the event of a data feed malfunction or mispricing, the collateral is paid out to compensate the affected parties for their loss. Governance over the API3 network and its parameters (staking yield, data feeds selection, and grants) is controlled by the API3 participants who stake their DAO tokens.

Thus, users participating in API3 are incentivized to launch as many data feeds as possible, provided those data feeds are secure, as insecure data feeds result in a direct financial cost to them, driving adoption in the form of collateral payouts (Apis & Benligiray, 2020).

In this incentive model, we again see the alignment of capital, labor, and consumers. Staking API3 tokens, which is putting up capital, entitles purchasers to do work (labor) in selecting data feeds and financially backing them. This aligns those putting up capital and labor that generates value by combining them into the same party. Finally, the consumers of those services are decentralized applications themselves that produce value by making claims and thereby surfacing problematic data feeds, which increases the data feed quality of the entire network.

DAOS: ILLUSION OR REALITY?

As it has been mentioned throughout the chapter, the central advantage of a DAO is to solve existing problems in corporations and organizations, which are mostly related to management and organizational issues of the corporations and organizations, with top-down structures that end up invalidating or devaluing contributions that come from the bottom of the pyramid and not from the top. The impossibility of power games arising is another advantage. Because of its autonomous structure, once the rules are established, the DAO executes them without the need for management. Everything happens as it is and when it is supposed to happen. And then, there is transparency as one of the major advantages of DAOs.

Everything that happens within the organization stays on the blockchain forever. Every individual who holds a stake in a DAO has a say in how the funds will be spent and managed. All stakeholders have equal responsibility.

However, there are some drawbacks associated with this system. DAOs are very much in their infancy. They are not only still lacking actual finished software solutions, but, in many ways, they also still lack some of the basic science required to understand the full dynamic through which self-organizing social systems can work in a stable, safe, and sustainable fashion. DAOs are in a experimental phase, as their enthusiasts try to understand the parameters and dynamics needed for them to reliably create value (Chohan, 2017).

There are some dangers and weaknesses associated with DAOs. Many things can go wrong with badly designed social systems. One of the first large-scale DAOs was hacked at the cost of millions of dollars (Finley, 2016). A single vulnerability (such as a logic error, an incorrect mathematical operation, or systemic flaw) can effectively destroy the DAO. The code in the DAOs is visible to the entire ecosystem, and any attempt to patch vulnerabilities are made more difficult by the universal visibility of all attempted fixes, which can be fronton for opportunistic exploitation (Chohan, 2017). The author has created a protocol himself, called Immunefi, specifically for safely surfacing and disclosing these vulnerabilities and protecting DAOs at large.

Governance and legal issues are also present. In terms of governance, there is a problem in terms of the voting processing on DAO-related modifications. BitShares is a clear example of this situation. BitShares was a decentralized platform designed to create a more effective payment network, however, it has been faced with low participation, a lack of engagement by members (Chohan, 2017). Shareholder participation in DAOs is an issue (Blog, 2020).

Legally speaking, DAOs are associated with indeterminacy. The legal status of DAOs is still not very explicit. This may have repercussions in terms of openness to adoption of and participation in this decentralized organization (Blog, 2020). This is a factor that cannot be overlooked. In the past, several similar organizational structures have been ruled by the U.S. Securities and Exchange Commission as illegal (Chohan, 2017).

The risks of voter manipulation are another issue that has been debated. It is critical that safeguards exist so that voter groups do not program machinations against the DAO machine. This horizontal accountability will be a necessary feature to preserve the democratic nature of the crypto-anarchist, thinking underlying the DAO (Chohan, 2017).

Several distributed systems for organizational management already exist, as presented in this chapter. Although DAOs are still experimental in nature, their potential should not be underestimated. They will only grow as the underlying technology develops and our understanding of distributed self-organizing systems matures. The blockchain and new distributed models of governance can play a major role providing a trust infrastructure - platforms and off-the-shelf organizational solutions to massive social systems -, the type that would be required to develop functional global institutions. Further research should focus on building on existing foundations to propose theoretical and practical solutions for DAO functionality in light of the above challenges.

CONCLUSION

The world is changing rapidly, and the internet is entering rapidly into a new technologic era as Web 2.0 gives way to an emerging set of BTs. They offer many attractive new technological economics and social innovations that will transform many fields from finance and insurance to energy and healthcare. However, the most fantastic thing about this technology is, as one commentator noted, an "institutional technology" at the heart of social organizations and institutions; namely, the question of how we work together by exchanging value within a trusted environment (Allen, Berg, Markey-Towler, Novak, & Potts, 2020).

The blockchain is a technology that enables automated trust and the automated frictionless value exchange. This capacity to automate social institutions' essential workings with increased interconnectivity means that one increasingly has the technological means to create massive organizations that are truly distributed and automated, something never seen before. The DAOs demonstrate this potential to revolutionize human social institutions.

At the core of these distributed organizations, there is the idea that groups are about value, which some form of a token can measure. With distributed ledgers, markets are created out of tokens representing whatever value system the organization is based around. It is this value token organization that regulates the system and defines anyone's position within the group.

In this chapter, the concept of DAO and its evolution was presented. It demonstrates the innovative side of DAOs and how promising they are, especially at the business and organizational level, and how it can promote an autonomous, self-managed, transparent, more efficient, secure, and democratic organization.

Current examples of DAO, including Bitcoin, Ethereum, Yearn Finance, and API3, were also introduced to the reader. It is fundamental to underly that these are not unique examples; there are many similar projects in the blockchain space operating in the same way, and many of those have similar growth patterns. However, these four examples are harbingers of an unexpected future enabled by blockchain technologies, one where products owned by their users compete head-to-head with corporations for market share.

This new kind of economic structure is the rarely noticed novel use case of BT. It is not only that it facilitates a new way to store and transfer value and data; it is that protocols and DAOs are fundamentally new ways of coordinating work, and several early examples have proved to be effective at creating vast amounts of wealth and value for users. Nevertheless, it is also because of their novelty that one must be aware that there is still a lot to learn, that many mistakes will be made and that these systems still have a lot to prove before DAOs are fully adopted by humanity.

REFERENCES

Agrawal, A., Catalini, C., & Goldfarb, A. (2014). Some simple economics of crowdfunding. *Innovation Policy and the Economy*, *14*, 63–97. Advance online publication. doi:10.1086/674021

Apis, D., & Benligiray, B. (2020). *Decentralized APIs for Web 3.0*. Academic Press.

Arslanian, H., Fischer, F., Arslanian, H., & Fischer, F. (2019). Blockchain As an Enabling Technology. In The Future of Finance. doi:10.1007/978-3-030-14533-0_10

Becker, C. (2020). *Financial services powered by Ethereum smart contracts grow exponentially.* Investec. https://www.investec.com/en_za/focus/innovation/financial-services-powered-by-ethereum-smart-contracts-grow-exponentially-in-2020.html

Biersteker, T. J., & Weber, C. (2011). The social construction of state sovereignty. In State Sovereignty as Social Construct. doi:10.1017/CBO9780511598685.001

Bruland, K., & Mowery, D. C. (2004). *Innovation through time.* Georgia Institute of Technology.

Buterin, V. (2013). A next-generation smart contract and decentralized application platform. *Etherum,* 1–36.

CoinDesk. (2021). *Bitcoin.* Www.Coindesk.Com. https://www.coindesk.com/price/bitcoin

CoinMarketCap. (2020a). *Ethereum.* https://coinmarketcap.com/currencies/ethereum/

CoinMarketCap. (2020b). *yearn.finance.* https://coinmarketcap.com/currencies/yearn-finance/

Cuneta, M. (2017). *The Big Bitcoin Battle: What I Found Out About Bitcoin VS BCash.* Hackernoon. https://medium.com/hackernoon/the-big-bitcoin-battle-what-i-found-out-about-bitcoin-vs-bcash-d9ebca8d370e

De Filippi, P. (2016). The interplay between decentralization and privacy: the case of blockchain technologies. *Journal of Peer Production.*

Economist, T. (2015). The promise of the blockchain: The trust machine'. *The economist, 31,* 27.

Edwood, F. (2020). *Cryptocurrency On-Ramps and Off-Ramps, Explained.* Cointelegraph. https://cointelegraph.com/explained/cryptocurrency-on-ramps-and-off-ramps-explained

Faridi, O. (2020). *12 Billion in Decentralized Application (dApp) Transactions Processed during Q2 2020, with Ethereum (ETH) Accounting for 82% of "Created Value": Report.* Crowded Media Group.

Greif, A. (2006). Family structure, institutions, and growth: The origins and implications of western corporations. *The American Economic Review, 96*(2), 308–312. Advance online publication. doi:10.1257/000282806777212602

Hill, T. P. (1977). On goods and services. *Review of Income and Wealth, 23*(4), 315–338. Advance online publication. doi:10.1111/j.1475-4991.1977.tb00021.x

Hyduchack. (2020). *API Tools Offer Easier KYC/AML Compliance.* Aver. https://medium.com/goaver/api-tools-offer-easier-kyc-aml-compliance-e852a0c52902

Iansiti, M., & Lakhani, K. R. (2017). The truth about blockchain. Harvard Business Review.

Ivan on Tech. (2020). *A Closer Look - What is Yearn Finance and YFI?* Ivan on Tech Academy.

Jim Sergent. (2020). *Apple is first $2 trillion US company. What that would look like in iPhones.* USA Today. https://eu.usatoday.com/in-depth/money/2020/08/19/apple-2-trillion-company-worth-what-looks-like-iphones/3353398001/

Kroll, J. a, Davey, I. C., & Felten, E. W. (2013). The Economics of Bitcoin Mining, or Bitcoin in the Presence of Adversaries. *The Twelfth Workshop on the Economics of Information Security (WEIS 2013).*

Lecarme, L. (2019). *What Is the Early Adopters Advantage in Crypto?* The Startup. https://medium.com/swlh/what-is-the-early-adopters-advantage-in-crypto-4ee18984f707

Li, Y. (2019). Emerging blockchain-based applications and techniques. In Service Oriented Computing and Applications. doi:10.100711761-019-00281-x

Liquid. (2020). *Bitcoin price history & future of the fastest-growing asset class.* Beginner Guide. https://blog.liquid.com/bitcoin-price-history

Maher, M. E., & Andersson, T. (2005). Corporate Governance: Effects on Firm Performance and Economic Growth. SSRN *Electronic Journal.* doi:10.2139srn.218490

Morgan, G. (2009). *Globalization, multinationals and institutional diversity.* Academic Press.

Nakamoto, S. (2009). *Bitcoin: A Peer-to-Peer Electronic Cash System.* Cryptography Mailing List. Https://Metzdowd.Com

Nakamura, Y., Zhang, Y., Sasabe, M., & Kasahara, S. (2020). Exploiting Smart Contracts for Capability-Based Access Control in the Internet of Things. *Sensors (Basel)*, *20*(6), 1793. doi:10.339020061793 PMID:32213888

Namasudra, S., Deka, G. C., Johri, P., Hosseinpour, M., & Gandomi, A. H. (2020). The Revolution of Blockchain: State-of-the-Art and Research Challenges. *Archives of Computational Methods in Engineering.* Advance online publication. doi:10.100711831-020-09426-0

Pomeranz, K. (2001). *The World's First Corporations.* The Globalist. https://www.theglobalist.com/the-worlds-first-corporations/

Romano, D., & Schmid, G. (2017). *Beyond Bitcoin: A Critical Look at Blockchain-Based Systems.* Cryptography. doi:10.3390/cryptography1020015

Saiedi, E., Broström, A., & Ruiz, F. (2020). Global drivers of cryptocurrency infrastructure adoption. *Small Business Economics.* Advance online publication. doi:10.100711187-019-00309-8

SFOX. (2018a). *From Crowdfunded Blockchain to ICO Machine: An Ethereum Price History.* SFOX Inc.

SFOX. (2018b). *Miners, Developers, and Users: The Checks and Balances of Bitcoin.* https://www.sfox.com/blog/miners-developers-and-users-the-checks-and-balances-of-bitcoin/

Sims, A. (2020). Blockchain and Decentralised Autonomous Organizations (DAOs): The Evolution of Companies? SSRN *Electronic Journal.* doi:10.2139srn.3524674

Smith, K. (2019). *Ethereum losing share as dapp developers choose other networks.* Brave New Coin.

Szabo, N. (1997). Formalizing and Securing Relationships on Public Networks. *First Monday*, *2*(9). Advance online publication. doi:10.5210/fm.v2i9.548

Team, C. E. (2019). *What are Communication APIs and why are they needed?* CEQUENS. https://www.cequens.com/story-hub/what-are-communication-apis-and-why-are-they-needed

Thorneycroft, R. (2020). *The Role of APIs in Modern Commerce.* Profound. https://www.profound.works/digital-transformation/application-programming-interfaces-for-headless-ecommerce/

Tomescu, A., & Devadas, S. (2017). Catena: Efficient Non-equivocation via Bitcoin. *Proceedings - IEEE Symposium on Security and Privacy*. 10.1109/SP.2017.19

Transformation, T. C. (2010). Corporations in the Modern Era. *Tuitt, 2006*, 280–332.

Tuwiner, J. (2020). *What is Bitcoin Mining and How Does it Work?* Buy Bitcoin Worldwide. https://www.buybitcoinworldwide.com/mining/

Volety, T., Saini, S., McGhin, T., Liu, C. Z., & Choo, K. K. R. (2019). Cracking Bitcoin wallets: I want what you have in the wallets. *Future Generation Computer Systems*, *91*, 136–143. Advance online publication. doi:10.1016/j.future.2018.08.029

Weber, M. (1978). *Economy and society: An outline of interpretive sociology* (Vol. 1). Univ of California Press.

Werbach, K. (2018). *The blockchain and the new architecture of trust*. MIT Press. doi:10.7551/mitpress/11449.001.0001

Wood Gavin. (2014). *Ethereum: A Secure Decentralised Generalised Transaction Ledger*. Ethereum Project Yellow Paper.

Yang, X., Chen, Y., & Chen, X. (2019). Effective scheme against 51% attack on proof-of-work blockchain with history weighted information. *Proceedings - 2019 2nd IEEE International Conference on Blockchain, Blockchain 2019*. 10.1109/Blockchain.2019.00041

yearn.finance. (2021). *Introduction to Yearn*. https://docs.yearn.finance

Yermack, D. (2015). Is Bitcoin a Real Currency? An Economic Appraisal. In *Handbook of Digital Currency*. Bitcoin, Innovation, Financial Instruments, and Big Data; doi:10.1016/B978-0-12-802117-0.00002-3

Zheng, Z., Dai, H.-N., Tang, M., & Chen, X. (Eds.). (2020). *Blockchain and Trustworthy Systems: First International Conference, BlockSys 2019, Guangzhou, China, December 7–8, 2019, Proceedings*. Springer Nature.

Zheng, Z., Xie, S., Dai, H. N., Chen, X., & Wang, H. (2018). Blockchain challenges and opportunities: A survey. *International Journal of Web and Grid Services*. doi:10.1504/IJWGS.2018.095647

Chapter 6
Combining E–Commerce and Blockchain Technologies to Solve Problems and Improve Business Results:
A Literature Review

Albérico Travassos Rosário
https://orcid.org/0000-0003-4793-4110
GOVCOPP, IADE, Universidade Europeia, Portugal

ABSTRACT

The internet and digital transformation have changed our relations with the market. These technologies have been developing continuously, creating opportunities for new business models, and e-commerce has grown overwhelmingly worldwide, changing the consumption process of a large part of the world's population. Companies are increasingly using blockchain technology to improve and create new global trading business models. Blockchain had its first application in cryptocurrencies, but it has quickly become a major solution in all sorts of activity sectors, providing increased security in commercial transactions. An important question is how the blockchain can leverage e-commerce in solving problems and improving business results. It was concluded that blockchain could leverage e-commerce in the four fundamental areas of (1) e-commerce financial transactions, (2) e-commerce supply chain management, (3) e-commerce forecasting and contractual relations, and (4) e-commerce transactions systems' trust and credibility.

BACKGROUND AND INTRODUCTION

The cumulative, transformative impacts of the advent of the Internet and the ever-increasing ubiquity of novel digital technologies on the very nature of contemporary human life are undoubtedly incomparable in magnitude to any other effects of the plethora of notable, drastic developments that have transpired

DOI: 10.4018/978-1-7998-7363-1.ch006

throughout the history of human existence. The most profound effects of the Internet and digitalization are, in this regard, arguably most manifest and apparent in the ways these new modalities of social connection have impacted the realm of the conduct of business worldwide. More specifically, the Internet and digital technologies continue to have a significant transformative effect on the patterns and tendencies of modern consumption and how new businesses market their offerings. Extant empirical research demonstrates, in this regard, that the Internet as a medium of marketing has multiple times the influence on consumers than traditional mediums like print media and television (Cochoy et al., 2017). Consumers rely increasingly on the Internet in different ways to make different decisions, including purchasing ones.

From the perspective of modern companies, the Internet has proven to improve marketing strategies effectively and approaches in diverse areas, including the conduct of marketing research, customer service and experience provision, product distribution, and problem-solving (Cochoy et al., 2017). The efficiency and performance in contemporary organizations brought by Internet marketing's intrinsic value give them a massive flow of information, new products, services development, and bolstered market transparency (Cochoy et al., 2017). The sum of new opportunities to organizations brought by the Internet and digital ways has unfolded over recent history through several distinct paths.

One unique path has been the fast development of electronic commerce. E-commerce refers to digital applications acting "as a trading bridge between merchants and purchasers" in an 'online' environment (Kathuria et al., 2019, p.1). The present proliferation of e-commerce companies best shows the rising importance in the modern consumer's life, "there are more than three million companies worldwide engaged in e-commerce," with notable examples of highly successful e-commerce giants like Amazon, Alibaba, and eBay (Kathuria et al., 2019). Driven by rapid advancements in e-commerce and Internet technologies, online shopping has drastically transformed how consumers to shop and buyers trade, mainly through the introduction of unprecedented levels of speed, efficiency, and convenience.

Another essential path that the Internet and the digital world have evolved in commerce has been blockchain technology. This technology can be described generically as constituting "a fully distributed system for cryptographically capturing and storing a consistent, immutable linear event log of transactions between network actors" (Marten & Kai, 2017, p.3). Based on the definition above alone, it is clear that blockchain technology, underpinned by the pervasive penetration of novel cloud-connected digital devices in addition to cloud-based data analytics and storage capabilities, can be potentially disrupted by technical innovations in the age of digitalization—current blockchain use cases in the digitalization of asset ownership evidence this fact. The technology is increasingly demonstrated and seen as a reliable modality for contract ownership and management and for conducting nearly unimpeachable but distributable audit trails through the mediums of distributed cryptocurrencies (Kathuria et al., 2019). The programmable and highly flexible provisions of blockchain technology, particularly concerning payment and transaction platforms, facilitate a broad spectrum of novel financial instruments.

More importantly, the feasibility of combining e-commerce and blockchain technologies is evident from the descriptions and definitions mentioned before. For instance, being a given fact that electronic payments and transactions are an indispensable part of e-commerce systems, it is reasonable to appreciate the possible integration of blockchain technology into e-commerce (Zhao & O'Mahony, 2020). Surprisingly, current digital innovations have failed to generate new applications that leverage e-commerce with blockchain technology. Moreover, to the best of knowledge verified as an author, it is thought that it does not provide a unified framework under which incorporating blockchain into e-commerce and vice versa is achievable. Against this backdrop, the main focus of this discussion is filling the gap mentioned above in the literature. This work wants to build an epistemological basis for that integration by exploring a research question regarding the potential ways in which blockchain technology can leverage e-commerce. It achieves the stated objective through a comprehensive and in-depth review of extant and emerging literature on the subjects of interest and, through thematic analysis, identifies four distinct pieces of the rationale for combining blockchain and e-commerce.

METHODOLOGICAL APPROACH

As stated before, this work's purpose is to get an exploratory review of a vast and literature to the over-arching research question at hand, particularly about answering the inquiry on how blockchain technology can leverage e-commerce. A literature review is a research methodology within the field of business research that is exceptionally consistent with this study's fundamental objective because it offers an evidence-based approach to evaluating the collective evidence available in a particular area of business inquiry (Synder, 2019; Rosário et al., 2021). More specifically, to bolster the methodological rigor and thoroughness of the research evidence available along the lines of this paper's research question, the study utilizes the integrative approach to the literature review process. Synder (2019) defines the integrative approach as one that has a different purpose relative to a traditional, systematic, and semi-systematic review of literature in that it aims to "assess, critique, and synthesize the literature on a research topic in a way that enables new theoretical frameworks and perspectives to emerge" (p.335). In the context of this paper, the aim is to facilitate a collated body of evidence that supports the emergence of theoretical frameworks, perspectives, and paradigms for the integration of blockchain technology and e-commerce.

The study continues as follows: (i) definition of the research question; (ii) study location; (iii) selection and evaluation of studies; (iv) analysis and synthesis; (v) presentation of results; and (vi) discussion and conclusions of the results. This methodology ensures that the review is comprehensive, auditable, and replicable and answers specific research questions (Rosário et al., 2021; Rosário & Cuz, 2019; Sacavém et al., 2019).

Under the said choice of research design, the articles whence the desired evidence is derived were retrieved and collected via an extensive, systematic search of the literature on the SCOPUS database. It was chosen because it is one of the most relevant peer-review databases in the scientific and academic environment.

Accordingly, the search strategy implemented the two key search terms of "e-commerce" and "block-chain" combined through the "AND" Boolean operator. The search was further delimited to articles published until November 2020 and to the scholarly subject area of business.

Overall, the search strategy yielded a total of 51 articles. This pool of eligible studies was subjected to further assessments of relevance and quality. Reading through the titles, abstracts, and reference pages of each article in the pool of studies allowed for narrowing the sample down to 44 articles, with the remainder excluded based on a pre-specified threshold of pertinence. Subsequent application of the criteria in a standardized quality appraisal checklist for literature reviews facilitated the exclusion of a further eight studies on the grounds of methodological rigor. Generally, a sample of 36 studies cited within the reference section at the end of this paper emerged from the literature search and assessment processes. Of the 36 publications selected, 3 in open access and others 33, 27 in conference, eight articles, and one book chapter.

PUBLICATION DISTRIBUTION

Peer-reviewed articles on the subject can be tracked since 2016. 2020 was the year with the most significant number of peer-reviewed articles, reaching 11. Figure 1 summarizes the peer-reviewed literature published until 2020.

The publications were sorted out as follows: Proceedings Of The International Conference On Electronic Business Iceb (7); Proceedings 2018 IEEE 15th International Conference On E-Business Engineering Icebe 2018 (6); Proceedings 2020 International Conference On E-Commerce And Internet Technology Ecit 2020 (5); Lecture Notes In Business Information Processing and Proceedings 14th IEEE International Conference On E-Business Engineering Icebe 2017 Including 13th Workshop On Service-Oriented Applications Integration And Collaboration Soaic 207, topped with 3 publications; Computer Law And Security Review; Electronic Commerce Research And Applications; Technological Forecasting And Social Change; Technology In Society (2); 2020 2nd Conference On Blockchain Research And Applications For Innovative Networks And Services Brains 2020; Conference Proceedings Of The 7th International Symposium On Project Management Ispm 2019; Handbook Of Blockchain Digital Finance And Inclusion Volume 1 Cryptocurrency Fintech Insurtech And Regulation; Picmet 2018 Portland International Conference On Management Of Engineering And Technology Managing Technological Entrepreneurship The Engine For Economic Growth Proceedings the with 1 publication each.

We can say that a growing interest in publications on entrepreneurship is emerging.

Figure 1. Documents by year
Source: own elaboration

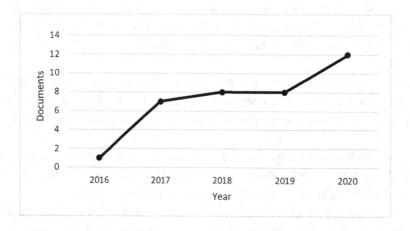

Table 1 analyzes the Scimago Journal & Country Rank (SJR), the best quartile, and the H index by publication. The Technological Forecasting and Social Change is the most quoted publication with 1,820 (SJR), Q1, and H index 103. Of 13 publications, six are not yet indexed in the SJR, the best quartile, and the H index per publication.

As shown in Table 1, the significant majority of articles on blockchain and e-commerce are not yet indexed.

Table 1. Scimago journal and country rank impact factor.

Title	SJR	Best Quartile	H Index
Technological Forecasting and Social Change	1,820	Q1	103
Electronic Commerce Research and Applications	1,240	Q1	69
Computer Law and Security Review	1,070	Q1	32
Technology in Society	0,570	Q2	47
Lecture Notes in Business Information Processing	0,260	Q3	44
Proceedings 14th IEEE International Conference on E Business Engineering Icebe 2017 Including 13th Workshop On Service Oriented Applications Integration And Collaboration Soaic 207	0,170	-*	5
Proceedings of The International Conference on Electronic Business Iceb	0,110	-*	6
Picmet 2018 Portland International Conference on Management of Engineering and Technology Managing Technological Entrepreneurship the Engine For Economic Growth Proceedings	-*	-*	9
Proceedings 2018 IEEE 15th International Conference on E Business Engineering Icebe 2018	-*	-*	-*
Proceedings 2020 International Conference on E Commerce and Internet Technology Ecit 2020	-*	-*	-*
2020 2nd Conference on Blockchain Research and Applications for Innovative Networks and Services Brains 2020	-*	-*	-*
Conference Proceedings of the 7th International Symposium on Project Management Ispm 2019	-*	-*	-*
Handbook of Blockchain Digital Finance and Inclusion Volume 1 Cryptocurrency Fintech Insurtech And Regulation	-*	-*	-*

Note: *data not available.
Source: own elaboration

The subject areas covered by the 36 scientific articles were: Business, Management and Accounting (36); Computer Science (30); Decision Sciences (19); Engineering (10); Economics, Econometrics, and Finance (6); Social Sciences (5); Mathematics (3); Psychology (2); Environmental Science (1).

The most quoted article was "A Blockchain-Based Supply Chain Quality Management Framework" from Chen et al. (2017) with 58 quotes published in the paper presented at the Proceedings - 14th IEEE International Conference on E-Business Engineering, ICEBE 2017 - Including 13th Workshop on Service-Oriented Applications, Integration, and Collaboration, SOAIC 2 with 0,170 (SJR), the best quartile (data not available) and with H index (5). The published article focuses on improving supply chain quality management by adopting blockchain technology, proposing a blockchain framework on supply chain quality management.

In Figure 2, we see the evolution of quotes from articles published between 2015 and 2020. The number of quotes shows positive net growth with an R^2 of 77% for 2015-2020, with 2020 reaching 66 citations.

The h-index was used to measure the productivity and impact of the published work, based on the largest number of articles included that had at least the same number of quotes. Of the documents considered for the h-index, 23 have been cited at least 23 times.

In Table 2 in the Appendix, citations of all scientific articles until 2020 are analyzed; 18 documents were not cited until 2020 (2018, 8; 2019, 52; and 2020, 66), with a total of 126 citations.

Figure 2. Evolution of citations between 2015 and 2020.
Source: own elaboration

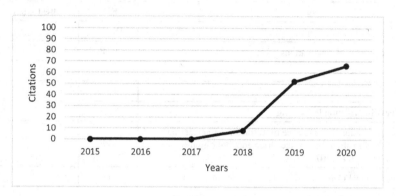

Table 3 in the Appendix examines the self-quotation of documents until 2020. Of articles, 36 were self-quotation for a total of 15 self-quotation "Design of evaluation system for digital education operational skill competition based on blockchain" was self-quoted four times.

Of the scientific papers, 18 have not been quoted until the writing of this study.

In Figure 3, a bibliometric study was carried out to investigate and identify indicators on the dynamics and evolution of scientific information using the main keywords. The study of bibliometric results using the scientific software VOSviewe, aims to identify the main research keywords in studies of blockchain, e-commerce.

The research of the analyzed articles: blockchain, e-commerce, electronic commerce., and the linked keywords can be seen in Figure 4, making it possible to clear the network of keywords that appear together / linked in each scientific article, allowing to know the topics analyzed by the research and identify future research trends. In Figure 5, a profusion of co-citations with a unit of analysis of cited references.

LITERATURE ANALYSIS: THEMES AND TRENDS

The publications were analyzed and revealed the emergence of four prominent themes in answer to the comprehensive research question of this study, as subsequent sections will show. Generally, we sustain that blockchain can leverage e-commerce in four fundamental areas, electronic e-commerce, financial transactions; e-commerce supply chain management, e-commerce forecasting, and contractual relations; and the trust and credibility of e-commerce transactions and systems. The majority of studies were focused on the last thematic area of concern try.

Blockchain Can Leverage and Enhance Various Aspects of E-Commerce Supply Chains

A tangible application of blockchain technology in e-commerce emerged from the literature about leveraging the blockchain in e-commerce supply chain systems and processes. Chu et al. (2017) begin their exploration of the potential of blockchain in improving both e-commerce and traditional supply chain, noting the problems associated with extant technological interventions for the advanced supply chain

Figure 3. Network of all keywords

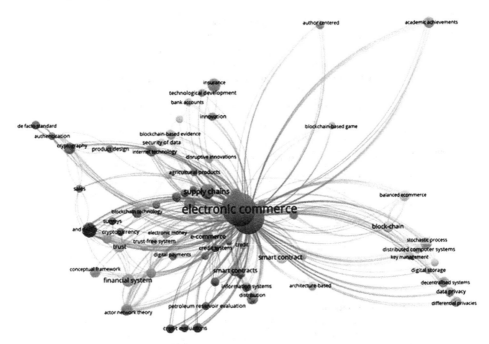

management. The authors subsequently proposed a conceptual framework for incorporating blockchain technology into contemporary supply chain management, calling this alternative "blockchain-based supply chain management" (Chen et al., 2017, p.172). All in all, the authors articulate a compelling case for implementing blockchain-based e-commerce supply chain management, providing concrete evidence of how such leveraging can improve e-commerce supply chains by, among other ways, solving current challenges of informational asymmetries in production processes, high costs, and limitations to decentralized supply chain quality management.

Figure 4. Network of linked keywords

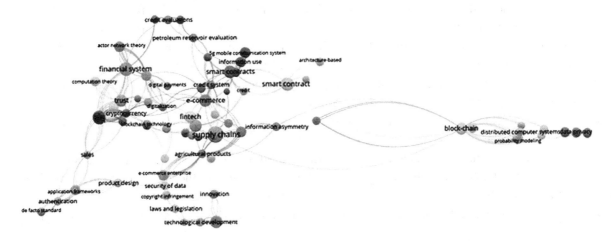

Figure 5. Network of co-citation

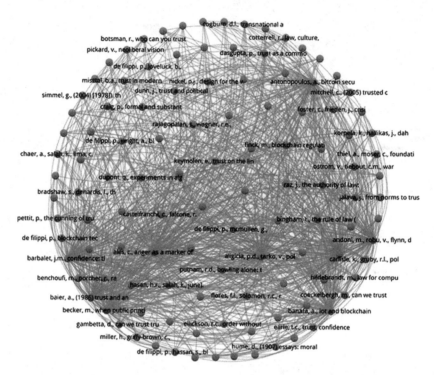

Hu et al. (2020) dig deeper into this matter but in the more specific context of China and the coronavirus pandemic. The authors validate the practical utility of blockchain-powered supply chain in resolving some of the critical problems that have been curtailing the growth and development of China's online retail market, namely "the problems of information asymmetry, and unclear market responsibilities and traceability of product information in B2C (business-to-consumer) sales" (Hue et al., 2018, p.335). The article notes that blockchain technology presents three unique capabilities particularly feasible to the resolution of the challenges mentioned above, including a distributed storage architecture, consistency algorithm, and lightweight digital signature algorithm (Hu et al., 2020). Nevertheless, Hu et al. (2020) observe that these advantages and capabilities, notwithstanding blockchain, are currently difficult to leverage in the desired path described caused by issues with reliability, authenticity, and integrity of information transmitted along with the blockchain network. The authors, therefore, propose an alternative that addresses the issues highlighted in the case of traceability of the products of the e-commerce operations of mask enterprises during the COVID-19 pandemic and find that blockchain technology can be leveraged to improve the quality of supply chain management through the context-specific integration of lightweight cryptography (Hu et al., 2020). Subsequent testing of the blockchain-based supply chain revealed that it achieved secure collaborative computing, peer-to-peer communication, and identity-based authentication.

Jemel & Sehrouchini (2017) undertook an experimental study to demonstrate the superiority of supply chain management solutions that leverage blockchain technology over the extant alternatives of cloud computing. The authors observe that the integration of cloud storage solutions into supply chains offers a meaningful and more efficient way of decentralizing information across various nodes of the supply chain, this intervention still possesses difficulties of encrypted data such as access control management challenges (Jemel & Sehrouchni, 2017). Accordingly, the authors propose a blockchain-based alternative with proven evidence of success in securely and legitimately facilitating decentralized access control in a multi-chain process (Jemel & Sehrouchni, 2017). Furthermore, Xie and He (2019) and Xie & Xiao (2020) conduct extensive assessments of blockchain technology used in the supply chain management of China's agricultural sector. Through practical experimentation with alliance chain Hyperledge technology, Xie and He (2019) show that blockchain can decentralize agricultural supply chains to facilitate the traceability and quality of "agricultural products from farmlands to table" (p.3).

Similarly, Xie and Xao (2020) find that blockchain-based supply chains can resolve the problems faced by producers and suppliers in the agricultural sector concerning information asymmetries in supply chain processes that often result in huge losses for farmers. Keller & Kessler (2018) also built a blockchain-powered supply chain management prototype that includes the Hyperleger Composer and Fabric frameworks. Although the prototype was implemented successfully and met all the pre-specified conditions and criteria, the outstanding question that lingered post-experimentation concerned the "maturity of the technologies to use in a productive environment" (Keller & Kessler, 2018, p.8). Nevertheless, the articles above offer a compelling use case of blockchain-based supply chains extensible to the e-commerce context.

Given the numerous advantages of leveraging blockchain technology in supply chain management, the outstanding question is why it is currently the case that widespread adoption of these technologies is lacking in the e-commerce industry and elsewhere. In the specific case of the Thai automotive industry, Supranee & Rotchanakitmnuai (2017) explore this line of inquiry and conclude that, once again, the challenge of leveraging blockchain technology is primarily an issue of technology acceptance. Specifically, the authors establish that acceptance boils down to two sets of predictive factors, namely inter-organizational trust and relationship, and the influence of the perceived benefits of blockchain in the automotive industry. The predictive set of perceived benefits has a positive and statistically significant relationship with acceptance, according to the authors, whereas that of inter-organizational trust and relationships has a negative and statistically significant relationship (Supranee & Rotchanakitmunai, 2017). These findings are also replicated by Wanitcharakkhakul and Rotchanakitumuai (2017). Their evaluation of the use of blockchain technology in the medical sector to manage electronic health records revealed that the system's perceived benefits, relative advantages, and trustworthiness were the most significant factors that influence acceptance of the blockchain-based information supply and management systems. Generally, both articles on the drivers affecting the adoption of blockchain-based management solutions highlight the need for focused research into technology acceptance concerning supply chain management and the integration of blockchain technologies therein, with specific reference to the e-commerce industry.

Blockchain Can Facilitate and Enhance Financial Transactions in E-Commerce

As stated in the introductory sections of this work, one of the strongest areas of blockchain technology application presently is in financial technology (fintech) and blockchain's intrinsic capacity to promote higher levels of innovation along these lines. As a business operation with an ever-increasing need for efficient electronic transactions, e-commerce could hugely benefit from introducing blockchain technology to its transaction systems and processes. In their systematic review of literature, Dula & Chuen (2018) corroborate this assertion by finding that one of the trends associated with "the internet and the ascent of e-commerce in the late 1990s" is the corresponding "significant growth in non-traditional non-bank" person-to-person (P2P) payment methods. The authors state that the inconvenience of traditional P2P payment mechanisms and modalities through tools like Western Union was the need that led to the invention of newer, faster, and more efficient solutions like PayPal (Dula & Chuen, 2018). Presently, blockchain-powered payment platforms can provide an even more convenient alternative, but these are distinguished from extant P2P mechanisms in one important way, especially the latter's subjection to regulations concerning electronic fund transfers. Albayati et al. (2020) say one of the reasons the integration of blockchain payment systems into e-commerce is yet to materialize is the "low acceptability of these technologies among consumers" (p.1). The researchers built a conceptual integration model consisting of the conventional technology acceptance model and external variables related to blockchain adoption. The two most significant proximal factors influencing consumers' adoption of blockchain technologies are regulatory support and experience (Albayati et al., 2020). The fundamental implication of the research by Albayati et al. (2020) is that increased governmental intervention into the e-commerce sector and increased consumer education and engagement by e-commerce companies regarding blockchain technology can facilitate higher adoption rates of blockchain payment platforms in e-commerce. Islam et al. (2019) explore an additional difficulty associated with integrating blockchain technologies into e-commerce, namely the instability of the fintech solutions that blockchain platforms deliver, which often manifest in the form of so-called "blockchain splits." The researchers highlight the need to leverage blockchain payment systems in e-commerce to be founded on extensive research into the role that human and non-human actors within the blockchain network play in contributing to the said splits. Additionally, Muller et al. (2020) assert that a core factor complicating the ability of blockchain to leverage e-commerce payment systems are lock-in effects inherent to the currently "centralized e-commerce platforms," and which "originate from the situation in which a centralized platform offers a variety of value propositions towards content creators and consumers" (p.1). The author proposes that blockchain can be utilized to solve this challenge by facilitating the development of electronic payment applications that offer 'smart' e-commerce contractual relations, thereby decentralizing e-commerce platforms and distributing value propositions among different actors said platforms.

Regardless of technology acceptance and diffusion challenges currently experienced in e-commerce and concerning blockchain technologies, extant NPD (new product development) metrics indicate that the e-commerce and the financial industry consider blockchain payment platforms as a promising prospect in leveraging the blockchain in e-commerce. Hsieh & Li (2017) came to this conclusion exploring the integration of e-commerce and blockchain through venture capitalism. The research found that a "total of 4,730 Fintech companies had founded from Crunchbase database," an emerging, open-source blockchain platform, and that "more than $200 billion" in funding had been released and allocated for the specific purpose of developing a blockchain-powered e-commerce payment system from the database aforementioned (Hsieh & Li, 2017, p.6). Su & Wang (2020) offer up yet another compelling use case of blockchain-based supply chains in e-commerce through a comparable application of blockchain technology to the supply chains of a "digital bulk commodities service platform" (p.341). The authors find that leveraging the blockchain in such supply chains has demonstrable benefits in reducing business operation risks, rebuilding the supply chain credit system, and improving customer service efficiency (Su & Wang, 2020). Notably, the case study is highly pertinent to this paper's exploration because e-commerce is, by nature, underpinned by supply chain modes dealing in bulk commodities. Therefore, the compelling value proposition of a blockchain technology-powered e-commerce system of electronic payments warrants additional research exploration as an important area in the inquiry regarding leveraging the blockchain in e-commerce.

Blockchain Can Leverage and Enhance E-Commerce Forecasting and Smart Contracting

Another important subject for leveraging e-commerce by blockchain that emerged from the analytical review of literature involved the potential application of blockchain technology to the development of smart contract relations, mainly by the automation of business processes through the reduction of paper-work and the elimination of intermediaries. Almassoud et al. (2018) explore how such smart contracts can be achieved by integrating artificial intelligence (AI) into the blockchain technologies underpinning typical business processes and systems in the real-life context. The authors find that the integration of AI with blockchain technology through adequately prepared, pre-specified rules and policies can lead to the creation of a smart contract with self-learning AI capabilities, which ensure that the contracts are not only legally binding but also accommodate the necessary adaptations for environmental issues (Almasoud et al., 2018). The same authors highlight the need for additional research into the development of standard blockchain architecture, yet to be constructed, that would allow for the technological automation of busi-ness processes in various industries, including e-commerce, facilitated by tech innovations like AI. Cao et al. (2020) explore the Chinese insurance industry to identify the drivers characterizing the current trend of so-called 'InsurTech' and finds that the insurance industry emphasizes the technological innovation on blockchain technology, particularly recognizing the technology's potential towards automation and 'smart' contractual relations. Additionally, Ferrer-Gornilla et al. (2019) examine another important, potential contribution of blockchain technology for-e-commerce transactions in the specific domain of electronic contracts. The authors find that by facilitating smart, and automated e-commerce contracts, blockchain technology provides "a new way to address classic problems such as double-spending, as well as problems such as fairness" (Ferrer-Gomila et al., 2019, p.1).

Moreover, the research reviewed reveals several other empirical benefits that naturally arise from blockchain's leveraging of e-commerce in the context of smart contracts and automation of business processes. For example, through a case study of the digital media ecosystem, Li et al. (2018) find that a media ecosystem "operated autonomously on a smart contract-based consortium blockchain" can deliver numerous benefits for users, including supporting their respective benefits, reducing brokerage, identifying accidence-raised liabilities, and doing a fair review to inspire product quality (p.201). These benefits are extensible to users of the conventional e-commerce system. Li et al. (2018) corroborate these benefits in credit systems that are also applicable to the e-commerce context. They show that the introduction of blockchain-powered autonomy capabilities with self-regulating and programmable smart contracts into existing credit systems can resolve current problems due to separate brokerage processes, insufficient supporting information, centralized and static evaluation models, and non-pertinence. Wang (2020a) and Wang (2020b) also demonstrate the tremendous potential of blockchain technology for SME and individual credit systems. Wang et al. (2020a) find that blockchain technology powers multiple tools for the creation of an enhanced, distributed credit evaluation system for SMEs capable of executing "intelligent protocols and distributed features to provide credit records through unchangeable timestamps and distributed ledger," correcting the problems existing in centralized credit systems for SMEs (p. 248). Wang (2020b) explores the context of personal credit evaluation systems and the chal-lenges that the fast development of financial systems combined with personal credit evaluation bears on traditional credit evaluation models, including excessive centralization, data transmission lags, and fake data identification. The exploration demonstrates that a newer blockchain-based personal credit evaluation model with decentralized data sources can solve these outstanding issues by, among other ways, outperforming traditional statistical credit models.

Concerning the predictive analytical potential of blockchain technology, moreover, Lee et al. (2019) undertake empirical research on whether users of blockchain-based games engage in such activity for pure enjoyment or also speculative purposes. The authors find that "it remains unclear whether users play Blockchain-based games just for fun or as a form of speculation," and therefore highlights the need for additional research on the e-commerce use case of blockchain in facilitating predictive analytics and general forecasting of consumer behavior, which could be potentially transformative for contemporary e-commerce practice (Lee et al. 2019, p.141).

In the more context-specific interests of this work, Kabi & Franquiera (2019) provides the most compelling, empirical proposition concerning the potential of smart e-commerce contracts whose construction is achieved through the autonomy capabilities delivered by blockchain technology. The authors focus specifically on the cost-reduction benefits associated with the said novel contracts. They develop a "proof-of-concept system that implements a distributed online marketplace using the Ethereum framework, where buyers and sellers can engage in e-commerce transactions without the need for a large central entity coordinating the process" (Kabi & Franquiera, 2019, p.1). After analyzing the costs of use for high volume users of the proposed system, the authors observe that the smart contract system does indeed significantly reduce the costs of use in relative comparison to the costs accrued by users of eBay and Amazon (Kabi & Franquiera, 2019). More importantly, the findings of this study validate the value of additional research into the ability to utilize Ethereum and other blockchain modalities in creating a distributed on-chain markets.

Nevertheless, the analysis yet again returns to the recurrent question of why blockchain in achieving smart contractual relations in e-commerce and other digital environments is not pervasive despite the self-evident positive use cases. Grounded theory research by de Graaf (2019) provides a paradigm for explaining this current reality by demonstrating that the issue yet again boils down to the absence of laws and regulations to govern smart contracts on the blockchain arena appropriately. The author attributes this absence of a practical regulatory framework to two primary reasons, including, firstly, the oppositional direction of the competing interests relating to "trust in people versus trust in code;" and, secondly, technical and practical obstacles that inhibit the application of Internet laws on smart contracts in a meaningful manner (de Graaf, 2019, p,10). This finding highlights the need for additional research into how programmers in the e-commerce industry can work collaboratively with legal and legislative practitioners to create better blockchain-powered smart contracts.

Blockchain Can Leverage E-Commerce Systems to Bolster Systemic Trust and Credibility

As shown in a previous section of this work, the vast majority of the literary contributions encompassed in this review focused on how blockchain technology can leverage e-commerce to achieve enhanced trust and credibility of the latter systems, thereby promoting the adoption of the integrated approach that incorporates both e-commerce and blockchain under a unified framework. Generally, the articles reviewed in this sub-section of the paper can be subdivided further into four thematic categories: firstly, those that provide use-case examples of blockchain technology leveraging e-commerce to enhance trust and credibility in systems. The second category consists of those articles that question and critique the said use-cases, whereas the third consists of those that detail how blockchain technologies can inherently overcome the criticisms cited in the second category of articles aforementioned. Finally, the fourth category encompasses those that highlight the knowledge and practice gaps outstanding, which must be achieved before blockchain can fully address the criticisms leveled against it in the context of its utility in bolstering the trusted credibility of e-commerce systems.

The study by De Filippi et al. (2020) falls into the category of articles seeking to demonstrate the use-case validity of blockchain' leveraging of e-commerce to enhance trust and credibility in e-commerce systems. The authors describe blockchain technology as a 'confidence machine' that "relies on cryptographic rules, mathematics, and game-theoretical incentives in order to increase confidence in the operations of a computational system" (De Filippi et al., 2020, p.6). Similarly, Huang & Chiang (2017) demonstrate how blockchain technology is the foundation of any sound RegTech system and how the technology achieves such status by comprising a long-lasting and irrefutable chain of trust through tracking the credit of organizations. Moreover, Elisa et al. (2019) constructed a model of an e-government information system based on a consortium of blockchain technology that facilitates the secure sharing of information. Cumulatively, the 'use-case articles' create the rationale of the power of blockchain as a so-called trustless technology to bolster the trust, confidence, and credibility of systems; benefits that are generalizable to the context of e-commerce systems.

However, the second category of articles introduced earlier pokes holes into the rationale of blockchain technology as the core driver of trustless systems with high degrees of credibility. Hawlitschek et al. (2020) mention three main reasons why the rational aforementioned is logically fallacious. The authors assert that blockchain technology does not inherently resolve all trust issues in real-life human interactions. The proponents of blockchain tend to underestimate the value of intermediaries and brokers for transactions and overestimate the power of blockchain to cut out such intermediaries (Hawlitschek et al., 2020). The authors also say that arguments in favor of blockchain's value in building trust and confidence in system interactions tend to overstate consumers' preference for blockchain technology. The criticism towards blockchain's supposed impermeability to security breaches is supported by the empirical findings of Hsieh, Chung, and Chi's "probability model for analysis of attacks on blockchain," which finds that blockchain-based systems are indeed vulnerable to attacks that can result in significant to extreme losses (2016, pp.352-355). The cumulative import of the critical perspective presented by the studies in this second category emanates from the fact that they are instrumental in allowing objective analysis of what remains unknown about blockchain technology.

Nevertheless, there is a large spectrum of studies related to the third category defined and described above that enumerates and demonstrates how blockchain, both inherently and by incorporating external variables, resolves most of the criticism in a practical context. Kapassa et al. (2020) demonstrate how using blockchain-based infrastructure incorporating smart contracts can eliminate security weaknesses of e-commerce systems operating in the 5G network environment. These smart contracts eliminate the bulk of security problems by validating all marketplace-oriented transactions, facilitating provenance tracking and accountability within the 5G ecosystem, among other provisions (Kapassa et al., 2020). Similarly, Li et al. (2019) found that blockchain technology can enhance intellectual protection in mobile digital intellectual property transactions by "enabling the recording and tracking of digital asset ownership, usage rights, usage records," and ensuring "the accuracy and verifiability of relevant documents" (p. 504). An e-commerce setting means blockchain technology enabling real-time paperless trading with smart contracts to bill, verify, maintain, store, and transfer transaction data between service requesters and providers. Li et al. (2017) model this proposition using the blockchain-based Balanced Commerce system that resolves trust issues relating to business expenses, fake products, profit-sharing, and user privacy on e-commerce platforms. Wu & Li (2018) extend the use of blockchain-based evaluation systems in the educational setting and demonstrates how the same concept applies to e-commerce, where it can be utilized to evaluate and improve constructive competition on e-commerce platforms. Lastly, Liu et al. (2018) develop a blockchain-based information system for data-sharing among government departments. The authors find that the system addresses outstanding data privacy issues in government information by enhancing the responsiveness, credibility, and security of information between government departments.

Moreover, the common consensus in the category of articles addressing the perquisites involved in blockchain addressing the criticisms leveled against its value in enhancing trust is that the vast majority of outstanding issues can be addressed by developing effective regulatory frameworks to underpin the technology's deployment. In an extensive case study review of the South Korean policy context, for example, Son & Sheikh (2018) find that regulators have a significant role in influencing the extent to which the e-commerce sector achieves the trust-related benefits leveraged by blockchain technology. Sung (2020) provides an example of such desired adaptive regulatory mechanisms by exploring a unique and emerging reality underpinning the increasingly pervasive global e-commerce industry and the digital era more broadly. The author's perspective, in this regard, encompasses the regulatory context and matters of legal dispute resolution about issues such as copyright infringements and other pains for which e-commerce users may require legal remedies. Sung (2020) explicitly examines the concept of Internet Courts in China, a novel innovation instituted to address some of the issues mentioned above and the role that blockchain technologies face therein.

Notably, the article observes that one of the critical limitations of administering 'digital justice' is the generation of solid and reliable evidence in legal proceedings, given the problems of data security and trust facing the centralized databases in which such evidence is stored (Sung, 2020). The author then examines how blockchain technology is increasingly considered one of the most effective ways for guaranteeing the trustworthiness of evidence pertinent to e-commerce disputes. However, questions remain outstanding regarding the possibility of a judicial paradigm that balances among the competing interests in matters of judicial access, namely cost, time, and correctness.

CONCLUSION

This extensive literature review began with the primary purpose of providing an answer for a specific research question regarding how blockchain technology can leverage e-commerce. After a systematic search of literature and analysis of the results so-retrieved, four major themes were identified in response to the research question, namely that blockchain can: leverage e-commerce in electronic transactions enhance several aspects of the e-commerce supply chain management, leveraging smart contracts and predictive analytics in e-commerce, and provide practical tools to bolster the trust, credibility, transparency, security, and privacy of e-commerce transactions and information flows. The most crucial factor is the foundation grounds for future researches raised by this exposition. These include research questions relating to what blockchain in leveraging e-commerce implies for: the theory and practice of technology acceptance, theories and models of technology readiness, a practical regulatory framework for the incorporation of blockchain technology into e-commerce, and research on the empirical potential, strengths, and limitations of blockchain in the context of e-commerce.

ACKNOWLEDGMENT

The author would like to express his gratitude to the Editor and the Referees. They offered precious suggestions or improvements. The author was supported by the GOVCOPP Research Center of Universidade de Aveiro.

REFERENCES

Albayati, H., Kim, S. K., & Rho, J. J. (2020). Accepting financial transactions using blockchain technology and cryptocurrency: A customer perspective approach. *Technology in Society, 62*, 101320. Advance online publication. doi:10.1016/j.techsoc.2020.101320

Almasoud, A. S., Eljazzar, M. M., & Hussain, F. (2018). Toward a self-learned smart contracts. *Proceedings - 2018 IEEE 15th International Conference on e-Business Engineering, ICEBE 2018*, 269-273. 10.1109/ICEBE.2018.00051

Cao, S., Lyu, H., & Xu, X. (2020). InsurTech development: Evidence from chinese media reports. *Technological Forecasting and Social Change, 161*, 120277. Advance online publication. doi:10.1016/j.techfore.2020.120277

Chen, S., Shi, R., Ren, Z., Yan, J., Shi, Y., & Zhang, J. (2017). A blockchain-based supply chain quality management framework. *Proceedings - 14th IEEE International Conference on E-Business Engineering, ICEBE 2017 - Including 13th Workshop on Service-Oriented Applications, Integration and Collaboration, SOAIC 207*, 172-176. 10.1109/ICEBE.2017.34

Cochoy, F., Hagberg, J., & Niklas, S. (2017). *Digitalizing Consumption: How devices shape consumer culture. Publisher*. Routledge. doi:10.4324/9781315647883

De Filippi, P., Mannan, M., & Reijers, W. (2020). Blockchain as a confidence machine: The problem of trust & challenges of governance. *Technology in Society, 62*, 101284. Advance online publication. doi:10.1016/j.techsoc.2020.101284

de Graaf, T. J. (2019). From old to new: From internet to smart contracts and from people to smart contracts. *Computer Law & Security Review, 35*(5), 105322. Advance online publication. doi:10.1016/j.clsr.2019.04.005

Dula, C., & Chuen, L. K. D. (2018). Reshaping the financial order. Handbook of blockchain, digital finance, and inclusion, volume 1: Cryptocurrency, FinTech, InsurTech, and regulation (pp. 1-18) doi:10.1016/B978-0-12-810441-5.00001-4

Elisa, N., Yang, L., Li, H., Chao, F., & Naik, N. (2019). Consortium blockchain for security and privacy-preserving in E-government systems. *Proceedings of the International Conference on Electronic Business (ICEB)*, 99-107.

Ferrer-Gomila, J., Francisca Hinarejos, M., & Isern-Deyà, A.-P. (2019). A fair contract signing protocol with blockchain support. *Electronic Commerce Research and Applications, 36*, 100869. Advance online publication. doi:10.1016/j.elerap.2019.100869

Hawlitschek, F., Notheisen, B., & Teubner, T. (2020). A 2020 perspective on "The limits of trust-free systems: A literature review on blockchain technology and trust in the sharing economy". *Electronic Commerce Research and Applications, 40*, 100935. Advance online publication. doi:10.1016/j.elerap.2020.100935

Hsieh, K., & Li, E. Y. (2017). Progress of fintech industry from venture capital point of view. *Proceedings of the International Conference on Electronic Business (ICEB)*, 303-307.

Hsieh, M., Chung, M., & Chi, Y. (2016). A probability model for analysis of attacks on blockchain. *Proceedings of the International Conference on Electronic Business (ICEB)*, 352-355.

Hu, J., Deng, J., Gao, N., & Qian, J. (2020). Application architecture of product information traceability based on blockchain technology and a lightweight secure collaborative computing scheme. *Proceedings - 2020 International Conference on E-Commerce and Internet Technology, ECIT 2020*, 335-340. 10.1109/ECIT50008.2020.00084

Huang, G. K. J., & Chiang, K. -. (2017). RegTech evolution: The TrustChain. *Proceedings of the International Conference on Electronic Business (ICEB)*, 308-311.

Islam, A. K. M. N., Mäntymäki, M., & Turunen, M. (2019). Why do blockchains split? an actor-network perspective on bitcoin splits. *Technological Forecasting and Social Change, 148*, 119743. Advance online publication. doi:10.1016/j.techfore.2019.119743

Jemel, M., & Serhrouchni, A. (2017). Decentralized access control mechanism with temporal dimension based on blockchain. *Proceedings - 14th IEEE International Conference on E-Business Engineering, ICEBE 2017 - Including 13th Workshop on Service-Oriented Applications, Integration and Collaboration, SOAIC 207*, 177-182. Retrieved from www.scopus.com doi:10.1109/ICEBE.2017.35

Kabi, O. R., & Franqueira, V. N. L. (2019). *Blockchain-based distributed marketplace.* doi:10.1007/978-3-030-04849-5_17

Kapassa, E., Touloupos, M., Kyriazis, D., & Themistocleous, M. (2020). *A smart distributed marketplace.* doi:10.1007/978-3-030-44322-1_34

Kathuria, S., Grover, A., Perego, V. M. E., Mattoo, A., & Banerjee, P. (2019). *Understanding E-Commerce.* World Bank Group.

Keller, T., & Kessler, N. (2018). Yet another blockchain use case-the label chain. *Proceedings - 2018 IEEE 15th International Conference on e-Business Engineering, ICEBE 2018*, 187-194. 10.1109/ICEBE.2018.00037

Lee, J., Yoo, B., & Jang, M. (2019). *Is a blockchain-based game a game for fun, or is it a tool for speculation? an empirical analysis of player behavior in crypokitties.* doi:10.1007/978-3-030-22784-5_14

Li, Q., Xu, M., Fang, M., Yang, M., & Guo, Y. (2019). A conceptual framework for data property protection based on blockchain. *Proceedings of the International Conference on Electronic Business (ICEB)*, 501-505.

Li, S. (2018). An author-centered media blockchain ecosystem. *Proceedings - 2018 IEEE 15th International Conference on e-Business Engineering, ICEBE 2018*, 201-206. 10.1109/ICEBE.2018.00039

Li, Y., Liang, X., Zhu, X., & Wu, B. (2018). A blockchain-based autonomous credit system. *Proceedings - 2018 IEEE 15th International Conference on e-Business Engineering, ICEBE 2018*, 178-186. 10.1109/ICEBE.2018.00036

Li, Y., Xue, S., Liang, X., & Zhu, X. (2017). I2I: A balanced ecommerce model with creditworthiness cloud. *Proceedings - 14th IEEE International Conference on E-Business Engineering, ICEBE 2017 - Including 13th Workshop on Service-Oriented Applications, Integration and Collaboration, SOAIC 207*, 150-158. 10.1109/ICEBE.2017.31

Liu, L., Piao, C., Jiang, X., & Zheng, L. (2018). Research on governmental data sharing based on local differential privacy approach. *Proceedings - 2018 IEEE 15th International Conference on e-Business Engineering, ICEBE 2018*, 39-45. 10.1109/ICEBE.2018.00017

Marten, R., & Kai, S. (2017). A blockchain research framework–What we (don't) know, where we go from here, and how we will get there. *Business & Information Systems Engineering, 59*(6), 385–409. doi:10.100712599-017-0506-0

Muller, M., Janczura, J. A., & Ruppel, P. (2020). DeCoCo: Blockchain-based decentralized compensation of digital content purchases. *2nd Conference on Blockchain Research and Applications for Innovative Networks and Services*, 152-159. Retrieved from www.scopus.com doi:10.1109/BRAINS49436.2020.9223299

Rosário, A., & Cruz, R. (2019). Determinants of Innovation in Digital Marketing, Innovation Policy and Trends in the Digital Age. *Journal of Reviews on Global Economics, 8*, 1722–1731. doi:10.6000/1929-7092.2019.08.154

Rosário, A. T., Fernandes, F., Raimundo, R. G., & Cruz, R. N. (2021). Determinants of Nascent Entrepreneurship Development. In A. Carrizo Moreira & J. G. Dantas (Eds.), *Handbook of Research on Nascent Entrepreneurship and Creating New Ventures* (pp. 172–193). IGI Global. doi:10.4018/978-1-7998-4826-4.ch008

Sacavém, A., Cruz, R., Sousa, M., & Rosário, A. (2019). An integrative literature review on leadership models for innovative organizations, innovation policy and trends in the digital age. *Journal of Reviews on Global Economics, 8*, 1741–1751. doi:10.6000/1929-7092.2019.08.156

Snyder, H. (2019). Literature review as a research methodology: An overview and guidelines. *Journal of Business Research, 104*, 333–339. doi:10.1016/j.jbusres.2019.07.039

Son, W., & Sheikh, N. J. (2018). Assessment of electronic authentication policies using multi-stakeholder multi-criteria hierarchical decision modeling. *PICMET 2018 - Portland International Conference on Management of Engineering and Technology: Managing Technological Entrepreneurship: The Engine for Economic Growth, Proceedings*. 10.23919/PICMET.2018.8481798

Su, L., & Wang, H. (2020). Supply chain finance research in digital bulk commodities service platform based on blockchain. *Proceedings - 2020 International Conference on E-Commerce and Internet Technology, ECIT 2020*, 341-344. 10.1109/ECIT50008.2020.00085

Sung, H. (2020). Can online courts promote access to justice? A case study of the internet courts in China. *Computer Law & Security Review, 39*, 105461. Advance online publication. doi:10.1016/j.clsr.2020.105461

Supranee, S., & Rotchanakitumnuai, S. (2017). The acceptance of the application of blockchain technology in the supply chain process of the Thai automotive industry. *Proceedings of the International Conference on Electronic Business (ICEB), 252-257.*

Wang, W. (2020a). A SME credit evaluation system based on blockchain. *Proceedings - 2020 International Conference on E-Commerce and Internet Technology, ECIT 2020,* 248-251. 10.1109/ECIT50008.2020.00064

Wang, W. (2020b). Exploring personal credit evaluation model based on blockchain. *Proceedings - 2020 International Conference on E-Commerce and Internet Technology, ECIT 2020,* 163-166. 10.1109/ECIT50008.2020.00043

Wanitcharakkhakul, L., & Rotchanakitumnuai, S. (2017). Blockchain technology acceptance in electronic medical record system. *Proceedings of the International Conference on Electronic Business (ICEB),* 53-58.

Wu, B., & Li, Y. (2018). Design of evaluation system for digital education operational skill competition based on blockchain. *Proceedings - 2018 IEEE 15th International Conference on e-Business Engineering, ICEBE 2018,* 102-109. 10.1109/ICEBE.2018.00025

Xie, C., & He, D. (2019). Design of traceability system for quality and safety of agricultural products in e-commerce based on blockchain technology. *Proceedings of the 7th International Symposium on Project Management, ISPM 2019,* 26-31.

Xie, C., & Xiao, X. (2020). Research on decision support system of E-commerce agricultural products based on blockchain. *Proceedings - 2020 International Conference on E-Commerce and Internet Technology, ECIT 2020,* 24-27. 10.1109/ECIT50008.2020.00013

Zhao, S., & O'Mahony, D. (2020). Applying Blockchain Layer2 Technology to Mass E-Commerce. *IACR Cryptol. ePrint Arch., 2020,* 502.

APPENDIX

Table 2. Overview of document citations period £2015 to 2020

Documents		£2015	2016	2017	2018	2019	2020	Total
lnsurTech development: Evidence from Chinese media reports	2020	-	-	-	-	-	-	-
Can Online Courts Promete Access to Justice? A Case Study of ...	2020	-	-	-	-	-	-	-
DeCoCo: Blockchain-based Decentralized Compensation of Digit...	2020	-	-	-	-	-	-	-
Blockchain as a confidence machine: The problem of trust &; am ...	2020	-	-	-	-	-	2	2
Accepting financial transactions using blockchain technology ...	2020	-	-	-	-	-	2	2
Application architecture of product information traceability ...	2020	-	-	-	-	-	-	-
A SME credit evaluation system based on blockchain	2020	-	-	-	-	-	-	-
Research on decision support system of E-commerce agricultur ...	2020	-	-	-	-	-	-	-
Exploring personal credit evaluation model based on blockcha ...	2020	-	-	-	-	-	-	-
Supply chain finance research in digital bulk commodities se ...	2020	-	-	-	-	-	-	-
A 2020 perspective on "the limits of trust-free systems: A 1...	2020	-	-	-	-	-	2	2
A smart distributed marketplace	2020	-	-	-	-	-	-	-
Why do blockchains split? An actor-network perspective on Bi ...	2019	-	-	-	-	-	9	9
From old to new: From internet to smart contracts and from p ...	2019	-	-	-	-	-	-	-
A fair contract signing protocol with blockchain support	2019	-	-	-	-	1	4	5
Consortium blockchain for security and privacy-preserving in ...	2019	-	-	-	-	-	-	-
A conceptual framework for data property protection based on ...	2019	-	-	-	-	-	-	-
Design of traceability system for quality and safety of agri ...	2019	-	-	-	-	-	-	-
Is a Blockchain-Based Game a Game for Fun, or Is lt a Toei f...	2019	-	-	-	-	-	2	2
Blockchain-based distributed marketplace	2019	-	-	-	-	1	3	4
An Author-Centered Media Blockchain Ecosystem	2018	-	-	-	-	-	-	-
Toward a Self-Learned Smart Contracts	2018	-	-	-	-	-	1	1
Yet Another Blockchain Use Case-The Label Chain	2018	-	-	-	-	-	-	-
Design of Evaluation System for Digital Education Operationa ...	2018	-	-	-	-	5	5	10
A Blockchain-Based Autonomous Credit System	2018	-	-	-	-	3	2	5
Research on Governmental Data Sharing Based on Local Differe ...	2018	-	-	-	-	-	-	-
Assessment of electronic authentication policies using multi ...	2018	-	-	-	-	1	-	1
Reshaping the Financial Order	2018	-	-	-	-	1	-	1
Decentralized Access Centrei Mechanism with Temporal Dimensi...	2017	-	-	-	1	6	4	11
121: A Balanced Ecommerce Model with Creditworthiness Cloud	2017	-	-	-	2	3	1	6
A Blockchain-Based Supply Chain Quality Management Framework	2017	-	-	-	5	27	16	58
Blockchain technology acceptance in electronic medical recor ...	2017	-	-	-	-	-	1	1
RegTech evolution: The TrustChain	2017	-	-	-	-	-	-	-
Progress of Fintech industry from venture capital point of v ...	2017	-	-	-	-	-	-	-
The acceptance of the application of blockchain technology i ...	2017	-	-	-	-	4	2	6
A probability model for analysis ofattacks on blockchain	2016	-	-	-	-	-	-	-
	Total	-	-	-	8	52	66	126

Source: own elaboration

Table 3. Overview of document citations period £ 2015 to 2020

Documents		£2015	2016	2017	2018	2019	2020	Total
InsurTech development: Evidence from Chinese media reports	2020	-	-	-	-	-	-	-
Can Online Courts Promete Access to Justice? A Case Study of ...	2020	-	-	-	-	-	-	-
DeCoCo: Blockchain-based Decentralized Compensation of Digit...	2020	-	-	-	-	-	-	-
Blockchain as a confidence machine: The problem of trust &;am ...	2020	-	-	-	-	-	-	-
Accepting financial transactions using blockchain technology ...	2020	-	-	-	-	-	-	-
Application architecture of product information traceability ...	2020	-	-	-	-	-	-	-
A SME credit evaluation system based on blockchain	2020	-	-	-	-	-	-	-
Research on decision support system of E-commerce agricultur ...	2020	-	-	-	-	-	-	-
Exploring personal credit evaluation model based on blockcha ...	2020	-	-	-	-	-	-	-
Supply chain finance research in digital bulk commodities se ...	2020	-	-	-	-	-	-	-
A 2020 perspective on "the limits of trust-free systems: A 1...	2020	-	-	-	-	-	-	-
A smart distributed marketplace	2020	-	-	-	-	-	-	-
Why do blockchains split? An actor-network perspective on Bi ...	2019	-	-	-	-	-	3	3
From old to new: From internet to smart contracts and from p ...	2019	-	-	-	-	-	1	1
A fair contract signing protocol with blockchain support	2019	-	-	-	-	-	-	-
Consortium blockchain for security and privacy-preserving in ...	2019	-	-	-	-	-	-	-
A conceptual framework for data property protection based on ...	2019	-	-	-	-	-	-	-
Design of traceability system for quality and safety of agri ...	2019	-	-	-	-	-	-	-
Is a Blockchain-Based Game a Game for Fun, or Is lt a Toei f...	2019	-	-	-	-	-	-	-
Blockchain-based distributed marketplace	2019	-	-	-	-	-	-	-
An Author-Centered Media Blockchain Ecosystem	2018	-	-	-	-	-	-	-
Toward a Self-Learned Smart Contracts	2018	-	-	-	-	-	-	-
Yet Another Blockchain Use Case-The Label Chain	2018	-	-	-	-	-	-	-
Design of Evaluation System for Digital Education Operationa ...	2018	-	-	-	-	2	2	4
A Blockchain-Based Autonomous Credit System	2018	-	-	-	-	2	1	3
Research on Governmental Data Sharing Based on Local Differe ...	2018	-	-	-	-	-	-	-
Assessment of electronic authentication policies using multi ...	2018	-	-	-	-	-	-	-
Reshaping the Financial Order	2018	-	-	-	-	-	-	-
Decentralized Access Centrei Mechanism with Temporal Dimensi...	2017	-	-	-	-	-	-	-
121: A Balanced Ecommerce Model with Creditworthiness Cloud	2017	-	-	-	-	1	2	3
A Blockchain-Based Supply Chain Quality Management Framework	2017	-	-	-	-	-	1	1
Blockchain technology acceptance in electronic medical recor ...	2017	-	-	-	-	-	-	-
RegTech evolution: The TrustChain	2017	-	-	-	-	-	-	-
Progress of Fintech industry from venture capital point of v ...	2017	-	-	-	-	-	-	-
The acceptance of the application of blockchain technology i ...	2017	-	-	-	-	-	-	-
A probability model for analysis of attacks on blockchain	2016	-	-	-	-	-	-	-
	Total	-	-	-	-	5	10	15

Source: own elaboration

Section 3
Blockchain Healthcare

Blockchain political-economic implications for patients and providers.

Chapter 7
Application of Technology in Healthcare:
Tackling COVID–19 Challenge – The Integration of Blockchain and Internet of Things

Andreia Robert Lopes
Hovione Farmaciencia, Portugal

Ana Sofia Dias
ISEG, Lisbon School of Economics and Management, Portugal

Bebiana Sá-Moura
ISEG, Lisbon School of Economics and Management, Portugal

ABSTRACT

The COVID-19 pandemic has disrupted healthcare worldwide and laid several fundamental problems that will have to be tackled to ensure high-quality healthcare services. This pandemic has represented an unparalleled challenge for healthcare systems and poses an opportunity to innovate and implement new solutions. Digital transformation within healthcare organizations has started and is reshaping healthcare. Technologies such as blockchain and IoT can bring about a revolution in healthcare and help solve many of the problems associated with healthcare systems that the COVID-19 crisis has exacerbated. In this chapter, IoT and blockchain technologies were discussed, focusing on their main characteristics, integration benefits, and limitations, identifying the challenges to be addressed soon. The authors further explored its potential in describing concrete cases and possible applications for healthcare in general and specifically for COVID-19.

DOI: 10.4018/978-1-7998-7363-1.ch007

INTRODUCTION

Coronaviruses are a large family of viruses that can cause mild to severe respiratory tract infections in humans. In 2002 and 2012, with SARS (Severe acute respiratory syndrome) and with MERS (Middle East Respiratory Coronavirus), respectively, the world had the first glimpse of the potential impact of this family of viruses. In the first crisis, the SARS-CoV virus capacity of human-to-human transmission, the lack of preparation within hospitals for infection control, and international air travel enabled global dissemination of this pathogenic agent. SARS-CoV was initially detected in Guangdong province in China in late 2002, and it constituted the first known significant pandemic caused by a coronavirus, with 8,096 cases and 774 deaths reported in over 30 countries in five continents (Cheng et al., 2007). MERS-CoV was isolated from a patient who died in Saudi Arabia in September 2012, and since then, there have been multiple outbreaks that have amounted to 2564 conðrmed cases of the Middle East respiratory syndrome 881 associated deaths. It has been reported in 27 countries, although most cases (80%) have been in Saudi Arabia. One of the most striking features is that this virus seems to have a case-fatality ratio of almost 35% (Al-Omari et al., 2019).

However, the worst was yet to come. In late 2019, in Wuhan in China, an initial outbreak of a new virus spread rapidly to other areas of China (Chahrour et al., 2020). In a few weeks, this virus had spread to other countries, and as of 1st February 2020, the World Health Organization (WHO) declared CO-VID-19 a Public Health Emergency of International Concern, and on 11th March 2020, the Coronavirus SARS-CoV-2 outbreak was declared a worldwide pandemic. As of January 2021, the virus has spread globally, with 89,416,559 confirmed cases of COVID-19, including 1,935,028 deaths. For the first time in history, a health crisis shut down the entire planet. Lockdowns and mobility restrictions imposed to control the spread of the virus and alleviate pressure on strained health care systems worldwide have had an enormous impact on economic growth and pushed millions of people into unemployment and poverty. The novel coronavirus pandemic has revealed deep underlying problems in health care systems across the world, and political, and healthcare authorities should swiftly address its impact in the longer term. Dealing with the impact of this health crisis, working on disease surveillance and prevention of new similar threats, and reconfiguring healthcare systems enabling them to deliver the best care while handling potential new crises are vital areas that must be tackled.

The COVID-19 challenge has undoubtedly been a catalyst for change. COVID-19 has dramatically accelerated digitalization and the adoption of new technology. This chapter aims to explore how block-chain combined with IoT could have played an essential role throughout the COVID-19 crisis in the healthcare system and pinpoint possible future applications.

BACKGROUND

Internet of Things (IoT)

The Internet of Things (IoT) is the real result of an applied principle: if you connect every tangible "thing" to the Internet, you create a network of shared data components.

Internet of Things refers to the ubiquitous network of interconnected objects capable of information storage and exchange using embedded sensors, actuators, and other devices. The IoT is a revolutionary technology which facilitates data-driven decision making by monitoring and managing objects in real-time. According to Kevin Ashton, the then executive director of the Auto-ID Center, he coined the term *"Internet of Things"* in 1999 while working on a presentation for Procter & Gamble in the context of RFID (Radio-Frequency Identification) supply chains (*RFID JOURNAL* |, n.d.).

The meaning of IoT is connecting systems and devices that, until now, have not been connected. The IoT is made up of things or devices connected by the internet that can take in information and talk to each other, sharing information back and forth. The connected things use sensors to absorb the information. The sensors input data into a large, intelligent system comprised of smaller smart systems.

The data is obtained through devices, vehicles or patients and are sent via protocols, i.e. communication channels, such as MQTT, Rest API, Coap or Custom, to a Cloud, and are stored in a database or they are received by an application that records and works on the same data.

The expanded definition of IoT is the upgrade of mobile, home and embedded applications to become part of a network of connected physical devices that all have sensors that both import and export data. The devices, using embedded sensors, gather data about the environment in which they are operating and how they are being used. The sensors are integrated into every physical device, from electrical appliances (fridges, stoves, furnaces), to lights (home lighting, traffic lights, car lights), to smartphones and tablets to barcodes on non-electrical items (pill bottles, boxes). The devices then share the data in real time about their operational state through the Cloud to an IoT platform where there is a universal language by which all IoT devices communicate. The gathered data is then dumped, or integrated, and data analytics is performed. Data analytics is drawing valuable insights and information from masses of raw data. Data analytics is now mostly automated, with algorithms performed by Artificial Intelligence (AI) software that clean, sort, and generally make sense of the vast amounts of data that IoT devices provide. With a far higher capacity for computation than humans, Internet of Things technologies can analyze enormous amounts of data in seconds. Valuable information and insights are then pulled from the data without the aid of human beings. The information is then shared with human users and other IoT devices. The Internet of Things leads to better healthcare outcomes, more efficient manufacturing, optimization of energy production and consumption, more effective use of natural resources and lowered waste production in addition to a host of other benefits. In terms of advantages of using IoT, it allows a dynamic control of the industries, an improvement in the relationship between people and technology and essentially an easy access to data.

Regarding data privacy, the concern with the protection of data stored on the internet is increasing, and therefore it is necessary to have control of the legal and regulatory part, technical control by the open-source, social ethic and Market Self- Regulation.

IoT and Healthcare Market

The internet of things is also described as a network of physical devices that uses connectivity to enable the exchange of data. In addition, in healthcare field, IoT is used for data collection, analysis for research, and monitoring electronic health records which contains personally identifiable information, protected health information, and for other machine-generated healthcare data. Further, IoT applications in healthcare facilitate important tasks such as improving patient outcomes and taking some burden off health practitioners. IoT enabled devices to have made remote monitoring in the healthcare sector possible, unleashing the potential to keep patients safe and healthy, and empowering physicians to deliver superlative care.

IoT Healthcare market can be broadly divided into three components - Medical devices, Systems & software, and Services. Software & system segment dominates global IoT Healthcare market. Some of the leading technologies facilitating integration of IoT in healthcare domain are RFID, mHealth, Telemedicine and Bluetooth Low Energy. Growth of the market is fueled by increasing prevalence of chronic diseases, rising number of geriatric populations globally and higher efficiency provided by use of IoT in healthcare. Other factors such as availability of high-speed internet and favorable government regulatory policies are also expected to boost market growth. However, certain limitations of IoT in healthcare segment poses challenges to industry growth. Some of these are lack of interoperability, privacy and security concerns and lack of regulatory oversight.

Companies operating in the segment, both medical device manufacturers and IT companies are developing innovative products and services such as, Cognitive solution to diabetes management by Medtronic and IBM, Medical data exchange by Cisco and Philips Medical dispensing service, amongst others.

The growing of IoT in healthcare segment is anticipated due to the use of technologically advanced medical devices. Adoption of IoT services in healthcare leads to introduction of technologically advanced connected medical devices which help in remote patient monitoring and clinical care in general. Furthermore, it provides new possibilities for personalized healthcare with the use of leading healthcare applications such as Health tracker apps, Healthcare wearable, Telemonitoring and smart homes, Electronic health records, etc. The next decade may well see a revolution in the treatment and diagnosis of disease. The IoT has opened up a world of possibilities in medicine: when connected to the internet, ordinary medical devices can collect invaluable additional data, give extra insight into symptoms and trends, enable remote care, and generally give patients more control over their lives and treatment.

The global internet of things in healthcare market was valued at $113.75 billion in 2019 and is expected to reach $332.67 billion by 2027, registering a CAGR of 13.20% from 2020 to 2027. The major factors that contribute toward the growth of the internet of things in healthcare market include technological advancements, rising incidence rates of chronic diseases such as COPD, genetic diseases, respiratory diseases, and others, better accessibility to high-speed internet, implementation of favorable government regulatory policies. Furthermore, growing demand for cost-effective treatment and disease management, increased adoption of smart devices and wearables, increasing interest in self-health measurement, and reduced healthcare cost with advanced and cost effectives IoT in healthcare products and solutions. Moreover, rising interest of the startup companies in IoT healthcare industry such as MedAngelONE, Amiko, SWORD health, and Aira, is expected to boost the market growth. However, factors such as high costs associated with IoT infrastructure development, data privacy and security issues, lack of awareness among public in developing regions, and limited technical knowledge are expected to impede the market growth. Various factors such as government initiatives to support IoT platform, improvement in healthcare infrastructure in developing countries, and high R&D spending are expected to boost the market growth.

The pandemic has caused change in providers willingness to implement IoT solutions which helped in diagnosing the virus using internet of things. Furthermore, IoT technology is playing a growing role in helping authorities to prevent the further spread of COVID-19, while also treating those that have been infected. IoT, specifically and especially when combined with other transformative technologies such as Cloud and Artificial intelligence (AI). This led to wide range of applications of IoT in healthcare during this crisis. For instance, in 2020, patients and staff at a field hospital in Wuhan, China, wore bracelets and rings synced with an AI. This platform from CloudMinds the Beijing-based operator of cloud-based systems for intelligent robots to provide constant monitoring of vital signs, including temperature, heart rate, and blood oxygen levels during Covid-19 pandemic (Chamola et al., 2020). In addition, in India, the mobile application named as aarogya setu app, launched by the Union Health ministry on April 2, 2020 which helps users identify whether they are at a risk of COVID-19 infection (Nagori, 2021). Therefore, Covid-19 has uplifted the demand of internet of things in healthcare market and provides opportunities for the manufacturers in various applications in the healthcare domain during the forecast period.

The segmentation of the internet of things in healthcare market is performed based on application, component, end user, and region. Based on component, the market is segmented into devices, system & software and services (Table 1). The devices segment is further segmented into implantable sensor devices, wearable sensor devices, and other sensor devices. System & software segment are further categorized into network layer, database layer, and analytics layer. Moreover, services segment covers architecture, consulting, and application development services. Based on application, the market is segmented into patient monitoring, clinical operation & workflow optimization, connected imaging, fitness & wellness measurement, and drug development. Based on end user, global internet of things in healthcare market is segmented into healthcare providers, patients, healthcare payers, research laboratories of pharmaceutical & biotechnology companies, and government authorities. The market has been analyzed across four regions namely North America, Europe, Asia-Pacific, and LAMEA (Figure1).

In 2019, North America accounted for a major share of the internet of things in healthcare market size and is expected to continue this trend owing to rapid technological advancements, increasing investments from top players, supportive governmental rules, rise in prevalence of chronic disease patient population and increase in demand for cost effective disease treatment. However, Asia-Pacific is expected to witness growth at significant rate during the forecast period, by registering a CAGR of 17.40%. This is mainly due to rapidly changing healthcare infrastructure in the developing countries such as India and China, large patient population, rising public awareness, and increasing healthcare spending.

Figure 1. Iot in healthcare market by region.
Adapted from (Telugunta & Choudhary, 2020)

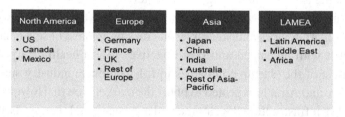

The service segment held the major market share of internet of things in healthcare in 2019, owing to growing demand for uninterrupted data flows to boost the efficiency of the medical systems, enhance security, and improve informed decision-making in real-time. However, the devices segment is estimated to be the fastest growing segment in the global internet of things in healthcare market during forecast period owing to the advancements of the wearable sensor devices, implanted sensor devices and other stationary devices. Among these devices, wearable device is the highest growing devices market. This is attributed to a surge in awareness to adopt the wearable devices, an increase in trend of self-monitoring and analysis health data. In addition, medical wearable devices can also help measure information such as blood pressure, cholesterol, blood sugar, and others, which resulted in a boost in the growth of the devices market during the forecast period.

The global internet of things in healthcare market is highly competitive, and prominent players have adopted various strategies for garnering maximum market share. These include collaboration, product launch, partnership, and acquisition. Major players operating in the market include Apple Inc., Cisco Systems Inc., GE Healthcare Ltd., Google (Alphabet), International Business Machines Corporation, Medtronic PLC, Microsoft Corporation, Proteus Digital Health, Koninklijke Philips N.V., QUALCOMM Incorporated, and Abbott Laboratories

By application, the patient monitoring segment is accounted for the highest revenue generator in 2019, owing to as patient monitoring enables data from devices to be collected and made available to healthcare professionals in real-time. Internet of Things in Healthcare services segment holds a dominant position in 2019 (Telugunta & Choudhary, 2020).

Table 1. Iot in healthcare market segmentation.

Application	Component	End User
Patient Monitoring	Sensor devices: - Implantable - Wearable - Others	Healthcare Providers
Clinical Operation and Workflow Optimization	Systems and Software: - Network Layer - Database Layer - Analytics Layer	Patients
Clinical Imaging	Services: - Architecture (system integration) - Consulting - Application Development	Healthcare Payers
Fitness and Wellness Measurement		Research Laboratories
Drug Development		Government Authority

Adapted from (Telugunta & Choudhary, 2020)

Blockchain

The first time a concept like blockchain was introduced was in 1991, when Stuart Haber and W. S. Stornetta (Haber & Stornetta, 1991) described a cryptographically secured chain of blocks for time stamping digital documents. Later, in 2000 Stefan Konst introduced his theory of cryptographic secured chains and identified strategies for its implementation (Konst & Wätjen, 2000). But the most important contribution to blockchain, came only in 2008, in a white paper written by Satoshi Nakamoto, a person or group of people, whose identity is still not known. Nakamoto introduced Bitcoin, a peer-to-peer electronic cash system that allowed for two parties to make a transaction overcoming the need for a trusted third party (Nakamoto, 2008). In January 2009, Nakamoto mined the first block of bitcoin and some days later, the first transaction took place: a man called Hal Finney received 10 bitcoins from Nakamoto. Later, in 2013, Vitalik Buterin introduced in a white paper, a new blockchain-based distributed computing platform, Ethereum, that featured a scripting functionality, called smart contract (Buterin, 2014). Blockchain and Bitcoin are concepts that are intertwined and often have been mistaken as the same, but in fact Blockchain is the technology behind Bitcoin, and its impact has surpassed Bitcoin and other cryptocurrencies and has affirmed itself as a groundbreaking technology far reaching into very different domains. Blockchain 1.0 was in fact focused on transactions, blockchain 2.0 initiated in 2013 with Ethereum and smart contracts and includes different applications in the financial area. In the last few years, the introduction of different platforms that aim to overcome the problems of Bitcoin and Ethereum, these are already part of Blockchain 3.0 and aim for global utilization of the technology. Blockchain can be defined as a decentralized database structured in blocks, each containing a certain amount of information and distributed through a chain (the ledger), and hence the name Blockchain. It is an immutable and distributed ledger that ensures data integrity (Nakamoto, 2008).

A block consists of two parts: the block header and the block body. The block header includes a block version, a parent block hash, a merkle root, a timestamp, bits and nonce. The block body is where the information about the transaction is stored. The information is organized in a Merkle tree, that is a binary tree containing cryptographic hashes, that enables all the information to be verified extremely efficiently and rapidly (Merkle, 1990) by producing an overall fingerprint of the transaction that occurred in the blockchain. In very simple terms, the Merkle Tree takes an enormous number of transaction IDs and runs them through a mathematical process that results in one 64-character code, which is called the Merkle Root, that is present at the Block Header also reducing the amount of data that has to be maintained for verification purposes (Figure 2).

Figure 2. Blockchain structure.
Adapted from (Liang, 2020)

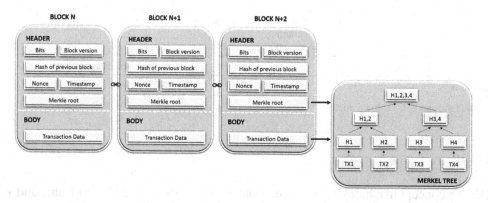

To achieve its goals, blockchain relies heavily on cryptography. In fact, the digital signatures based on asymmetric encryption are the ones used in blockchain networks. The utilization of public key cryptosystems for digital signatures was first suggested by Diffie and Hellman (Diffie & Hellman, 1976). Blockchain uses public key cryptosystems; in fact, every node of the network receives two different sets of keys: a public and a private key. Before a node initiates the transaction, it signs it with its own private key. The other nodes in the network will be then able to verify the authenticity of the transaction by using the public key.

Another key feature of the blockchain is the Hash function, which is the process of taking an input string of any length and turning it into a cryptographic fixed output. The hash function is deterministic which means that it should originate the exact same hash for the same message. The primary identifier of a block is its cryptographic hash, which works like a digital fingerprint. Ideal hashing functions should have the following properties:

- **Pre-Image Resistance:** one important aspect of secure cryptographic hash functions is that they are one-way, which means that no algorithm can produce the original input. It is very hard for a hash value to be decoded since all possible combinations will have to be tried before that, which poses a computational problem that is hard to solve. This feature provides a layer of security to any transaction.
- **Collision Resistance:** that means that it should be hard to find two different inputs that originate the same hash. Majority of current cryptographic hash functions are designed to be collision resistant, but that does not mean that they in fact are; collisions occur but they are typically very hard to find.
- **Second Pre-Image Resistance:** refers to the property in which it is computationally infeasible to find any second input that has the same output as a given input.

The peer-to-peer network is also essential for blockchain technology. This network involves a large number of computers, and each of these peers performs a specific task within the network to facilitate the activities of the blockchain eliminating problems related to the vulnerability of centralized servers while using different cryptographic methods to ensure the security of the network.

Blockchain miners are special nodes in that network that are responsible for securing and validating transactions. Mining is the process by which new transactions records (blocks) are added to the ledger (the blockchain). This process is intentionally designed to be challenging and resource-intensive and the miner that solves that complex mathematical puzzle is rewarded. The miner presents the new block that must be verified by the other nodes of the network and only if they reach a consensus the block is added.

In summary, someone requests a transaction that online is represented as a block. The block is broadcasted through a P2P network consisting of different nodes. These nodes are responsible for validating the transaction in a process called mining. The first miner to validate the new block is rewarded and the block is added to the blockchain which provides an unalterable, transparent record of all transactions. The transaction is then completed.

Blockchain has the following key features that are summarized below:

- **Decentralization:** this is one key feature of blockchain but also one of its main advantages. In conventional centralized systems the transaction needs to be validated by a central authority, in blockchain the validation is through the P2P network which means that both system and the data are resistant to technical failures and malicious attacks, and since the network includes sometimes thousands of nodes and each node has a local copy of the ledger there is no single point of failure.
- **Trustless System:** in blockchain there is no need for a central authority to validate the transaction. Moreover, the different nodes don´t need to trust one another. In fact, by distributing the transaction across the ledger and relying on a consensus to ensure its validity, blockchain overcomes the need for a trustworthy environment. By cutting the intermediaries it also reduces the costs and transaction fees.
- **Transparency and Immutability:** Each transaction is recorded on the Blockchain and is available to every node in a public network making it a transparent system. Since each block is linked

to the previous one through the hash function, any attempt to change the content will affect all the other subsequent blocks that are replicated over different nodes, making it almost tamper-proof.

- **Traceability:** The distributed and transparent nature of the blockchain allows for it to be easily traced back to its origin. Every block header has a timestamp which records the time when the block is created. Nodes can therefore verify and trace the origin of the previous blocks.
- **Non-Repudiation:** Every transaction is cryptographically signed with a private key and since the private key is specific for its owner, the transaction cannot be denied by its initiator.
- **Anonymity:** Every node or user can interact with the network using a self-generated address that keeps the identity of the participant protected, overcoming the need for a central party to have users´ information.

Blockchain and Healthcare Market

Blockchain is already changing our lives from the way all citizens make transactions, manage assets, vote, and even listen to music to the way it is transforming financial institutions, companies and governments, among others. Likewise, blockchain also has the potential to completely change the landscape of healthcare.

The WHO (World Health Organization) Constitution states that "…the highest attainable standard of health as a fundamental right of every human being". Access to affordable and efficient healthcare services is essential for human wellbeing and it is a driver of long-term economic growth as well as societal development. The healthcare industry is one of the fastest-growing industries despite still being characterized as old-fashioned, overly complex, and impenetrable, mostly due to an inefficient and outdated infrastructure.

The European healthcare systems are currently facing several challenges associated with population aging. In fact, the costs associated with delivering healthcare rise faster than the GDP of each one of the European countries, which is not sustainable in the long run. Moreover, the current pandemic is adding pressure to an already pressured system which will have consequences in years to come.

It is of the utmost importance to identify and implement solutions that will strengthen healthcare systems, contributing to their sustainability with the goal of promoting better health of the citizens. Government, consumers, payers, providers will have to reimagine how care is delivered and leverage technology to reduce cost while improving or maintaining quality of the services.

Blockchain presents itself as one interesting technology that can help face some of these challenges. While the adoption of blockchain in the healthcare industry was slow in comparison to other industries, this has steadily been changing. In fact, according to a new research study published by Global Market Insights, Inc, global Blockchain Technology in Healthcare market is set to reach a value of USD 1,636.7 million by 2025 (Bhutani & Wadhwani, 2017). Its impact in the industry is widespread and its applications will only increase in the next few years. Figure 3 highlights some examples of possible application of blockchain in different domains of healthcare.

One example of this utilization of blockchain in healthcare is its role in the improvement of medical record management. New technological solutions are essential to improving patients care while reducing associated costs. Current healthcare information systems have serious problems and challenges which include fragmented patient data, centralized systems that can be used as single points of attack, and the lack of patient-oriented services.

Figure 3. Overview of applications of blockchain in the healthcare sector (Weinberg, 2019)

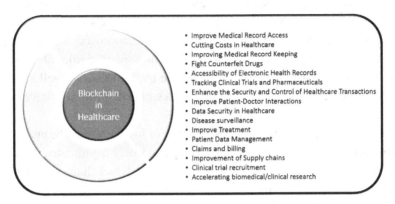

One important step towards improving healthcare has been the introduction of electronic health records (EHR) which enables doctors to easily store, view, share, and update patient records (Shuaib et al., 2019). EHRs may include very different formats of files, including images, videos, text among others that pertain to clinical data (laboratory results, imaging data and even measurements of vital signs) but also billing information and other general details that when handled incorrectly can cause very serious issues. Costs associated with EHR adoption, implementation, and maintenance of technological infrastructure necessary as well as concerns about privacy and security have been identified as problematic (Menachemi & Collum, 2011).

Moreover, data generated in healthcare settings is growing rapidly, with healthcare data suffering from various challenges, including interoperability between systems and fragmented data. In fact, patients go to different healthcare facilities and there must be exchange of the medical records, which is often hindered by different EHR systems used between institutions.

Although the EHRs are individual, patients do not control the EHRs themselves, where they are stored nor who has access to them and therefore, they are regarded with some suspicion. Generally, within institutions, the EHRs are stored in a centralized infrastructure, which by itself constitutes a risk (McDermott et al., 2019).

Blockchain has the potential to transform healthcare and help solve some of these issues by making electronic health records more efficient, secure and intermediate free. Blockchain will empower the patients to take initiative and be at the center of decision regarding their health and what happens to their data Due to its nature and for the reasons explained in previous sections, blockchain will increase system security, data privacy and security as well as improving interoperability of health data .

Blockchain for Internet of Things (BIoT) and Healthcare Market

As previously described in this chapter both Blockchain and Internet of Things are highly disruptive technologies that if integrated can open an infinite number of new possibilities. The integration of blockchain technology is often seen as the solution for the privacy and reliability concerns of Internet of Things but there are several other benefits associated with this integration:

1. **Improving Security:** The IoT devices are very easily compromised, and in fact in the past there have been several instances in which they have been the target of distributed denial-of-service (DDoS) attacks (Kolias et al., 2017). Contrary to IoT, blockchain has a decentralized architecture in which the nodes have to reach a consensus for a transaction to be approved and added to the ledger, there is no single authority responsible for approving or setting specific rules about the transactions. By combining blockchain with IoT you could eliminate traffic flows as well as single point failure, but also it would facilitate overcoming the need for a single institution to have control over the vast amount of data generated by IoT (Atlam et al., 2018).

2. **Increasing Reliability and Traceability:** Reliability of IoT data could be guaranteed by the several cryptographic mechanisms that Blockchain exploits, namely asymmetric encryption algorithms, hash functions and digital signature (Wang et al., 2018). Blockchain will ensure that data in the chain is immutable and can identify any tampering that may occur.

3. **Enhancement of Interoperability between IoT Systems:** One of the critical issues in IoT is that the different proprietary IoT platforms and systems are still not interoperable (Noura et al., 2019). Blockchain can improve the interoperability of these systems by converting the heterogeneous data from different devices and extracting, processing, transforming, and storing the data into a blockchain.

4. **Reducing Costs:** Blockchain utilizes a peer-to-peer structure without need for a central point of control, which reduces business expenses. The existing IoT solutions are expensive due to this centralized architecture which requires high infrastructure and maintenance costs.

5. **Accelerated Data Change:** The smart contracts are another relevant feature of Blockchain, that could record and manage all IoT interactions, which could be used to accelerate data exchange and enable processes between IoTs while removing the middleman. The contract clauses can be embedded in smart contracts and they are executed automatically when the specified conditions are satisfied (Viriyasitavat et al., 2019).

Reflecting about all the benefits of Blockchain and IoT (BIoT), the areas that can be apply and take advantage of this technology are infinite. BIoT has already been applied in several areas like food industry, pharmaceutical industry, healthcare, etc. It can help increase data legitimacy or reliability and provide distributed identity, authentication, and authorization mechanisms without the need for central authorities (Reyna et al., 2018).

Practical Applications

This section aims to describe some practical applications of Blockchain of Internet of Things (BIoT) in Healthcare helping face the challenges and make people and healthcare professionals life´s better.

Remote Healthcare Systems

The increase of the elderly population worldwide translates into a series of healthcare concerns, mostly related with the increase of chronic diseases every year. The senior patients visit the doctor routinely to be diagnosed and receive treatment. Besides that, when the senior patients don't stay hospitalized, they need help at home from healthcare professionals that work in the community. Therefore, remote healthcare has become extremely important. With this technology and new medical devices, patients can be monitored for a long period of time, increasing their quality of life and gaining more autonomy.

The devices that compose the remote health system are a combination of IoT and wearable technology because they are efficient and convenient. The patient wears several different physiologically sensible sensors that can be worn or implanted to measure vital signs in real life, such as blood pressure, heart rate and temperature(Pham et al., 2018). This data is sent to a centralized server, usually through a mobile phone, who collects and sends the sensor data. Healthcare professionals can access and analyze this information, preventing the need for face-to-face appointments, which is more convenient to the patient.

However, all of this is based on IoT which leads to several questions and concerns about security and privacy of data specially because the IoT architecture could be a target for non-expected hacking attacks. This can be dangerous because health information is one of the most sensitive types of data. The privacy of this data must be maintained while the EHR needs to be manageable by the healthcare teams and the patient itself.

Since the number of medical devices capable of monitoring the patient (IoT devices) has increased in the last couple of years, the privacy and security of patients is becoming an increased concern topic. To protect personal data, this BIoT project uses blockchain-based smart contracts for managing patient's information and medical devices (Pham et al., 2018). Some projects used the Ethereum protocol to create a remote healthcare system that integrates healthcare professionals and patients. This system provides a connection between the medical devices and its sensors, that generates the information about the patient's health, and directly stores the information on blockchain. Because of that, the system reduces the size of the blockchain as well as saving the amount of coins needed for transactions. This fact is especially interesting because abnormal data from the patients' sensors can trigger an emergency contact to the doctor and hospital for immediate treatment which in some cases could be lifesaving.

The author of the project already tested it with a verified smart contract on Ethereum Protocol on an experiment environment with real devices, and it works well at small scale (Luan Pham, 2018).

So, to summarize this application of BIoT in Remote Healthcare, the authors propose several changes to improve the remote system:

1. **To ensure the privacy and security of patient data:** Using a smart contract.
2. **A processing mechanism that filters the data from sensors before writing to blockchain**: Alerts the healthcare providers about abnormal data collected.
3. **With a highly secure system based in blockchain technology**: A GPS was incorporated to locate the patient in an emergency situation (Pham et al., 2018).

BIoT and Pharmaceutical Supply Chain (PSC)

Enyinda & Tolliver defined the Pharmaceutical Supply Chain (PSC) as a channel by which medicines have been shipped at the appropriate place and at the proper time (Enyinda & Tolliver, 2009).

Current PSC present numerous challenges as:

- Rapid demand changes in the market, fierce competition that puts pressure on margins of the products.
- Extensive supply chains increase the risks of data manipulation (too many suppliers for example).

- Ineffective supply chain risk management: the lack of monitoring or not having the right tools to do it.
- Lack of end-to-end visibility.
- Obsolescence of technologies.

Additionally, the pharmaceutical market faces the challenge of counterfeit pharmaceutical products. According to around 30% of the total medicine sold in Africa, Asia, and Latin America is counterfeit which could have major implications in citizens´ health and lives and a huge economic impact for the pharmaceutical industry. In fact, according to the same organization, the counterfeit market represents 200 billion dollars per year. Therefore, pharma companies and distributors are looking for new solutions that could improve supply chain security and traceability and therefore tackle this major issue (Jamil et al., 2019)Implementing electronic records based on blockchain technology will increase the traceability and auditability of pharmaceutical products.

When analyzing these challenges, it is important to understand the solutions that BIoT offers to this entire process. In a practical way, many things can be done to improve the supply chain. In terms of traceability, (the ability to monitor events and metadata associated with a product), blockchain technology can bring auditability, a full audit trail of data, creating a record of all the traces of the product. On compliance, (the standards and controls provide the evidence that regulatory conditions are met), blockchain brings immutability when all the operations are time and place proof, with only one source of data. Pharmaceutical companies are increasingly under pressure with regulatory issues, so this particular area is crucial to the system. On flexibility, (the ability to adapt to events or issues, without significantly increasing operational costs), blockchain offers smart contracts, a way to track data in real time along the supply chain. And at last, on stakeholder management, (an effective governance in place to enable communication, risk, reduction and trust among the involved parties), blockchain provides disintermediation, enable peer-to-peer interactions based on digital signatures (Kehoe et al., 2017)

But implementing BIoT is difficult because it is such a disruptive innovation, and the different stakeholders have to make the effort to invest in human and financial resources to implement BIoT. The investment must be made along the supply chain, from the raw material suppliers to the hospitals but also pharmacies to ensure that the product that the consumer is buying is in the best possible conditions.

Some practical examples of strategies that companies are adopting to improve the process, include:

- Using a "sealed" smart device to authenticate the goods. This sealed devices uniquely identify the object on which they are attached.
- If it's not possible to attach sensors to the good itself, it can be put on the packaging to track the goods through the supply chain.
- In the healthcare industry supply chain could be helpful to track and secure medical supplies. Combining IoT sensors with blockchain, to collect and capture information will help certifying the authenticity, and viability of the supplies through the entire supply chain and will help detect potential frauds and manipulations (Laurent, 2017).

Overall, the major advantages of the BIoT are: ensuring that all the stakeholders are at the same level, and through decentralization increase security and reliability. It's a chain that brings more trust to all of the participants, with real time information updates. Integrated blockchain-IoT can enable trust, transparency and visibility by tracking the material from the origin to end customers (Laurent, 2017).

Our country's healthcare system, hospital and primary health care, is not yet prepared to implement such a new technology because they don't have the human or financial resources needed to do it.

BIoT on Clinical Trials Research

According to a study by Tufts Center for the Study of Drug Development, it costs more than $2.6 billion to bring a drug to market and the clinical development is an important part of those costs (DiMasi et al., 2016).

Clinical trials are notoriously complex and expensive and serious challenges must be overcome to ensure their success. These challenges include patient recruitment and retention, rising costs to meet regulatory policies, monitoring complexity and issues related to data privacy and security. Moreover, data is typically obtained exclusively at clinical settings and real-world data is missing, often skewering results.

The utilization of IoT in clinical trials is still in its early stage. The Asthma Mobile Health Study was a good example of how a clinical research observational study was performed using a smartphone. It was a study that involved 7,593 participants from across the United States. Tasks such as recruitment, consent, and enrollment, that are generally resource intensive and costly were conducted remotely via smartphone. The platform that was developed for the study enabled the collection of clinical, environmental, and passive biometric data providing important findings on asthma care and research (Chan et al., 2017). Similarly, the mPower, was a clinical observational study about Parkinson disease conducted solely through an app interface in a phone. Enrolled subjects were requested to answer questions but also perform specific tasks that were recorded by the sensors in the phone. This app enabled the collection and monitoring of information about the daily changes in Parkinson's disease symptom severity as well as potentially assessing the effect of medication (Bot et al., 2016). Although the utilization of IoT in the recruitment as well as in the long distancing monitoring in real life, is very interesting, one important challenge to overcome, that is highlighted by (Chan et al., 2017), is data security which could potentially be tackled by the blockchain technology. Collecting and analyzing real-world evidence is fundamental for phase IV studies, to understand the long-term efficacy of drugs, track possible non-expected effects on patients' health and wellbeing or even identify new therapeutic indications, likewise the integration of blockchain and IoT could be key for this activity.

Clinical trial research could profit from blockchain main benefits, namely transparency, immutability, disintermediation, auditability, and trust. Even though, the advantages are obvious there are very few examples in which the blockchain technology has been used by the pharmaceutical industry in clinical trials, which might be due to lack of regulatory instructions or a clear position on the matter from the responsible agencies, in addition to a general lack of knowledge about the technology which hinders its acceptance.

Blockchain could help in the recruitment of patients and their engagement which is a key success factor for clinical trials. It could be used for the patient to give consent to participate in the trial, archiving the informed consent through cryptographic validation in an unalterable and transparent way, that upon any change to the trial protocol needs to be accepted and validated again by the patient (Benchoufi et al., 2018). Data integrity and provenance are key in clinical trials. Sponsors and clinical sites must prove the origin and integrity of all the data to the regulatory agencies which can be ensured by blockchain. Data management is key to ensure the success of the clinical trial and blockchain has been proposed to improve software systems used for clinical data management. Multiple projects exist in that realm, namely: Medvault, Gem Health Network, BitHealth, among others (Omar et al., 2020).

One example of the integration of the two technologies is the solution offered by InnoME, Essentim and Cryptowerk that enables IoT data acquisition and allows for easy blockchain-based digital notarization. The solution can be used to collect important raw data using sensors in combination with measurement equipment, to ensure the integrity of clinical trial data from IoT devices, to detect changes to any data set being able to trace it back to the origin, to track all drugs used in clinical trials according to regulatory agencies demands, and to instantly verify the identity and experience of all the clinical research staff involved in the study (Cryptowerk, 2018). .).

Another example of a combination of IoT and Blockchain is the digital health application proposed by Angeletti et al, that confers a secure way to control the flow of personal data in the recruitment of participants for clinical trials. Blockchain technology is employed to guarantee that all personal data is only shared with the right stakeholders when the subject is enrolled in the clinical trial, ensuring privacy and confidentiality. Moreover, they use IoT devices potentially at the subject´s homes to collect relevant data that can be used in clinical trial recruitment process, to pre-screen for suitable candidates that match the inclusion criteria (Angeletti et al., 2017).

There are no magic bullets that will solve the clinical development challenges, but technology will certainly play a part. IoT is used widely in Healthcare, for example in remote monitoring, but not so often in clinical development. On the other hand, the potential of Blockchain for clinical trials is recognized but very few examples of real application exist. The combination of these technologies can open new avenues and contribute, for the successful, timely and cost-efficient implementation of clinical trials therefore accelerating the discovery of new innovative therapies that can change people´s lives.

SOLUTIONS AND RECOMMENDATIONS

In this section the authors explore how BIoT could have been used during the COVID-19 pandemics, to address a lot of the problems in the healthcare industry and how it can be used in its aftermath.

Remote Healthcare System on COVID-19

The SARS-CoV-2 pandemic is a real-life example about the importance of collecting patient's information because data is the key to fully comprehend the disease, the dissemination, and the consequences of the infection. But sharing the information worldwide must avoid breaking national and international data sharing regulations. Patients' privacy is mandatory and a major concern. However, detailed information such as blood oxygen level, heart rate and medication doses can be gathered by integrating medical devices (Medical IoT).

Having a decentralized process with blockchain could help and solve the privacy and security issues. Like the example before, blockchain supports real-time data sharing. And uploading the medical devices data remotely directly to a blockchain based system, can eliminate data forging and mutation, maintaining the trust in the numbers, improving the trust between stakeholders and protecting patient's privacy (Kalla et al., 2020).

In recent times, the outbreak of several viral infections across the world, including Ebola and Zika virus, have raised attention to a potential global health threat. Globalization enables spreading of infectious diseases (Chattu et al., 2019). Unfortunately, these examples were just a glimpse of what was yet to come. In late 2019, a new coronavirus started spreading in Wuhan in China. The SARS-CoV-2 epidemic has changed the global landscape and its impact is yet to be fully understood. This global pandemic crisis has highlighted the importance of effective and reactive surveillance mechanisms. It is of the utmost importance to spot the threat early and immediately report it to the health authorities to start preventive measurements. National health systems are ultimately responsible for the surveillance of infectious diseases, but these tasks are spread through many independent agencies, which then report back to a centralized information system. The process is slow, inefficient, and complex. Blockchain and IoT could help these independent agencies to collect, access and manage surveillance data and receive it in real time in a secure way enabling a faster and more informed response.

BIoT on PSC in COVID-19

In a previous chapter, the authors described that blockchain and IoT technology can be used to deal with many problems and gaps on PSC. With the COVID-19 pandemic, many of these issues became even more obvious. During this pandemic crisis, the world has watched healthcare systems struggle with shortage of pharmaceuticals, personal protective equipment, medical devices, and medical supplies. The rapid escalation in demand meant traditional procurement processes were no longer suitable; identifying new vendors and swiftly reallocating the supplies was essential. But instead of finding innovative solutions, countries, states, hospitals ended up fighting each other for the supplies and in many cases overpaying for them (Mirchandani, 2020).

Moreover, many factories had to interrupt or decrease their production activities, in some cases because of the lockdown, in others because they were simply not prepared (equipped and designed) to the "new normal" of social distancing and using protective equipment. The import and export of goods suffered a big impact and caused the disruption of global supply and demand.

The complexity and fragmentation of the conventional supply chains could be tackled with blockchain and IoT. Blockchain has the capacity to connect pharmaceutical suppliers and customers, while maintaining a secure record of each transaction which protects every party and ensures transparency and immutability across supply chains. It was proposed to increase the use of technology to improve forecasting, to reduce the complexity of the distribution system, and to utilize the resources effectively (Kumar & Pundir, 2020). Also, Blockchain can increase trust among stakeholders, because they can build the supply chain together, and not just be dependent on each other. That is the major difference with a blockchain implementation. It supports auditability, provenance, and transparency, based on smart contracts with high level of access restrictions and automation (Kalla et al., 2020).

COVID-19 is having a huge impact in majority of companies, nevertheless some are more resilient, adapting, and able to tackle this issue. It all depends on how companies prepare for the unknown. The BIoT and new digital technologies can improve the communication between stakeholders, anticipate disruptions and reconfigure themselves appropriately to mitigate major impacts.

According to Kumar and Pundir there are benefits of implement BIoT in a traditional PCS changing some of the standards in this area (Table 2).

BIoT on Clinical Trials: The COVID-19 Impact

COVID-19 pandemics might be a driver for the implementation of new technologies in clinical trials. This pandemic has represented an unparalleled challenge for clinical research but also poses an opportunity to

Table 2. Benefits of integrating blockchain-IoT in supply chain

Activity in PSC	Blockchain	IoT	Benefits
Manufacturing the product	Registration of product with unique id and generation of a new block with product ID in the blockchain network	Product ID is scanned and transferred to the cloud	Transparency, Trust, Product details and Data security
Transported to distributor/ warehouse	Generation of smart contract block, Verification of manufacturer's contract, generation of transaction ID, product id and block ID verification	Path tracking and product ID verification GPS and smart devices (camera,sensors, temperature control, etc.) enabled track	Visibility,Traceability,Reliability, Quality tracking,Transparency, Trust, Immutability
Received at distribution center warehouse	Verification of contract of the supplier, transaction ID, product ID, and block ID	Track the location of the product and update the specified quantity (information is stored in the cloud)	
Distribution center/ warehouse to retailers /hospitals	Enabled the verification of product ID and order ID	Helps in continuous tracking of products till it reaches to the final customers	

Source: (Kumar & Pundir, 2020)

innovate and implement new solutions that will enable fast, simple and cost-effective clinical development up to the standards expected by the regulatory agencies while having the patients´ interest at heart.

In the past few months, COVID-19 pandemic has disrupted the healthcare industry and the clinical trials are no exception. Since the beginning of 2019, thousands of clinical trials were either put on hold or experienced delays, as clinical sites were often overwhelmed with COVID-19 patients and resources were scarce (van Dorn, 2020). Moreover, the COVID-19 posed a risk for those patients that were enrolled in these trials and had to frequently visit the clinical sites, which was especially serious since many of these patients are already populations at risk. Many patients have discontinued participation and others are less likely to participate in any ongoing trials. These challenges will most likely persist till effective vaccines are widely available and therefore new strategies will have to be implemented to overcome this situation, in fact according to FDA Guidance on the Conduct of Clinical Trials of Medical Products during COVID-19 Pandemic, alternative methods for safety assessments could be implemented when necessary and feasible, which could include virtual visits, remote monitoring, and the use of electronic data sources (Fda & Cder, 2020). The use of mobile devices, smartphones, wearables, and IoT technology can produce real time, high quality data overcoming possible errors associated with human data collection while blockchain would ensure its integrity and security. Moreover, IoT would enable continuous monitoring, generating larger data pools which can be used to better assess the efficacy of a drug, its potential side effects, as well as its overall impact on patient's quality of life.

Related to COVID-19 research, there are currently 4274 clinical trials registered in ClinicalTrials.gov. In less than one year, researchers have identified and characterized a novel virus, developed diagnostics tools, proposed treatment protocols, and tested the efficacy of therapies and vaccines in clinical trials. Similarly, to other therapeutic areas, IoT in combination with Blockchain could also play an important role in these clinical trials by enabling virtual patient recruitment, consent, and data collection. Despite the hard times, valuable lessons have been learned on clinical development, pinpointing the main obstacles to overcome, and developing and implementing new strategies to streamline the process.

FUTURE RESEARCH DIRECTIONS

Blockchain technology can be applied to all industries (Makridakis & Christodoulou, 2019). And can be completely disruptive in so many ways for the business. It's not a surprise that many startups are using Blockchain to solve many of the company's issues.

However, BIoT is still is its early stage and the future brings challenges that need to be overcome. Some of these include:

- **Scalability:** the large number of nodes of IoT can be a difficulty, since blockchain scales poorly as the number of nodes in the network increases.
- **Processing Power and Time:** blockchain encryption algorithms required a high demand computing power. And some of the IoT devices do not have the computer power necessary to run these algorithms.
- **Storage**: Blockchain eliminates the need for a central server because it stores all transactions in a decentralized way, storing the data from the ledger in the system nodes. The distributed ledger will increase in size as time passes. Many IoT devices don't have a large storage capacity.
- **Lack of Skills:** Blockchain is a new technology and very few people have profound knowledge and experience with it. On the other hand, IoT devices exist everywhere. Therefore, efficient and productive integration of blockchain and IoT is only possible when experts of the different areas are more knowledgeable about the advantages and pitfalls of each.
- **Legal and Compliance**: Blockchain permits to connect different people from different places without having any legal or compliance code to follow, and this can be a serious issue to manufacture and services providers. This can be a barrier to implementing blockchain in many businesses.
- **Naming and Discovery**: Blockchain and IoT are two separate technologies that were not created with integration as main purpose, which means that nodes were not meant to find each other in the network (Atlam et al., 2018).

According to Makridakis and Christodoulou, the future of blockchain can move in two directions. The first will include all the applications requiring decentralized and super secured networks like smart contracts. In the future, there will be no alternative than to use blockchain with all these applications. The other direction is the use of blockchain with AI that when combined can substantially add value. Blockchain and AI can be used synergistically to improve the safety of big data and decentralizing who holds it. Now big data is centralized and owned almost exclusively by Google or Facebook. By using IoT and AI, people could preserve their own data and choose how and for who their information would be available. "At least, Blockchain and AI can cooperate on cybersecurity by combining AI and blockchain together to create a double shield against cyberattacks by training ML algorithms to automate real-time threat detection and to continuously learn about the behavior of attackers, while decentralized blockchains can minimize the inherent vulnerability of centralized databases" (Makridakis & Christodoulou, 2019).

Data Privacy

The explosion of IoT adoption is bound to threat its user´s privacy and pose significant data protection risks. The IoT devices constantly collect and share a lot of information that includes personal data, location, health data, users activities, amongst others, which means that data protection is a must have feature in all IoT systems. In healthcare, ensuring patients data privacy and security is of the utmost importance.

In this context and at the European level, the General Data Protection Regulation (GDPR), has been adopted on 14 April 2016, and came into force on the 25th of May 2018. This legislation set new rules that aim to facilitate the free movement of personal data between the EU's various Member States but also to protect and regulate data privacy. GDPR applies to any organization that holds or processes data of EU citizens. According to Article 5, the principles for personal data are: lawfulness, fairness and transparency, purpose limitation, data minimization, accuracy, storage limitation and accountability. GDPR includes a specific part dedicated to health data; it states that personal data concerning health should include all data pertaining health status (mental or physical) of an individual, in the past, present and future, as well as genetic and biometric data regardless of its source. Much of this data is nowadays obtained through technology, including IoT devices (*General Data Protection Regulation (GDPR) – Official Legal Text*, n.d.).

Some of the major issues about IoT according to the GDPR are transparency, consent, privacy. Companies are required to give customers or patients full access to their own personal data, specify how personal data is collected and used and offer clear opt-out options, and when it happens report data breaches (*Ethical IoT: GDPR, Personal Data, and Maintaining Consumer Trust*, n.d.). Importantly, users must provide consent and it needs to be informed, freely given, specific, and it requires an affirmative action. IoT companies must ensure that their devices strictly collect only the data that is necessary for fulfilling the relevant purpose, fulfilling the GDPR's principles of data minimization and purpose limitation. Moreover, they must ensure the right to be forgotten, meaning the IoT device must erase all data that it holds about an individual when requested to do so for example upon consent withdrawal (El-Mousa, 2018).

Although the application of blockchain to IoT could help manage some of these issues, for example consent could be achieved using smart contracts (Kouzinopoulos et al., 2018) and blockchain would be essential to provide security and privacy, blockchain is not devoid of challenges in what concerns to GDPR. The first one is accountability; GDPR assumes that there is a data controller, a natural or legal person, public authority, agency or other body, that must be able to demonstrate compliance with GDPR, but blockchains are distributed databases, so the allocation of responsibility and accountability is complex. The other challenge relates to the fact that according to GDPR data can be modified or erased when required to comply with legal requirements and can only be stored for a limited period of time except for public interest, scientific or historical research purposes or statistical purposes, but the information stored in Blockchain is immutable and perpetual as a way of ensuring integrity of the data (*Blockchain and the General Data Protection Regulation Can Distributed Ledgers Be Squared with European Data Protection Law?*, n.d.).

GDPR has been introduced only recently, and emerging technologies might not have been taken in account when developing it. But COVID-19 has pushed forward these new technologies, including blockchain and IoT, as part of solutions to tackle a lot of the pandemic associated challenges, therefore the authors consider that there needs to be further clarification by the lawmakers in order to accommodate the societal demand for innovation and unlock the full potential of the technologies while ensuring the privacy of citizens data.

CONCLUSION

In this paper, the authors reflected on the importance of blockchain and IoT technologies in the healthcare system, focusing on its application or possible future applications during the COVID-19 crisis and its aftermath. These two technologies were not created to be used together and are used separately in the healthcare industry to tackle different issues. The IoT industry has been on the market for some decades now, and the number of medical devices that allow data collection and interconnection remotely increases exponentially every year. Nevertheless, the security problems due to the IoT architecture must be handled to ensure better privacy and security. Blockchain technology will help overcome these issues associated with IoT. The three cases explored in this article demonstrate the potential of integrating these two technologies in the healthcare sector. As the world faces COVID-19 pandemics consequences, it is of the utmost importance to understand how Blockchain for Internet of Things (BIoT) could make industries more resilient and help the public health systems cut costs while delivering the best care.

REFERENCES

Al-Omari, A., Rabaan, A. A., Salih, S., Al-Tawfiq, J. A., & Memish, Z. A. (2019). MERS coronavirus outbreak: Implications for emerging viral infections. *Diagnostic Microbiology and Infectious Disease*, *93*(3), 265–285. Advance online publication. doi:10.1016/j.diagmicrobio.2018.10.011 PMID:30413355

Angeletti, F., Chatzigiannakis, I., & Vitaletti, A. (2017). The role of blockchain and IoT in recruiting participants for digital clinical trials. *2017 25th International Conference on Software, Telecommunications and Computer Networks (SoftCOM)*, 1–5. 10.23919/SOFTCOM.2017.8115590

Atlam, H. F., Alenezi, A., Alassafi, M. O., & Wills, G. B. (2018). Blockchain with Internet of Things: Benefits, Challenges, and Future Directions. *International Journal of Intelligent Systems and Applications*, *10*(6), 40–48. doi:10.5815/ijisa.2018.06.05

Benchoufi, M., Porcher, R., & Ravaud, P. (2018). Blockchain protocols in clinical trials: Transparency and traceability of consent. *F1000 Research*, *6*, 66. doi:10.12688/f1000research.10531.5 PMID:29167732

Bhutani, A., & Wadhwani, P. (2017). *Blockchain Technology Market 2019-2025 | Global Report*. https://www.gminsights.com/industry-analysis/blockchain-technology-market

Blockchain and the General Data Protection Regulation Can distributed ledgers be squared with European data protection law? (n.d.). doi:10.2861/535

Bot, B. M., Suver, C., Neto, E. C., Kellen, M., Klein, A., Bare, C., Doerr, M., Pratap, A., Wilbanks, J., Dorsey, E. R., Friend, S. H., & Trister, A. D. (2016). The mPower study, Parkinson disease mobile data collected using ResearchKit. *Scientific Data*, *3*(1), 160011. Advance online publication. doi:10.1038data.2016.11 PMID:26938265

Buterin, V. (2014). *A next generation smart contract & decentralized application platform*. Academic Press.

Chahrour, M., Assi, S., Bejjani, M., Nasrallah, A. A., Salhab, H., Fares, M. Y., & Khachfe, H. H. (2020). A Bibliometric Analysis of COVID-19 Research Activity: A Call for Increased Output. *Cureus*. Advance online publication. doi:10.7759/cureus.7357 PMID:32328369

Chamola, V., Hassija, V., Gupta, V., & Guizani, M. (2020). A Comprehensive Review of the COVID-19 Pandemic and the Role of IoT, Drones, AI, Blockchain, and 5G in Managing its Impact. *IEEE Access: Practical Innovations, Open Solutions*, 8, 90225–90265. Advance online publication. doi:10.1109/AC-CESS.2020.2992341

Chan, Y. F. Y., Wang, P., Rogers, L., Tignor, N., Zweig, M., Hershman, S. G., Genes, N., Scott, E. R., Krock, E., Badgeley, M., Edgar, R., Violante, S., Wright, R., Powell, C. A., Dudley, J. T., & Schadt, E. E. (2017). The Asthma Mobile Health Study, a large-scale clinical observational study using ResearchKit. *Nature Biotechnology*, 35(4), 354–362. doi:10.1038/nbt.3826 PMID:28288104

Chattu, V. K., Nanda, A., Chattu, S. K., Kadri, S. M., & Knight, A. W. (2019). The emerging role of blockchain technology applications in routine disease surveillance systems to strengthen global health security. In Big Data and Cognitive Computing (Vol. 3, Issue 2, pp. 1–10). MDPI AG. doi:10.3390/bdcc3020025

Cheng, V. C. C., Lau, S. K. P., Woo, P. C. Y., & Yuen, K. Y. (2007). Severe Acute Respiratory Syndrome Coronavirus as an Agent of Emerging and Reemerging Infection. *Clinical Microbiology Reviews*, 20(4), 660–694. Advance online publication. doi:10.1128/CMR.00023-07 PMID:17934078

Cryptowerk. (2018). *Using Blockchains and IoT to Record Clinical Trial Data*. Retrieved January 22, 2021, from https://cryptowerk.com/blockchains-iot-clinical-trial-data

Diffie, W., & Hellman, M. (1976). New directions in cryptography. *IEEE Transactions on Information Theory*, 22(6), 644–654. doi:10.1109/TIT.1976.1055638

DiMasi, J. A., Grabowski, H. G., & Hansen, R. W. (2016). Innovation in the pharmaceutical industry: New estimates of R&D costs. *Journal of Health Economics*, 47, 20–33. doi:10.1016/j.jhealeco.2016.01.012 PMID:26928437

El-Mousa, F. (2018). *GDPR Privacy Implications for the Internet of Things*. https://www.researchgate.net/publication/331991225

Enyinda, C. I., & Tolliver, D. (2009). Taking Counterfeits out of the Pharmaceutical Supply Chain in Nigeria: Leveraging Multilayer Mitigation Approach. *Journal of African Business*, 10(2), 218–234. Advance online publication. doi:10.1080/15228910903187957

Ethical IoT, GDPR, Personal Data, and Maintaining Consumer Trust. (n.d.). Retrieved April 17, 2021, from https://www.aeris.com/news/post/ethical-iot-gdpr-personal-data-and-maintaining-consumer-trust/

FDA & CDER. (2020). *Conduct of Clinical Trials of Medical Products During the COVID-19 Public Health Emergency Guidance for Industry, Investigators, and Institutional Review Boards Preface Public Comment*. https://www.fda.gov/regulatory-

General Data Protection Regulation (GDPR) – Official Legal Text. (n.d.). Retrieved April 17, 2021, from https://gdpr-info.eu/

Haber, S., & Stornetta, W. S. (1991). How to Time-Stamp a Digital Document. In *LNCS* (Vol. 537). Springer-Verlag.

Jamil, F., Hang, L., Kim, K., & Kim, D. (2019). A Novel Medical Blockchain Model for Drug Supply Chain Integrity Management in a Smart Hospital. *Electronics (Basel), 8*(5), 505. doi:10.3390/electronics8050505

Kalla, A., Hewa, T., Mishra, R. A., Ylianttila, M., & Liyanage, M. (2020). The Role of Blockchain to Fight Against COVID-19. *IEEE Engineering Management Review, 48*(3), 85–96. Advance online publication. doi:10.1109/EMR.2020.3014052

Kehoe, L., O'Connell, N., Andrzejewski, D., Gindner, K., & Dalal, D. (2017). *When two chains combine Supply chain meets blockchain*. https://www2.deloitte.com/tr/en/pages/technology/articles/when-two-chains-combine.html

Kolias, C., Kambourakis, G., Stavrou, A., & Voas, J. (2017). DDoS in the IoT: Mirai and other botnets. *Computer, 50*(7), 80–84. doi:10.1109/MC.2017.201

Konst, S., & Wätjen, D. (2000). *Sichere Log-Dateien auf Grundlage kryptographisch verketteter Einträge*. http://publikationsserver.tu-braunschweig.de/get/64933

Kouzinopoulos, C. S., Giannoutakis, K. M., Votis, K., Tzovaras, D., Collen, A., Nijdam, N. A., Konstantas, D., Spathoulas, G., Pandey, P., & Katsikas, S. (2018, September 14). Implementing a Forms of Consent Smart Contract on an IoT-based Blockchain to promote user trust. *2018 IEEE (SMC) International Conference on Innovations in Intelligent Systems and Applications, INISTA 2018*. 10.1109/INISTA.2018.8466268

Krawiec, R. J., Housman, D., White, M., Filipova, M., Quarre, F., Barr, D., Nesbitt, A., Fedosova, K., Killmeyer, J., Israel, A., & Tsai, L. (2017). *Blockchain: Opportunities for Health Care*. Academic Press.

Kumar, S., & Pundir, A. K. (2020). *Blockchain–Internet of things (IoT) Enabled Pharmaceutical Supply Chain for COVID-19*. Academic Press.

Laurent, P. (2017). *Continuous interconnected supply chain Using Blockchain & Internet-of-Things in supply chain traceability*. Academic Press.

Liang, Y. C. (2020). Blockchain for dynamic spectrum management. In *Signals and Communication Technology* (pp. 121–146). Springer. doi:10.1007/978-981-15-0776-2_5

Makridakis, S., & Christodoulou, K. (2019). Blockchain: Current challenges and future prospects/applications. In Future Internet (Vol. 11, Issue 12). MDPI AG. doi:10.3390/fi11120258

McDermott, D. S., Kamerer, J. L., & Birk, A. T. (2019). Electronic Health Records- A Literature Review of Cyber Threats and Security Measures. *International Journal of Cyber Research and Education, 1*(2), 42–49. doi:10.4018/IJCRE.2019070104

Menachemi, N., & Collum. (2011). Benefits and drawbacks of electronic health record systems. *Risk Management and Healthcare Policy*, *47*, 47. Advance online publication. doi:10.2147/RMHP.S12985 PMID:22312227

Merkle, R. C. (1990). *One Way Hash Functions and DES.*, doi:10.1007/0-387-34805-0_40

Mirchandani, P. (2020). Health Care Supply Chains: COVID-19 Challenges and Pressing Actions. In Annals of internal medicine (Vol. 173, Issue 4, pp. 300–301). NLM (Medline). doi:10.7326/M20-1326

Nagori, V. (2021). "Aarogya Setu": The mobile application that monitors and mitigates the risks of COVID-19 pandemic spread in India. *Journal of Information Technology Teaching Cases*. doi:10.1177/2043886920985863

Nakamoto, S. (2008). *Bitcoin: A Peer-to-Peer Electronic Cash System*. www.bitcoin.org

Noura, M., Atiquzzaman, M., & Gaedke, M. (2019). Interoperability in Internet of Things: Taxonomies and Open Challenges. *Mobile Networks and Applications*, *24*(3), 796–809. doi:10.100711036-018-1089-9

Omar, I. A., Jayaraman, R., Salah, K., Yaqoob, I., & Ellahham, S. (2020). Applications of Blockchain Technology in Clinical Trials: Review and Open Challenges. *Arabian Journal for Science and Engineering*. Advance online publication. doi:10.100713369-020-04989-3

Pham, H. L., Tran, T. H., & Nakashima, Y. (2018, December). A Secure Remote Healthcare System for Hospital Using Blockchain Smart Contract. *2018 IEEE Globecom Workshops (GC Wkshps)*. doi:10.1109/GLOCOMW.2018.8644164

Piscini, E., Dalton, D., & Kehoe, L. (2017). *Blockchain & Cyber Security. Let's Discuss*. https://www2. deloitte.com/tr/en/pages/technology-media-and-telecommunications/articles/blockchain-and-cyber.html

Reyna, A., Martín, C., Chen, J., Soler, E., & Díaz, M. (2018). On blockchain and its integration with IoT. Challenges and opportunities. *Future Generation Computer Systems*, *88*, 173–190. Advance online publication. doi:10.1016/j.future.2018.05.046

RFID Journal. (n.d.). Retrieved January 22, 2021, from https://www.rfidjournal.com/

Telugunta, R., & Choudhary, S. (2020). *Internet of Things (IOT) in Healthcare Market Size, and Growth 2027*. https://www.alliedmarketresearch.com/iot-healthcare-market

van Dorn, A. (2020). COVID-19 and readjusting clinical trials. *Lancet*, *396*(10250), 523–524. doi:10.1016/S0140-6736(20)31787-6 PMID:32828180

Viriyasitavat, W., da Xu, L., Bi, Z., & Pungpapong, V. (2019). Blockchain and Internet of Things for Modern Business Process in Digital Economy—The State of the Art. *IEEE Transactions on Computational Social Systems*, *6*(6), 1420–1432. doi:10.1109/TCSS.2019.2919325

Wang, H., Zheng, Z., Xie, S., Dai, H. N., & Chen, X. (2018). Blockchain challenges and opportunities: A survey. *International Journal of Web and Grid Services*, *14*(4), 352. doi:10.1504/IJWGS.2018.10016848

Weinberg, B. (2019). *14 Major Real Use Cases of Blockchain in Healthcare | OpenLedger Insights*. https://openledger.info/insights/blockchain-healthcare-use-cases/

Zimprich, S. (2019). *Data Protection and Blockchain - Security & Trust in Digital Services - Issues - dotmagazine*. https://www.dotmagazine.online/issues/security-trust-in-digital-services/data-protection-and-blockchain

KEY TERMS AND DEFINITIONS

Block: Blocks are records, which together form a blockchain. Each block contains a record of a transaction that is locked in chronological order and secured using cryptography. Each block contains, among other things, a record of recent transactions, and a reference to the block that came immediately before it.

Blockchain of Internet of Things: The integration of the two technologies. Blockchain will help solve some of the security issues typically associated with Internet of Things.

Blockchain Technology: Decentralized, distributed ledger that records transactions, tracks assets and builds trust.

Clinical Trial: A research study in which one or more human subjects are prospectively assigned to one or more interventions (which may include placebo or other control) to evaluate the effects of those interventions on health-related biomedical or behavioral outcomes.

COVID-19: Coronavirus disease is an infectious disease caused by a newly discovered coronavirus SARS-COV-2. The first case was detected in Wuhan, in China and quickly spread to a worldwide pandemic.

Internet of Things: Ubiquitous network of interconnected objects capable of information storage and exchange using embedded sensors, actuators, and other devices.

Pharmaceutical Supply Chain: A channel by which medicines have been shipped in the right quantity, with acceptable quality, at the appropriate place and costumers and at the proper time, and with optimum cost to be consistent with health system's objectives.

Chapter 8
Electronic Health Record Patient Portals and the Blockchain Technology

Jorge Tavares

NOVA IMS, Universidade Nova de Lisboa, Portugal

ABSTRACT

The electronic health records (EHR) patient portals are an integrated eHealth technology that combines an EHR system and a patient portal, giving patients access to their medical records, exam results, and services, such as appointment scheduling, notification systems, and e-mail access to their physician. EHR patient portals empower patients to carry out self-management activities and facilitate communication with healthcare providers, enabling the patient and healthcare provider to access the medical information quickly. Worldwide governmental initiatives have aimed to promote the use of EHR patient portals. The implementation of EHR patient portals encompasses several challenges, including security, confidentiality concerns, and interoperability between systems. New technological approaches like blockchain could address these issues and enable a successful worldwide implementation of EHR patient portals.

INTRODUCTION

The world is changing fast, and the healthcare environment is facing a more significant challenge. The warning signs are that the number of patients with chronic diseases is projected to grow by 45% between 2007 and 2025, and the workforce will be 10% smaller (Alpay et al., 2010; Tavares & Oliveira, 2016b). Hence, a new reality is emerging where there will be fewer healthcare professionals available in the future to support patients. The Covid-19 pandemic presented the world with its first big challenge of the digital age, and the countries that had their health systems more prepared, including from the digital standpoint, in general, had a better response to Covid-19 (Morris et al., 2020).

The Electronic Health Records (EHR) Patient Portals are an integrated eHealth Technology that combines an EHR system and a Patient Portal, which give patients access to their medical records, exam results, and services, such as appointment scheduling, notification systems, and e-mail access to their

DOI: 10.4018/978-1-7998-7363-1.ch008

physician (Osborn et al., 2013; Tavares & Oliveira, 2018). EHR Patient Portals empower patients to carry out self-management activities and facilitate communication with healthcare providers, enabling the patient and healthcare provider to easily access the medical information (Gordon & Hornbrook, 2016). This convenience is making the use of the healthcare system more effective and sustainable, not only from the patient care viewpoint but also from the national health systems perspective, due to the lack of human resources and increasing healthcare costs, that can be better managed with the progressive use of digital tools in healthcare. (Alpay et al., 2010; McKee et al., 2012; Metaxiotis et al., 2004).

The challenge of an older patient population with chronic diseases is now joined by the Covid-19 pandemic (Morris et al., 2020). The Covid-19 pandemic only reinforced the weakness of the traditional healthcare systems and the need for digitalization (Morris et al., 2020; Petracca et al., 2020). Many healthcare providers already implemented online video consultation and e-prescriptions via their EHR Patient Portals (Morris et al., 2020; Petracca et al., 2020), avoiding unnecessary travel of people to healthcare centers during pandemic times. The digitalization of healthcare will also allow populations living in remote areas to access more immediate healthcare support (Jordanova & Lievens, 2011; Rho et al., 2015).

Many governments worldwide, including European Union and the United States, promote the use of EHR Patient Portals to increase the efficiency of healthcare systems and give access and control to the patient to their data (Blumenthal & Tavenner, 2010; Commission, 2004). Blockchain is a technology that enables the ownership of virtual property or data to be determined beyond doubt and eliminates the need for a central ledger (Hoberman & Safari, 2018a). This technology also enables transactions' security, efficiency, and transparency, which can be viewed as critical features in a relationship between a patient and their healthcare provider. Showing how blockchain can improve and enhance healthcare, EHR Patient Portals will be addressed further in this chapter.

Methodology

The present study aims to describe how blockchain technology can be helpful to improve the current usage of EHR Patient Portals instead of presenting an extensive review about the structure or technical details of EHR Portals or blockchain technology. To achieve this goal, we searched scientific literature, between the years 2000 and 2021, in the following databases: Scopus, Web of Science, Google Scholar, and IGI global database. The leading search topics were: a) EHR Patient Portals projects; b) blockchain AND EHR; c) blockchain technology in healthcare; d) EHR security AND blockchain AND cyber-attacks. Two hundred and thirty-five references with potential interest were identified and reviewed, and from those, thirty-nine were referenced in this chapter.

BACKGROUND

EHR Patient Portals

To better comprehend the definition of EHR Patient Portals, it is critical to have a clear view of the technologies that support them. The first one is the Patient Portal, healthcare-related online applications that allow patients to interact and communicate with their healthcare providers to perform tasks such as asking healthcare-related questions, scheduling appointments, and requesting prescription refills

(Weingart et al., 2006). The second one is the EHR system, a software platform that physicians' offices and hospitals use to create, store, update, and maintain EHRs for patients (Angst & Agarwal, 2009).

EHR means a repository of patient data stored in digital form that must be exchanged securely. It contains retrospective, concurrent, and prospective information, and its primary purpose is to support continuing, efficient, and quality integrated health care (Hayrinen et al., 2008). EHRs may include a range of data, such as medical records, radiology images, vital signs, laboratory test results, and personal statistics like age and weight (Angst & Agarwal, 2009; Tavares & Oliveira, 2017)

Table 1 provides an overview of the differences and commonalities between the traditional EHR system and the enhanced EHR Patient Portal.

Table 1. Definition, differences, and communalities between EHR patient portals and EHR systems

	EHR Patient Portal	**EHR System**
Definition	Web based application that combines an EHR System with a Patient Portal that enables several functionalities such as: request prescription refills, schedule medical appointments, email messaging and disease management information areas. Currently EHR Patient Portals can also offer mobile versions.	It is an IT platform for realizing the mechanisms of creating, using, storing, and retrieving an EHR. EHR Systems have to be based on an architecture that enables them to be communicable, comprehensive, useful, and ethically compliant.
Differences	• The aim of the EHR Patient Portal is to give patient access to their clinical data and to enable the communication between the patients and the healthcare providers. • Patient centered technology	• The EHR System focus is to provide access to clinical integrated information to the healthcare professionals. • Healthcare professional centered technology.
Communalities	Both technologies use EHR. The main building block of an EHR Portal is the EHR System that with their interoperability capability may enable EHR Patient Portals to communicate.	

Adapted from Tavares & Oliveira (2016b)

EHR Patient Portals have received significant attention at the governmental level worldwide. In the United States, the support given to EHRs, via a meaningful use program, led the federal government to commit unparalleled resources to support the adoption of EHRs through incentive payments that can reach up to $27 billion over ten years (Angst & Agarwal, 2009; Blumenthal & Tavenner, 2010; Tavares & Oliveira, 2016a). EHR Patient Portals are a relevant topic not only in the United States but also in Europe. One of the most successful implementations in Europe is the Sundhed portal in Denmark, with a coverage of more than 20% of the Danish population (Gheorghiu & Hagens, 2017; Tavares & Oliveira, 2018).

Still, the implementation of EHR Patient Portals is made of successes, but security is also a concern for governments and health authorities worldwide. EHRs contain sensitive information that should be securely protected from falling into the wrong hands. The EHR Patient Portal from the Portuguese National Health Service (NHS), in its new release, already provides a higher level of security (2-factor authentication) to increase security and reassure confidence to their users, since it provides broader access to the patients to their clinical information data across NHS hospitals and healthcare centers (Tavares & Oliveira, 2018). Another topic that can also reduce the adoption of EHR Patient Portals is patients' concerns over EHR confidentiality. They are not only related to unauthorized access of the data from entities outside of the organizations (hackers), but also if within the healthcare organization, people who have access to the patient data are not the right authorized people, or how the data is shared with other healthcare organizations and private health insurance companies (Angst & Agarwal, 2009). It has been demonstrated that confidentiality concerns are a first barrier to the initial adoption of EHR Patient Portals, but they should not impact the ongoing usage (Angst & Agarwal, 2009).

EHR Patient Portals project using a multi-country approach like the European Patients Smart Open Services (EpSOS) initiative, which the European Union Commission promoted, failed a broad implementation (Tavares & Oliveira, 2016b). EpSOS focused on developing a practical information and communication technology infrastructure to secure access to patient information, including EHR, among different European countries. At the time of the project execution in 2014, different confidentiality protection laws among the different European countries made sharing EHR data between countries a legal issue challenging to solve (Grossman, 2014; Milberg et al., 2000; Tavares & Oliveira, 2016b). The General Data Protection Regulation (GDPR) that was adopted in 2016 and became enforceable during May 2018 (Markham, 2018) is a regulation in European Law on data protection and privacy in the European Union (EU) and the European Economic Area (EEA). The GDPR's primary aim is to give individuals control over their data and simplify the regulatory environment by unifying the regulation within the EU (Markham, 2018). If, at the time of EpSOS implementation, the GDPR law was in place, some of the regulatory aspects of data sharing between countries would have been easier to deal with. Still, perceptions connected with confidentiality and security concerns related to the IT infrastructure supporting EHR Portals are not solved only by new laws. Another particularly challenging topic during the EpSOS project is connecting and sharing information between different EHR Patient Portals (system interoperability). This issue equally affects systems within the same country or between countries (Tavares & Oliveira, 2016b).

Interoperability refers to the capacity to share information between systems. The interoperability level can be increased if the systems agree on the structure of data to be exchanged. This feature is often called functional interoperability, with which the only objective is to transfer information so that it is humanly readable by the receiver (Bisbal & Berry, 2011). However, the total goal is that two systems that need to share data agree on precisely the structure of the information to be exchanged, and more crucially, on the meaning of all the information to be shared, and this is the aim of semantic interoperability (Bisbal & Berry, 2011; Tavares & Oliveira, 2016b). Presently, semantic interoperability can be attained via standardization of data models, clinical data structure, and terminologies (This approach can be exemplified by current standardization efforts at CEN (standard EN-13606, known as EHRCom) as well as HL7 (RIM version 3) (Goeg et al., 2015; Tavares & Oliveira, 2016b).

Implementing EHR Patient Portals encompasses several challenges, including issues related to security, confidentiality concerns, and interoperability between systems. New technological approaches like blockchain could address these issues and enable a successful and worldwide implementation of EHR Patient Portals. The next section of this chapter provides an overview of blockchain technology and how it can support new digital tools in healthcare, particularly with EHR Patient Portals.

EHR AND BLOCKCHAIN TECHNOLOGY

A blockchain is, in its essence, a growing list of records, called blocks, that are linked together using cryptography (Hoberman & Safari, 2018a). Each block contains a cryptographic hash of the previous block, a timestamp, and transaction data (Hoberman & Safari, 2018a). Differently from traditional methods, blockchain allows peer-to-peer transfer of digital assets. All the transactions happen in a decentralized manner (Hoberman & Safari, 2018a). The characteristics of blockchain include transparency decentralization, immutability, and auditability (Monrat et al., 2019), making transactions safer and tamper-proof (Hoberman & Safari, 2018a; Monrat et al., 2019).

A Blockchain digital ledger is a buildup of records called blocks used to record transactions across systems so that any block cannot be altered retroactively without the modification of all subsequent blocks. This feature allows all the participants to check and audit transactions effectively (Hoberman & Safari, 2018b). A blockchain database is run in an autonomous manner using a peer-to-peer network and a shared timestamping server. They are validated by collaboration (Hoberman & Safari, 2018a), and this type of approach facilitates robust workflow where members' doubt regarding data security is minimal. Blockchain usage eradicates the feature of unlimited reproducibility from a digital asset and checks that each unit was transferred only once (Hoberman & Safari, 2018a; Monrat et al., 2019).

We can consider three types of blockchains that can be used in EHR Patient Portals: public, private, and consortium (Omar et al., 2020). Looking specifically to public blockchains, decentralized networks, all transactions can be verified by anyone, and their consensus mechanisms are also open for everyone to participate. Bitcoin is a well-known example of a public blockchain (Hoberman & Safari, 2018a). The openness concept of the public blockchain networks makes it difficult for a malicious entity to control the network where the EHRs are stored (Ismail et al., 2020; Omar et al., 2020). If this concept of openness gives a sense of more transparency and security; the characteristics of the data that is store in an EHR, that deals with sensitive topics, and the need to ensure a safe and private connection between the patient and the healthcare providers, may result that this may not be the best option for healthcare sensitive data. Another type of blockchains is the Private blockchains, also known as permissioned blockchains (Hoberman & Safari, 2018a; Omar et al., 2020). They do not allow all entities to join the network and they supervise and control reading and writing operations into the blockchain (Hoberman & Safari, 2018a; Omar et al., 2020). Financial or healthcare organizations often use this type of blockchain to ensure efficiency and auditability (Omar et al., 2020). Private blockchains provide a solution to solve critical issues related to EHR data, such as privacy and compliance. Unlike the public blockchain, only authorized or designated organizations/ entities can join the EHR Patient Portal wherein EHR data are stored, thereby ensuring security and data privacy (Ismail et al., 2020; Omar et al., 2020). This option is standard in the USA, where the regulatory environment allows private healthcare institutions, like healthcare insurance companies, to manage patients' data (Angst & Agarwal, 2009).

The last consortium to be discussed is known as the hybrid blockchain. In hybrid blockchains, the ledger is distributed only to permitted participants, while the consensus mechanism is controlled by selected servers using rules that are agreed upon by all participants in the network (Hoberman & Safari, 2018a; Omar et al., 2020). As a result, the network is partly decentralized. The significant advantages of consortium blockchain platforms are that their consensus mechanism consumes less computational effort when compared with a public blockchain, there is not only one single entity controlling all the network like with the permissioned blockchains, and this platform is more flexible and ensures greater privacy compared to the public blockchain (Hoberman & Safari, 2018a; Omar et al., 2020). The concept of hybrid blockchain seems to be able to keep the confidential relationship between the patients and their healthcare providers when exchange data between them, allowing at the same time the patient to retain rights to whom and how to share their information. This convenience is aligned with GDPR's primary aim to give individuals control over their data. One of the factors that was identified as a barrier to the adoption of EHR Patient Portals in the USA is the use of private EHR networks where access to their "own patient data" was restricted by the individual himself (Angst & Agarwal, 2009). Another advantage of hybrid blockchains is that when they are associated with smart contracts, they can filter the amount of data to be available or kept private between the different stakeholders of a network regarding specific and individual patient records (Kamel Boulos et al., 2018). Smart contracts are an algorithm of code that is kept, executed, and verified on a blockchain and can act on patient data sharing, either through storing the information itself or instructions on the entities than accessing that information (Kamel Boulos et al., 2018).

When an EHR Patient Portal integrates several institutions within an organization, at the national level, or even with data sharing between countries, data integrity is of the utmost importance. Data integrity in a blockchain network is guaranteed by authenticating each transaction using a consensus algorithm. If there is a situation of error detection in a chain, it is feasible to trace back and pinpoint the error's origin alongside the person accountable for inserting this information (Ismail et al., 2020; Kamel Boulos et al., 2018; Omar et al., 2020). It is possible to identify and correct errors because blockchain networks have a very efficient traceability mechanism. As mentioned before, using blockchain technology can increase security and data privacy in the EHR Patient Portals. This safety can be guaranteed more efficiently as each patient has an encrypted address that is mapped to his/her identity. Then the patient agrees to provide their private keys to a designated physician or healthcare institution, keeping control of their medical data and the number of healthcare providers that can access it (Kamel Boulos et al., 2018; Omar et al., 2020).

EHR Patient Portals serve as a repository for valued health information, an asset to both the patients and criminals (Alharam et al., 2017). Medical data contains sensitive information that, for different reasons, individuals may not wish to be revealed as this may cause personal embarrassment, discrimination, or damage to their professional reputation (Alharam et al., 2017; Chen & Lambright, 2016). For these reasons, cyber-attacks may cause irreparable damages to patients, healthcare institutions, and society in general. One of the most significant known healthcare cyber-attack occurred in Singapore in 2018; hackers have stolen personal healthcare data belonging to 1.5 million people, approximately a quarter of the Singapore population (BBC, 2018). The Prime Minister of Singapore, who survived twice cancer (BBC, 2018), was explicitly and repeatedly targeted. These cyber-attacks are frequent, and not all are disclosed to the public. In 2017, a hacking group named Lazarus crippled the UK's National Health Service (NHS) and other healthcare organizations worldwide (BBC, 2018). These risks are not unnoticed by governments.

Acknowledging the unique and severe nature of electronic health records, the United States Congress founded the Health Care Industry Cybersecurity Task Force under the Cybersecurity Information Sharing Act of 2015, intending to review cybersecurity risks in the healthcare industry (Farringer, 2019). Interestingly the findings in the United States position the cybersecurity in healthcare considerably weaker when compared to (Peng et al., 2021) other industries, and unless some general system redesign is achieved that increases security, the cyber-attacks will continue to cause damage (Farringer, 2019). Blockchain technology is addressing this problem, like using secure encryption schemes for EHR sharing in blockchain with auspicious results (Peng et al., 2021). One of the criticisms of blockchain in decentralized systems is the computational effort. Nonetheless, recent studies have shown that blockchain technology can be up to 50% faster than conventional data security and storage (Nagasubramanian et al., 2020; Peng et al., 2021).

The previously mentioned studies provide additional evidence on how blockchain technology can protect EHR Patient Portals. Still, the fundamental nature of blockchain technology is by itself an excellent way to protect patient data against cyber-attacks (Pandey & Litoriya, 2020). With multiple medical authorities planning to have digital medical passports and immunity certificates to cope with the Covid-19 pandemic and to allow safe sharing of information between healthcare institutions and countries, security and data integrity play a fundamental role (Hasan et al., 2020). Smart contracts have been written and tested successfully to maintain a digital medical identity for test-takers that help prompt, trusted response directly by the relevant medical authorities (Hasan et al., 2020). Blockchain technology can help increase the security and data integrity related to information sharing between countries during the Covid-19 pandemic, dealing with many critical issues, including cyber-attacks (Hasan et al., 2020; Petracca et al., 2020).

CONCLUSION

The use of Blockchain technology can improve EHR Patient Portals in specific topics. Some of them were also identified as potential weaknesses or areas to improve. The well-known security against external attacks from malicious entities given by the well-designed architecture of blockchain networks benefits the data integrity when an exchange between different stakeholders happens within the network (Hoberman & Safari, 2018a; Omar et al., 2020).

Data integrity in a blockchain network is guaranteed by authenticating each transaction using a consensus algorithm, making it feasible to trace back and pinpoint the origin of errors. These features improve users' trust when using this technology in healthcare, mainly dealing with critical and sensitive patient data. Blockchain enables better communication between systems with full traceability and data integrity. The topic of confidentiality is also critical for the patients and healthcare institutions, and the usage of hybrid networks with smart contracts could be an excellent approach with a high level of security that filters the access of the individual patient data within the network, allowing the information to be shared with whom needs to have access.

The European General Data Protecting Regulation (GDPR) initiative that aims to give individuals control over their data can also benefit from blockchain technology to implement their goals. This review demonstrated that blockchain technology could be an effective solution for topics related to areas that require improvement in the implementation and roll-out of EHR Patient Portals, such as system security, data integrity, confidentiality concerns, and better interoperability between systems. Particularly during the Covid-19 pandemic, blockchain technology can increase the safety of the electronic health data transfer between institutions and countries, keeping data integrity a priority.

Finally, it should be emphasized that security and data integrity are of the utmost importance for digital medical passports and immunity certificates.

REFERENCES

Alharam, A. K., & El-Madany, W. (2017). The Effects of Cyber-Security on Healthcare Industry. *IEEE GCC Conference and Exhibition GCCCE*.

Alpay, L. L., Henkemans, O. B., Otten, W., Rovekamp, T. A. J. M., & Dumay, A. C. M. (2010). E-health Applications and Services for Patient Empowerment: Directions for Best Practices in The Netherlands. *Telemedicine Journal and e-Health, 16*(7), 787–791. doi:10.1089/tmj.2009.0156 PMID:20815745

Angst, C. M., & Agarwal, R. (2009). Adoption of electronic health records in the presence of privacy concerns: The elaboration likelihood model and Individual Persuasion. *Management Information Systems Quarterly*, *33*(2), 339–370. doi:10.2307/20650295

BBC. (2018). *Singapore personal data hack hits 1.5m, health authority says*. BBC News. Retrieved Feb 25th 2021 from https://www.bbc.com/news/world-asia-44900507

Bisbal, J., & Berry, D. (2011). An Analysis Framework for Electronic Health Record Systems Interoperation and Collaboration in Shared Healthcare. *Methods of Information in Medicine*, *50*(2), 180–189. doi:10.3414/ME09-01-0002 PMID:19936438

Blumenthal, D., & Tavenner, M. (2010). The "Meaningful Use" Regulation for Electronic Health Records. *The New England Journal of Medicine*, *363*(6), 501–504. doi:10.1056/NEJMp1006114 PMID:20647183

Chen, Q., & Lambright, J. (2016). Towards Realizing a Self-Protecting Healthcare Information System. *Proceedings International Computer Software and Applications Conference*. 10.1109/COMPSAC.2016.264

Commission, E. (2004). e-Health - making healthcare better for European citizens: An action plan for a European e-Health Area. Brussels: European Commission

Farringer, D. R. (2019). Maybe If We Turn It Off and Then Turn It Back On Again? Exploring Health Care Reform as a Means to Curb Cyber Attacks. *The Journal of Law, Medicine & Ethics*, *47*(4, SUPPL), 91–102. doi:10.1177/1073110519898046 PMID:31955693

Gheorghiu, B., & Hagens, S. (2017). Use and Maturity of Electronic Patient Portals. *Studies in Health Technology and Informatics*, *234*, 136–141. PMID:28186030

Goeg, K. R., Cornet, R., & Andersen, S. K. (2015). Clustering clinical models from local electronic health records based on semantic similarity. *Journal of Biomedical Informatics*, *54*, 294–304. doi:10.1016/j.jbi.2014.12.015 PMID:25557885

Gordon, N. P., & Hornbrook, M. C. (2016). Differences in Access to and Preferences for Using Patient Portals and Other eHealth Technologies Based on Race, Ethnicity, and Age: A Database and Survey Study of Seniors in a Large Health Plan. *Journal of Medical Internet Research*, *18*(3), e50–e50. doi:10.2196/jmir.5105 PMID:26944212

Grossman, L. A. (2014). The rise of the empowered consumer: In recent decades, the FDA has allowed people to take a more active role in their health care. *Regulation*, (4), 34.

Hasan, H. R., Salah, K., Jayaraman, R., Arshad, J., & Omar, M. (2020). Blockchain-Based Solution for COVID-19 Digital Medical Passports and Immunity Certificates. *IEEE Access: Practical Innovations, Open Solutions*, *8*, 222093–222108. doi:10.1109/ACCESS.2020.3043350

Hayrinen, K., Saranto, K., & Nykanen, P. (2008). Definition, structure, content, use and impacts of electronic health records: A review of the research literature. *International Journal of Medical Informatics*, *77*(5), 291–304. doi:10.1016/j.ijmedinf.2007.09.001 PMID:17951106

Hoberman, S., & Safari, O. R. M. C. (2018a). *Blockchain Explanation, Usage, and Impact*. Technics Publications. https://library.villanova.edu/Find/Record/2246337/Description

Hoberman, S., & Safari, O. R. M. C. (2018b). Blockchainopoly: How Blockchain Changes the Rules of the Game. Technics Publications.

Ismail, L., Materwala, H., Karduck, A. P., & Adem, A. (2020). Requirements of Health Data Management Systems for Biomedical Care and Research: Scoping Review [Review]. *Journal of Medical Internet Research, 22*(7), 16. doi:10.2196/17508

Jordanova, M., & Lievens, F. (2011). *Global Telemedicine and eHealth (A synopsis). E-Health and Bioengineering Conference*. EHB.

Kamel Boulos, M. N., Wilson, J. T., & Clauson, K. A. (2018). Geospatial blockchain: Promises, challenges, and scenarios in health and healthcare. *International Journal of Health Geographics, 17*(1), 25. doi:10.118612942-018-0144-x

Markham, K. (2018). *A practical guide to the general data protection regulation (GDPR)*. Law Brief Publishing, Ltd.

McKee, M., Karanikolos, M., Belcher, P., & Stuckler, D. (2012). Austerity: A failed experiment on the people of Europe. *Clinical Medicine, 12*(4), 346–350. doi:10.7861/clinmedicine.12-4-346 PMID:22930881

Metaxiotis, K., Ptochos, D., & Psarras, J. (2004). E-health in the new millennium: A research and practice agenda. *International Journal of Electronic Healthcare, 1*(2), 165–175. doi:10.1504/IJEH.2004.005865 PMID:18048218

Milberg, S. J., Smith, H. J., & Burke, S. J. (2000). Information privacy: Corporate management and national regulation. *Organization Science, 11*(1), 35–57. doi:10.1287/orsc.11.1.35.12567

Monrat, A. A., Schelén, O., & Andersson, K. (2019). A Survey of Blockchain From the Perspectives of Applications, Challenges, and Opportunities. *IEEE Access: Practical Innovations, Open Solutions, 7*, 117134–117151. doi:10.1109/ACCESS.2019.2936094

Morris, D., Solon, L., Simpson, J., Read, O., & Abel, J. (2020). *Tech powered healthcare: a strategic approach to implementing technology in health and care*. PricewaterhouseCoopers.

Nagasubramanian, G., Sakthivel, R. K., Patan, R., Gandomi, A. H., Sankayya, M., & Balusamy, B. (2020). Securing e-health records using keyless signature infrastructure blockchain technology in the cloud. *Neural Computing & Applications, 32*(3), 639–647. doi:10.100700521-018-3915-1

Omar, I. A., Jayaraman, R., Salah, K., Simsekler, M. C. E., Yaqoob, I., & Ellahham, S. (2020). Ensuring protocol compliance and data transparency in clinical trials using Blockchain smart contracts. *BMC Medical Research Methodology, 20*(1), 224. doi:10.118612874-020-01109-5 PMID:32894068

Osborn, C. Y., Mayberry, L. S., Wallston, K. A., Johnson, K. B., & Elasy, T. A. (2013). Understanding Patient Portal Use: Implications for Medication Management. *Journal of Medical Internet Research, 15*(7), 204–215. doi:10.2196/jmir.2589 PMID:23823974

Pandey, P., & Litoriya, R. (2020). Securing and authenticating healthcare records through blockchain technology. *Cryptologia, 44*(4), 341–356. doi:10.1080/01611194.2019.1706060

Peng, X. Z., Zhang, J. Q., Zhang, S. B., Wan, W. N., Chen, H., & Xia, J. Y. (2021). A Secure Signcryption Scheme for Electronic Health Records Sharing in Blockchain. *Computer Systems Science and Engineering*, *37*(2), 265–281. doi:10.32604/csse.2021.014557

Petracca, F., Ciani, O., Cucciniello, M., & Tarricone, R. (2020). Harnessing Digital Health Technologies During and After the COVID-19 Pandemic: Context Matters. *Journal of Medical Internet Research*, *22*(12), e21815. Advance online publication. doi:10.2196/21815 PMID:33351777

Rho, M. J., Yoon, K. H., Kim, H. S., & Choi, I. Y. (2015). Users' perception on telemedicine service: A comparative study of public healthcare and private healthcare. *Multimedia Tools and Applications*, *74*(7), 2483–2497. doi:10.100711042-014-1966-6

Tavares, J., & Oliveira, T. (2016a). Electronic Health Record Patient Portal Adoption by Health Care Consumers: An Acceptance Model and Survey. *Journal of Medical Internet Research*, *18*(3), e49. doi:10.2196/jmir.5069 PMID:26935646

Tavares, J., & Oliveira, T. (2016b). Electronic Health Record Portals Definition and Usage. In C.-C. Maria Manuela, M. Isabel Maria, M. Ricardo, & R. Rui (Eds.), *Encyclopedia of E-Health and Telemedicine* (pp. 555–562). IGI Global. doi:10.4018/978-1-4666-9978-6.ch043

Tavares, J., & Oliveira, T. (2017). Electronic Health Record Portal Adoption: A cross country analysis. *BMC Medical Informatics and Decision Making*, *17*(1), 1–17. doi:10.118612911-017-0482-9 PMID:28679423

Tavares, J., & Oliveira, T. (2018). New Integrated Model Approach to Understand the Factors That Drive Electronic Health Record Portal Adoption: Cross-Sectional National Survey. *Journal of Medical Internet Research*, *20*(11), e11032. doi:10.2196/11032 PMID:30455169

Weingart, S. N., Rind, D., Tofias, Z., & Sands, D. Z. (2006). Who uses the patient Internet portal? The PatientSite experience. *Journal of the American Medical Informatics Association: JAMIA*, *13*(1), 91–95. doi:10.1197/jamia.M1833 PMID:16221943

Chapter 9
A Concrete Way to Develop Clinical Research in a Fair Way to the Users/Patients Using Blockchain Technology

João Fonseca-Gomes

Instituto de Medicina Molecular João Lobo Antunes, Portugal

Denise Francisco

Instituto de Medicina Molecular João Lobo Antunes, Portugal

João Mota Sequeira

ISEG, Lisbon School of Economics and Management, University of Lisbon, Portugal

ABSTRACT

Blockchain is being explored as a potential solution to many problems in areas other than the one created initially: cryptocurrency. Blockchain technology allows the authenticity of data, security in transactions, and privacy without the need for a third party. For that main reason, one of the growing interests concerns its application in healthcare, namely in clinical research. Multiple pain points of clinical research might benefit from the implementation of blockchain technology. This chapter shows some examples in which this technology is already implemented, identifying the advantages of its use. One of those advantages is clinical research, with the possibility of the patients managing their own clinical data and being properly rewarded for that. Research about clinical data monetization for patients is currently limited, and this chapter also proposes a hypothetical scenario of health data monetization workflow.

DOI: 10.4018/978-1-7998-7363-1.ch009

INTRODUCTION

Generically, it is widely established that Science is made of reliable data. Unfortunately, over the past years, there is a tendency for an increase in research misconduct, data fraud, and lack of transparency. (Benchoufi et al., 2017, 2019; Gupta, 2013). Inevitably, this tendency can disrupt one of the essential characteristics of clinical research: trust. Combining the incorruptibility of blockchain technology with clinical research might be a powerful tool to re-establish trust in clinical data. Moreover, the introduction of this technology may allow patients to possess their clinical data and decide to share it in exchange for a token representing some benefit. This study describes a way to develop clinical research in a fair way to patients using blockchain technology. This chapter also discusses the main advantages of blockchain-based technologies in clinical research and the challenges of their implementation. On the other hand, it explores data monetization to benefit the patient using smart contracts. Pros and challenges of blockchain implementation in clinical trials for the patient and the healthcare industries and society were also discussed.

BLOCKCHAIN TECHNOLOGY OVERVIEW

In October 2008, Satochi Nakamoto introduced a peer-to-peer electronic cash system: The Bitcoin (Nakamoto, 2008). He/she proposed a way to make transactions between two parties without the need of going through a financial institution. Nakamoto realized that digital signatures would not solve the need of a trusted third part to avoid double-spending transactions. The solution proposed was a peer-to-peer network. Timestamps transactions hashed and saved on an ongoing chain former a record of data that can no longer be edited or removed (Nakamoto, 2008). Although it was been explored in other systems, to date, cryptocurrencies are still the most commonly recognized use of blockchain technology. This technology have been described in several ways, the most generally accepted is: a peer-to-peer (P2P) distributed ledger technology (Laure A. Linn, 2016). This means that blockchain works as a system where each member in the network (node) stores an identical copy of the ledger. Each node gives their contribution on the collective process of validation and certification of the data recorded. The advantage of this decentralised P2P architecture is the lack of a central server to guarantee trust. When happens to occur a record of a digital transaction it has to be evaluated through algorithms by each member of the distributed network. The update of a new transaction on a shared ledger occurs only if the majority of the members vote as a valid process. When a consensus is reached all the other nodes updated themselves and that information can no longer be edited or deleted.

The security of the process is guarantee through the usage of cryptographic keys and signatures. Privacy is protected in the blockchain using a system of a key pair for each member: a public key and a private key. Zhuang and colleagues refer to the private key as a signature and a public key as a bank account. To understand how this key pair works, a new transaction by an user might be considered. All the other members of the blockchain can see the public key of that user, but it keeps the private key hidden. Although the private key is not accessible, it is possible to check if the public key and the signed private key of the transaction match. If they not match the transaction will be voted down by the users and discarded. (Yan Zhuang et al., 2019) In addition, to being digitally signed the information contained in the transaction is encrypted to guarantee authenticity and accuracy. Transactions are stored into blocks that are added in a chronological order to a chain. Each block contains a unique code called hash. It also contains the hash of the prior block of chain (Laure A. Linn, 2016). The overview of the process is schematized in Figure 1.

Figure 1. Overview of how blockchain technology operates. It starts with a user request of transaction that can be cryptocurrency or other data; The transaction is signed with user's private key and then the other nodes can verify the transaction using user's public key as it is shared to the network; Transaction is included in a block and nodes compete to had a cryptographic hash value for the block; The block is added to the blockchain where all the transactions are stored; The block added is now immutable and permanent – making a change would require an huge computing power; The transaction is executed and the process concluded (adapted from Chen et al, 2019)

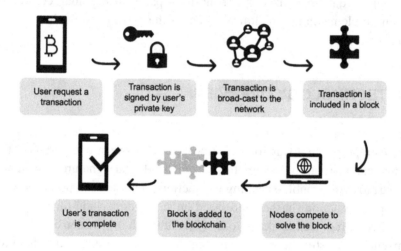

Authenticity of the data, security and privacy are the fundamental keys for the success of this technology. Accordingly, their potential has been increasingly explored as it is possible to observe by the number of publications presented on the *Pubmed* database for the past few years (Figure 2).

Blockchain can be presented as a "public chain" or a "private chain". In the public chain all the users can join the system, see and participate on the validation process of all transactions. In this chain the stability of the blockchain depends on the number of participating nodes. The higher is the number of users the higher is the confidence on the consensual process of a transaction validation. Bitcoin is one of the most recognized examples of a public chain. (Yu Zhuang et al., 2018).

On the other hand, "private chains" are chains with limited access since only the users that have permission can join the system. To be part of a private system, participants have to install a genesis block – the first block of the chain. This first block is responsible of determine the characteristics of that private chain and they are different for each blockchain. This means that they can only be acquired be the creators. The creators have the power to manage the permissions to join the chain, some authors suggest that unlike public chain this private chain is not a fully decentralized chain (Yu Zhuang et al., 2018).

Another feature of blockchain technology is the creation of smart contracts. Nick Szabo was the first proposing distributed ledger systems to regulate contracts in 1994 (Szabo & The, 2015). Smart contracts are programing codes protocols that are self-executable stablishing restrictive rules in the same way of

Figure 2. Representation of evolution observed regarding publication of manuscripts focusing both "blockchain" (data obtained from Pubmed database, data available online at 11ᵗʰ November, 2020)

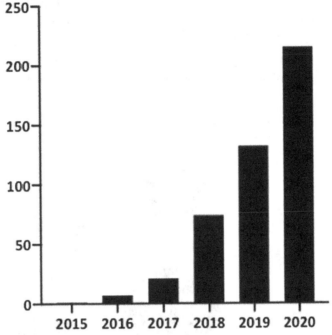

the traditional contract document. It has obligations, benefits or penalties for all the parties involved. All the users on blockchain have to follow the coded consensus protocol to make transactions. Contracts are programed as conditioned events that looks like "IF Condition 1 AND Condition 2… AND Condition N (are met) THEN DO this ELSE DO that". (Benchoufi et al., 2019) Smart contracts do not require a third-party intermediate to verify if the conditions are met and apply the consequences. In that way, it is reduced failure points and costs (Yu Zhuang et al., 2018).

Prementioned characteristics highlight the many promises that blockchain presents for the future. One of the biggest potentials is combining blockchain with Big Data. In that way, users could be in their control of data and transactions and could also trust that transactions will be executed following protocol commands. At the same time, blockchain technology avoids the introduction of unreliable information, increasing the authenticity of data. On the other hand, the possibility of having an identical copy of the information in different servers avoid the need of having one big central server. For that main reasons, blockchain contributes to collect more and real data (Karafiloski & Mishev, 2017).

BLOCKCHAIN-BASED TECHNOLOGY ON CLINICAL RESEARCH: A NEW WORLD OF ADVANTAGES, APPLICATIONS AND LIMITATIONS

Before considering the possible application and importance of blockchain in clinical research, it is essential to understand the concept behind this particular field, together with all the subtopics inside this bigger umbrella. Actually, it is not so uncommon that clinical research and clinical trials or clinical research and medical care are considered the same. However, clinical trials and medical care are just small elements among many others included in the clinical research field, together with health services, mental health, education, outcomes, epidemiology, physiology and pathology itself (Figure 3). In this way, in a broader manner, clinical research is often considered as the study of health and illness in people, including not only the translation of pre-clinical studies (basic research) into clinical ones, but also the scientific groundwork for prevention, diagnosis and treatment of pathologies (Institute of Medicine (US) Forum on Drug Discovery Development and Translation, 2010; Tunis et al., 2002; U. S. Food & Drug, 2020).

Figure 3. Summary of all elements constitutive of clinical research field

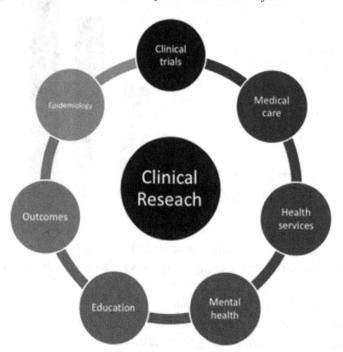

Over the last decades, it is becoming clear that, although all the efforts, evolution, development, maturity, experience and, in some cases, success, clinical research has a multiplicity of pain points that delay its effectiveness around the world. Some of the main limitations that underlie the quality of clinical research are related with the subjectivity behind the studies, together with misconduct, error, frauds, hard traceability, lack of integration of lateral information (such as cultural or environmental data) and also personal or company interests (George & Buyse, 2015; Goldacre et al., 2018; Gupta, 2013; House of Commons Science and Technology Committee, 2018; Ioannidis, 2005). Therefore, it is easily and directly understandable that the clinical research field might really benefit from advances in technology and, more particularly, from the implementation of blockchain technology. Supporting this suggestion, it is becoming noticeable an increase of studies focusing both topics in the more recent years (Benchoufi et al., 2017, 2019; Benchoufi & Ravaud, 2017; Nugent et al., 2016; Pane et al., 2020; Park et al., 2019; Yan Zhuang et al., 2019). Actually, as shown in Figure 4, it is totally clear that in the last few years there has been an impactful growth in research articles that connect "Blockchain" and "Clinical Research" in its scopes. More importantly, this growth is being supported in scientific and technological experiments already planned or finished all over the world (Abdel-Basset et al., 2020; Dai et al., 2018; Hirano et al., 2020; Marbouh et al., 2020; Maslove et al., 2018; Nugent et al., 2016; Pane et al., 2020; Roman-Belmonte et al., 2018; Wong et al., 2019). Anyway, it should be mentioned that this growth can be even bigger, because only one particular database (Pubmed) was considered and certainly there are studies being developed in these days, which were not reported in their planification stage. Nevertheless, the next paragraphs will demonstrate some applications of blockchain technologies already being implemented, being only a part of all the possible applications of this *new era* of knowledge focusing clinical research.

Figure 4. Representation of evolution observed regarding publication of manuscripts focusing both "blockhain" and "clinical research" (data obtained from Pubmed database, data available online at 11th November, 2020)

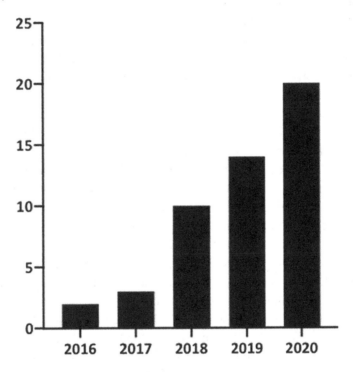

Some Examples of Blockchain-based Technologies in Clinical Research

One significant example regarding the unmeasurable impact of blockchain technology in clinical research nowadays is related with the easy adaptation of its concept for many elements of our days. In particular, this disruptive technology might be converted into learning and knowledge to better handle the COVID-19 crisis, together with other technological elements. Even considering the surprise and complexity of COVID-19 pandemic, blockchain technology is already being implemented to fight the health, societal and economic consequences that arose in the last few months (Abdel-Basset et al., 2020; Fusco et al., 2020; Hau & Chang, 2020; Marbouh et al., 2020; Nandi et al., 2021). Actually, only regarding the health issues caused by this pandemic crisis, several authors indicate that blockchain-based technology might have several potential uses, allowing 1) the implementation of a reliable data tracker, 2) promotion of confidentiality and transparency regarding track donations and fundraising activities (by an increased public awareness) and also as a 3) simplification of clinical trial processes for therapeutics drugs and vaccines (Hau & Chang, 2020; Marbouh et al., 2020). As a consequence, in this context, blockchain systems also allow the elaboration of a decentralized tracking system that incorporates data from several authoritative and public sources (such as World Health Organization, the Center for Disease Control, and the Institute for Health Metrics and Evaluation). Finally, this system will improve the trust among all the stakeholders, ensuring data integrity, security, transparency and its traceability, which may promote faster solutions for the pandemics of our days (Marbouh et al., 2020).

Another example regarding the direct application of blockchain technology in clinical research regarding COVID-19 pandemic is the result of the work produced at Emerge. Emerge is a Toronto-based blockchain startup that developed and launched an app (*Civitas*) that, by using blockchain technology, intends to assist local authorities in controlling the COVID-19 occurrence, being already implemented in Latin America countries (e.g. Honduras). This particular software associates each person identification with its corresponding and personal blockchain record, without disclosing their identity. Therefore, this data is only accessed by the user and the healthcare provider (mainly doctors, locals' government or national healthcare system), ensuring the privacy and confidentiality. In addition, this app can help to minimize the spread of the virus, by 1) unrevealing whether a person has left his home or his job, 2) tracking the evolution of health issues or even 3) monitoring their symptomatology. In return, *Civitas* is able to send medical reports to the users (which might include medication to be followed, if necessary) or indicate the best and safest days to go out for essentials (Marbouh et al., 2020; Wright, 2020).

As mentioned before, together with national and local authorities, the scientific community is implementing new and totally disruptive technologies in several different areas in science, and in clinical research in particular. Interestingly, one of the main fields that are taking advantage of blockchain technology concerns the clinical trials (Benchoufi et al., 2017; Dai et al., 2018; Drosatos & Kaldoudi, 2019; Gordon & Catalini, 2018; Hirano et al., 2020; Maslove et al., 2018; Rao, R.; Jain, 2019; Roman-Belmonte et al., 2018; Shae & Tsai, 2017; Verde et al., 2019; Wong et al., 2019; Yan Zhuang et al., 2019) . Actually, even though all the outstanding development and experience in clinical trials, in the recent years it is becoming urgent to handle the increased complexity, longevity and cost of clinical trials, as well as higher regulatory hurdles (Gefenas et al., 2017; Institute of Medicine (US) Forum on Drug Discovery Development and Translation, 2010; Pane et al., 2020; Satia, 2017). Therefore, the interaction between blockchain technology (and all the respective applications and capabilities) with the design, implementation and post-validation of clinical trials is being noticed in a clear way.

Briefly, a clinical trial includes the demonstration of safety and efficiency (without relevant side effects) of a particular medication and/or medical device, being an obligatory requirement before accessing the market. Considering the strong impact upon health, all these trials must be strictly and minutely prepared, conducted and analyzed. Clinical trials include four different phases, reaching more responsibility and integrating a greater number of patients in each phase. Therefore, it is easy to understand how complex and highly labor-intensive might be to manage a single clinical trial, from its design until the final report (Gefenas et al., 2017; Institute of Medicine (US) Forum on Drug Discovery Development and Translation, 2010; Satia, 2017). Actually, human-induced errors and/or data falsification (whether accidental or intentional) might compromise that the clinical protocol to be followed is being correctly used. Its implementation should occur in the safest, fastest and most transparent way possible to the stakeholders included in the entire network (Marbouh et al., 2020; Rao, R.; Jain, 2019; Satia, 2017). Indeed, it is shocking that an intentional fabrication of particular data in research is confirmed by around

17% of authors of clinical trials (George & Buyse, 2015; Gupta, 2013). As a consequence, there is not surprising that one of the greatest medical challenges of our time is related to the poor reproducibility of clinical research, due to several factors, including lack of data sharing and some misconduct concerning switched outcomes during the trial analysis (George & Buyse, 2015; Gupta, 2013; House of Commons Science and Technology Committee, 2018; Ioannidis, 2005).

In this way, and as indicated above, blockchain technology opened new perspectives that might provide the groundwork to ensure all the basic issues needed to a successful clinical trial. Actually, there are three particular widely-recognized researchers that are in the pole position of this journey of using Blockchain technology into clinical trials. They are already responsible for some scientific reviews arguing that this disruptive technology is a "game changer for improving transparency" of clinical trials (Benchoufi et al., 2017, 2019; Benchoufi & Ravaud, 2017). Namely, this new technology might allow the 1) real time recording of clinical data provided by researchers and/or clinicians, 2) reducing trial timelines, 3) warranting regulatory compliance and 4) increasing accuracy and data sharing between the scientific experts (Figure 5). Blockchain technology is also often considered as the "guardian of the integrity of the existence of events and their correct chronological order", being possible to prevent some "after-the-fact" modifications, as switched outcomes are an example or, if they exist, identify and trace who was the responsible (Benchoufi et al., 2019). In addition, clinical trials design, implementation and analysis might also benefit from blockchain technology regarding the safety and privacy of participants, by tracking who accessed (and when) the datasets (Benchoufi & Ravaud, 2017; Darryl G. Glover & Jan Hermans, 2017; Nugent et al., 2016). In that cases, it is even possible to design and apply a transparency index for all tracked events and to validate work streams by Smart Contracts, guaranteeing a *timestamping* and *timeordering* of the events, as well as its inspection by different stakeholders of the agreement (see Benchoufi et al., 2019 for a complete characterization and design of complex and complete clinical trials encoded in blockchain).

Figure 5. Association of the main advantages regarding blockchain-based technologies and the central consequences achieved by its use in the design, implementation and process of clinical trials

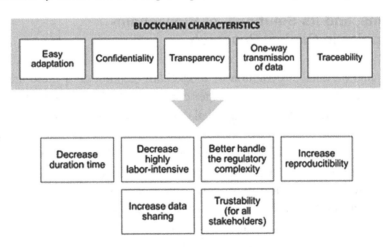

Nowadays, there are already implemented several prototypes of clinical trials using blockchain architecture, such as TrialChain, which uses public Ethereum blockchain, and also Hyperledger, which is a popular private blockchain prototype (Benchoufi et al., 2019; Cachin, 2016; Dai et al., 2018; Wong et al., 2019). Just as an example, Hyperledger platform was recently used in a clinical trial for breast cancer in Japan, for data validation and verification with an impactful positive feedback. This particular study also concluded that the limited cost of the tested system contributes to the sustainability of health care services, since it counteracts the increasing costs of monitoring clinical trials by the traditional methods with disruptive ant promising set of technologies (Hirano et al., 2020). Although the existence of public blockchain solutions might be most well accepted (due to the consequent data incorruptibility), in some cases private blockchains might also be important for certain uses. The storage and accessibility of different data is one of several examples regarding the ambiguous choice between public and private domains: personal data might be stored on a private blockchain decipherable only by agreed-upon parties and, on the other hand, public blockchain might storage metadata and/or proof of concept data, which might be verifiable by anyone able to read encrypted objects (hashes), allowing a remoted audition of the clinical-trial data work-stream (Benchoufi et al., 2019; Pane et al., 2020). In line with this, it is being expectable that the number of these attempts to validate the relevance of blockchain technology in clinical trials will grow exponentially.

Another example of the utility of blockchain technology regarding clinical research is related with postmarket surveillance of medical devices. At a first view, it might seem that this topic is not directly related with clinical research. However, an implementation of new medical devices is totally dependent on reviewing the standard medical devices already on the market and its updating and/or replacement for better and more complete devices. In that way, having in mind the complexity and the increasingly regulatory requirements from Health Authorities, a system that guarantees a fast, efficient and reliable evaluation of medical devices is a crucial need for better clinical health care (Pane et al., 2020).

Finally, highlighting the outstanding importance of blockchain technology, there are also some other prototypes that uses this concept to develop drug verification systems (such as Mediledger, operated by Chronicled) or systems that guarantee to the patients more control regarding their own health recordings (such as Embleema) (Benchoufi et al., 2019). Next representation intends to summarize the main applications of blockchain technologies already being used in the context of clinical research (Figure 6).

Major Limitations, and Its Solutions, of Blockchain-based Technologies in Clinical Research

Giving the novelty and permanent evolution of blockchain technologies, there are some limitations that should be addressed in further studies to better comprehend all the possibilities and implications regarding its use in clinical research. The empirical data reported in several original papers related to proof of concept trials indicate that some obstacles might be overcome, in order to establish a concrete, understandable and accessible system for all the intervenient of the built network. Actually, a very recent work developed by Chang Lu and colleagues indicated that the health care consumers did not demonstrate a significant increase in their willingness to become owners of health data and share the data with third parties, via blockchain technologies. This concern exhibited by the participants was mainly associated with the irrevocability of data access and the fear of losing the private keys, which might be reflected into a more difficult access to medical care. But, interestingly, small modifications in the construction of the blockchain-based system were well-accepted by the participants and increased its willingness in adopting this system, such as: 1) the possibility of a private key recovery system, 2) the compensation of data sharing through a "health wallet" hosted by the national authorities or 3) the opportunity of using the

Figure 6. List of some contexts in which blockchain technology is being crucial to better and faster develop clinical research studies

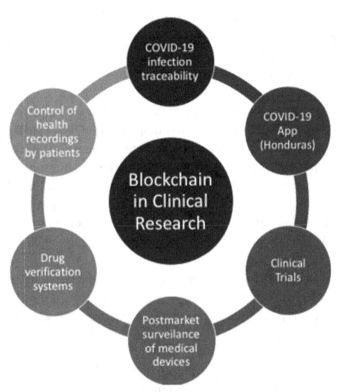

shared data for collective good (Lu et al., 2020). Other authors also indicate that all the stakeholders must collaborate with a blockchain technology expert to clear some potential obstacles in the implementation of the new system and, for that, it is needed to increase and boost the knowledge and formation of more experts (Pane et al., 2020). On the other hand, in a blockchain-based clinical trial for breast cancer, the authors also exhibited some concerns related to the scalability of the system, indicating that is urgent to evaluate whether multiple clinical trials performed in a single technological system might be conducted. In addition, they also indicated that, in a near future, it will be important to confirm the possibility and feasibility of collecting data via multiple devices (such as using personal smartphone, PC or Internet of Things) in a simultaneous way, which may promote the spreading of virtual clinical trials (breast cancer). Finally, only as a reference to have in mind, it would be also crucial to: 1) develop systems that are able to storage and process health data that, in some cases, include very big size files (such as lab tests, pathology results, prescriptions, fMRI and others) (Linn & Koo, 2016) and 2) guarantee an equal and fair access for this disruptive technology all over the world, to circumvent possible differences of medical care admission in both developed and undeveloped countries.

Although some limitations that still persist and were briefly mentioned above, it is unmeasurable the impact that blockchain-based technologies may have in the next few years. Indeed, all the applications already in practice, together with others not mentioned before, show that we are already living the future and we must be ready for all the challenges that will appear soon to exploit and maximize the opportunities created.

DATA MONETIZATION

Firstly, it is important to understand how a consumer (or, in this case, a patient, since it corresponds to the health data of consumers) can monetize his data. For that, it is important to understand how the concept of data monetization is created. Data monetization is the process of using data to obtain economic benefits, which includes, not only the cash flow in (data selling), but also all the actions that brings value to the company (Gartner, 2019).

Regarding its methods, data monetization can be classified in two aspects: 1) Internal or Indirect when data is used to take strategical decisions in the company to get better business performance and 2) External or Direct when data is shared and the company obtains beneficial terms from business partners, information bartering, selling data outright or offering information products and services (Gartner, 2019).

Some years ago, the concept of data monetization were not considered in the existing Value Chain, although, some strategies could be taken with the influence of the Company Data (Weil, 1985). However, year after year with digitization of end-to-end process, data has become the main source of value, so it was important to do some changes in the Value Chain. Therefore, new chain models were created and Data Chain Values were developed (Faroukhi et al., 2020).

With data being part of the Value Chain, there was a bigger concern in having better data available for analysis and some problems as high volume, velocity and variety starting to be a concern (Mittal, 2013). In that way, to solve this problem, Big Data emerged and, again, a new chain model was created: Big Data Value Chain. As a consequence, organizations rely in Big Data to extract valuable insights (Curry, 2016).

Although data monetization is not a recent concept, the introduction of Big Data and Big Data Value Chain ideas increased data monetization interest. Actually, using Big Data theory, data monetization can now provide exponential economic benefits (Hacker & Petkova, 2016). Regarding data, it might be classified into different classes inside Big Data Value Chain (Figure 7) (Faroukhi et al., 2020).

Figure 7. Big data value chain – a new insight
(adapted from Faroukhi, 2020)

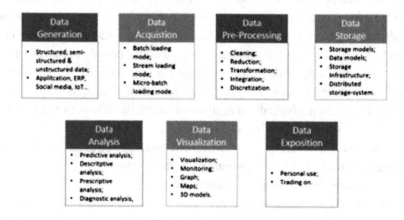

Analyzing step by step the process of data in Big Data Value Chain, data can be generated passively or actively by humans, systems or sensors and with heterogeneous formats. Data generated must be transformed from is capture point to a storage infrastructure (Hu et al.,2014). After the acquisition and considering that noisy and redundant data might be present (affecting the final data), it might be necessary to clean, reduce, transform, integrate or discretize part of the total data (Adnan & Akbar, 2019).

Next, a huge amount of data must be prepared to be stored. Therefore, it is necessary that the system have reliable storage space and allow powerful access for data analysis. For that, there are four different pillars in this topic that should be addressed: storage models, data models, storage infrastructure and distributed processing infrastructure (Hu et al., 2014). Then, the pre-processed and stored data is analyzed to find correlations, identify patterns and create actionable insights, being extremely important to have methods of visualization to communicate insights in a compelling and comprehensible way (Faroukhi et al., 2020). Finally, the last phase is data exposition in which data is shared and/or exposed, and may have a personal use or a trading one (Moro Visconti et al., 2017).

Importantly, for all the phases indicated above, it should be used the described "Big Data Analytics Tools", commonly referred as the 7 Vs: Volume, Velocity, Variety, Veracity, Value, Variability and Visualization (Khan et al., 2014).

Considering the main advantages provided from Blockchain technology (such as security, transparency, decentralization and flexibility), it is possible to cover the flaws of Big Data. Therefore, in this particular case, blockchain technology might be beneficial regarding data integrity, preventing malicious activities, real times analysis and manage data sharing (Dhanalakshmi & Babu, 2019).

After this preliminary description of data monetization in the perspective of a Business world, now we should do the transition to the Consumer/Patient case. There is a multiplicity of ways that blockchain technology might be used by Consumers/Patients to monetize his data, such as the implementation of smart contracts. This Smart Contract might be signed between the patient and, for example, Pharmaceutical Industry, Government Organizations, Healthcare Professionals and Health Players. Every time that some of the organizations above access the Patient Data, this one earns the tokens contracted.

Going back some years, in 2008, an important step regarding monetization and blockchain technology was concluded with the development of Bitcoin. This is a peer-to-peer version of electronic cash that allows online payments without intermediaries, through hashing the transactions into an ongoing chain of hash-based proof-to-work forming a record that cannot be changed without redoing the proof-of-work (Nakamoto, 2008). Since then, 29 healthcoins were already created, the tokens contractualized between Patient and health entities should be one of those 29 healthcoins (*CryptoSlate*, 2020).

Data Monetization Upon Clinical Research Field

"There is no healthcare without management, and there is no management without information" – Director of the Brazilian National Health Service (Bram et al., 2015).

Nowadays, it is crucial to study a particular population to identify and tackle their main needs and limitations. Actually, the clinical research is a great example regarding the importance of the data collected, being important for many purposes, such as: identification of health trends and epidemics, tracking of immunization coverage, targeting of health research efforts and interventions, allocation of healthcare resources, education of healthcare professionals, management of staffing requirements and reduction of wait times and increased patient volume at local clinics (Bram et al., 2015).

In the last few decades, there are already numerous examples regarding the importance of data sharing to treat severe diseases, as we will present now and were previously reported by Bram and colleagues (Bram et al., 2015). In Peru, for example, data sharing using an online platform software (Open MRS) was important to track the resistance of *M. tuberculosis* before, during and after the clinical treatment, identifying regional health trends. In addition, an electronic medical record program allowed the government to detect problems and get a better a strategy in the allocation of resources to the areas hit by *M. tuberculosis* (Fraser & Blaya, 2010; Soto Cabezas et al., 2020).

In Uganda, an integrated disease surveillance strategy implementation led to a 30% increase in the reporting of diseases cases from clinics, which were consequently used to identify the spread of several diseases (Bram et al., 2015).

Also, in Africa, the data sharing was particularly important for the implementation of vaccination programs, such as for polio and MMR (Clements et al., 2008). For that, it was crucial the creation of Global Immunization and Vision Strategy by the WHO and UNICEF, which were responsible for the integration of immunization efforts with the surveillance of health interventions (Brown et al., 2011). Again, only through the sharing of personal data by competent entities was possible to reduce the heavy burden of several diseases. More than sharing data, it is needed to trust in the data, to have reliable data. In particular, there are some sensitive diseases which really need this transparency combined with confidentiality, such as Ebola HIV, since its transmission is often a result of modifiable social behaviors (Bram et al., 2015).

Finally, in Kenya, researchers implemented and electronic medical records system that allowed the aggregation of patient data for community members who visited the clinic. As a result, the Health Professionals (nurses and doctors) spent 58% less time with patients, making possible to do more consultations per day. As a consequence, it also had beneficial effects for patients, who got a 38% reduction in their wait times, and for the economy, since those individuals could return to their daily jobs or roles as caregiver sooner (Rotich et al., 2003).

All these examples mentioned above show better and understandable data are important for the health players get more information and therefore, to have more effectiveness with less resources possible (cash, human or material). In the most part of the examples indicated above, people provide their health Data relatively easily, but those cases are very severe (namely, AIDS and Tuberculosis). Importantly, data sharing is important not only in such severe cases, but also in "day to day" situations, which might be converted into value, health benefits for the patients, possibility to have a monetization and benefits for all the health players, with more, better and real time data, allowing a better management of their resources.

In any case, it should be mention that, like happens for all chains, there are some pros and some challenges that must be solved.

Regarding clinical trials, volunteer payments has been raised a lot of discussion for many years, mainly due to the ethical concerns. According to EU legislation, no incentives or financial inducements should be given to participants of clinical trials except compensation (European Parliament, 2001). The compensation is not a standard, however, is used in many clinical trials and can be given through the reimbursement of expenses, vouchers or money. Reimbursement can cover travel expenses, meals, accommodation or loss of income. On the other hand, compensation can be a payment/benefit for the participation in the clinical trial or when a participant suffers any harm from the clinical trial. In agreement with EU legislation, the compensation has to be approved by the respective Ethics Committee of the trial and discriminated at informed consent form. Importantly, EU legislation states that a subject cannot be financially influenced to participate in the clinical, which is a reason for an ongoing debate about how much compensation can influence decisions and how this perception is different depending on financial situation of the patients (Parliament, 2014). Compensation values varies a lot between the studies. A cohort study about Wilson disease in London can give to the participant patients a payment up to 7000 euros for the commitment and time dispensed to the clinical trial (Trials4us, 2020b). At the same medical facility, for a study regarding type 2 diabetes a participant can receive about 1000 euros for the participation (Trials4us, 2020a). The amount of the compensation depends on time involved to participate in the clinical trial, on the phase of the trial and consequently the risks involved. However, this money is not a payment for participants data, is literally a compensation for the time dispensed and not a valorization of clinical data.

For the Patient who provides access to his health data, this new concept of data monetization brings an important fact to the table: the opportunity that the Patient have to monetize his data, to have Benefit Economics with his own data. A major advantage for the Patient is that the data sharing with the maximum possible people becomes possible to understand better the global health problems, being possible to track diseases evaluation, the groups of risk, the geographical origin, the best treatments, etc. Briefly, data sharing itself might allow to evaluate, in the best possible way, the respective disease and to allocate the best existing resources to treat or even hill persons with those illness. So, one advantage, would be a better diagnosis and the chance to get the more effectiveness treatment (Bram et al., 2015). In addition, there is a clear possibility to better treat numerous diseases with an unmeasurable impact on social aspects. Anyway, this should be interpreted in a cautious way, since it could be that people would not be conformable to share their data. For that, it would be important to insecure that data would not be accessible for everyone, being even possible to have several levels of anonymity.

Data monetization brings to the table the chance to have, not only social benefits, but also an important impact upon Economics. Actually, through the signing of a smart contract with all Entities who needs personal data for their development (Pharmaceutical Industries, Government Organizations, Healthcare Professionals and Health Players), the Patient will ensure that when his data get used, he will be rewarded by it. Therefore, as main advantages, the Patient can get better analysis and treatment, as well as an economical benefit.

However, there are some challenges that must be solved, one of the majors is the fear that people have to share their personal data. Again, to tackle this possible limitation it is necessary to deeply explain that blockchain technology really protects the encoded information, together with all the remaining benefits possible to get. As an example, in the current days, we may refer the smartphone application *StayAway Covid*. This app was developed and launched in Portugal with the purpose of help to track the COVID pandemics. Briefly, someone who had been in contact with an infected person would be noticed and should take the respective precautions earlier, which will positively impact upon all society. However, this app was installed for a small portion of total population (accordingly with explanations of Health Minister of Portugal, Mrs. Marta Temido, at 27th October there was less than 2,5M downloads and only a little bit more than 500 codes) (Lusa, 2020a). In addition, the problem got even bigger when the government talk about the obligation of the use of the app in some cases (Lusa, 2020b). Probably, if there was a Monetization in this process, the app could be more successful with the respective health, social and economic consequences.

Although the world has an exponential development, technologically speaking, nowadays this is not accessible to everyone due to the access of light, internet or, a major part of the cases, access to technological equipment (Bram et al., 2015).

Analyzing Pros and Challenges for the Pharmaceutical Industry, Government Organizations, Healthcare Professionals and Health Players, these ones are always in search of the best possible data. With this system working, the data collected will be better and in real time, providing more effectiveness and operational management, making possible to have Economical Benefits. Indeed, it will allow that the actions will be directed to the problem itself, providing a best management of the resources (material and human) that will allow more money savings. Data is a business of Millions nowadays, the entities above spend a lot of money to get the data that they need, most part of it is gotten through intermediaries, that will no longer exist with the use of blockchain technology, and the payment is done by tokens to the consumer/patient (Bram et al., 2015). Again, there are some challenges that should be handled. First of all, the scalability of this system might be a problem, since it will take a huge initial investment to provide the infrastructure needed in a global scale (Shovlin et al., 2013). In addition, it will be necessary to create incentive mechanisms to those who are the data collectors and those ones who have more interactions with the Patients (Bram et al., 2015).

FUTURE RESEARCH DIRECTIONS

In order to explain, in the best possible way, the concrete impact that this technology might have in Clinical Research Field, a hypothetical scenario of using blockchain-based technologies and data monetization in Clinical Research will be presented next. In summary, it is related to a new concept of a chain that goes from the patient giving his data to receive the tokens contracted:

Patient A had an asthmatic episode and Doctor B received him and then proceeded to a medical examination. Doctor B produces a Medical Report that indicates that Patient A has Asthma, automatically this Medical Report is generated (and it is encrypted with Patient's private key). Doctor B may suggest admission to a clinical trial, leaded by Doctor B, who informs the patient about the all the issues regarding the clinical trial and, in an automatic way, the consent information and the protocol are created. Considering previous studied, it is selected the best dose to treat the Patient A, ensuring that there is real time registration of clinical progression and adverse effects. Finally, clinical data is processed, stored, analyzed and encrypted. For every time that data is accessed/exported, the Patient A receives the tokens contracted, being those tokens possibly used to buy drugs, to pay clinical exams or even transacted to his family or friends. It should be mentioned that this example is not totally described in the literature references used. It is, therefore, a construction of a possible scenario, considering the concepts and possibilities that those references support.

This example was just a preliminary presentation of a possible, and expectable, healthcare world in the next few years/decades. Considering that projections ruined in 2017 suggest that 55 percent of healthcare applications will have adopted blockchain for commercial deployment by 2025, it is understandable the prioritization that blockchain-based technologies has gained in the last years (Elflein, 2017). As an example, it should be highlighted the case of Medtronic, an American-Irish registered medical device company that operates in 140 countries and employs over 104,950 people. This company is known by its string position worldwide and blockchain has being obtained a notorious importance for that. Accordingly, in one interview Tim Paffel, a senior principal IT technologist at Medtronic stated that "the first player to identify the ultimate use case where data integration and efficiency are achievable together will have tremendous opportunity to impact the healthcare industry", and also "all of us are working toward a better future, and blockchain [distributed ledger] is - and will become - a very smart path forward" (Medtronic, 2020).

CONCLUSION

The last few years indicated that all of us are already living in a healthcare blockchain ecosystem. Up until now, all the studies regarding the use of blockchain-based technologies in clinical research produced a considerable conceptual and empirical set of data, emphasizing the possible application of this disruptive technology. Even considering some limitations indicated in this chapter, it is inevitable that the immediate costs of designing and implementing blockchain-based technologies in a global way for the healthcare system are insignificant when compared with the beneficial consequences from a long-term perspective. Indeed, it is becoming clear that the maturation and maximization of blockchain technology opportunities overcome, by far, some challenges that have been addressing by some authors. Therefore, the synergic operation between blockchain technology, clinical research, and data monetization will allow unpredictable revenues and benefits in social, economic, political, and organizational aspects.

ACKNOWLEDGMENT

This research received no specific grant from any funding agency in the public, commercial, or not-for-profit sectors.

REFERENCES

Abdel-Basset, M., Chang, V., & Nabeeh, N. A. (2020). An intelligent framework using disruptive technologies for COVID-19 analysis. *Technological Forecasting and Social Change*, *120431*. Advance online publication. doi:10.1016/j.techfore.2020.120431 PMID:33162617

Adnan, K., & Akbar, R. (2019). An analytical study of information extraction from unstructured and multidimensional big data. *Journal of Big Data*, *6*(1), 91. Advance online publication. doi:10.118640537-019-0254-8

Benchoufi, M., Altman, D., & Ravaud, P. (2019). From Clinical Trials to Highly Trustable Clinical Trials: Blockchain in Clinical Trials, a Game Changer for Improving Transparency? *Frontiers in Blockchain*, *2*, 23. doi:10.3389/fbloc.2019.00023

Benchoufi, M., Porcher, R., & Ravaud, P. (2017). Blockchain protocols in clinical trials: Transparency and traceability of consent. *F1000 Research*, *6*, 66. doi:10.12688/f1000research.10531.1 PMID:29167732

Benchoufi, M., & Ravaud, P. (2017). Blockchain technology for improving clinical research quality. In Trials (Vol. 18, Issue 1, p. 335). BioMed Central Ltd. doi:10.118613063-017-2035-z

Chen & Jarrel. (2019). Blockchain in Healthcare: A Patient-Centered Model. *Biomedical Journal of Scientific & Technical Research*, *20*(3), 15017–15022. PMID:31565696

Bram, J. T., Warwick-Clark, B., Obeysekare, E., & Mehta, K. (2015). Utilization and Monetization of Healthcare Data in Developing Countries. *Big Data*, *3*(2), 59–66. doi:10.1089/big.2014.0053 PMID:26487984

Brown, D. W., Burton, A., Gacic-Dobo, M., Karimov, R. I., Vandelaer, J., & Okwo-Bele, J. (2011). A mid-term assessment of progress towards the immunization coverage goal of the Global Immunization Vision and Strategy (GIVS). In BMC Public Health (Vol. 11). doi:10.1186/1471-2458-11-806

Cachin, C. (2016). *Architecture of the hyperledger blockchain fabric*. https://pdfs.semanticscholar.org/f852/c5f3fe649f8a17ded391df0796677a59927f.pdf

Clements, C. J., Nshimirimanda, D., & Gasasira, A. (2008). Using immunization delivery strategies to accelerate progress in Africa towards achieving the Millennium Development Goals. In Vaccine (Vol. 26, Issue 16). doi:10.1016/j.vaccine.2008.02.032

CryptoSlate. (2020). https://cryptoslate.com/cryptos/healthcare/

Curry, E. (2016). The big data value chain: Definitions, concepts, and theoretical approaches. In New Horizons for a Data-Driven Economy: A Roadmap for Usage and Exploitation of Big Data in Europe. doi:10.1007/978-3-319-21569-3_3

Dai, H., Young Phd, P., Js, T., Md, D., Gong, G., Kang Phd, M., Krumholz, H. M., Sm, M. D., Schulz, W. L., & Jiang, L. (2018). *TrialChain: A Blockchain-Based Platform to Validate Data Integrity in Large, Biomedical Research Studies*. https://github.com/ComputationalHealth/TrialChain

Dhanalakshmi, S., & Babu, G. C. (2019). An Examination Of Big Data And Blockchain Technology. *International Journal of Innovative Technology and Exploring Engineering*, *8*(11), 2278–3075. doi:10.35940/ijitee.K2497.0981119

Drosatos, G., & Kaldoudi, E. (2019). Blockchain Applications in the Biomedical Domain: A Scoping Review. *Computational and Structural Biotechnology Journal*, *17*, 229–240. doi:10.1016/j.csbj.2019.01.010 PMID:30847041

Elflein, J. (2017). Projected distribution of healthcare blockchain adoption worldwide 2017-2025. *Statista Website*. https://www.statista.com/statistics/759208/healthcare-blockchain-adoption-rate-in-health-apps-worldwide/

European Parliament. (2001). EU Clinical Directive 2001/20/EC of the European Parliament and of the Council of 4 April 2001 on the approximation of the laws, regulations, and administrative provisions of the Member States relating to the implementation of good clinical practice. *Official Journal of the European Communities*.

Faroukhi, A. Z., El Alaoui, I., Gahi, Y., & Amine, A. (2020). Big data monetization throughout Big Data Value Chain: A comprehensive review. *Journal of Big Data*, *7*(1), 1–22. doi:10.118640537-019-0281-5

Fraser, H. S. f., & Blaya, J. (2010). Implementing medical information systems in developing countries, what works and what doesn't. *AMIA ... Annual Symposium Proceedings / AMIA Symposium. AMIA Symposium, 2010*.

Fusco, A., Dicuonzo, G., Dell'atti, V., & Tatullo, M. (2020). Blockchain in healthcare: Insights on CO-VID-19. *International Journal of Environmental Research and Public Health*, *17*(19), 1–12. doi:10.3390/ijerph17197167 PMID:33007951

Gartner. (2019). *Data Monetization - Gartner Information Technology Glossary*. Gartner IT Glossary. https://www.gartner.com/en/information-technology/glossary/data-monetization

Gefenas, E., Cekanauskaite, A., Lekstutiene, J., & Lukaseviciene, V. (2017). Application challenges of the new EU Clinical Trials Regulation. In European Journal of Clinical Pharmacology (Vol. 73, Issue 7, pp. 795–798). Springer Verlag. doi:10.100700228-017-2267-6

George, S. L., & Buyse, M. (2015). Data fraud in clinical trials. *Clinical Investigation*, *5*(2), 161–173. doi:10.4155/cli.14.116 PMID:25729561

Glover, D. G., & Hermans, J. (2017). Improving the Traceability of the Clinical Trial Supply Chain | Applied Clinical Trials Online. *Applied Clinical Trials*, *26*(12). https://www.appliedclinicaltrialsonline.com/view/improving-traceability-clinical-trial-supply-chain

Goldacre, B., DeVito, N., Heneghan, C., Irving, F., & Bmj, S. B. (2018). undefined. (2018). Compliance with requirement to report results on the EU Clinical Trials Register: Cohort study and web resource. *BMJ (Clinical Research Ed.)*, *362*. https://www.bmj.com/content/362/bmj.k3218

Gordon, W. J., & Catalini, C. (2018). Blockchain Technology for Healthcare: Facilitating the Transition to Patient-Driven Interoperability. *Computational and Structural Biotechnology Journal*, *16*, 224–230. doi:10.1016/j.csbj.2018.06.003 PMID:30069284

Gupta, A. (2013). Fraud and misconduct in clinical research: A concern. *Perspectives in Clinical Research*, *4*(2), 144. doi:10.4103/2229-3485.111800 PMID:23833741

Hacker, P., & Petkova, B. (2016). Reining in the Big Promise of Big Data: Transparency, Inequality, and New Regulatory Frontiers. SSRN *Electronic Journal*. doi:10.2139srn.2773527

Hau, Y. S., & Chang, M. C. (2020). Healthcare Information Technology Convergence to Effectively Cope with the COVID- 19 crisis. *Health Policy and Technology*. Advance online publication. doi:10.1016/j.hlpt.2020.10.010 PMID:33163353

Hirano, T., Motohashi, T., Okumura, K., Takajo, K., Kuroki, T., Ichikawa, D., Matsuoka, Y., Ochi, E., & Ueno, T. (2020). Data validation and verification using blockchain in a clinical trial for breast cancer: Regulatory sandbox. *Journal of Medical Internet Research*, *22*(6), e18938. doi:10.2196/18938 PMID:32340974

House of Commons Science and Technology Committee. (2018). *Research integrity: clinical trials transparency Tenth Report of Session 2017-19 Report, together with formal minutes relating to the report.* www.parliament.uk/science

Hu, H., Wen, Y., Chua, T. S., & Li, X. (2014). Toward scalable systems for big data analytics: A technology tutorial. *IEEE Access: Practical Innovations, Open Solutions*, *2*, 652–687. Advance online publication. doi:10.1109/ACCESS.2014.2332453

Institute of Medicine (US) Forum on Drug Discovery Development and Translation. (2010). Transforming Clinical Research in the United States: Challenges and Opportunities. In *Medical Journal of Malaysia* (Vol. 62, Issue 4). National Academies Press (US). https://www.ncbi.nlm.nih.gov/books/NBK50888/

Ioannidis, J. P. A. (2005). Why Most Published Research Findings Are False. *PLoS Medicine*, 2(8), e124. doi:10.1371/journal.pmed.0020124 PMID:16060722

Karafiloski, E., & Mishev, A. (2017). Blockchain solutions for big data challenges: A literature review. *17th IEEE International Conference on Smart Technologies, EUROCON 2017 - Conference Proceedings, July*, 763–768. 10.1109/EUROCON.2017.8011213

Khan, M. A. U. D., Uddin, M. F., & Gupta, N. (2014). Seven V's of Big Data understanding Big Data to extract value. *Proceedings of the 2014 Zone 1 Conference of the American Society for Engineering Education - "Engineering Education: Industry Involvement and Interdisciplinary Trends", ASEE Zone 1 2014*. 10.1109/ASEEZone1.2014.6820689

Laure, A., & Linn, M. B. K. (2016). Blockchain For Health Data and Its Potential Use in Health IT and Health Care Related Research. *ONC/NIST Use of Blockchain for Healthcare and Research Workshop*, 1–10. 10.5455/aim.2019.27.284-291

Linn, L. A., & Koo, M. B. (2016). *Blockchain For Health Data and Its Potential Use in Health IT and Health Care Related Research*. Academic Press.

Lu, C., Batista, D., Hamouda, H., & Lemieux, V. (2020). Consumers' Intention to Adopt Blockchain-based Personal Health Records (PHR) and Data Sharing: Focus-group Study (Preprint). *JMIR Formative Research*, 4(11), e21995. Advance online publication. doi:10.2196/21995 PMID:33151149

Lusa, A. (2020a). *Covid-19: Portugal já fez 3,2 milhões de testes e "app" de rastreio soma 2,4 milhões de 'downloads.'* https://www.lusa.pt/article/S8LuGAwMQ7SQaypC08jvETMSZM5iuSI1/covid-19-portugal-já-fez-3-2-milhões-de-testes-e-app-de-rastreio-soma-2-4-milhões-de-downloads

Lusa, A. (2020b). StayAway Covid obrigatória abre "graves questões" de privacidade. *RTP Notícias - Economia*. https://www.rtp.pt/noticias/economia/stayaway-covid-obrigatoria-abregraves-questoes-de-privacidade_n1267109

Marbouh, D., Abbasi, T., Maasmi, F., Omar, I. A., Debe, M. S., Salah, K., Jayaraman, R., & Ellahham, S. (2020). Blockchain for COVID-19: Review, Opportunities, and a Trusted Tracking System. In Arabian Journal for Science and Engineering (p. 1). Springer Science and Business Media Deutschland GmbH. doi:10.100713369-020-04950-4

Maslove, D. M., Klein, J., Brohman, K., & Martin, P. (2018). Using Blockchain Technology to Manage Clinical Trials Data: A Proof-of-Concept Study. *JMIR Medical Informatics*, 6(4), e11949. doi:10.2196/11949 PMID:30578196

Medtronic. (2020). Blockchain in healthcare - Meaningful innovation. *Medtronic website*. https://www.medtronic.com/us-en/transforming-healthcare/meaningful-innovation/science-behind-healthcare/blockchain-in-healthcare.html

Mittal, A. (2013). Trustworthiness of Big Data. *International Journal of Computers and Applications*, *80*(9), 35–40. Advance online publication. doi:10.5120/13892-1835

Moro Visconti, R., Larocca, A., & Marconi, M. (2017). Big Data-Driven Value Chains and Digital Platforms: From Value Co-Creation to Monetization. SSRN *Electronic Journal*. doi:10.2139srn.2903799

Nakamoto, S. (2008). *Bitcoin: A Peer-to-Peer Electronic Cash System*. Www.Bitcoin.Org doi:10.1162/ARTL_a_00247

Nandi, S., Sarkis, J., Hervani, A. A., & Helms, M. M. (2021). Redesigning Supply Chains using Blockchain-Enabled Circular Economy and COVID-19 Experiences. *Sustainable Production and Consumption*, *27*, 10–22. doi:10.1016/j.spc.2020.10.019 PMID:33102671

NugentT.UptonD.CimpoesuM. (2016). Improving data transparency in clinical trials using blockchain smart contracts. *F1000Research, 5*. doi:10.12688/f1000research.9756.1

Pane, J., Verhamme, K. M. C., Shrum, L., Rebollo, I., & Sturkenboom, M. C. J. M. (2020). Blockchain technology applications to postmarket surveillance of medical devices. *Expert Review of Medical Devices*, *17*(10), 1–10. doi:10.1080/17434440.2020.1825073 PMID:32954855

Park, Y. R., Lee, E., Na, W., Park, S., Lee, Y., & Lee, J. H. (2019). Is blockchain technology suitable for managing personal health records? Mixed-methods study to test feasibility. *Journal of Medical Internet Research*, *21*(2), e12533. doi:10.2196/12533 PMID:30735142

Parliament, E. (2014). *Regulation (EU) No 536/2014 of the European Parliament and the Council*. Official Journal of the European Union.

Rao, R., & Jain, H. (2019). Improving Integrated Clinical Trial Management Systems through Blockchain. *Genetic Engineering & Biotechnology News*.

Roman-Belmonte, J. M., De la Corte-Rodriguez, H., & Rodriguez-Merchan, E. C. (2018). How blockchain technology can change medicine. In Postgraduate Medicine (Vol. 130, Issue 4, pp. 420–427). Taylor and Francis Inc. doi:10.1080/00325481.2018.1472996

Rotich, J. K., Hannan, T. J., Smith, F. E., Bii, J., Odero, W. W., Vu, N., Mamlin, B. W., Mamlin, J. J., Einterz, R. M., & Tierney, W. M. (2003). Installing and implementing a computer-based patient record system in sub-saharan Africa: The Mosoriot Medical Record System. *Journal of the American Medical Informatics Association: JAMIA*, *10*(4), 295–303. Advance online publication. doi:10.1197/jamia.M1301 PMID:12668697

Satia, M. C. (2017). Global challenges in conducting clinical trials. *Journal of Clinical Trials*. https://www.longdom.org/proceedings/global-challenges-in-conducting-clinical-trials-56064.html

Shae, Z., & Tsai, J. J. P. (2017). On the Design of a Blockchain Platform for Clinical Trial and Precision Medicine. *Proceedings - International Conference on Distributed Computing Systems*, 1972–1980. 10.1109/ICDCS.2017.61

Shovlin, A., Ghen, M., Simpson, P., & Mehta, K. (2013). Challenges facing medical data digitization in low-resource contexts. *Proceedings of the 3rd IEEE Global Humanitarian Technology Conference, GHTC 2013*. 10.1109/GHTC.2013.6713713

Soto Cabezas, M. G., Munayco Escate, C. V., Escalante Maldonado, O., Valencia Torres, E., Arica Gutiérrez, J., & Yagui Moscoso, M. J. A. (2020). Perfil epidemiológico de la tuberculosis extensivamente resistente en el Perú, 2013-2015. *Revista Panamericana de Salud Pública, 44*, 1. Advance online publication. doi:10.26633/RPSP.2020.29 PMID:32973891

Szabo, N., & The, I. (2015). Smart Contracts. *Building Blocks for Digital Markets., c*, 1–11.

Trials4us. (2020a). *Clinical Trials - C19040 Cohort 4.* https://www.trials4us.co.uk/ongoing-clinical-trials/caucasian-type-2-diabetic-male-and-female-patients-aged-18-to-65-c19040-part-1/

Trials4us. (2020b). *Clinical Trials - C19048 Cohort 2.* https://www.trials4us.co.uk/ongoing-clinical-trials/male-and-female-patients-with-wilson-disease-c19048/

Tunis, S., Korn, A., & Ommaya, A. (2002). Definitions of Clinical Research and Components of the Enterprise. In *The Role of Purchasers and Payers in the Clinical Research Enterprise: (p. Appendix V).* National Academies Press. https://www.ncbi.nlm.nih.gov/books/NBK220717/

U.S. Food & Drug. (2020). *What Are the Different Types of Clinical Research?* https://www.fda.gov/patients/clinical-trials-what-patients-need-know/what-are-different-types-clinical-research

Verde, F., Stanzione, A., Romeo, V., Cuocolo, R., Maurea, S., & Brunetti, A. (2019). Could Blockchain Technology Empower Patients, Improve Education, and Boost Research in Radiology Departments? An Open Question for Future Applications. In Journal of Digital Imaging (Vol. 32, Issue 6, pp. 1112–1115). Springer New York LLC. doi:10.100710278-019-00246-8

Weil, K. E. (1985). PORTER, Competitive advantage, creating and sustaining superior performance. *Revista de Administração de Empresas, 25*(2). doi:10.15900034-75901985000200009

Wong, D. R., Bhattacharya, S., & Butte, A. J. (2019). Prototype of running clinical trials in an untrustworthy environment using blockchain. *Nature Communications, 10*(1), 917. doi:10.103841467-019-08874-y PMID:30796226

Wright, T. (2020). *Blockchain App Used to Track COVID-19 Cases in Latin America.* https://cointelegraph.com/news/blockchain-app-used-to-track-covid-19-cases-in-latin-america

Zhuang, Y., Sheets, L. R., Shae, Z., Chen, Y. W., Tsai, J. J. P., & Shyu, C. R. (2019). Applying Blockchain Technology to Enhance Clinical Trial Recruitment. *AMIA ... Annual Symposium Proceedings. AMIA Symposium, 2019*, 1276–1285.

Zhuang, Yu., Sheets, L., Shae, Z., Tsai, J. J. P., & Shyu, C. R. (2018). Applying Blockchain Technology for Health Information Exchange and Persistent Monitoring for Clinical Trials. *AMIA ... Annual Symposium Proceedings. AMIA Symposium, 2018*, 1167–1175.

KEY TERMS AND DEFINITIONS

Big Data: Data rapidly generated, in large scale and from multiple sources, mainly characterized by the 3 Vs: Volume, Velocity, and Variety.

Chain Value: A business model that describes the set of activities that a company carries out to deliver a valuable product or service in order to generate value.

Clinical Research: Study of health and illness in people, including not only the translation of pre-clinical studies (basic research) into clinical ones, but also the scientific groundwork for prevention, diagnosis, and treatment of pathologies.

Clinical Trial: Set of studies focusing the demonstration of safety and efficiency (without relevant side effects) of a particular medication and/or medical device, being an obligatory requirement before accessing the market.

Data Monetization: Process of using data to obtain economic benefits, which includes, not only the cash flow in (data selling), but also all the actions that brings value to the company.

Smart Contract: A contract programmed with protocol codes that are self-executable stablishing restrictive rules in the same way of the traditional contract document. It has obligations, benefits, or penalties for all the parties involved.

Token: Type of virtual currency that resides on their own blockchains and represents an asset or utility.

Chapter 10
Data Security in Clinical Trials Using Blockchain Technology

Marta de-Melo-Diogo

ISEG, Lisbon School of Economics and Management, University of Lisbon, Portugal

Jorge Tavares

NOVA IMS, Universidade Nova de Lisboa, Portugal

Ângelo Nunes Luís

ISEG, Lisbon School of Economics and Management, University of Lisbon, Portugal

ABSTRACT

Blockchain technology in a clinical trial setting is a valuable asset due to decentralization, immutability, transparency, and traceability features. For this chapter, a literature review was conducted to map the current utilization of blockchain systems in clinical trials, particularly data security managing systems and their characteristics, such as applicability, interests of use, limitations, and issues. The advantages of data security are producing a more transparent and tamper-proof clinical trial by providing accurate, validated data, therefore producing a more reliable and credible clinical trial. On the other hand, data integrity is a critical issue since data obtained from trials are not instantly made public to all participants. Work needs to be done to establish the significant implications in security data when applying blockchain technology in a real-world clinical trial setting and generalized conditions of use to establish its security.

INTRODUCTION

Since its discovery, Blockchain is emerging as an innovative technology to provide data transactions and storage in an effective, secure, and timely manner system. This technology has been applied to many sectors of activity, potentializing its features and improving processes and business mindsets.

The health sector is no exception, and many uses of this technology have been reported. Blockchain's full applicability in healthcare is still underway, and many optimizations are needed to be made, not

DOI: 10.4018/978-1-7998-7363-1.ch010

only from a technology development perspective but also concerns about ethical and data protection regulation are raised and need improvement.

It is considered essential to mention that the interest in the applicability of blockchain systems in the healthcare sector has been increasing since 2016. More specifically, the number of published articles related to Blockchain in the Pubmed bibliographic database has increased drastically in 2018 (only five studies were published in 2016 and only 16 in 2017), reflecting the potential and growing interest of these systems in the healthcare sector (Mackey et al., 2019). Only 4% of these studies were related to clinical trials, and 32% were related to healthcare data (Mackey et al., 2019).

Particularly in clinical trials, this technology is yet to reach its full potential. Nevertheless, considering the dimension and complexity of a clinical trial network and process interlined, blockchain technology might improve data sharing, management, and access to all key players. However, identifying the risks and threats of applying this technology in such an environment is still amiss, and work needs to be done to establish them in a realistic scenario setting.

Therefore, the purpose of this chapter is to map the current use of blockchain systems in clinical trials, particularly data security managing systems, and its characteristics, such as applicability, interests of use, limitations, and issues, as reported throughout the literature review.

BACKGROUND

Although variations of term have been used before, Blockchain came around in 2008 when this technology was created by Satoshi Nakamoto to support and securely record Bitcoin cryptocurrency transactions (Meunier, 2018; Monrat et al., 2019). Since then, the interest in this technology has increased and soon was applied into other areas of interested such as government, manufacturing, finance, healthcare and distribution (Monrat et al., 2019).

Blockchain is an advanced data structure, designed for storing and sharing information, composed by a growing chain of blocks organized by chronological order (Agbo et al., 2019)(S Chen, Hannah et al., 2019). Each block stores information with digital signatures in a decentralized and distributed network, it allows to record a transaction by binding different blocks connected with chains (S Chen, Hannah et al., 2019) (Abu-elezz et al., 2020) (Monrat et al., 2019). This transaction is validated by a consent algorithm, and therefore, needs no third-party validation to complete an action. The chain continues to grow as new transactions are built and blocks are added into it (Omar, Jayaraman, Salah, Yaqoob, et al., 2020).

Unlike traditional methods, blockchain enables peer-to-peer transfer of digital assets without any intermediaries. All the transactions occur in a decentralized manner that eliminates the requirement for any intermediaries to validate and verify the transactions. Every transaction is regulated by the participants who store and share the information throughout the private key: an unique and individual signature linked to each transaction recorded (S Chen, Hannah et al., 2019).

The digitalization era is reaching almost every industry and is expected that the Distribution Ledger Technology, where technologies such as blockchain, artificial intelligence and Internet of Things are inserted, to reach a market value of $60.7 billion by 2024 (Smetanin et al., 2020).

The features of blockchain, include (Hussien et al., 2019):

- Decentralization, access of information through third parties with multiple copies in multiple locations;

- Consent, the consensus algorithm created controls the access and distribution within a network;
- Immutability: once the information has entered a blockchain no longer can be changed or altered; a
- Auditability and transparency, every transaction information and signature can be traced; interoperability, different systems are connected and communicate in an autonomous manner.

The blockchain platform is distinguished by its key characteristics enabling it to be a promising disruptive technology that reduces the emphasis on traditional data management systems (Omar, Jayaraman, Salah, Yaqoob, et al., 2020). The blockchain is poised to innovate and transform a wide range of applications, including goods transfer (supply chain), digital media transfer (sale of art), remote services delivery (travel and tourism), platforms for example, moving computing to data sources and distributed credentialing.

Healthcare systems are complex and multi-dimensional organizations, involving multiple professionals whin different functions and degrees of access information, multiple organizations of different sectors of activities such as regulatory agencies, insurance companies, suppliers, technical supports and many others. Providing care to a patient involves many professionals and actions, therefore is important that health records are available and updated in time to provide the accurate and appropriate care to each patient at all times. On the other hand, it is also important that every patient owns is medical record and has fully knowledge of the parties that have been granted access to the very same.

Data security and ownership represent two of the most sensitive topics of today's generation. In fact, since the approval of General Data Protection Regulation in 2016 in European Union, when it comes to medical records these two topics became even more important and prominent. Besides this, managing patient data integrity is one of the major concerns for the healthcare industry, combining the need to access each patient characteristics and complete medical records at any time.

The introduction of blockchain systems in healthcare might be the solution to some of the concerns raised in data security and medical records accessibility and might the solution to gather and improve communications and data sharing between every player in the healthcare systems.

Concerning blockchain applications in healthcare, blockchain benefits are the following (Agbo et al., 2019)(Hasselgren et al., 2020):

- Decentralization: Healthcare access is spread to multiple players, such as doctors, hospitals, health insurance companies, pharmacies, etc. This feature of blockchain allows access to multiple stakeholders in a timely manner and provides information sharing in real time.
- Transparency: Given the security and transparency of transactions, information systems and storing systems are very reliable, and therefore provide a solid source of information for healthcare stakeholders. This feature is very important for example, when submitting information to regulatory agencies.
- Data verifiability: every transaction can be check for its integrity and validity. This information is important for healthcare records validation, insurance claim verification and in pharmaceutical supply chain to detect contrafact products.
- Transparency and trust: given the amount of information stored and that every transaction is record, blockchain provide for healthcare providers and stakeholders an ambient of trust and transparency since every information is available to consult.

- Robustness: The blockchain storage method guarantees that data is available and prevented from loss.
- Data ownership: given the levels of access and control of access of a blockchain, through this data storage system, patients are able to a more detailed control of the availability of their medical records to third parties.
- Data security and privacy: once an information has entered in a blockchain it is extremely difficult to alter through maleficent intentions. Additionally, every transaction is recorded in chronological order and is also traceable by its time stamp and user responsible for that action.

Concerning healthcare, blockchain systems can be applied in different areas such as (PwC, 2018) (Deloitte, 2020)(S Chen, Hannah et al., 2019)(Tan et al., 2020) (Smetanin et al., 2020) (Omar, Jayaraman, Salah, Yaqoob, et al., 2020)(Monrat et al., 2019):

- Supply chain: products status can be checked by the supplier at all times. This includes information regarding the transportation route, and more importantly, about controlled factors such as temperature and humidity throughout the transportation, contributing for a better monitorization and assuring the quality and safety of the products delivered. This contribution is especially important when it comes to products that need refrigeration, such as vaccines and biological products. Blockchain systems also improve security and authenticity of the products delivered, tacking the issue of distribution of falsified drugs.
- Precision medicine and medical records: the access of multiple players in healthcare to medical records of a patient in real time not only can improve the care provided, and can also potentiate the uses of precision medicine, since the patient medical records and genomic data can by easy shared between doctors and researchers.
- Data management: Gathering medical records, expenses and reports concerning a medical treatment could be time consuming and an extensive process. Blockchain can improve this field since data sharing would be available and updated by the multiple players making the communication between them more efficient, for example between a hospital and an insurance company.
- Electronic prescription: electronic prescription would be improved by blockchain systems, given the ability of the information can be spread throughout the different services such as hospital-doctor-patient-pharmacy. Patient electronic devices can be also updated with app to monitor the adhesion to therapy, giving precious information to the doctor and pharmacist about the success of the treatment in a timely manner.
- Regulatory compliance: given the security and data authenticity provided by blockchain systems, regulatory compliance and monitorization of records by the regulatory agencies can be improved and in case of no compliance, actions could be performed in a timely manner.
- Research and development: clinical research data throughout every step of a clinical trial could be actively monitored, the information shared between multiple stakeholders have a high classification of security and authenticity, logistical processes can also be improved, such as patient recruitment, payments, consent and authorization, etc.

It is clear that Blockchain technology can bring many improvements for the healthcare sector, in fact, by 2022 it is expected that the blockchain market in healthcare sector is valued in $500 million and those investment would be in the clinical trial management, improvement of sharing electronic records and fulfilling regulatory compliance (Hasselgren et al., 2020).

One of the essential uses of blockchain in the healthcare is, undoubtedly the clinical trials, the theme of this chapter. Specifically, the key features of blockchain technology, such as data provenance, transparency, decentralized transaction validation, and immutability, may contribute to overcome data management issues in clinical trials (Omar, Jayaraman, Salah, Yaqoob, et al., 2020). Areas of clinical trials where blockchain represents an improvement also include patient recruitment, medical data sharing and privacy, data integrity, consent traceability and transparency, as mentioned before (Omar, Jayaraman, Salah, Yaqoob, et al., 2020).

On the other hand, another important topic in authenticity in clinical trials is related to data management. Data could be altered or lost which could represent a major problem in a clinical trial setting creating an untrustworthy environment. In fact, 80% of the assays submitted to FDA are not reproductible due to the presence of various errors, such as fraud, data misrepresentation, and trial misconduct (Petre & Haï, 2018). This is one of the factors that contributes to data obtained from clinical trials not being immediately made public to key-players.

Taking all of this into consideration, to further explore the benefits, disadvantages, threats and opportunities of blockchains in clinical trials in data management, a review as conducted to map this information.

Review Methods

Research Objective

There are several studies reporting the advantages and disadvantages and applicability of blockchains in clinical trials, however the knowledge of those characteristics when applied to data security in clinical trials is lacking.

The role of this review is to map the current utilization of blockchain systems in clinical trials, particularly the data security managing system and its characteristics, such as applicability, interests of use, limitations and issues, as reported in literature.

In this section we report the methodology applied to conduct this review including the selection process.

Research Protocol

To identify potentially relevant publications a search was conducted on November 8th, 2020 in the following online bibliographic databases: PubMed, Science Direct and Google Scholar.

Backward-reference list checking was conducted to identify other relevant references.

The search was conducted using several combination of search terms in order to establish first the amount of information available related to blockchain and to clinical trials or health care sector, and secondly directly related to data security provided by a blockchain in a clinical trial setting. Therefore, several search terms were used and ultimately the search words used to retrieve studies from databases has: "blockchain" AND "Healthcare" AND "Clinical trials" AND "data security".

Data Base Selection Criteria

Search was conducted simultaneously in three data bases: PubMed, Science Direct and Google Scholar.

Pubmed database was considered, as it is one of the leading databases in healthcare content. Google Scholar database was chosen in order to bring different background and variability content sources. Science Direct database was chosen considering the high percentage of peer-review content.

Eligibility Criteria

In this review were included studies and review studies that reported the advantages and disadvantages of use of blockchain in clinical trials particularly in the data security optic. For the purpose of this study were excluded studies that merged blockchain and other technologies not related to the theme of this chapter and that targeted blockchain uses in healthcare other than clinical trials.

Information from magazines with peer-review, newspapers, conference abstracts and book chapters were excluded from this review. Were included studies from 2017 onwards since no relevant information before that year has found in the literature associated with blockchain and its uses in clinical trials.

Additionally, studies that were written in languages other than French and English were excluded. This criteria was established given the authors proficiency in the selected languages.

The study eligibility criteria are described in Table 1.

Table 1. Eligibility criteria of studies included in this work

Inclusion Criteria	Studies that address benefits and/or threats of blockchain in Clinical trials
	Studies from 2017 onwards
	Studies reported in English or French
Exclusion Criteria	Information from magazines, newspapers, conference abstracts and book chapters
	Studies that merged blockchain and other technologies not relevant to the theme of the chapter
	Studies that targeted other uses of blockchain in healthcare other than clinical trials

Study Selection Process

As mentioned above, studies were retrieved from multiple bibliographic databases resulting from a process divided into four phases: (i) screening phase, were multiple search words were used to establish the amount of studies related to the theme; (ii) identification phase, were the citations were retrieved from the several databases; (iii) screening phase, where titles and abstracts of citations were screened to select or exclude articles; (iv) duplicates screening phase, were the citations whom were considered as relevant during screening phase were checked for duplicates; (v) eligibility phase, where the full-texts of articles were read to assess their relevancy to this study.

Data Extraction and Data Synthesis

A summary of the included studies related to the theme of this review were extracted from the selected citations and the articles were categorized by the type of publication. The year of publication was also extracted from thc articles.

Search Findings

The number of articles retrieved and consequent process of studies search and selection is described in Figure 1.

Figure 1. Study selection and research process.

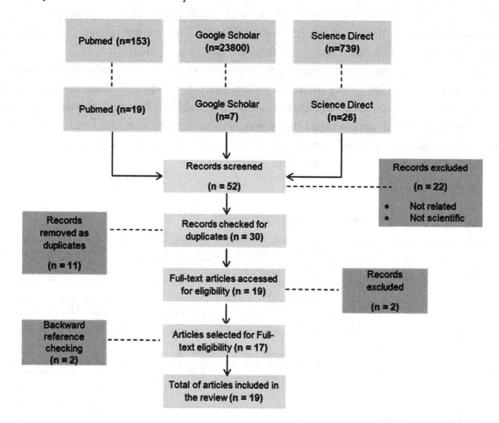

As a result from the initial search with search terms "blockchain" AND "healthcare", a total of 24692 results were obtained gathered from the three bibliographic databases used. After a combination of different search words, as described in Table 2, the search words used ("blockchain" AND "healthcare" AND "clinical trials" AND "data security") produced a total of 52 records to be screened considering the inclusion and exclusion criteria mentioned above. Therefore, these records were screened through their title and abstract and 22 were excluded considering the fact they were not related to the theme or not scientific content. Afterwards, the records were checked for duplicates and 11 records were deleted. A number of 19 records were gathered to check its full text for eligibility and 17 records were considered relevant.

Backward reference was partially conducted to gather additional studies relevant to the theme. Overall, 20 studies were included in this review.

Table 2. Results obtained using the several search terms across the three bibliographic databases (Pubmed, Science Direct and Google Scholar)

Search Terms	Number of Results (n)
"blockchain" AND "Healthcare"	24692
"blockchain" AND "Healthcare" AND "Clinical trials"	1534
"blockchain" AND "Healthcare" AND "Clinical trials" AND "security"	1130
"blockchain" AND "Healthcare" AND "Clinical trials" AND "data security"	52
"blockchain" AND "clinical trials"	19[1]

List of the Articles Reviewed

- Abu-elezz et al., (2020) - The benefits and threats of blockchain technology in healthcare: A scoping review
- Angeletti et al., 2017 - The role of blockchain and IoT in recruiting participants for digital clinical trials
- Benchoufi et al., 2017 - Blockchain protocols in clinical trials: Transparency and traceability of consent
- Benchoufi et al., 2019 - From Clinical Trials to Highly Trustable Clinical Trials: Blockchain in Clinical Trials, a Game Changer for Improving Transparency?
- Benchoufi & Ravaud, 2017. Blockchain technology for improving clinical research quality.
- Choudhury et al., 2019 - A Blockchain Framework for Managing and Monitoring Data in Multi-Site Clinical Trials
- Drosatos & Kaldoudi, (2019) - Blockchain Applications in the Biomedical Domain: A Scoping Review
- Hirano et al., 2020 - Data Validation and Verification Using Blockchain in a Clinical Trial for Breast Cancer: Regulatory Sandbox
- Kamel Boulos et al., 2018 - Geospatial blockchain: promises, challenges, and scenarios in health and healthcare
- Mackey et al., 2019 - 'Fit-for-purpose?' – challenges and opportunities for applications of blockchain technology in the future of healthcare
- Maslove et al., 2018 - Using Blockchain Technology to Manage Clinical Trials Data: A Proof-of-Concept Study
- Monrat et al., 2019 - A survey of blockchain from the perspectives of applications, challenges, and opportunities.
- Omar, Jayaraman, Salah, Simsekler, et al., 2020 - Ensuring protocol compliance and data transparency in clinical trials using Blockchain smart contracts
- Omar, Jayaraman, Salah, Yaqoob, et al., 2020 - Applications of Blockchain Technology in Clinical Trials: Reviewand Open Challenges
- Petre & Haï, 2018 - Opportunities and challenges of blockchain technology in the healthcare industry
- Radanovic et al., 2018 - Opportunities for Use of Blockchain Technology in Medicine

- Tandon et al., 2020 - Blockchain in healthcare: A systematic literature review, synthesizing framework and future research agenda
- Wong et al., 2019 - Prototype of running clinical trials in an untrustworthy environment using blockchain
- Yan Zhuang et al., 2019 - Applying Blockchain Technology to Enhance Clinical Trial Recruitment
- Yu Zhuang et al., 2018 - Applying Blockchain Technology for Health Information Exchange and Persistent Monitoring for Clinical Trials

Characteristics of the Selected Studies

As presented in Figure 2, more than 50% of the studies selected for this article were published afterwards the year of 2019 (5 published in 2019 and 6 published in 2020, therefore 11 of 19 studies selected). Additionally, 4 of the selected studies were published in 2018 and only 3 studies were published in 2017.

Figure 2. Distribution of included studies by year of publication.

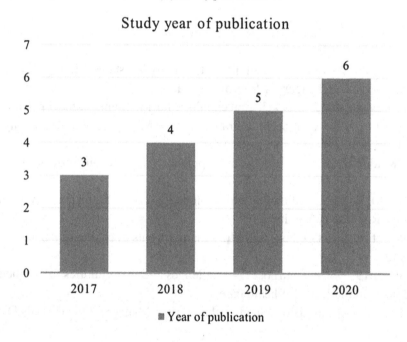

As presented in Figure 3 the selected studies for this article have a heterogenous distribution if the type of publication is considered. In fact, 3 of the studies were classified as articles, 4 as research articles, 4 as reviews, 1 as a paper, 2 as editorials, 1 as method article, 4 as research articles and 3 as proof of concept work.

Figure 3. Study type of publication

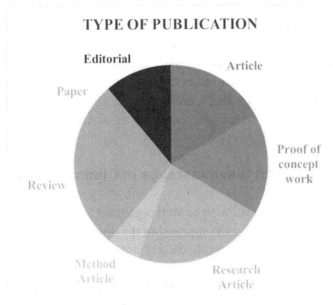

Summary of the Included Studies

Several citations enumerate the major benefits and threats of blockchain technology application in a healthcare system, including in a clinical trial setting (Abu-elezz et al., 2020) (Drosatos & Kaldoudi, 2019) (Petre & Haï, 2018) (Tandon et al., 2020) (Choudhury et al., 2019) (Omar, Jayaraman, Salah, Yaqoob, et al., 2020) (Angeletti et al., 2017) (Kamel Boulos et al., 2018)(Mackey et al., 2019) (Tandon et al., 2020)(Benchoufi et al., 2017; Yan Zhuang et al., 2019) (Yu Zhuang et al., 2018). They reflect that this technology adds significant value through improved efficiency, access control, technological advancement, privacy protection, and security of data management processes. However, in general, there are also some disadvantages mentioned related to high implementations costs, need for robust systems and specialized human resources, difficulty of scalability and data security and protection issues.

Several studies develop and implement blockchain systems in hypothetical real-life clinical trials. Omar, Jayaraman, Salah, Simsekler, et al (2020) propose a blockchain-based framework for clinical trial data management, using Ethereum smart contracts, concluding that the use of these systems assures data integrity, transparency, and traceability of the process in a clinical trial. Wong et al (2019) proposes a blockchain-based system to make data collected in the clinical trial process immutable, traceable, and potentially more trustworthy, and its resilience to data tampering. Maslove et al. (2018) explores the role of blockchain in supporting clinical trials data management and develop a proof-of-concept implementation of a patient-facing and researcher-facing system. Hirano et al (2020) validate a system that enables the security of medical data in a clinical trial using blockchain technology.

Tandon et al (2020) addresses the concerns for the improvement of regulatory compliance and security. Several important aspects are highlighted, particularly that further work needs to be done to address blockchain systems vulnerabilities and robustness, data privacy and authentication in shared storages.

BLOCKCHAIN IN CLINICAL TRIALS

As mentioned before, the interest of the applicability of blockchain systems in the healthcare sector has been increasing since 2016. In fact, this growing interest was also palpable through the research made for this chapter in Pubmed database, using the search words "blockchain" AND "healthcare" 153 results were obtained. This represents an increase of about 139% of the number of citations published in this database since 2018. Additionally, using the search words "blockchain" and "clinical trials" in Pubmed database 19 citations were obtained, which also represents an increasing number of citations since 2018 related to clinical trials and blockchain systems.

Blockchain Advantages and Disadvantages in Clinical Trials

Clinical trials require data and information to be well organized and categorized for the submission of the findings to the regulatory agency for the approval of the drug in test. Such compliance can be time consuming and resource consuming considering the amount of data, number of individuals and entities involved, and therefore it is a process particularly prone to human and system errors.

Blockchain can be the solution for the majority of errors that happen in clinical trials. Therefore, this technology can solve human errors such as: inconsistent data entry (transcription and transposition errors) and missing signatures/authorizations and system errors such as loss of data. Having a blockchain system that allows, in real time, the users in the network to verify, identify and solve the errors, can be a major improvement in clinical trials.

In fact, the most pressing challenges in clinical trials include access and management of clinical trial data; data integrity and provenance for clinical trial processes for regulatory purposes; updating and maintaining patient consent; and patient recruitment and enrolment, reproducibility of results, protocol compliance and data sharing (Mackey et al., 2019) (Omar, Jayaraman, Salah, Simsekler, et al., 2020).

Blockchain systems have the ability of transforming this process by revolutionizing the way data is stored, transmitted and managed throughout the network of participants, investigators and entities engaged in a clinical trial. Therefore, blockchain can lead to the structuration of a global community gathering all the key player involved in a clinical trial setting, such as researchers and patient communities, social networks and Internet of Things data flows with features of individual granularity, decentralization and security and with transparent interactions to ensure easier and more transparent analysis (Benchoufi & Ravaud, 2017). An additional asset is the possibility of a closer monitorization of patient health data tracking and health status (Abu-elezz et al., 2020).

Disadvantages of blockchain system in clinical trials are related to organizational difficulties, such as installations and transactions costs, operability issues and the need of specialized technical resources to manage these systems scalability issues, authorization and security issues, high energy consumption, and slow processing speeds. It is important to emphasize that the interoperability is also one of the major challenges for the blockchain adoption due to the lack of trust between healthcare organizations and lesser number of IT (Information Technology) professionals available to implement the technology. Lack of sufficient technical skills while implementing blockchain technologies may lead to disastrous consequences (Abu-elezz et al., 2020).

The principal advantages and disadvantages of the utilization of blockchain technology in clinical trials is summarized in Table 3.

Table 3. Advantages and disadvantages of blockchain technology used in clinical trials

Advantages	Monitorization
	Transparency
	Immutability
	Decentralization
	Real-time consent
	Real time access to all key players involved
Disadvantages	General access to all key players (need to constrain access depending on its user)
	Implementation system difficulties
	Need of specialized technical resources
	High levels of protection needed
	Implementation costs
	Scalabilities difficulties
	Appropriate software and hardware

Advantages of Blockchain Applied to Data Security in Clinical Trials

Considering the four main assets of blockchain systems in a clinical trial setting monitorization, transparency, immutability, and decentralization, blockchain technology might also prove to be useful in supporting or even supplanting the traditional data infrastructure used in clinical trials. Blockchain enables to establish a permanent record agreed upon by all participating parties, therefore has a tremendous potential to mitigate some of the threats related to data validity.

Taking all of this into consideration, in a real-world setting blockchain technology might have the following characteristics in terms of data security:

- Establish a more difficult precedent to falsifications or adulterations of data, since every transaction is monitored, time-stamped, transparent and in real time;
- Enables permanent recordings, a very desirable asset for clinical trial auditing;
- More compatibility between the results presented to the regulatory agency and later published in scientific publications;
- More efficient volunteer recruitment and protocol attribution;
- More accurate access and recording of data;
- Overall, less time consuming and more, efficient process of data recording, processing and storage.

Ultimately, blockchain systems in terms of data security, specifically, address the questions of data validity, integrity and reproducibility and therefore stands to achieve more confidence and veracity in the results obtained in a clinical trial (Maslove et al., 2018).

Types of Blockchain and Their Applicability in Clinical Trials

Blockchain can be applied in the healthcare sector due to its many characteristics such as immutability, decentralization, traceability and transparency (Abu-elezz et al., 2020). This technology has a potential in protecting sensitive information such as patient related information (medical records and personal information). Therefore, these characteristics have the most relevant interest in the clinical trials setting.

The potential of the Blockchain applicability to clinical trials relies on the type of Blockchain technology used. As described by Abu-elezz et al., (2020) there are three different design types considering their access permissions: public (permissionless), private (permissioned) and hybrid blockchains. Public blockchains allow anyone to participate and allow a complete transparent view to anyone participating in it, and there is no control by any single user on identity. On the other hand, private blockchains are only open for those who are invited to join the network, but nevertheless, the process remains transparent for everyone included in the network. Finally, it is important to characterize the third different type of blockchain. Hybrid Blockchains are a type of blockchains that are flexible because they allow the users to choose the data they want to be made available for the public and the data they want to be kept private for them (Abu-elezz et al., 2020) . To be easily understood, they can be seen as a public blockchain where a private network is hosted, where all of the users only have access to the data that is available for them. Taking all of this into consideration, hybrid blockchains associated with smart contracts could represent a solid method to use in a clinical trial setting since it has the possibility to select a specific amount of data to be available or kept private to the public, as previously mentioned (Kamel Boulos et al., 2018). This platform is more flexible compared to other types of blockchain because it enables the consensus mechanisms to be controlled by selected users in a decentralized manner, which in other hand, makes its structure more vulnerable to information (Omar, Jayaraman, Salah, Yaqoob, et al., 2020).

Smart Contracts

Another major contribution of blockchain technology in a clinical trial setting is the ability to provide in real time consent by the patient to protocol alterations by the sponsor (Petre & Haï, 2018). This process is followed through smart contracts.

Smart contracts are a type of code that is stored, executed, and verified on a blockchain, and also has the ability to act on clinical data sharing, either through storing the data itself or instructions on who can access that data (Maslove et al., 2018)(Kamel Boulos et al., 2018). Smart contracts can play several roles, including encoding the business logic for an application, ensuring that preconditions for action are met before itis executed, and enforcing permissions for an action. As described by Maslove et al. (2018), smart contracts run on a blockchain, they have unique characteristics compared with other types of software. First, the program itself is recorded on the blockchain, which imparts the blockchain's characteristic permanence and resistance to censorship. Second, the program can control blockchain assets. Third, the program is executed by the blockchain, meaning it will always execute as written and no one can interfere with its operation.

Since Smart Contracts all transactions follow rigorous protocols under secure conditions, their use has the possibility to ensure data provenance and create immutable audit trails, and potentially add more integrity and confidence to a clinical trial, by reducing, prevent and detect fraudulent activities and errors (Yu Zhuang et al., 2018).

Benchoufi & Ravaud (2017), described a Smart Contract example applied to a clinical trial setting. In their example, each of the clinical trial steps (trial protocol setup, patient enrollment, data collection, trial monitoring, data management, data analysis, study report, diffusion of results) as described in Figure 4, can be chained together in a preceding order, consolidating a transparent trial and preventing *a posteriori* reconstruction or beautification of data by granting several levels of access. This example represents a piece of code that holds a programmatically written contract between as many parties as needed, without any trusted third party, and that executes algorithmically according to the terms provided by the contracting parties, making the process more automatic, transparent and less prone to falsifications (Benchoufi & Ravaud, 2017).

Blockchain Systems Protection Against Liabilities

Blockchain technology allows the users to track more closely and in real time, the series of events occurring in clinical trials. This is crucial when we are talking about security and protection. By tracing and controlling the processes of clinical trials, Blockchain can prevent frauds or at least discourage them, because they become traceable and averted. But this technology cannot protect against every threat, such as data invention or data falsification since it only protects the information with time stamps and traceability once the information has entered the system (Benchoufi et al., 2019).

Other threats to the validity of clinical trials data stand to undermine the veracity of a clinical trial. These threats could be defined as internal, when they occur within the users of a blockchain, or external, when they came from outside the network of blockchain users, for example in a cyber-attack.

Maslove et al (2018) identified some of these threats. Data can be altered or lost, either accidentally or by nefarious intent; there is a risk that the published analysis is not a true representation of the analysis that was initially planned due for example to lack of monitorization resulting in a bias of the information presented to the regulatory agencies and later published in scientific publications; and lastly, data may be fabricated, manipulated, or duplicated by researchers committing outright fraud.

Some of the functionalities of the Blockchain technology like timestamping, time-ordering and the smart contracts can define a roadmap, that helps tracking errors and frauds. Clinical trials can benefit a lot from using these roadmaps (Benchoufi et al., 2019).

Omar, Jayaraman, Salah, Simsekler, et al., (2020) developed a blockchain-based solution and simulated several data mistakes or internal malicious attempts. These were stopped since the recorded data is validated using consensus algorithms resulting in a tamper-proof system.

As described by Omar, Jayaraman, Salah, Simsekler, et al., (2020) one of the biggest threats to the blockchain technology are the selfish mining external attacks. Blockchains are vulnerable to 51% of these attacks. This generally occurs when malicious blocks are higher than honest blocks in a network. As a result, one of the possibilities is that a new block gets attached to the malicious chain. This strategy is called selfish mining because selfish miners keep their blocks private and reveal them to the public only when the private chain is longer than the current public chain, and thus, it may be accepted by all miners in the network (Omar, Jayaraman, Salah, Simsekler, et al., 2020).

SOLUTIONS AND RECOMMENDATIONS

Clinical trials require data and information to be well organized and categorized for the submission of the findings to the regulatory agency for the approval of the drug in test. Such compliance can be time and resource consuming considering the amount of data, number of individuals and entities involved, and therefore it is a process particularly prone to human and system errors.

In fact, the most pressing challenges in clinical trials include access and management of clinical trial data; data integrity and provenance for clinical trial processes for regulatory purposes; updating and maintaining patient consent; patient recruitment and enrolment, reproducibility of results, protocol compliance and data sharing.

From the review conducted it is possible to point out that the operational benefits of implementing a blockchain technology to conduct a clinical trial are hardly contestable. Indeed, this technology solves many logistical constrains in terms of data sharing, communication between each involved parties and data storage and traceability.

Blockchain certainly represent a technology capable of managing and improving the information system in the healthcare sector and, particularly, in the clinical trial area, by allowing a more transparent, real time and authentic process when submitting a new drug for regulatory approval. Blockchain allows several levels of optimization regarding the organization aspects of a clinical trial (number of participants, number of departments and their areas of action) and in an individual level (the patient has more control and monitorization of his own progression), also.

Reproducibility and data integrity are crucial factors in a clinical trial setting. Regulatory agencies not only shall be able to trace back and identify the players responsible for any information in a clinical trial environment, but also be able to trust the validity of that content. In fact, 80% of the assays submitted to FDA are not reproductible (Petre & Haï, 2018). Blockchain improves the traceability of data and therefore stands to tackle this issue.

Blockchain offers a valuable contribution in addressing this problem since every transaction is validated using consensus algorithms and identity signatures with identification and date stamps.

Notwithstanding, blockchain cannot address a problem that still could affect the integrity and veracity of a clinical trial. In fact, if the information itself introduced in a software is wrong or misleading, this technology cannot address this issue. Blockchain, only, can track this wrong data and timestamp it. There is yet a need to find a solution within the design and operational side of a clinical trial to tackle this question.

Considering the four main assets of blockchain systems in a clinical trial setting, monitorization, transparency, immutability, and decentralization, blockchain technology might also prove useful in supporting or even supplanting the traditional data infrastructure used in clinical trials. Blockchain enables to establish a permanent record agreed upon by all participating parties, therefore has a tremendous potential to mitigate some of the threats related to data validity.

Disadvantages of blockchain system in clinical trials are related to organizational difficulties, such as installations and transactions costs, operability issues and the need of specialized technical resources to manage these systems scalability issues, authorization, security issues, high energy consumption, and slow processing speeds.

Overall, this technology has the ability of producing a clinical trial more transparent and tamper proofing by providing authentic validated data, and therefore, producing a more reliable and credible clinical trial. Nevertheless, there are some technical issues that need to be overcome, such as scalability, implementation costs, the need of technical resources and processing difficulties of implementation and operation. Solving all these issues, we can expect blockchain technology to be fully adopted in clinical trials, with substantial improvements.

FUTURE RESEARCH DIRECTIONS

Work needs to be done to establish the major implications in security data when applying blockchain technology in a real-word clinical trial setting and in generalized conditions of use, since as we move forward through the several phases of a clinical trial more data, more participants and more complexity of results are expected and thereby there is a need of a robust and reliable system to maintain the necessary trust levels to present the findings of a clinical trial to support the process of drug approval to a regulatory agency.

On a regulatory level, it is also important that key regulatory agencies such as FDA and EMA, provide guidelines to construct a blockchain managing system in clinical trials, in order to establish uniformity between the several systems used by different companies and guarantee the overall compliance with ethical, regulatory and safety requirements of a clinical trial.

Covid-19 pandemic lockdown revolutionized the use of technology and overall ability to distance and virtual communication in healthcare. Because of the pandemic, in one year, technology evolved exponentially, in a way never seen before. Given this opportunity, the bases of a digital revolution in healthcare are in order. However, it is important to take into consideration the technology literacy of healthcare professionals and volunteers in clinical trials. In fact, in a survey conducted by HSCB to Bitcoin users about Blockchain, 80% of the percentage of consumers that are familiarized with the term didn't know or fully understand the concept (Radanović & Likić, 2018). Therefore, digital education and technological formation of each player in clinical trials should be a priority to the implementation of blockchain systems. This is essential for the correct adoption of the technology in the clinical trials and if it doesn´t happen, the errors that will occur, can be disastrous.

On the other hand, considering the high level of investment and the need of technological specialized work force to design and run a blockchain system, investments and grants should be also created to incentivize not only the adoption of these systems, but also to educate specialized work force. There aren´t many specialized professionals that know how to work with this technology and that fully understand it, so, this digital formation must be given to the healthcare professionals, in order to have the best results possible. Of course, this formation involves a large investment, so this must be taken into consideration.

Lastly, considering the importance and impact of the data stored in a clinical trial not only on a regulatory level but also on a personal level considering the number of volunteers involved, additional work shall also be made to establish the security of a blockchain system applied in a clinical trial setting to external hazards such as cyber-attacks.

CONCLUSION

Ultimately, blockchain systems represent a technology capable of managing and improving the information organization system in the healthcare sector, specifically in the clinical trial area, by allowing a more transparent, real-time, and exact process when submitting a new drug for regulatory approval.

Blockchain allows several optimization levels regarding the organizational aspects of a clinical trial (number of participants, number of departments, and their areas of action) and individual level (the patient has more control and monitorization of his progression). These advantages also reflect data security optic since this technology can produce a more transparent and tamper-proofing clinical trial by providing accurate, validated data, producing more reliable and credible outcomes from the research conducted in a clinical trial. Nevertheless, some technical issues need to be overcome, such as scalability, implementation costs, the need for technical resources, and processing difficulties of implementation and operation of blockchain technology.

ACKNOWLEDGMENT

This research received no specific grant from any funding agency in the public, commercial, or not-for-profit sectors.

REFERENCES

Abu-elezz, I., Hassan, A., Nazeemudeen, A., Househ, M., & Abd-alrazaq, A. (2020). The benefits and threats of blockchain technology in healthcare: A scoping review. *International Journal of Medical Informatics*, *142*(August), 104246. doi:10.1016/j.ijmedinf.2020.104246 PMID:32828033

Agbo, C., Mahmoud, Q., & Eklund, J. (2019). Blockchain Technology in Healthcare: A Systematic Review. *Health Care*, *7*(2), 56. doi:10.3390/healthcare7020056 PMID:30987333

Angeletti, F., Chatzigiannakis, I., & Vitaletti, A. (2017). The role of blockchain and IoT in recruiting participants for digital clinical trials. *2017 25th International Conference on Software, Telecommunications and Computer Networks, SoftCOM 2017*. 10.23919/SOFTCOM.2017.8115590

Benchoufi, M., Altman, D., & Ravaud, P. (2019). From Clinical Trials to Highly Trustable Clinical Trials: Blockchain in Clinical Trials, a Game Changer for Improving Transparency? *Frontiers in Blockchain*, *2*(December), 1–6. doi:10.3389/fbloc.2019.00023

Benchoufi, M., Porcher, R., & Ravaud, P. (2017). Blockchain protocols in clinical trials: Transparency and traceability of consent. *F1000 Research*, *6*, 66. doi:10.12688/f1000research.10531.1 PMID:29167732

Benchoufi, M., & Ravaud, P. (2017). Blockchain technology for improving clinical research quality. *Trials*, *18*(1), 1–5. doi:10.118613063-017-2035-z PMID:28724395

Chen, Jarrell, Carpenter, Cohen, & Huang. (2019). Blockchain in Healthcare: A Patient-Centered Model. *Biomedical Journal of Scientific & Technical Research*, *20*(3), 15017–15022. PMID:31565696

Choudhury, O., Fairoza, N., Sylla, I., & Das, A. (2019). A Blockchain Framework for Managing and Monitoring Data in Multi-Site Clinical Trials. *ArXiv*, 1–13.

Deloitte. (2020). *Intelligent drug discovery About the Deloitte Centre for Health Solutions*. Author.

Drosatos, G., & Kaldoudi, E. (2019). Blockchain Applications in the Biomedical Domain: A Scoping Review. *Computational and Structural Biotechnology Journal, 17*, 229–240. doi:10.1016/j.csbj.2019.01.010 PMID:30847041

Hasselgren, A., Kralevska, K., Gligoroski, D., Pedersen, S. A., & Faxvaag, A. (2020). Blockchain in healthcare and health sciences—A scoping review. *International Journal of Medical Informatics, 134*(May), 104040. doi:10.1016/j.ijmedinf.2019.104040

Hirano, T., Motohashi, T., Okumura, K., Takajo, K., Kuroki, T., Ichikawa, D., Matsuoka, Y., Ochi, E., & Ueno, T. (2020). Data validation and verification using blockchain in a clinical trial for breast cancer: Regulatory sandbox. *Journal of Medical Internet Research, 22*(6), 1–21. doi:10.2196/18938 PMID:32340974

Hussien, H. M., Yasin, S. M., Udzir, S. N. I., Zaidan, A. A., & Zaidan, B. B. (2019). A Systematic Review for Enabling of Develop a Blockchain Technology in Healthcare Application: Taxonomy, Substantially Analysis, Motivations, Challenges, Recommendations and Future Direction. *Journal of Medical Systems, 43*(10), 320. Advance online publication. doi:10.100710916-019-1445-8 PMID:31522262

Kamel Boulos, M. N., Wilson, J. T., & Clauson, K. A. (2018). Geospatial blockchain: Promises, challenges, and scenarios in health and healthcare. *International Journal of Health Geographics, 17*(1), 1–10. doi:10.118612942-018-0144-x PMID:29973196

Mackey, T. K., Kuo, T. T., Gummadi, B., Clauson, K. A., Church, G., Grishin, D., Obbad, K., Barkovich, R., & Palombini, M. (2019). "Fit-for-purpose?" - Challenges and opportunities for applications of blockchain technology in the future of healthcare. *BMC Medicine, 17*(1), 1–17. doi:10.118612916-019-1296-7 PMID:30914045

Maslove, D. M., Klein, J., Brohman, K., & Martin, P. (2018). Using Blockchain Technology to Manage Clinical Trials Data: A Proof-of-Concept Study. *JMIR Medical Informatics, 6*(4), e11949. doi:10.2196/11949 PMID:30578196

Meunier, S. (2018). Blockchain 101: What is Blockchain and How Does This Revolutionary Technology Work? What is Blockchain and How Does This Revolutionary Technology Work? In *Transforming Climate Finance and Green Investment with Blockchains*. Elsevier Inc. doi:10.1016/B978-0-12-814447-3.00003-3

Monrat, A. A., Schelén, O., & Andersson, K. (2019). A survey of blockchain from the perspectives of applications, challenges, and opportunities. *IEEE Access: Practical Innovations, Open Solutions, 7*, 117134–117151. doi:10.1109/ACCESS.2019.2936094

Omar, I. A., Jayaraman, R., Salah, K., Simsekler, M. C. E., Yaqoob, I., & Ellahham, S. (2020). Ensuring protocol compliance and data transparency in clinical trials using Blockchain smart contracts. *BMC Medical Research Methodology, 20*(1), 1–17. doi:10.118612874-020-01109-5 PMID:32894068

Omar, I. A., Jayaraman, R., Salah, K., Yaqoob, I., & Ellahham, S. (2020). Applications of Blockchain Technology in Clinical Trials: Review and Open Challenges. *Arabian Journal for Science and Engineering*. Advance online publication. doi:10.100713369-020-04989-3

Petre, A., & Haï, N. (2018). Opportunités et enjeux de la technologie blockchain dans le secteur de la santé. *Medecine Sciences, 34*(10), 852–856. doi:10.1051/medsci/2018204 PMID:30451661

PwC. (2018). A Prescription for Blockchain and Healthcare: Reinvent or be Reinvented. *PriceWaterhouseCoopers*, 19. www.pwc.com/us/en/health-industries.html%0A©

Radanović, I., & Likić, R. (2018). Opportunities for Use of Blockchain Technology in Medicine. *Applied Health Economics and Health Policy*, *16*(5), 583–590. doi:10.100740258-018-0412-8 PMID:30022440

Smetanin, S., Ometov, A., Komarov, M., Masek, P., & Koucheryavy, Y. (2020). Blockchain evaluation approaches: State-of-the-art and future perspective. *Sensors (Switzerland)*, *20*(12), 1–20. doi:10.339020123358 PMID:32545719

Tan, L., Tivey, D., Kopunic, H., Babidge, W., Langley, S., & Maddern, G. (2020). Part 2: Blockchain technology in health care. *ANZ Journal of Surgery*, *90*(12), 2415–2419. doi:10.1111/ans.16455 PMID:33236489

Tandon, A., Dhir, A., Islam, N., & Mäntymäki, M. (2020). Blockchain in healthcare: A systematic literature review, synthesizing framework and future research agenda. *Computers in Industry*, *122*, 103290. Advance online publication. doi:10.1016/j.compind.2020.103290

Wong, D. R., Bhattacharya, S., & Butte, A. J. (2019). Prototype of running clinical trials in an untrustworthy environment using blockchain. *Nature Communications*, *10*(1), 1–8. doi:10.103841467-019-08874-y PMID:30796226

Zhuang, Y., Sheets, L. R., Shae, Z., Chen, Y. W., Tsai, J. J. P., & Shyu, C. R. (2019). Applying Blockchain Technology to Enhance Clinical Trial Recruitment. *AMIA ... Annual Symposium Proceedings. AMIA Symposium*, *2019*, 1276–1285.

Zhuang, Yu., Sheets, L., Shae, Z., Tsai, J. J. P., & Shyu, C. R. (2018). Applying Blockchain Technology for Health Information Exchange and Persistent Monitoring for Clinical Trials. *AMIA ... Annual Symposium Proceedings. AMIA Symposium*, *2018*, 1167–1175.

KEY TERMS AND DEFINITIONS

Blockchain: A decentralized, distributed ledger technology that records the provenance of a digital asset.

Clinical Trial: A research study performed in people that are aimed at evaluating a medical, surgical, or behavioral intervention.

Data Security: The process of protecting data from unauthorized access and data corruption throughout all lifecycle.

Decentralization: The transfer of control of an activity or organization to several local offices or authorities rather than one single one.

Immutability: The state of not changing or being unable to be changed.

Traceability: The quality of having an origin or course of development that may be found or followed throughout all lifecycle.

Transparency: The quality of operating in such a way that it is easy for others to see what actions or changes are performed.

Chapter 11
Blockchain and Clinical Data Economics:
The Tokenization of Clinical Research in the EU

Ana Pêgo

Centro de Estudos de Doenças Crónicas (CEDOC), NOVA Medical School, Universidade NOVA de Lisboa, Lisbon, Portugal

Inês Graça Raposo

ISEG Executive Education, Lisbon School of Economics and Management, University of Lisbon, Portugal

Mitchell Loureiro

Immunefi, Portugal

ABSTRACT

Clinical research evolved side-by-side with technology, leading to exponential data generation contributing to social and economic development. Nevertheless, data storage, integrity, and privacy concerns have emerged, raising trust issues regarding data sharing. This chapter will demonstrate how blockchain technology (BT) can address these problems and help optimizing processes, minimize costs, and monetize data. It will explain why these models are not fully explored and how cryptocurrencies are advantageous compared to traditional currency. Worldwide examples of companies developing network infrastructures that rely on private players will be provided, and European cases, where consortium models that count with different partners to build health blockchain infrastructures are being developed, will be discussed. Considering the business models to be addressed under the European Union (EU) jurisdiction, a hypothetical BT-based healthcare model with potential application in the EU scenario will also be highlighted.

DOI: 10.4018/978-1-7998-7363-1.ch011

INTRODUCTION

In 1956, IBM launched IBM 305 RAMAC, the first computer with a hard drive weighing over 900 kg, but this supercomputer could only hold around five megabytes of data (Bhushan, 2018; Lesser & Haanstra, 2000). In 2007, 51 years after the first computer, a hard disk drive (HDD) reached one terabyte size, while only two years later, that capacity doubled. Ten years later, the largest commercially available HDD can store at least 15 terabytes. Electronics have increasingly become much smaller, powerful, and cheaper. The American businessman, engineer, and co-founder and chairman *emeritus* of Intel Corporation, Gordon Moore, had predicted this exponential growth in 1965, saying that a computer processor speed would double every two years (Moore, 1998). It can be perceived how accurate Moore's Law was, as technology exponentially evolved as predicted.

Nowadays, data and technology are a crucial part of our daily life. Simple actions, such as calling someone on the phone, or even paying for lunch using a bank card, rely on digital technology. It is safe to say that humans would not be able to grow on a scientific, industrial, and economic basis as effectively as we did if it was not for the advancements in technology. As human civilization demanded, technology got more intricate and subtle, becoming almost imperceptible.

Digital technology has evolved in every sector, and the healthcare field is not an exception. Clinical research has grown side-by-side with technology development, leading to an exponential increase in data generation and analytics worldwide. Clinical trials are a significant part of the clinical research world. Nevertheless, it is essential to note that clinical research comprises a continuum of studies involving healthy people, patients, diagnostic clinical data (such as biopsies), or specific populations (with a particular pathology, per example). It includes biomedical research, observational studies, translational research, genetic diagnosis, health promotion, real-world evidence (RWE) studies, and even health services research (outcomes and economic analysis) (Coorevits et al., 2013; Salber, 2002). All these steps are under the umbrella of the "clinical research" concept, having the common goal of contributing to disease prevention, diagnosis, and treatment. Therefore, massive amounts of data are generated, analyzed, stored, and accessed daily to achieve this objective.

Along with the clinical research data exponential, several social and economic opportunities have emerged. The use of the most up-to-date and trustworthy clinical data in the healthcare sector provides an advantage to all involved parties, including patients, researchers, pharmaceutical companies, and even the government (PwC Portugal, 2019). Regarding patients, early access to innovative therapies is one of the most significant benefits of a better quality of life. On the scientific community side, clinical research leads to knowledge acquisition, scientific publications, higher recognition by other entities, and collaborations. From a governmental perspective, clinical research can boost economic development.

Moreover, access to better therapies can significantly reduce healthcare expenses while creating an attractive environment for international investment entry that boosts the national economy. Unfortunately, all this potential is not fully explored, partially due to the lack of data reproducibility (Eisner, 2018; Resnik & Shamoo, 2017). Additionally, data sharing, personal data privacy concerns, and patient enrolment also present significant challenges for contemporary clinical research and its development (Benchoufi & Ravaud, 2017). All these factors lead to trust issues between the parties involved in this data-sharing system, and blockchain technology (BT) has emerged as a viable solution.

The Birth of Blockchain: A New Technological Era

In 1990, Leslie Lamport described a consensus model called "Paxos protocol." *Paxos* is an algorithm used to reach consensus among a set of computers that communicate via an asynchronous network (where data is not transmitted and received simultaneously). (Lamport, 1998). In 1991, Stuart Haber and W. Scott Stornetta published a paper called "How to timestamp a digital document." They presented practical procedures for timestamp digital documents in a non-editable way, guaranteeing their reliability (Haber & Stornetta, 1991). These concepts were the basis for the establishment of what was going to be called the blockchain network. BT was developed to be a digital network to store data in a trustable way. Once data is created, broadcasted, and verified on a peer-to-peer network, a "block" of information is generated. Besides not requiring the involvement of a third party, only authorized users with the correct key can modify the data, namely accessing and changing its information, within the block (Drescher, 2017). When generating several blocks of information, these are subsequently linked to each other, in an unbreakable "chain," being impossible to modify one without impacting the others (Wust & Gervais, 2018; Zheng et al., 2018). This sequence means every blockchain-based chain is in constant expansion. Bitcoin, Ethereum, and Hyperledger are well-known examples of these chains (Paik et al., 2019). Once a change is allocated to a block, the whole chain requires review and validation, being, therefore, impossible for mutated data to pass unnoticed. If there is an attempt to interfere with a transaction or block, approved members and validation tools work together to confirm or reject the new data.

BT was primarily implemented in the fields of economics and cryptocurrencies. A cryptocurrency is a digital asset that was originated to work as an exchange medium in which individual coin ownership records are stored in a ledger - a digital "records book" (Greenberg, 2011). Bitcoin, the first decentralized cryptocurrency, is the result of the successful application of BT. A decentralized currency is independent of financial institutions, meaning allowing the transfer of wealth or ownership of any commodities without a third party (Tardi, 2020). However, Bitcoin is just one of the many protocols using blockchain (Zheng et al., 2018). With its progress, BT is expected to expand its disruptive potential to tokenize and decentralize not only a currency but also other business assets, as stocks or titles (Lee, 2019). In its purest form, blockchain can offer clinical research a safe and secure system for data sharing, guaranteeing data integrity and validity, preventing fraud, and protecting healthcare data, *i.e.*, increasing the confidence in its procedures, results, and data interpretation (van der Waal et al., 2020). Although it requires some investment, there are plenty of opportunities to leverage this technology to optimize clinical research procedures (Kassab et al., 2019). Hence, blockchain reduces the time associated with study development and minimizes the associated costs (Nofer et al., 2017).

Throughout this chapter, several blockchain applications in the healthcare sector will be presented, demonstrating the potential of BT not only for process optimization and cost minimization but also for data monetization in clinical research. Several reasons why these models have not been fully explored so far will be addressed. The benefits of cryptocurrency, in contrast to the traditional currency, will also be highlighted. Finally, different practical examples of worldwide investments in developing network infrastructures that rely on private players, such as Capgemini and Nebula Genomics, will be presented. An overview of the European Union (EU) perspective will also be presented, at the national (CareChain) and international (MyHealthMyData) level, with developed consortium models that count with different partners as the way of building health BT-based infrastructures. Considering the business models to be addressed and the possibilities under EU jurisdiction, a hypothetical BT-based healthcare model with potential application in the EU scenario, will also be proposed.

BLOCKCHAIN TECHNOLOGY FOR IMPROVING CLINICAL RESEARCH QUALITY

The current premise is the more data the merrier. More data collection is equivalent to broader analysis, and, therefore, more knowledge (Woods, 2013). However, this is a misleading idea, as the increase of gathered data per study also increases the difficulty in ensuring data integrity. At all scope of clinical research, from basic biomedical research to RWE studies, the impossibility of science reproducibility is recurrent (Colhoun et al., 2003; Vandenbroucke, 2004). A study conducted at Stanford University, in California, indicates that 80% of studies are not reproducible due to misconduct or fraud (Ioannidis, 2005). Even when researchers are aware of data falsification, they do not report it, and this is problematic (Fanelli, 2009, 2012; Habermann et al., 2010). In fact, the negative consequences of such actions are enormous, as a data falsification report would have critical implications in the reputation of pharmaceutical companies, state entities, and any type of sponsors (George & Buyse, 2015).

Before the commercialization of an innovative medicine or medical device, it is mandatory to know the underlying side-effects and if it indeed provides a therapeutic benefit, comparing to the current treatments. Without those conclusions, no medicine can get marketing authorization. To make this decision, market access competent authorities and clinicians require highly specific scientific and clinical data from all kinds of clinical research studies. Nevertheless, most medicines fail during the research progress. Although the drug approval success rates vary according to the therapeutic area, one of the broadest and more recent statistical studies on the topic indicates that only 13.8% of human-tested medicines get to the market (Wong et al., 2019). Several reasons are responsible for this phenomenon. One of them is the inability to prove efficacy and/or safety, due to over-selective eligibility criteria (Fogel, 2018). When the eligibility criteria are exceedingly specific, researchers might encounter difficulties in finding suitable patients. A snowball effect is then created, as three more problems emerge. By having broader groups, less targeted, the results are likely unrealistic. Second, when the market-access competent authorities analyze both marketing authorization and financial processes, they usually conclude that there is not enough proof of an added therapeutic value for the target population. Finally, when the medicine starts to be commercialized and used by real-world patients, low efficacy or even safety issues can be revealed (Hill et al., 2008).

Another reason explaining the lower percentage of drug approval than excepted is the enrollment process. At the beginning of a clinical study, a potential patient learns about its purpose and underlying conditions, such as safety, healthcare data treatment, and confidentiality. The recruiting team clarifies any questions and/or concerns of the participant before he/she agrees to enroll in the study. All terms are accepted upon signing a study contract, called informed consent form (ICF), allowing the conduction of the under-study healthcare intervention or disclosure of healthcare data in an anonymized form (T. C. Davis et al., 1998). Nevertheless, the patient has the right to withdraw at any moment, even if it implies the annulation of that patient's data, due to lack of time-points, per example. Although the participants are not obliged to justify the withdrawal, it has been reported that lack of information is one of the most common reasons (Rosbach & Andersen, 2017). This situation gets worse when participants do not observe an immediate health improvement, believe they were assigned to the control group, and, therefore, perceive that the study will not be beneficial to them. Besides the lack of trust in the clinical research procedure, various difficulties have been encountered in understanding the ICF, especially in what concerns legal terms (Bostock & Steptoe, 2012; Hosely, 2020; Krieger et al., 2017). Other major concerns of the participants include data sharing, re-use for marketing purposes (rather than science), discrimination, individual re-identification, and exploitation of data for profit (Mello et al., 2018). In the end, if the data collected up to the moment of withdrawal are not sufficient to establish a significant outcome result, the collection of those data is not viable. This leads to an increased cost for the sponsor, as another participant enrollment process is needed. Since this is not always doable, the consequently low sampling compromises market approval due to a lack of statistically significant results. As a result, the company loses time and money, making this kind of activity less stimulating to invest in.

Increasing clinical research quality, by increasing reproducibility, and empowering both research communities with secure data sharing and patient with tools guaranteeing their privacy are aims that the BT can help achieve (Benchoufi & Ravaud, 2017).

Using BT for Clinical Trials Development

BT involves a decentralized, secure tracking system for any data exchange that can occur with a peer-to-peer network, enabling data sharing on the researcher side. On the patient side, it ensures transparency. Hence, BT can be the basis for better-quality clinical research methodology (Benchoufi & Ravaud, 2017). During a clinical trial, significant data and metadata are produced. It is necessary to ensure its integrity, traceability, and historicity. BT allows the time-stamping of each transaction (Gipp & Meuschke, 2009; Schulz et al., 2010). Thus, the existence of data becomes provable while the data remain confidential and incorruptible. This allows the construction of a reliable clinical study (Benchoufi & Ravaud, 2017). Also, within the data collection process, clinical trial steps can be chained together so that each step depends on its predecessor. This is accomplished through Smart Contracts (Radanović & Likić, 2018), which are protocols that are automatically executed when the terms and conditions provided by the different parties are met, without the need for the involvement of a third party. For instance, the Smart Contracts-enclosed chain of blocks can guarantee that the planned methodology has been respected. A correct performance would show that the study was well conducted (Benchoufi & Ravaud, 2017; Cong & He, 2019).

BT in clinical research is no longer just an idea, as there are already ongoing projects using this technology. For example, the Triall Foundation is developing the first clinical trials employing blockchain. Partnering with Sphereon, this company is improving verifiability and operational efficiency in clinical trials (Rakesh Joshi, 2020). The consortium's Verial application, a clinical document management solution, has been used in a phase-II clinical trial. Overall, Verial is a blockchain-based document management solution that can ensure integrity, authenticity, traceability, and immutability in clinical trial research (Omar et al., 2020). Another example is the multinational corporation Capgemini. As previously mentioned, patients' enrollment and trial completion highly depend on the recruitment and research team, particularly on their expertise and empathy to correctly explain all steps and implications of the study. To help with this, Capgemini developed a BT-based simple consent management platform. It allows the disclosure of confidential information about the study in a secure way. Patients are provided with a simple consent document, as a new version of the ICF, that can be read on a tablet, smartphone, or computer. This tool includes a protocol description, informative videos, and an interactive quiz to ensure that the patient has a complete understanding of the process. After a validated and successful patient enrollment, the ICF is made available via a cloud system on the patient's devices, being easily accessed at any moment. If a new and updated ICF is required, then the same method is used. Also, all consent records are automatically populated within an immutable database, contributing to the development of secure and reliable time-stamped audit trails (Javier Moreno, n.d.).

BT in Academia

Regarding research institutes, they could also take advantage of this technology. They can use data stored in the BT network to conduct cutting-edge research to find patients of interest for potential studies (Radanović & Likić, 2018). Besides, the conceptual model of BT with a peer-to-peer network exists in the scientific world. Peer review is a standard procedure when talking about the publication of scientific papers. However, and here lies the problem, it is not a standardized process (D'Andrea & O'Dwyer, 2017). A peer review does not always achieve good quality control of the work due to high variability in both theory and practice (Roman-Belmonte et al., 2018). The scientific community does not blame the concept, recognizing that scientific papers should be corrected and moderated by experts in the field. The research world blames how journals and publishers put them into practice (Mulligan et al., 2013). BT may help re-invent the peer-review system making it more efficient, fair, and objective when compared to the currently used system (Tennant et al., 2017).

All BT features highlighted above have shown the potential of this technology in organizing a more transparent methodology and contributing to the generation of clinical research data with integrity and transparency. By optimizing the current procedures and by removing the need for third parties to manage the transaction and keep records, BT can massively reduce the costs of clinical research. Innovative companies should start focusing on the adoption of this technology to boost their projects and decrease their costs, in a long-term perspective. Besides these advantages, can the clinical research sector also start to make an economic profit from BT? This is a question that the authors will try to answer next.

VALUE EXCHANGE IN CLINICAL RESEARCH

Money is one of the bases of society. It promoted the development of the first large-scale societies in ancient times (Ingham, 1996). Throughout history, it was observed that the tendency was the requisition of a central figure or government to issue currency and coin. The argument rests on the economic efficiency of a currency, which is both uniform (one issuer) and stable (issued in economically suitable sums). The rationale for this centralization has weakened over time, and the main reason is the need for at least one intermediary. For each of these middlemen, a fee is associated to pay for a service, which is not guaranteed to be effective nor safe. Nevertheless, these players have been working with the power of being the only option for the customer. The need to receive monetary remuneration and have access to our data gives these intermediaries power. But, if they fail, the whole system collapses (Harford, 2019). What if they were not needed? The parties would surely benefit from the elimination of all the intermediary steps, simplifying the transaction process.

In 2008, the development of the Bitcoin network encouraged the creation of many new cryptocurrencies (Nakamoto, 2009). According to the CoinMarketCap, there are currently more than 7 800 cryptocurrencies; each one of them with a different use case and backstory (Freitas, 2020). The landscape is being turned upside down by the digital revolution, namely the issuance and circulation of private-label cryptocurrencies, and the prospect of central bank digital currencies. These new units are expected to transform the world as it is known. Digital currencies, especially cryptocurrency, can be seen as a convenient way of transacting with lower costs (or even none), no middleman, and at any time, being, therefore, considered the next step in this evolution (Yeung & Eichengreen, 2020).

At first glance, both traditional and crypto money are used to store and transfer value. Cryptocurrency, as well as traditional currency, is used to purchase goods and services. Both have their value dictated by supply, demand, work, shortage, and other economic factors, but cryptocurrency is a decentralized and global currency. It has no central point of control, meaning that it is out of the banks' control, and it is not supported by a central government. The BT used by cryptocurrencies, such as Bitcoin, is an open distributed ledger that records transactions. It was soon noticed that the underlying technology might have wider applications. It offered a completely new way for strangers to collaborate without needing to trust an intermediary or a centralized authority (Harford, 2019). Decentralization allows BT to have increased potential, greater security, and faster settlement. While these are the major cornerstones of the cryptocurrency system, they are also the weaknesses of the traditional financial systems (Kuo Chuen et al., 2017). Additionally, cryptocurrencies increase the financial awareness of consumers. They are the only individuals with access to the funds and full control over them.

Blockchain is a general-purpose technology. It can lower the cost of verifiable transactions and lower the barriers to create new marketplaces. By principle, BT might be useful in any situation where we currently trust some entity to manage data in ways that help us interact. Surprisingly or not, many situations fit this description (Catalini & Gans, 2016). Beyond the financial sector, BT has recently penetrated different domains. One field where this technology has great potential is clinical research, but its implementation is expensive. From hiring BT experts to establish a team that deals with the legal aspects, several expenses need to be considered (Azati, 2020). Despite the numerous opportunities mentioned previously, both at the optimization and reduction costs level, BT is only going to be adopted in clinical research if it provides an economic benefit. In other words, for companies and individuals to be willing to adopt BT, they will need the assurance that this will minimize the costs associated with clinical research and/or will result in a positive return on investment (Dijkman et al., 2015).

Currently, the focus is to create value through data - the monetization process - for all parties, companies, healthcare establishments, and patients. Experts believe that data itself will be developed into a valuable good, as customers will be eager to pay for their access (Bucherer & Uckelmann, 2011). In this section, several blockchain applications will be described, demonstrating the potential of BT for data monetization in clinical research. Further examples of healthcare-related data monetization are summarized in **Table 1** (appendix section).

Blockchain's Potential in the Clinical Market

The medical technology startup Longenesis is the first example. This decentralized medical record marketplace, founded in 2017, focuses on one very simple, yet not solved, problem in the pharma and healthcare environment. It aims to provide pharmaceutical companies, usually the largest clinical data consumers/acquirers, as well as hospitals and research institutions, the big data aggregators, a simpler communication system, essentially enabling data access and sharing between the two parties. Longenesis solved the technology and legislation issues by promoting an environment where both parties can directly exchange information, without intermediaries, enabling safe data curation as well as compliant consent-enabled biomedical data utilization for research. This platform allows individuals to store and monetize their health data, including blood test results, medical history, genetic profile, and other sensitive information in a blockchain-based marketplace. This would not be possible without some kind of incentive for all parties. Every piece of information provided is exchanged by LifePounds, a cryptocurrency that acts as rewards points and that can be spent on different services provided by the marketplace

(Dinh & Thai, 2018; Gammon, 2018). This data-sharing system allows the pharmaceutical industry or any research institution to query medical data, by directly request its access to the hospital or to the patients itself, for clinical trial recruitment or any proactive studies.

Several projects are also being established at the genetics level. From the simple curiosity to know more about their ethnic roots to the desire to know the probability of developing certain diseases, the genomic sequencing of individuals is getting popular. With this market opportunity, companies like 23andMe, MyHeritage, and AncestryDNA took the chance to monetize genetic data. Nevertheless, this trendy industry has inherent privacy concerns, as these companies are selling genetic sequencing access to third parties, including pharmaceutical companies (Swan, 2015). BT is also revolutionizing this business as BT-based genomics data-exchange platforms or networks are giving control of the patients' data to their primary owners (Diego et al., 2019). A practical example is Nebula Genomics, a startup founded in 2018. This company gathers data from genome sequencing of the human genome and uses the BT to allow individuals to sell access to their entire genome in exchange for a cryptocurrency called Nebula tokens (counters with no real economic value). This company permits individuals to sell their data to researchers around the world. Their main customer is the pharmaceutical industry. These data can, for example, provide new insights about who is at risk of developing certain diseases, and/or why those individuals are at risk. For individuals who do not have their genome sequenced, they can also make a profit by taking paid surveys about their health conditions. If a company is interested in their genomic information, it can subsidize the cost of the genomic sequencing of the individual (Dinh & Thai, 2018; Gammon, 2018; Maxmen, 2018).

Besides genomics, multiple projects are directing their attention to imaging (Diego et al., 2019). The development of blockchain-based marketplaces to promote data sharing between individuals and companies or academic researchers, in exchange for data interpretation and payment, is entering the oncology field, more specifically breast cancer. Hadley and colleagues at the University of California, San Francisco, launched a system called BreastWeCan, whose artificial intelligence (AI) algorithm was trained to detect cancer using mammograms obtained from more than 3 million women in the United States of America, with or without breast cancer. The goal is to classify tumors more efficiently than doctors do. The accuracy of the algorithm grows as it is trained on more and varied data. After completing the ICF and medical release, women can share their breast imaging and related clinical reports, to improve breast-cancer screening. With this appliance, patients gain control over information, which usually is only held by clinics, with the additional advantage of getting clinical interpretations of their risk of breast cancer, based on tissue density, age, and other known factors (BreastWeCan, n.d.; Maxmen, 2018).

A Token-Based Peer Review Model

As mentioned in the previous section, academia could also benefit from this technology. Peer-review is a common procedure; however, it is demanding, time-consuming, and relies on willing and hopefully capable members of the scientific field's community to conduct reviews voluntarily as a service. The review procedure is viable only if the available reviewers can manage the flow of submissions promptly (Avital, 2018). Additionally, it is not a standardized process (D'Andrea & O'Dwyer, 2017). The emergence of BT and the proliferation of cryptocurrencies are an opportunity for the development of a token-based peer review payment system to solve the current problems in the world of publication review. As has already been noted, cryptocurrencies use blockchain-based tokens that allow users to represent and exchange value and tangible externalities without the need for intermediation or central management. For example, an author would pay a submission fee. The reviewers would receive part of this contribution and the journal would receive another part. A smart contract would define how and when the submission fee is divided among the different members of the review team. BT would provide a secure, commonly shared ledger that records transactions of value to participants in an exchange network (Avital, 2018). BT can also permanently record the revision history (Choi & Seo, 2021). Despite being a quite simplistic description, this token-based model could eliminate "jammed review pipelines" while fairly controlling quality and spreading the equity generated through peer review.

The take-home message is that the adoption of BT by the clinical research world will enable conditional data sharing between parties that do not necessarily trust each other. This inevitably promotes data standardization, which can make the whole system a greater asset. In this network, patients can conditionally share personal data with clinical research-associated institutes (from academy or industry). Then the institutes can share the data, results, and conclusions within each other, and continuously improve scientific knowledge as it is nowadays. Using BT, the aforementioned startups standardize the data while guaranteeing their integrity, validity and privacy (Shrestha et al., 2020). Additionally, the creation of a marketplace that standardizes and creates clear and unbreakable rules facilitates the valuation of the data in bulk and distributing this value through all parties involved in the exchange. BT can build incentive schemes to boost the generation of clinical data that would not otherwise be possible. Once BT gets developed considering data monetization, individuals and companies will start better understanding the appliances of this system. The sooner investors promote this environment, the sooner a future where people will have a basic income by leasing out health data will emerge. Nevertheless, it is still fundamental to underline that these technological advances will require considerable responsibility. Some underlying legal and ethical questions are still needed to be answered (Gammon, 2018).

TOKENIZATION OF CLINICAL RESEARCH IN THE EU

Health data is one of the most valuable types of information (Mettler, 2016). Sadly, as it was mentioned, there are significant problems with the way that clinical data is handled. Patients commonly barely have control over their records, mainly due to difficult access and even control, since their data is being stored separately by every healthcare provider that they visit (doctors, hospitals, clinics). The same happens in the industry, where a great deal of data is stored in several incompatible data storehouses. If stored properly, these data could have been used more efficiently, promoting savings and medical breakthroughs (EUblockchain, 2019). However, the challenges are numerous. Every year, this industry invests billions of dollars in research and development, and most of that money is lost on products/services that do not reach the market (Wong et al., 2019). For this reason, conducting well-thought and targeted research based on a good data foundation is fundamental to optimize this investment. Conversely, accessing to reliable and private data is becoming more challenging. This is a significant problem worldwide, with the EU being no exception. Complex consent processes and centralized data storage increase data inaccessibility and vulnerability, as well as encourage fraud. Inside the EU borders, more than 193 million personal records were open to fraud and identity theft in 2015 (J. Davis, 2015). Additionally, medical records are worth up to ten times more on the black market than any other information (Humer & Finkle, 2014). BT can be a valuable instrument to overcome these hurdles.

In the EU, there are diverse difficulties to be overcome, and they require better solutions than at the national level. Centralization has contributed greatly to those problems. EU also knows that research and innovation are the future, and investment in these areas promotes smart, sustainable, and inclusive growth and jobs (Tom Lyons, 2020). Taking this into account, the EU launched the initiative Horizon 2020 (H2020), intending to guarantee that the EU develops first-class science, eliminates walls to novelty, and makes it easier for the public and private sectors to work together in delivering innovation. Bearing this in mind, within the framework of the EU's H2020, BT was not forgotten (Gassner, 2018). The H2020 initiative included a group of blockchain-related projects. For instance, under the eHealth Cybersecurity Research and Innovation effort, in 2018, there was a call for projects for improving cybersecurity in hospitals. Among the 40 submitted proposals, 15 included BT, and among the seven selected for funding, five contained a blockchain component (EUblockchain, 2019).

The following practical cases have the individual as the main character. With the help of blockchain, patients can store their health records and control access to them. This makes it easier for individuals to aggregate and have an overview of health-related information. Once combined, individuals can choose to take their data to market via BT-based patient-mediated health data exchanges. They can share, rent, or sell some of their health data to interested entities. These new models allow them to support research and monetize their health data privately. The data itself is never revealed nor leaves the possession of its owner. Thanks to BT and cryptoeconomics, there is a chance to apply behavioral economics and game theory to improve this process (EUblockchain, 2019).

MyHealthMyData (MHMD) project is the first example of how the EU has taken the lead in pioneering transnational approaches to healthcare (Santos Rutschman, 2018). In 2016, EU's H2020 awarded MHMD with an amount of 3.5 million euros. This project aimed to use BT to enable medical data to be stored and transmitted safely and effectively. The MHMD project is centered on the connection between organizations and individuals, encouraging hospitals to start making anonymized data available for open research, while prompting EU citizens to become the ultimate owners and controllers of their health data (Morley-Fletcher, 2017; MyHealthMyData, 2016a; Santos Rutschman, 2018). It is crucial to underline that, opposing to what was observed in previously mentioned cases, the MHMD model was conceptualized under a consortium model with the collaboration of different partners (MyHealthMyData, 2016b).

At the national level, the EU also has successful examples, including Estonia and Sweden. Estonia was an early adopter of this technology in its national infrastructure. Since 2012, Estonia's healthcare system has been revolutionized by BT (Heller, 2017). At the moment, 99% of patients have a countrywide digital record. Besides, all country's health care billing is handled electronically, and 99% of their prescriptions are digital. Additionally, each Estonian that has visited a doctor has an electronic medical record (EMR) that can be tracked. Identified by the ID card, the health information is saved securely and can be accessible by authorized individuals (e-estonia, n.d.; Santos Rutschman, 2018).

More recently, in 2017, Sweden also applied the consortium model by developing a blockchain health data platform called CareChain. It seeks to give individuals ownership and total control over their health information, deciding if they want to allow healthcare professionals and researchers access to their health records as well as to purchase services in a global marketplace. This consortium has a broad and diverse range of institutions that go from the government to hospitals and pharmacies (CareChain, n.d.; Santos Rutschman, 2018). Despite CareChain being the one developing the platform, the future idea is to have different entities contributing to the network. CareChain is also actively helping to reduce costs and complexity associated with the recruitment process of clinical trials, by creating ecosystems that facilitate the communication between volunteers and entities which are responsible for developing those studies (Leeming et al., 2019).

There is also PharmaLedger. The goal of its project is to build a platform that supports the design and adoption of blockchain-enabled solutions for the healthcare sector, using supply chain, clinical trials, and health data as case studies. An interesting feature of this project is that BT is used as a combination with exponentially growing technological innovations, including the Internet of Things (IoT) to solve the current challenges in the healthcare sector (EUblockchain, 2019; IMI, 2020). For instance, BT could be combined with the IoT to help ensure the authenticity of IoT-generated data along the data lifecycle, as well as more securely control devices remotely. It could be used to support health data markets for medical research and development (EUblockchain, 2019).

Overall, in the various examples presented, the main goal is to put personal health data in the hands of the patient, and also to foster/facilitate the interaction between organizations and individual data-owners. The examples also demonstrated that it is understood that blockchain is just one of the tools available. If combined with other technologies (such as IoT) BT will be able to fuel innovation in the old continent. At last, the Estonian example has showed that it is not something utopic, it is feasible and promotes process optimization.

Based on the previous ideas, and considering the European context, this chapter proposes a hypothetical health care blockchain model (**Figure 1**) with a potential application inside the EU. This BT model would mobilize data that is currently collected and stored in separate places, used by different stakeholders, and sometimes difficult to get access to, even by data owners (the patients). It would open up a major conceptual advance, via an incentive system, that flows to the owner of each data element based on its value. This arrangement could form the basis for a health-based cryptocurrency, with far-reaching implications (Krittanawong et al., 2020; Mamoshina et al., 2018). These types of initiatives can be highly effective, and policymakers must support such efforts. The world is changing, the blockchain race is happening, and old Europe will not want to be left out.

DISCUSSION

These days, blockchain is one of the key drivers behind innovation. However, it is far from being mainstream, mostly due to the direct and restrictive connection that society does between Bitcoin and BT. First impressions are important. Bitcoin's history and evolution, disruption, fluctuation, and volatility are making BT pay greatly for the early fame that Bitcoin and other cryptocurrencies helped to form (Campione, 2019). There is a need to erase these preconceptions surrounding BT and cryptocurrencies, which are distracting the world from their true potential: the possibility of developing a real business around it (Dinh & Thai, 2018). Clinical research is one of the sectors where blockchain would be more beneficial (Richie Etwaru, 2017).

Conceptually, BT is secure by design. Clinical research data contain personal and sensitive information that may be attractive to cybercriminals, and therefore it is crucial to sure the security of this ecosystem. Blockchain has been explored as one potential mechanism that would ensure the safety of this environment. Several benefits of this technology have already been mentioned, namely the promotion of an agreement without the involvement of a trusted mediator, thus, avoiding a single point of failure. This decentralized consensus also gives the patients control over their data. Data is complete, consistent, timely, accurate, and easily distributed when using BT. It assures completeness through smart contracts. Changes to the blockchain are visible to all members of the patient network, and all data insertions are immutable. Also, any unauthorized modifications can be detected (Benchoufi & Ravaud, 2017; Esposito et al., 2018).

By presenting a broad range of solutions, blockchain not only reduces the trial timeline, but also promotes cost minimization (Benchoufi & Ravaud, 2017). Cost minimization is extremely important for any company, and the pharmaceutical industry is not an exception. Every single year, billions of dollars are invested in research and development. However, most of the money spent is lost on products/services that do not even reach the market. This underlines the importance of conducting well-tough and targeted research, based on a good data foundation. While access to good data is getting harder due to complex consent processes, a new potential business emerged and BT-based startups have started to explore data monetization (Rama Rao; Himanshu Jain, 2019).

Many healthcare providers and multinational pharmaceutical companies are starting to get interested in the power that this technology underlies. Even outside the healthcare world, it is possible to find examples of companies who have understood the potential of this field. For instance, in 2019, Microsoft Technologies has made a great step towards clinical data monetization, by filing a patent named "Cryptocurrency System Using Body Activity Data". Based on the statement that patients are both data producers and storers, this patent describes the use of energy generated from human body activity to mine cryptocurrency (Ali Sina User, 2020).

Nevertheless, we cannot delude ourselves; there is a long way to go. To effectively start implementing BT in the healthcare sector, trust and satisfaction are a requirement for the users. As an emerging technology, BT is facing numerous obstacles that should not be forgotten and must be overcame. BT can also be somehow disruptive and requires a radical rethink and significant investment. In other words, it is necessary to develop a cost-benefit evaluation to understand the return on investment and any potential implications, both legal and financial (Esposito et al., 2018).

Scalability is an additional issue (Mazlan et al., 2020; Zheng et al., 2018). Blockchain was originally designed to record transaction data, which is relatively small in size and linear. Bitcoin, for example, has three to four transactions a second. Visa averages one to 600. To confirm these transactions, computers consume about as much electricity as Ireland (Altcointoday, 2017). Besides, blockchain was designed to record small and linear data, and healthcare data, such as imaging, can be large and complex. How well can blockchain storage manage this type of data is still uncertain (Esposito et al., 2018). In the future, the efforts should focus on storage optimization, or even blockchain redesigning (Mazlan et al., 2020; Zheng et al., 2018).

Another point to be considered is that as long as users are conducting transactions in a trusted ecosystem, there is no need for outside validation of operations, meaning that there is no need for mediators. However, blockchain does not allow integration with the external world. When a blockchain network needs to interact with other databases, intermediation with the external database is required. It is believed that middlemen will unlikely disappear completely, at least in the near future (Pavel Kravchenko, 2018).

In the specific context of clinical research, there is an abundance of uncertainties, and speculations about the potential of the BT (Mazlan et al., 2020). One of the questions regarding the usage of this technology is if the access of individuals (some of them with no scientific or medical background) is actually beneficial. While some are in favor of individuals having access to their own data, others think that they may read too much into it without appropriate medical guidance (Swan, 2015). Another question is what the actual value of data is. How much should patients be paid for their data and who defines that? The question of whether payment for personal clinical data for clinical trials would be a form of economic coercion to recruit participants also remains unanswered (Weigmann, 2015). Additionally, the current European legislation defines that "no undue influence, including that of a financial nature, [must be] exerted on subjects to participate in the clinical trial" (Regulation [EU] No 536/2014). In opposition to what occurs in the USA, where clinical research organizations can promote their studies as a possibility of making money by enrolling in them, the volunteers of Europeans clinical trials can only receive a (monetary or not) compensation for their participation. This might be something worth to revisit by governments, in order to guarantee the compliance of clinical research with individuals once BT is implemented.

Still focusing in the EU, when observed from a General Data Protection Regulation (GDPR) perspective, some legal uncertainties provide some insecurity when talking about this technology (Gassner, 2018). The centralization versus decentralization system and the mutability versus immutability of personal data are some of the concepts that create a branch between BT and the GDPR (M. Finck, 2018; Michèle Finck, 2019). While blockchain's data integrity and distributed storage/access can offer new opportunities for healthcare data management, these same features also pose challenges. Data integrity results in immutability. Once in the chain, alteration is not an option, and this is a problem when referring to healthcare/clinical data. Article 17 of the GDPR has strengthened the rights of individuals to request personal data to be erased. Therefore, anyone planning to use BT cannot ignore this legal obligation (M. Finck, 2018; Michèle Finck, 2019). With this in mind, governments must pay attention to these obstacles. While it is in their interest to continue protecting the interests of individuals, it should also be in their interest to keep developing the nations.

CONCLUSION

In this chapter, next-generation technologies in clinical research were presented, and innovative solutions were identified given their potential to accelerate biomedical research and give patients new tools to control and profit from their data. Specifically, the current status of BT in the EU and how it can impact the development of clinical research going forward was presented. Overall, it was found that one of the biggest problems related to clinical research is individuals' trust in the available tools, and there is an entire industry that suffers from the absence of trust.

Through this literature review, the authors concluded that blockchain could transform clinical research, bringing significant improvements in operational efficiency, data security, management, and cost reduction. However, it is essential to highlight that, despite being a technology where trust, immutability, and shared governance join forces for good, blockchain integration in healthcare systems creates some technical challenges. These include immaturity of the technology, scalability, interoperability, complex integration with existing healthcare systems, complexity, and even resistance from the different players (researchers, patients, funders), who may not embrace this technology due to a wrong technology perception (Campione, 2019).

It cannot be forgotten that blockchain only appeared ten years ago. One should expect some wrong moves and false starts. However, despite BT's controversy or doubts, human life data represents one of BT's most valuable and straightforward applications. Numerous trusted companies are already developing answers (Zhavoronkov & Church, 2019). Once the potential of these business models is demonstrated, perhaps, soon, blockchain can provide significant benefits to the industry, the economy, and the European society as a whole.

REFERENCES

Ali Sina User, I. A. (2020). The inevitable digitalization of the globe and the steps that are bringing us there. *New Europe*. https://www.neweurope.eu/article/the-inevitable-digitalization-of-the-globe-and-the-steps-that-are-bringing-us-there/

Altcointoday. (2017). *Bitcoin and Ethereum vs Visa and PayPal – Transactions per second - Altcoin Today*. Altcointoday.

Avital, M. (2018). Peer Review: Toward a Blockchain-enabled Market-based Ecosystem. *Peer Review : Toward a Blockchain-enabled Market-based Ecosystem, 42*, 646–653. Advance online publication. doi:10.17705/1CAIS.04228

Azati. (2020). *How Much Does It Cost To Develop Blockchain In 2020*. Azati. https://azati.ai/how-much-does-it-cost-to-blockchain/

Benchoufi, M., & Ravaud, P. (2017). Blockchain technology for improving clinical research quality. *Trials, 18*(1), 1–5. doi:10.118613063-017-2035-z PMID:28724395

Bhushan, B. (2018). Historical evolution of magnetic data storage devices and related conferences. Microsystem Technologies. doi:10.100700542-018-4133-6

Bostock, S., & Steptoe, A. (2012). Association between low functional health literacy and mortality in older adults: longitudinal cohort study. *BMJ, 344*(3), e1602–e1602. doi:10.1136/bmj.e1602

BreastWeCan. (n.d.). *Crowdsourcing earlier detection of breast cancer from patient imaging*. https://www.breastwecan.org/

Bucherer, E., & Uckelmann, D. (2011). Architecting the Internet of Things. *Architecting the Internet of Things*. doi:10.1007/978-3-642-19157-2_10

Campione, T. (2019). *The Blockchain Case: Can we trust the intermediary of trust?* PwC. https://blog.pwc.lu/blockchain-case-trust-the-intermediary-of-trust/

CareChain. (n.d.). *A joint effort to establish blockchain infrastructure and personal data management for health*. https://www.carechain.io/

Catalini, C., & Gans, J. S. (2016). Some Simple Economics of the Blockchain. SSRN *Electronic Journal*. doi:10.2139srn.2874598

Choi, D. H., & Seo, T. S. (2021). Development of an open peer review system using blockchain and reviewer recommendation technologies. *Science Editing, 8*(1), 104–111. doi:10.6087/kcse.237

Colhoun, H. M., McKeigue, P. M., & Smith, G. D. (2003). Problems of reporting genetic associations with complex outcomes. *Lancet, 361*(9360), 865–872. doi:10.1016/S0140-6736(03)12715-8 PMID:12642066

Cong, L. W., & He, Z. (2019). Blockchain Disruption and Smart Contracts. Review of Financial Studies. doi:10.1093/rfs/hhz007

Coorevits, P., Sundgren, M., Klein, G. O., Bahr, A., Claerhout, B., Daniel, C., Dugas, M., Dupont, D., Schmidt, A., Singleton, P., De Moor, G., & Kalra, D. (2013). Electronic health records: New opportunities for clinical research. *Journal of Internal Medicine*, *274*(6), 547–560. doi:10.1111/joim.12119 PMID:23952476

D'Andrea, R., & O'Dwyer, J. P. (2017). Can editors save peer review from peer reviewers? *PLoS One*, *12*(10), e0186111. Advance online publication. doi:10.1371/journal.pone.0186111 PMID:29016678

Davis, J. (2015). *7 Largest Data Breaches of 2015*. Healthcare IT News.

Davis, T. C., Holcombe, R. F., Berkel, H. J., Pramanik, S., & Divers, S. G. (1998). Informed consent for clinical trials: A comparative study of standard versus simplified forms. *Journal of the National Cancer Institute*, *90*(9), 668–674. Advance online publication. doi:10.1093/jnci/90.9.668 PMID:9586663

de Diego, S., Gonçalves, C., Lage, O., Mansell, J., Kontoulis, M., Moustakidis, S., Guerra, B., & Liapis, A. (2019). Blockchain-Based Threat Registry Platform. *2019 IEEE 10th Annual Information Technology, Electronics and Mobile Communication Conference (IEMCON)*, 892–898. 10.1109/IEMCON.2019.8936249

Dijkman, R. M., Sprenkels, B., Peeters, T., & Janssen, A. (2015). Business models for the Internet of Things. *International Journal of Information Management*, *35*(6), 672–678. doi:10.1016/j.ijinfomgt.2015.07.008

Dinh, T. N., & Thai, M. T. (2018). AI and Blockchain: A Disruptive Integration. *Computer*, *51*(9), 48–53. doi:10.1109/MC.2018.3620971

Drescher, D. (2017). Blockchain basics: A non-technical introduction in 25 steps. In Blockchain Basics: A Non-Technical Introduction in 25 Steps. doi:10.1007/978-1-4842-2604-9

e-estonia. (n.d.). *Healthcare*. https://e-estonia.com/solutions/healthcare/

Eisner, D. A. (2018). Reproducibility of science: Fraud, impact factors and carelessness. *Journal of Molecular and Cellular Cardiology*. doi:10.1016/j.yjmcc.2017.10.009

Esposito, C., De Santis, A., Tortora, G., Chang, H., & Choo, K. K. R. (2018). Blockchain: A Panacea for Healthcare Cloud-Based Data Security and Privacy? *IEEE Cloud Computing*, *5*(1), 31–37. doi:10.1109/MCC.2018.011791712

Etwaru, R. (2017). *Blockchain: Trust Companies: Every Company Is at Risk of Being Disrupted by a Trusted Version of Itself*. Dog Ear Publishing.

EUblockchain. (2019). *Feeling good: Healthcare data and the blockchain*. https://www.eublockchainforum.eu/news/feeling-good-healthcare-data-and-blockchain

Fanelli, D. (2009). How many scientists fabricate and falsify research? A systematic review and meta-analysis of survey data. *PLoS ONE*. doi:10.1371/journal.pone.0005738

Fanelli, D. (2012). Negative results are disappearing from most disciplines and countries. *Scientometrics*. doi:10.100711192-011-0494-7

Finck, M. (2018). Blockchains and Data Protection in the European Union. *European Data Protection Law Review*. doi:10.21552/edpl/2018/1/6

Finck, M. (2019). Blockchain and the General Data Protection Regulation : can distributed ledgers be squared with European data protection law? European Parliament.

Fogel, D. B. (2018). Factors associated with clinical trials that fail and opportunities for improving the likelihood of success: A review. *Contemporary Clinical Trials Communications*, *11*, 156–164. https://doi.org/10.1016/j.conctc.2018.08.001

Freitas, C. (2020). *How many cryptocurrencies are there?* Currency.Com. https://currency.com/how-many-cryptocurrencies-are-there

Gammon, K. (2018). Experimenting with blockchain: Can one technology boost both data integrity and patients' pocketbooks? *Nature Medicine*, *24*(4), 378–381. https://doi.org/10.1038/nm0418-378

Gassner, U. M. (2018). *Blockchain in EU e-health - blocked by the barrier of data protection?* Compliance Elliance Journal.

George, S. L., & Buyse, M. (2015). Data fraud in clinical trials. *Clinical Investigation*, *5*(2), 161–173. https://doi.org/10.4155/cli.14.116

Gipp, B., & Meuschke, N. (2009). *Decentralized Trusted Timestamping using the Crypto Currency Bitcoin Trusted Timestamping*. Academic Press.

Greenberg, A. (2011). Crypto currency. Forbes.

Haber, S., & Stornetta, W. S. (1991). How to time-stamp a digital document. *Journal of Cryptology*, *3*(2), 99–111. https://doi.org/10.1007/BF00196791

Habermann, B., Broome, M., Pryor, E. R., & Ziner, K. W. (2010). Research Coordinators' Experiences With Scientific Misconduct and Research Integrity. *Nursing Research*, *59*(1), 51–57. https://doi.org/10.1097/NNR.0b013e3181c3b9f2

Harford, T. (2019). *How important will blockchain be to the world's economy?* BBC News. https://www.bbc.com/news/business-48526666

Heller, B. N. (2017). Estonia, the Digital Republic. *New Yorker (New York, N.Y.)*, 1–25. https://www.newyorker.com/magazine/2017/12/18/estonia-the-digital-republic

Hill, N. S., Preston, I. R., & Roberts, K. E. (2008). Patients with Pulmonary Arterial Hypertension in Clinical Trials: Who Are They? *Proceedings of the American Thoracic Society*, *5*(5), 603–609. https://doi.org/10.1513/pats.200803-032SK

Hosely, M. (2020). *Retention in Clinical Trials – Keeping Patients on Protocols*. Academic Press.

Humer, C., & Finkle, J. (2014). *Your medical record is worth more to hackers than your credit card*. Philly.Com.

IMI. (2020). *PharmaLedger selects use cases to advance adoption of blockchain in healthcare*. https://www.imi.europa.eu/news-events/newsroom/pharmaledger-selects-use-cases-advance-adoption-blockchain-healthcare

Ingham, G. (1996). Money is a social relation. *Review of Social Economy*. doi:10.1080/00346769600000031

Ioannidis, J. P. A. (2005). Why most published research findings are false. *PLoS Medicine, 2*(8), e124–e124. https://doi.org/10.1371/journal.pmed.0020124

Joshi, R. (2020). *How Can Blockchain Be Implemented in the Life Sciences Ecosystem?* Technology Networks. https://www.technologynetworks.com/informatics/articles/how-can-blockchain-be-implemented-in-the-life-sciences-ecosystem-330614

Kassab, M. H., DeFranco, J., Malas, T., Laplante, P., Destefanis, G., & Graciano Neto, V. V. (2019). Exploring Research in Blockchain for Healthcare and a Roadmap for the Future. *IEEE Transactions on Emerging Topics in Computing, 6750*(c), 1–16. doi:10.1109/TETC.2019.2936881

Khezr, S., Moniruzzaman, M., Yassine, A., & Benlamri, R. (2019). Blockchain Technology in Healthcare: A Comprehensive Review and Directions for Future Research. *Applied Sciences (Basel, Switzerland), 9*, 1736. https://doi.org/10.3390/app9091736

Kravchenko, P. (2018). *Blockchain doesn't Eliminate Intermediaries and Never Will — It's a Fact.* Coinspeaker. https://www.coinspeaker.com/blockchain-doesnt-eliminate-intermediaries-and-never-will-its-a-fact/

Krieger, J. L., Neil, J. M., Strekalova, Y. A., & Sarge, M. A. (2017). Linguistic Strategies for Improving Informed Consent in Clinical Trials Among Low Health Literacy Patients. *Journal of the National Cancer Institute, 109*(3), djw233. https://doi.org/10.1093/jnci/djw233

Krittanawong, C., Rogers, A. J., Aydar, M., Choi, E., Johnson, K. W., Wang, Z., & Narayan, S. M. (2020). Integrating blockchain technology with artificial intelligence for cardiovascular medicine. *Nature Reviews. Cardiology, 17*(1), 1–3. https://doi.org/10.1038/s41569-019-0294-y

Kuo, C. D. L., Guo, L., & Wang, Y. (2017). Cryptocurrency: A New Investment Opportunity? *The Journal of Alternative Investments, 20*(3), 16–40. doi:10.3905/jai.2018.20.3.016

Lamport, L. (1998). The Part-Time Parliament. *ACM Transactions on Computer Systems.* doi:10.1145/279227.279229

Lee, J. Y. (2019). A decentralized token economy: How blockchain and cryptocurrency can revolutionize business. *Business Horizons.* doi:10.1016/j.bushor.2019.08.003

Leeming, G., Cunningham, J., & Ainsworth, J. (2019). A Ledger of Me: Personalizing Healthcare Using Blockchain Technology. *Frontiers in Medicine.* doi:10.3389/fmed.2019.00171

Lesser, M. L., & Haanstra, J. W. (2000). Random-Access Memory Accounting Machine. I. System organization of the IBM 305. *IBM Journal of Research and Development.* doi:10.1147/JRD.2000.5389196

Mamoshina, P., Ojomoko, L., Yanovich, Y., & Ostrovski, A. (2018). *Converging blockchain and next-generation artificial intelligence technologies to decentralize and accelerate biomedical research and healthcare Converging blockchain and next-generation artificial intelligence technologies to decentralize and accelerate.* doi:10.18632/oncotarget.22345

Maxmen, A. (2018). AI researchers embrace Bitcoin technology to share medical data. *Nature, 555*(7696), 293–294. https://doi.org/10.1038/d41586-018-02641-7

Mazlan, A. A., Daud, S. M., Sam, S. M., Abas, H., Rasid, S. Z. A., & Yusof, M. F. (2020). Scalability Challenges in Healthcare Blockchain System-A Systematic Review. *IEEE Access*. doi:10.1109/ACCESS.2020.2969230

Mello, M. M., Lieou, V., & Goodman, S. N. (2018). Clinical Trial Participants' Views of the Risks and Benefits of Data Sharing. *The New England Journal of Medicine*, *378*(23), 2202–2211. https://doi.org/10.1056/NEJMsa1713258

Mettler, M. (2016). Blockchain technology in healthcare: The revolution starts here. *2016 IEEE 18th International Conference on E-Health Networking, Applications and Services (Healthcom)*, 1–3. doi:10.1109/HealthCom.2016.7749510

Moore, G. E. (1998). Cramming More Components Onto Integrated Circuits. *Proceedings of the IEEE*, *86*(1), 82–85. https://doi.org/10.1109/JPROC.1998.658762

Moreno, J. (n.d.). *Blockchain for Life Sciences*. https://www.capgemini.com/de-de/service/blockchain-for-life-sciences/#nutzung-von-blockchains-fuer-die-einwilligungserklaerung-in-klinischen-studien

Morley-Fletcher, E. (2017). MHMD: My health, my data. *CEUR Workshop Proceedings*, 1810.

Mulligan, A., Hall, L., & Raphael, E. (2013). Peer review in a changing world: An international study measuring the attitudes of researchers. *Journal of the American Society for Information Science and Technology*. doi:10.1002/asi.22798

MyHealthMyData. (2016a). *A New Paradigm in Healthcare Data Privacy and Security*. http://www.myhealthmydata.eu/

MyHealthMyData. (2016b). *Consortium*. http://www.myhealthmydata.eu/consortium/

Nakamoto, S. (2009). *Bitcoin: A Peer-to-Peer Electronic Cash System*. Https://Metzdowd.Com

Nofer, M., Gomber, P., Hinz, O., & Schiereck, D. (2017). Blockchain. *Business & Information Systems Engineering*, *59*(3), 183–187. https://doi.org/10.1007/s12599-017-0467-3

Omar, I. A., Jayaraman, R., Salah, K., Yaqoob, I., & Ellahham, S. (2020). Applications of Blockchain Technology in Clinical Trials: Review and Open Challenges. *Arabian Journal for Science and Engineering*. doi:10.100713369-020-04989-3

Paik, H. Y., Xu, X., Bandara, H. M. N. D., Lee, S. U., & Lo, S. K. (2019). Analysis of data management in blockchain-based systems: From architecture to governance. *IEEE Access*. doi:10.1109/ACCESS.2019.2961404

PwC Portugal. (2019). *Ensaios Clínicos em Portugal*. Author.

Radanović, I., & Likić, R. (2018). Opportunities for Use of Blockchain Technology in Medicine. *Applied Health Economics and Health Policy*. doi:10.100740258-018-0412-8

Rao & Jain. (2019). *Improving Integrated Clinical Trial Management Systems through Blockchain*. Genetic Engineering & Biotechnology News. https://www.genengnews.com/insights/improving-integrated-clinical-trial-management-systems-through-blockchain/

Resnik, D. B., & Shamoo, A. E. (2017). Reproducibility and Research Integrity. *Accountability in Research*. doi:10.1080/08989621.2016.1257387

Roman-Belmonte, J. M., De la Corte-Rodriguez, H., & Rodriguez-Merchan, E. C. (2018). How blockchain technology can change medicine. *Postgraduate Medicine*. doi:10.1080/00325481.2018.1472996

Rosbach, M., & Andersen, J. S. (2017). Patient-experienced burden of treatment in patients with multimorbidity – A systematic review of qualitative data. *PLoS One*, *12*(6), e0179916. https://doi.org/10.1371/journal.pone.0179916

Salber, P. R. (2002). The role of purchasers in the clinical research enterprise.). . *Journal of Investigative Medicine*, *50*(3). doi:10.2310/6650.2002.33429

Santos Rutschman, A. (2018). *Healthcare Blockchain Infrastructure: a Comparative Approach*. Academic Press.

Schulz, K. F., Altman, D. C., & Moher, D. (2010). CONSORT 2010 Statement: Updated guidelines for reporting parallel group randomised trials. *Italian Journal of Public Health*. doi:10.4178/epih/e2014029

Shrestha, A. K., Vassileva, J., & Deters, R. (2020). A Blockchain Platform for User Data Sharing Ensuring User Control and Incentives. *Frontiers in Blockchain, 3*(October), 1–22. doi:10.3389/fbloc.2020.497985

Swan, M. (2015). Blockchain: Blueprint for a new economy. In Climate Change 2013 - The Physical Science Basis.

Tardi, C. (2020). *Decentralized Market*. Investopedia. https://www.investopedia.com/terms/d/decentralizedmarket.asp

Tennant, J. P., Dugan, J. M., Graziotin, D., Jacques, D. C., Waldner, F., Mietchen, D., Elkhatib, Y., Collister, B. L., Pikas, C. K., Crick, T., Masuzzo, P., Caravaggi, A., Berg, D. R., Niemeyer, K. E., Ross-Hellauer, T., Mannheimer, S., Rigling, L., Katz, D. S., Greshake Tzovaras, B., … Colomb, J. (2017). A multi-disciplinary perspective on emergent and future innovations in peer review. *F1000Research*. doi:10.12688/f1000research.12037.3

Tom Lyons, L. C. (2020). *Blockchain use cases in healthcare*. Academic Press.

van der Waal, M. B., dos S. Ribeiro, C., Ma, M., Haringhuizen, G. B., Claassen, E., & van de Burgwal, L. H. M. (2020). Blockchain-facilitated sharing to advance outbreak R&D. *Science, 368*(6492), 719–721. doi:10.1126cience.aba1355

Vandenbroucke, J. P. (2004). When are observational studies as credible as randomised trials? *Lancet*, *363*(9422), 1728–1731. https://doi.org/10.1016/S0140-6736(04)16261-2

Weigmann, K. (2015). The ethics of global clinical trials. *EMBO Reports*. doi:10.15252/embr.201540398

Wong, C. H., Siah, K. W., & Lo, A. W. (2019). Estimation of clinical trial success rates and related parameters. *Biostatistics (Oxford, England)*, *20*(2), 273–286. https://doi.org/10.1093/biostatistics/kxx069

Woods, D. (2013). How To Create A Moore's Law For Data. *Forbes*. https://www.forbes.com/sites/danwoods/2013/12/12/how-to-create-a-moores-law-for-data/?sh=22e2db0f44ca

Wust, K., & Gervais, A. (2018). Do you need a blockchain? *Proceedings - 2018 Crypto Valley Conference on Blockchain Technology, CVCBT 2018*. doi:10.1109/CVCBT.2018.00011

Yeung, B., & Eichengreen, B. (2020). From Commodity to Fiat and Now to Crypto: What Does History Tell Us? *Digital Currency Economics and Policy*. doi:10.1142/9789811223785_0003

Zhavoronkov, A., & Church, G. (2019). The Advent of Human Life Data Economics. *Trends in Molecular Medicine, 25*(7), 566–570. https://doi.org/10.1016/j.molmed.2019.05.002

Zheng, Z., Xie, S., Dai, H. N., Chen, X., & Wang, H. (2018). Blockchain challenges and opportunities: A survey. *International Journal of Web and Grid Services*. doi:10.1504/IJWGS.2018.095647

KEY TERMS AND DEFINITIONS

Artificial Intelligence: The simulation of human intelligence by machines programmed to think like humans.

Blockchain: A distributed ledger that allows the storage of digital data in a collection of blocks. A new block is added every single time a transaction occurs. These transactions are developed, transmitted, and validated on a peer-to-peer network.

Bitcoin: Digital cryptocurrency. The transactions are saved in the blockchain.

Cloud: Everything that can be accessed over the internet. When a file is in the cloud, it means it was stored on the internet and not in the hard drive of the computer.

Electronic Medical Records: The patient's treatment and medical history that is collected by the individual doctor and recorded in a digital format.

Informed Consent Form: A document sign by the participant of research study saying that he/she is aware of its purpose and that is participating willingly.

Internet of Things: Devices connected to the internet that can collect information by the user.

Token: a unit of cryptocurrency, similar to coin.

APPENDIX 1

Abbreviations

AI: Artificial Intelligence
BT: Blockchain Technology
EMR: Electronic Medical Records
EU: European Union
GDPR: General Data Protection Regulation
HDD: Hard Disk Drive
ICF: Informed Consent Form
IoT: Internet of Things
MHMD: MyHealthMyData
RWE: Real-world Evidence

APPENDIX 2

Figure 1. Monetization of clinical research data. In this blockchain model, a blockchain technology company uses blockchain to monetize data, empowering patients (data owners) to securely collect, organize, share, provide and/or trade their personal information [medical records, medical data obtained by the Internet of Things devices, and personal information]. Data produced are kept on blocks or cloud storage. Artificial intelligence helps blockchain to create intelligent virtual agents, which in turn can create new records automatically. In the case of medical records, the artificial intelligence system helps blockchain to reach maximum security (Khezr et al., 2019). Because the access to each data element is approved by its owner, patients in this model are enabled to select the providers, pharmaceutical companies, or researchers, who can access their data. This gives them full control but also full responsibility. The access to data would not be the only benefit for clinical research. Pharmaceutical companies would also be able to recruit suitable volunteers. Smart contracts would define rules and penalties in an agreement, enforce those rules, and this way, ensure a compliant patient enrolment. All consent records automatically would populate an immutable database. As a result, the motivation of patients in continuing the study would increase, and the cost for the sponsor would decrease. Patients would also have access to their profile in an application developed by the blockchain company, and that could be accessed over their cell phone, computer, or tablet. In that application, the data owner would be able to check the medical records, active contracts with data purchasers, and check their token balance. As observed in other business models, those tokens can be used as discounts in specific online stores. Other possible features are the engagement in challenges that have as a goal the improvement of the patient health index.

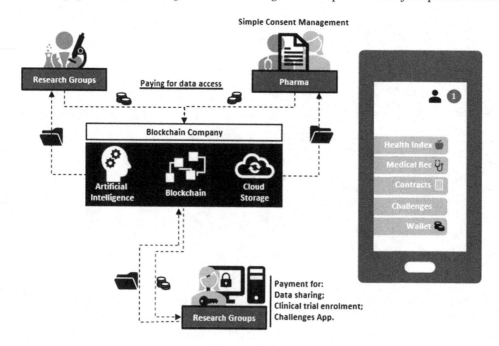

Table 1. Initiatives on the use of blockchain for clinical research sharing and data monetization.

Fields	Company	Location	Founded	Description	Data type	Currency	Website
General	Longenesis	Hong Kong, China	2017	-Direct communication between pharmaceutical companies and hospitals/research groups; -Safe data curation and utilization for research; -Individuals store and monetize their health data; -Financial rewards to lease the information.	Genome, blood test, surveys, phenotypic data, wearable device vital signs, vocal input, photograph, drug and supplement consumption, drug and treatment prescriptions, patients self-monitored experiments, and protocols already implemented in the platform.	LifePounds	https://longenesis.com/
	Doc.ai	California, USA	2016	-An app to collect and store health data and to generate personalized health insights; -Data can be shared with research companies for data trials in exchange for financial rewards.	Poly-omics data (phenome, genome/proteome, microbiome, etc).	Neuron tokens	https://doc.ai/
Genome	Encrypgen	Florida, USA	1985	-Peer-to-peer marketplace to protect, share, and remarket genomic data. -The individuals decide who they want to sell the information to and for how much.	DNA and phenotypic information.	DNA tokens	https://encrypgen.com/
	LunaDNA	California, USA	2017	-Community-owned platform for health research; -Anyone can join.	DNA.	Ownership shares in the organization	https://lunadna.com/
	Zenome	Moscow, Russia	2017	-It helps people to sell their genomic data without involving big companies	Genomic and personal data.	ZNA	https://zenome.io/
	Shivom	England, UK	2018	-Focus on building the largest genomic repository. -Consumers and donors have a platform to be able to securely store their data, share it, and if they want, to monetize it.	DNA and phenotypic information.	Shivom tokens	https://shivom.io/
	Nebula Genomics	California, USA	2018	-Access to genome sequencing, DNA data storage, analytics, sharing for financial rewards.	DNA and phenotypic data.	Nebula tokens	https://nebula.org/whole-genome-sequencing/
Imaging	BreastWeCan	Florida, USA	2018	-It allows patients to share their imaging and electronic health records and retain control over it.	Imaging and electronic health records.	Tokens	https://www.breastwecan.org/

Chapter 12
Dentacoin:
A Blockchain–Based Concept for Dental Healthcare

Rafael Duarte Pinto
ISEG, Lisbon School of Economics and Management, University of Lisbon, Portugal

Diana Madaleno Ferreira
ISEG, Lisbon School of Economics and Management, University of Lisbon, Portugal

Maria Teresa Barbosa
ISEG, Lisbon School of Economics and Management, University of Lisbon, Portugal

Margarida Chinita Nieto

ISEG, Lisbon School of Economics and Management, University of Lisbon, Portugal

Ana Filipa Funenga
ISEG, Lisbon School of Economics and Management, University of Lisbon, Portugal

Marta Sousa da Silva
ISEG, Lisbon School of Economics and Management, University of Lisbon, Portugal

Pedro Picaluga Nevado
ISEG, Lisbon School of Economics and Management, University of Lisbon, Portugal

ABSTRACT

Blockchain is a decentralized digital ledger of transactions shared amongst all participating web nodes, over which every data is recorded. Since the first blockchain was conceptualized in 2008, much research has been done to expand its applications to non-financial purposes. Dentacoin is the first cryptocurrency ever created worldwide that strives to create a dental industry community by rewarding people with a given token—Dentacoin cryptocurrency—for specific actions that have a desirable effect on the Dentacoin ecosystem. This concept aims to improve the global dental market by applying blockchain technology advantages and promoting intelligent prevention in dental healthcare. The purpose of this chapter is to review the concept of blockchain-based Dentacoin ecosystem, as it is expected that, in the future, this method will significantly improve dental health and oral hygiene habits, thus improving the quality of life for individuals resulting in overall health enhancement and increased longevity.

DOI: 10.4018/978-1-7998-7363-1.ch012

INTRODUCTION

Similar to how the Internet has changed the world by providing better and greater access to information, blockchain technology is ready to change the way people do business, promising a new dimension of conducting commercial transactions between untrusted entities (Yassine et al., 2020).

Although there are many severe objections to the use of this technology in the most critical and government-mediated financial exchanges, blockchain technology has several valuable resources of interest and research in the areas of e-business and e-commerce. In addition, the openness of distributed ledger technology also makes visibility ubiquitous, rather than leaving it entirely under the control of some chosen trusted parties. The mindset of a whole generation of traditional online exchange users will take some time to adapt to the new philosophy of open and decentralized exchanges. It is correct to say that users' sociocultural and economic backgrounds will play an important role in the final diffusion of this technology (Ghosh, 2019; Justinia, 2019).

Blockchain technology has a global extension and could connect users worldwide, allowing them to carry out transactions with encryption, data security, and decentralization. The implications of opening the transaction system to individual consumers and businesses are substantial. These transactions are carried out in many different types of markets and platforms. Because of its diversity, the perception of a particular transaction or contract may vary widely between users in different geographic regions and countries.

The implications of global blockchain technology research are multifaceted. First, the transactional transparency built into the openness of technology can be a double-edged sword. It is unlikely that an established institution's absence of coordination and intermediation will be interpreted uniformly by people of all cultures and lifestyles in all countries of the world.

The role played by trust in international supply chain transactions is still very unclear. Although an open market economy depends on its smooth functioning of formalized and explicit trust-based agreements and protocols, many essential business transactions have an informal nature based on trust relationships between companies in many developing and transitional economies in the world.

The problem of how two parties with different business structures and based on different economies worldwide can be linked together to carry out decentralized and trust-based transactions in the international market is highly unexplored (Ghosh, 2019).

BACKGROUND

Blockchain Technology: Concepts and Applications

Blockchain technology is one of the recent years' most significant technological innovations, particularly in digitalization secure asset ownership. This technology was founded upon the concept of a distributed ledger, decentralized cataloging, and accounting for large volumes of data. It is seen by many as a disruptive technology that will revolutionize business and redefine companies and economies (Ghosh, 2019). It is the underlying technology of Bitcoin and has come up with several promising potential applications, with an architecture that allows different and unique users to make transactions and presents the ability to create an unchangeable, secure record of those transactions (Mearian, 2019).

Blockchain is a network that works with secure chained blocks that can carry content along with a fingerprint. In this technology, the last block will contain the fingerprint of the previous one, plus its content, and with these two pieces of information, it will generate its own fingerprint (Prado, 2017).

It is a secure business network in which participants transfer value items through a distributed shared ledger, of which each participant has a copy and whose content is in constant synchronization with the others (Prado, 2017).

In this revolutionary technology, verification, identification, authentication, integrity, and immutability are guaranteed through cryptography, transparency, decentralized smart contracts, and smart ledgers (Yassine et al., 2020).

The capability to read blockchain data and submit new transactions is determined by access to transactions. Public blockchains allow all nodes to read blockchain data and propose new transactions, whereas private blockchains allow only nodes preregistered by a central authority to read blockchain data and submit new transactions (Table 1). Public blockchains offer permissioned or permissionless access to transaction validation. In permissionless blockchains, all nodes can validate transactions, while in permissioned blockchains, only nodes that have been preregistered can validate transactions (Beck et al., 2018).

Table 1. Blockchain typology

Access to Transactions	Access to Transaction Validation	
	Permissioned	**Permissionless**
Public	All nodes can read and submit transactions. Only authorized nodes can validate transactions.	All nodes can read, submit, and validate transactions.
Private	Only authorized nodes can read, submit, and validate transactions.	Not applicable

Source: (adapted from Beck et al., 2018).

Blockchain technology presents itself as a revolution that impacts the industrial and economic world. It is considered different from other digital platforms since blockchain is a decentralized system that allows each participant to regularly updated copies of the large register.

It is characterized by not having a central server but collaborative management, which protects against counterfeiting and other attacks. The system is entirely transparent. The entire transaction history can be consulted at any time by each internet user, enabling the traceability of each asset or product sold. This technology allows information to be registered in the blocks, and the information can no longer be changed or deleted. It is an electronic document that can have as much or more probative value as the paper. This system also offers a guarantee against piracy by multiplying the number of copies (Yassine et al., 2020).

The function of blockchain is to guarantee trust between companies and is called a "trust protocol." In addition, this technology has some other advantages, such as:

- **Privacy:** ensures adequate visibility to the network, as transactions can be verifiable. In blockchain technology, sensitive parts of the ledger can be hidden without impairing the verification of the block.

- **Smart Contract**: it is characterized by being a document that cannot be changed after writing. It is possible to sign contracts and authorize transactions according to the established terms.
- **Consensus:** transactions are verified by network participants and cannot be defrauded.

Moreover, blockchain is considered a technology with benefits for different sectors and businesses, including reducing the time to search for information, resolving disputes, and verifying transactions. It also includes reducing costs and mitigating fraud risks (Justinia, 2019).

Currently, there is a growing expectation that Blockchain technology will have a profound impact in many sectors. Blockchain has moved to a real-world implementation in a wide variety of sectors, such as supply chain management and Internet of Things (IoT), financial services, manufacturing transport, health, fashion, entertainment, and for different applications such as cybersecurity and digital forensics, partially evidenced by its evolution in the last decade (Justinia, 2019).

Blockchain technology is suitable in projects where there is the contribution of multiple stakeholders (trust is extremely required between parties) and a greater need for reliable tracking of activity and data to be reliable over time (Engelhardt, 2017).

This system has been applied to the public sector and academic institutes, which is why governments have been planning and developing blockchain in the public sector. For example, the company KPMG reports that in the first half of 2018, investment in the US fintech companies was $14.2 billion. In addition, blockchain has been applied to the public and private sectors, and more than 53% of Deloitte's survey respondents say that this technology is a priority for their organizations (Yassine et al., 2020).

Blockchain in Healthcare

Large volumes of digital transactions are acquired from online servers to feed various applications using blockchain technology. One of these applications is in healthcare.

For now, the development of Blockchain solutions in the healthcare field is dominated by prototypes, proof-of-concept efforts, and initial phases of project investments. The purpose of these prototypes is to solve existing problems focusing on public health, advanced research modalities, prescription monitoring, and the organization of patient data (Ghosh, 2019).

Recognizing the high sensitivity of health data related to the records of individual patients and medical professionals, discreet sharing and collaboration in intelligent medical systems have recently been made possible by intelligent use of Blockchain ledger (Ghosh, 2019). Thus, understanding the actual applications of blockchain can help explain how this technology works for the healthcare sector and what it can offer (Engelhardt, 2017).

Blockchain technology can also play an essential role in the pharmaceutical supply chain. A problem in this sector is delays and defaults in delivering goods and other logistical and data theft issues. A model was proposed to improve the blockchain's smart contracts with systems that aim to increase efficiency in managing logistics systems (hoping that this can be applied in the pharmaceutical supply chain).

Drug counterfeiting is a global problem that puts public health at risk and reduces research, development, and innovation incentives. The Blockchain system is considered a disruptive intervention in the drug supply chain, which aims to fight these risks (Justinia, 2019).

Healthcare and biomedical research can also benefit from this technology: reproducibility, data sharing, personal data privacy issues, and the difficulties of registering patients in clinical trials are significant medical challenges. Blockchain can provide better sharing of medical research, which can lead to new paths for biomedical research and drug treatment therapies to cure diseases. Blockchain can also be used to reward the sharing of computing and storage resources, facilitate decentralized data distribution and provide genome privacy. Due to the dynamic nature of biomedical evidence data, it is crucial to ensure adequate recovery and integrity of the collected data (Justinia, 2019).

On the other hand, blockchain is also used for insurers with innovative insurance products and services, increasing fraud detection and pricing efficacy and reducing administrative costs. The technology can be used to remove intermediaries by going directly to providers, and this can be used as the basis for more sophisticated Blockchain applications (Justinia, 2019).

As blockchain can eliminate intermediaries, transactions can happen in real-time with less cost and without loss of security, as they can be verifiable and auditable. Most importantly, the risk of fraud is reduced through smart contracts (Prado, 2017).

Cryptocurrencies

Cryptocurrency is encrypted decentralized digital money created by code purchased electronically through an exchange. These exchanges provide a platform for exchanging paper currencies (for example, Euro) into a digital currency used to purchase goods and services from certain suppliers. Cryptocurrencies can be used for quick payments and to avoid transaction fees. It can also be obtained as an investment. Most of the cryptocurrency market is shared between Bitcoin and Ethereum.

Bitcoin is the most used cryptocurrency and was the first application of blockchain technology. Regarding Ethereum, in just two years it has become the most prominent digital currency (Justinia, 2019). Blockchain technology forms cryptocurrency transactions in different types of network environments (Ghosh, 2019). Cryptocurrencies are becoming more common. Legal agencies, tax authorities, and legal regulators are trying to understand the concept of cryptocurrencies and where they can fit into existing regulations and legal structures (Royal & Voigt, 2017).

Cryptocurrencies facilitate the transfer of funds between two parties since there is no need for trusted third parties such as banks or credit cards. Transfers are guaranteed using public and private keys and different forms of incentive systems. In cryptocurrency systems, users have a public key, while the private key is known only by the owner's account, and this is the key used to sign transactions (Frankenfield, 2020). So, what are the benefits of cryptocurrencies over traditional money?

- Totally anonymous: it is possible to make purchases without anyone obtaining a single piece of personal information;
- Irreversible transactions: once a transaction is made, it is not possible to reverse the transaction without an agreement by both parties;
- Free of government supervision and managed by a peer-to-peer internet protocol that has the ability to validate each currency, confirming all subsequent transactions in the currency's history;
- No one else has access to a unique code;
- Cryptocurrency cannot be falsified.

The fact that the nature of cryptocurrency transactions is anonymous facilitates the occurrence of illegal activities, such as money laundering and tax evasion. At the same time, cryptocurrency lawyers value the anonymity of the system, citing privacy benefits, such as protection for activists living under repressive governments, the possibility of preserving value against inflation, and being easier to transport and share. It is important to emphasize that some cryptocurrencies are more private than others (Frankenfield, 2020).

Healthcare Cryptocurrencies

Healthcare cryptocurrencies are blockchain technology-based currencies. The adoption of Blockchain technology in the health sector offers an interoperable sharing of medical data between payers, patients, and healthcare professionals.

Some examples of possible uses for cryptocurrency in the hospital space include drug and equipment acquisitions, accommodations for family members around the hospital, and minor things like ordering entertainment to a patient's room.

Outside of the hospital, this cryptocurrency can also add fluidity to online consultations with doctors, keeping track of a patient's health, and purchasing medicines (TyN Magazine, 2020).

Healthcoin is an example of a healthcare cryptocurrency: the objective is to prevent new diabetes cases and reduce the symptoms of current patients. Healthcoin has an incentive system that tracks the lifestyle choices of the patient. As patients continue to make good choices, and after submitting biomarkers (like heart rate, weight, and sugar level) to a database run on the blockchain, an algorithm calculates the change or improvement in the individual's health. Based on that, such patients earn a certain amount of Healthcoins that can then be used to decrease insurance costs, recognize achievements, and show personal health improvement to health care professionals, friends, and family (Bennett, 2017).

Another example is Dentacoin, a cryptocurrency designed for the dentistry field, as will be discussed.

Ethereum Smart Contracts

Smart contracts are computer programs or transactions intended to automatically execute, control or document legally relevant events and actions according to the terms of a contract or agreement. These contracts are lines of code stored on a blockchain to be immutable and self-executing and can also interact with other smart contracts, websites, and humans, allowing for the emergence of programmable value transfer networks ("Internet of Value").

Since smart contracts can handle and transfer assets of considerable value, besides their correct execution, it is also crucial that their implementation is secure against attacks that aim at stealing or tampering with the transacted assets. Dentacoin smart contracts are computer protocols in the Ethereum blockchain that facilitate, verify, negotiate and conclude contracts between individuals and their contracting party. All smart contracts are connected to one "super-smart contract" (SSC), and if a smart contract cannot be fulfilled due to performance impossibility, then the SSC saves the patient's rights (Atzei et al., 2017).

Coins, Cryptocurrency, Tokens, and Token Economy

It is considered essential to acknowledge the difference between a traditional digital currency transaction and a cryptocurrency transaction. A traditional transaction requires money in any form in actual use or circulation as a medium of exchange, especially circulating banknotes and coins. It is a government-issued currency. On the other hand, a cryptocurrency transaction requires encryption techniques to regulate the currency units available. This kind of currency is non-physical (a realm where banknotes and coins do not exist) and it can only be transmitted via electronic means, usually accepting instantaneous transactions and borderless transfer of ownership (Abu Bakar et al., 2017).

A cryptocurrency requires the ownership of an independent blockchain, for instance as Bitcoin (BCN), Quantum (QTUM), and Ethereum (ETH). In contrast, a token does not have an independent blockchain network. Examples include Tron (TRX), IOS (EOS), and Dentacoin (DCN) (Yoo, 2020). A token is a quantified unit of value, generic and fungible, meaning that most blockchain projects use a token for implementing their own crypto-economics. In the simplest case, the token is the cryptocurrency itself (Dapp, 2018).

Tokens can also be classified into two different categories: the IOU token and the native token. An IOU token requires a centralized entity: it needs a guarantor that faithfully implements the token exchange. On the other hand, no guarantee subject is required to a native token (Bitcoin is an example) (Yoo, 2020). Table 2 summarizes these aspects.

Table 2. Types of tokens

Classification	Contents	Use Case
IOU token	I owe you. The guarantee of the exchange voucher gives value and is the same concept as the voucher. Needs a guarantor and it is centralized.	Tether
Native token	Characterized by no confidence; no guarantee subject is required. Token issue according to blockchain code rules, e.g., bitcoin compensation half-life.	Bitcoin

Source: (adapted from Yoo, 2020).

The Token Economic is a brand-new system of rewarding communities with a given token for specific actions that positively affect the community. There are three essential elements for this system to work: tokens, desirable behavior, and rewards. These economies' assessments are usually based on how 1) to induce the users' desirable behavior within the network; 2) to circulate the token within the blockchain; 3) to form a rule of distribution for the token; 4) to set its value (Yoo, 2020).

In the specific case of the Dentacoin, the user token is the Dentacoin (DCN) cryptocurrency. The desired behavior is that people become more effective in maintaining their oral health by rewarding them with a specified amount of DCN.

This brand-new system exists because blockchain allows creating monetary systems accessible by anyone on the Internet. So, local communities can create and design their own currencies and economic policies ("cryptoeconomics") tailored to their local needs. Therefore, bottom-up cryptocurrencies will, over time, democratize money supply and money governance in contrast to fiat currencies. So, for example, anyone can obtain and use Bitcoin, which means that traditional pricing mechanisms and exchange rate systems will be less relevant (Dapp, 2018).

In addition, personal artificial intelligence tools could create behavioral recommendations for users on managing their wallets. Thus, crypto-economic will power incentive systems on various platforms that focus on different externalities, and new ''token economies'' will be created, circulating within and between the platforms. As a result, this will create new sources of income, having their own built-in governance systems (Dapp, 2018).

Blockchain-Based Cryptographic Token Economics

In 2008, Bitcoin was the first application offering digital cash or "cryptocurrency" to its users by using blockchain technology. Then similar projects have created uncounted alternative cryptocurrencies, and several new exchanges have started allowing users to trade all these cryptocurrencies (Dapp, 2018).

Later, in 2013, there was the introduction of smart contracts by the Ethereum project, already described earlier in this chapter. Such decentralized applications (DApps) explore a new space to create a domain in specific applications and issue tokens on top of a blockchain platform (Dapp, 2018).

Then, in 2016, a Decentralized Autonomous Organization project started, a network based on smart contracts interaction (Dapp, 2018).

Technology and governance represent the critical challenges at the current stage of development through all these phases.

Blockchain economy seeks to evolute towards a decentralized form of decision-making; however, these approaches to technology are critically limited in magnitude and throughput performance, as well as the conceit of creating democratic structures on top of the digital applications or programs that exist and run on a blockchain (Dapp, 2018).

A blockchain is a distributed cryptographic ledger shared amongst all participating nodes, over which every data or transaction is recorded and collected in blocks found in a random process from the protocol (Barreiro-Gomez & Tembine, 2019).

When blockchains have cryptographic tokens, a user's utility function would be dependent on the number of tokens in circulation in the blockchain, the aggregated drives of users or entities, the network characteristics, and incentives to verifiers (miners, validators, and other stakeholders). A successful token must consider the variance-aware utility function per decision-maker to capture the risk of cryptographic tokens associated with the uncertainties of technology adoption, regulatory legislation, market volatility, financial economics, network, and the number of active participants security. All these aspects affect a token's demand and price. So, a well-designed token can provide significant incentives to the users and boost participation. Therefore, the transfers of cryptographic assets through a distributed digital ledger require verification to avoid duplicating or changing electronic files or data. For these matters, the blockchain network needs verifiers. The verification tasks are delegated to different members of the network. Trust does rely on the behavior of the network and its protocols; as a result, then reputation and token are designed to give incentives to verifiers and disincentives malicious nodes, allowing the selection of verifiers who are known for their excellent work in the blockchain and who do not necessarily need many native tokens. This feature enables better network security, minor delay, better supply, and a medium of exchange, enabling demand (Barreiro-Gomez & Tembine, 2019).

METHODOLOGY

The present chapter follows a case study methodology, issuing the use of Dentacoin in the dental care field. For this purpose, a narrative literature review methodology was used, considering information taken from the database Google Scholar, along with searches on the world wide web, mainly in business reviews, international journals articles, whitepapers, and searches in grey literature, such as google, institutional website, blogs, and specific technology and economy websites. The authors' research is based on a comprehensive literature review in business model innovation research, especially in blockchain technology implemented in the dental industry.

THE CASE OF DENTAL HEALTHCARE – A NOVEL BUSINESS MODEL FOR DENTISTRY

The companies that run their business on digital platforms cause a profound disruption to the existing traditional business models in many competitive industries. Those platforms integrate business models that create value by facilitating value exchanges between two or more interdependent groups (usually consumers and producers). That is why it is essential to introduce a fundamentally new platform-based business model established on blockchain technology with a new management mechanism for the dental industry and the first steps of its model implementation (Ostapenko, 2018).

The concept is built on the principles of self-organization of consumers actualizing their expectations in the new values. The values for consumers are (Ostapenko, 2018):

- Objective information about services and manufacturers (price, quality);
- Free diagnostics and preparation of insured contract (service selection, risk reduction);
- Logistics services (time, transportation, accommodation);
- The motivation of a loyal consumer (fair price, discounts for loyal customers, the opportunity of financial participation in business, and obtaining long-term benefits).

This business model for dentistry is based on objective feedback from consumers using blockchain technology; it tries to create a unified global information platform. In order to involve patients and clinics in this new model, incentives were created such as quality service at a fair price, inclusion in the management process, bonus and discount system, logistical facility, and participation in Dentacoin token systems (Ostapenko, 2018).

This model focus on the patient's needs is the driving engine of the Dentacoin concept. Contrary to the classical business model, with a platform-driven model based on blockchain technology, the self-organizing ecosystem of customers is the utmost force shaping and driving the industry towards long-term success. Thus, the platform supports the dental community by building and creating solutions devoted to improving the quality of dental care worldwide (Ostapenko, 2018).

However, the validation of this model in dentistry practice is one of the future challenges.

Phase 1 of the project was based on implementing a blockchain-based trusted review platform for Dentacoin users to use blockchain technology to connect dentists, patients, and suppliers. The idea is to provide and maintain a decentralized review platform based on Ethereum smart contracts, where actions such as writing reviews are rewarded by transferring cryptocurrency to patients that can use it to purchase dental services. Dentists also can be rewarded for participating through access to market research and using the cryptocurrency with manufacturers that accept it. Phase 2 consists of an incentive strategy to encourage patients to educate themselves about dental care through Dentacoin Apps and creating a global community. The third phase of the project plans to set up decentralized insurance contracts between patients and dentists that reward patients who perform a minimum of dental maintenance. The last phase plans to build up Dentacoin infrastructure for direct international trading between dentists and suppliers.

Slowly establishing its position, this blockchain technology already has clinics that accept payments in Dentacoin (Engelhardt, 2017).

The Dentacoin

Nowadays, dentistry is a growing, high-tech-oriented industry that is in a period of transformation. Consumers are becoming more astute purchasers of healthcare and seeking value for their spending. There are conflicts of interest between dentists and patients because the costs of acquiring are getting higher, which naturally leads to an increase in the costs for end customers (Ostapenko, 2018). Since the costs in dental medicine, whether for preventive or specific dental treatments, are increasing, many patients feel obligated to resort to less effective and adequate treatments, which in the long run could result in health issues, decrease the quality of life and even lead to self-esteem problems. In addition, dentists have had difficulty achieving efficiency in their work and seeing their role in the daily health care field recognized by the population (Dentacoin Foundation, 2020).

Due to the above-mentioned reasons, it has been emerging the need to develop a new business model for the dental industry with a concept of a self-organizing industry management system based on a blockchain platform, cryptocurrency, and reward for consumer target behavior (Ostapenko, 2018).

The first blockchain concept is designed to help make the global dental industry more affordable and accessible to everyone (Dentacoin Foundation, 2018). Following a decentralized, smart contract protocol, the Dentacoin token rewards users through a system that inspires community contribution. This project counts with a vast community of progressive dentists, software developers, and marketing specialists. It is a unique ecosystem that supports all stakeholders: patients, dentists, manufacturers, suppliers, labs, and insurance companies. All players are securely connected using an industry-specific cryptocurrency Dentacoin (DCN), and several Blockchain-based software tools (Dentacoin Foundation, 2018).

Dentacoin was created as the first and only cryptocurrency for the global dental industry. Although many people realized the high potential of this industry-specific currency, others were not wholly convinced and defined it as offering minimal optionality because only dentists will use it. Therefore, it is crucial to clarify the different possibilities to use this token because although the main focus is to serve dentists and patients worldwide, the currency can be used in multiple ways, just as any functional currency.

To help grow the Dentacoin Foundation, the Dentacoin Token was created. People who use and implement this platform receive Dentacoin Tokens as a reward, which they can later use to pay for their dental treatment or purchase dental products (Dentacoin Foundation, 2018). The participation of patients in developing this information platform has been encouraged from the industry-specific cryptocurrency named, Dentacoin (DCN) fund (Ostapenko, 2018).

Blockchain technology in Dentacoin serves a community that emphasizes the industry's challenges. It reveals the solutions for increasing the dental practice's efficiency, where there is nothing more valuable to the industry players than constant, trustworthy feedback from the patients, and this is how Dentacoin appears – Dentacoin community (Ostapenko, 2018).

By creating and implementing the first Ethereum-based blockchain platform for trusted dental treatment reviews, The Dentacoin Foundation will allow patients to share relevant information about their dental treatments and the entire process through this platform. At the same time, dentists will have access to the latest, precious data on market research and qualified feedback from the patient, which will allow them to improve the quality of care and create a local patient base. Thanks to the self-enforcing

Smart Contract, the Dentacoin review platform ensures optimal autonomy, trust, speed, and security (Ostapenko, 2018).

Dentacoin's primary purpose is to improve dental care quality worldwide, reduce treatment costs and create a global dental community. The most important strength for the Dentacoin Foundation is that all user contributions, such as reviews, recommendations, and trusted feedback, can create recognition in the dental industry and help other users to make better choices. With Dentacoin, patients can get access to better and affordable treatments and take control of their preventive dental care. Thus, creating and implementing the first blockchain-based platform in dentistry allows achieving a transformative change of a whole industry and greatly enriches both the theory and practice of healthcare (Dentacoin Foundation, 2018).

In this sense, it is possible to state that Dentacoin covers several challenges that the dental healthcare field undertakes in current business models. It motivates patients to achieve proper oral health while also allowing dentists to build strong relationships with patients, offering affordable and appropriate dental care. Another essential purpose is to allow everyone to access preventive dental care and better oral hygiene, avoiding more complex and expensive treatments (Dentacoin Foundation, 2020).

Thus, the goal is to provide a solution and support for the healthcare industry through a blockchain and not compete with other cryptocurrencies. In addition, the Dentacoin Foundation is also interested in evaluating the actual substance and value that can be created with a coin (Dentacoin) that is responsible for representing the health of all individuals (Dentacoin Foundation, 2018).

One of the most important strengths for The Dentacoin Foundation is that all user contributions, such as reviews, recommendations, rewards, payments, trusted feedback, create recognition in the dental industry (Dentacoin Foundation, 2018).

Dentacoin Cryptocurrency

Cryptocurrency is "money that lives on software platforms" (ClinicAll Healthcare, 2019). It is virtual money or tokens that exist online, any government does not endorse it, and it was built to be very secure.

Cryptocurrencies are irreversible, which means that after a cryptocurrency has been sent and the network has been confirmed, it cannot be retrieved. They also have varying stages of anonymity depending on which token is utilized, enabling anyone to open a wallet without identification. Cryptocurrencies are fast and globally accessible, whereby entries are immediately broadcast across the network and confirmed within a few minutes (Nel, 2018).

A "DCN" refers to one individual Dentacoin, and because it is an ERC20 token, it is configured to be used globally by all individuals, and its value is derived from the exchange with Ether. The symbol ʌ has been chosen to represent a DCN (Dentacoin Foundation, 2018).

The benefit of DCN is that patients earn these tokens for their contributions to the platform. They have real-world applications and can be used as payment for dental treatments from any Dentacoin partner dentists or clinics (Dentacoin Foundation, 2020).

Cryptocurrencies paint a future that is drastically different from the fiat-based world today. This painting is either exciting or unsettling, perhaps for the vast majority. The trend will be that we must be equipped with the best possible resources and become active in communities that further explore the technical applications of Dentacoin and other cryptocurrencies and their overall potential to disrupt virtually every market (Nel, 2018).

Dentacoin Usefulness

Not only the community of dentists can benefit from Dentacoin. As we further observe, potential users include, but are not limited to the people in need of dental treatment. The Dentacoin team presents a list of some cases where Dentacoin can be helpful (Dentacoin Team, 2019):

1. Rewards and bonuses: Dentacoin is used in apps that allow users to earn rewards for different activities, such as taking surveys on Dentacoin apps and submitting feedback to their dentists on Dentacoin Trusted Reviews, and maintaining proper oral hygiene through the 90-day Dentacare app challenge. It is also possible to reward dentists with DCN for their willingness to become partners and overall contribution and reward exceptional employee achievements.
2. Covering dental treatment costs: at some point in life, anyone will need dental treatment. Right now, more than 90 organizations in 23 countries accept Dentacoin as a method of payment.
3. Paying Dentacoin Assurance monthly fees: Dentacoin Foundation launched its first dental assurance program based on direct, smart contracts between patients and dentists. Though Dentacoin Assurance, patients are entitled to receive lifelong preventive care against affordable monthly fees paid exclusively in Dentacoin.
4. Paying for dental supplies and equipment: dentists can spend Dentacoin for their daily business needs, such as ordering dental materials (e.g., implants) or buying equipment, like mobile dental care chairs.
5. Spending it on various other goods and services: right now, it is possible not only to use the currency to pay for dental treatments but also it is possible to pay for various gift cards for clothes, food, and beverages, games, and entertainment, sporting goods, homes, and renovation, hotels, travels, directly with Dentacoin.
6. Trading it against other cryptocurrencies: it is possible to trade Dentacoin against hundreds of other cryptocurrencies on various international exchange platforms.
7. Exchanging it to traditional currencies: once most Dentacoin users are outside the crypto space, it is essential to say that Dentacoin can be exchanged to any traditional currency (e.g., USD, EUR, GBP), and thus used for any purpose needed. It involves a two-step approach for most currencies: first, to exchange DCN to BTC and exchange BTC to the national currency.
8. Holding it for later use and value multiplication: as more and more people use the currency, the more it contributes to the development of the Dentacoin Ecosystem, the more expected for its value grow. Therefore, many people prefer to securely store their tokens in wallets and expect a future value multiplication before they decide to pay with Dentacoin for services/goods or exchange it for another currency.

Dentacoin Ecosystem

The Dentacoin Ecosystem is a reward system that generates value for the whole dental industry (Dentacoin Team, 2019). The Dentacoin Currency is in the center of this modern ecosystem: this Ethereum-based utility token is used for rewards, payments, and exchange within the dental industry (Dentacoin Foundation, 2018).

The Dentacoin Assurance is the first smart contract-based dental assurance plan: it focuses on prevention and is exclusively paid in Dentacoin currency. The cycle is simple: the patient starts by installing one of the many existing Dentacoin Apps on their smartphone/tablet. The App promotes better oral care and rewards users for submitting feedback, taking surveys, and maintaining oral hygiene. This way, the patient receives Dentacoins for taking care of their dental health, concomitantly reducing their dental costs. Dentists can boost patient loyalty and prevention with free apps and a fast and innovative payment method (Dentacoin Foundation, 2018).

This system provides both health and financial benefits to all users. By dealing with smart contracts, the platform eliminates any third-party intervention, and as a result, a trusted review platform is provided to the users (Dentacoin Team, 2019).

Securely connected through Dentacoin blockchain-based software tools, dentists and patients are empowered to generate real value, exchange information, and improve global dentistry (Dentacoin Team, 2019).

According to the partners and from the first experiences gathered, Dentacoin is a highly beneficial tool for creating a community with patients and improving the service's quality by aligning it with their needs. It is like creating a "dental ecosystem" to benefit patients, dentists, manufacturers, suppliers, laboratories, and insurance companies (P. Grenzebach, 2017).

Among all Dentacoin network users worldwide are dental practices, dental labs, dental suppliers, and others. North America, Asia, and Europe stand out in partner locations accepting Dentacoin, which are around 1200 (Dentacoin Foundation, 2021).

All the benefits and transactions achieved in the Dentacoin platform are regulated and managed through the Dentacoin Apps. These Apps are designed to help dentists build a loyal patient base and access valuable market research data while simultaneously allowing users to earn Dentacoin (DCN) for their behavior concerning dental health care efforts. There are more than 200K active Dentacoin users (Dentacoin Foundation, 2021).

Trusted Reviews Platform

The Trusted Reviews system will have two different types of reviews: standard reviews that anyone can write and trusted reviews that patients can only write. The trusted reviews provide a higher reward (in DCN currency) than the standard ones. The Dentacoin community will primarily benefit from these trusted reviews because they have higher quality and reliability, which achieves an objective reference to each dentist's services, making them comparable (Dentacoin Foundation, 2018).

Dentacoin Trusted Reviews is the first Blockchain-based review platform on dental services, developed by the Dentacoin Foundation, for verified and rewarded dental reviews that help dentists improve their services and online presence and allows patients to raise their voices. It will operate through a self-executing Smart Contract and assure autonomy, speed, trust, and safety, thus mitigating any risks regarding manipulating the data (Dentacoin Foundation, 2018). The trusted reviews are written upon a unique invitation sent by a dentist to a patient, which can be recognized by the tag "Trusted Review."

Hence, some of the benefits of this technology include: transparent reviews, the impossibility to modify or manipulate data once on the blockchain, permanent data storage, market research value; patients will have access to the rating of each dentist and can make an informed choice when choosing one; every review is rewarded in Dentacoins. This incentive configuration strongly influences the quality of dental treatments and raises the responsibility between dentists and patients (Dentacoin Foundation, 2018).

It is important to note that this technology fills in two different gaps (Dentacoin Foundation, 2018).:

- The need dentists have to build strong relationships with patients and gaining valuable feedback / market research data to enhance their treatment plans and communications;
- Patients did not have a reliable source where different dentists can be compared through their ratings and reviews.

Dentacoin Apps

DentaVox

The DentaVox App is a collective intelligence tool: it rewards users for their honest opinions on a great diversity of dental health-related topics. At the same time, up-to-date, valuable market search data is created and used by dentists, suppliers, and manufacturers. It precisely consists of surveys on various healthcare subjects (between 8 and 100 questions). The DCN rewards are attributed depending on user efforts: smart mechanisms detect the concentration of the individual when answering the questionnaires, thus guaranteeing high-quality results (Dentacoin Foundation, 2018).

This app acts like an open space where users can give their honest opinions, get rewarded for doing so, and significantly influence the industry, as no one can ignore, delete or manipulate their answers. The statistics from each questionnaire are also visible for all registered users. Furthermore, DentaVox will allow businesses to conduct their own surveys based on a defined audience (Dentacoin Foundation, 2018).

Dentacare Mobile App

The Dentacare Mobile App aims to create lifelong dental care habits through an intensive 3-month program in a gamified experience. It acts through reminders, notifications, and valuable tutorials. Users will learn how to improve their dental hygiene and will ultimately acquire a healthy dental lifestyle. The app has tutorials about how to brush properly, floss, rinse and advises patients to take regular check-ups at the dentist. It is important to note that this app is also appropriate for children: developing good dental hygiene habits at a young age helps to prevent dental problems in the future (Dentacoin Foundation, 2018).

The initial program lasts for three months, as this is the average time slot needed for a particular activity to be part of our routine. Only after maintaining a proper routine during this period will users be rewarded with DCN tokens, which can later be used to pay for dental services, dental products, Dentacoin Assurance. Users can also store the DCN or trade it on exchange platforms (Dentacoin Foundation, 2018).

Dentacoin Wallet

Dentacoin Wallet App allows users to store, send and receive DCN tokens quickly and securely, and purchase DCN. Therefore, many people prefer to securely store their tokens in wallets and expect a future value multiplication before they decide to pay with DCN for services/ goods or exchange it for another currency.

The users have two main alternatives to create a Dentacoin wallet:

- Creating a wallet via Dentacoin Wallet App - it's user-friendly, easy-to-use and secure.
- Creating a wallet through a third-party provider supporting Dentacoin (DCN) currency.

Dentacoin Assurance

Dentacoin Assurance is the first dental assurance plan designed exclusively on smart contracts between patients and dentists. It is focused on prevention rather than complicated treatments and is paid only in DCN. These smart contracts are self-executing protocols on the Ethereum blockchain, ensuring optimal autonomy, trust, speed, and safety. In order contracting, both parties must agree with its conditions, and there is full freedom for them to be decided. Once the agreement is met, the contract becomes registered on the blockchain. This technology provides a shared, distributed ledger representing a single version of the truth and permanently in sync recording these contracts. All the contracting parties can consult the contract throughout the time that it is active. Also, one of the many characteristics of blockchain technology is that once the block is registered on the chain, it becomes immutable, so all the network users have anonymous information on the ledger at their disposable safely and free from manipulation. This kind of environment has no third parties to regulate them, but due to the value inherent with every single one of these contracts, they can be auditable on Github (UNECE, 2019). All smart contracts in existence will form part of a "super smart contract." "Super smart contracts" ensure that the patient is covered in the case of insolvency or death of the Dentist (Dentacoin Foundation, 2018). In Dentacoin's case, the smart contract between Dentist and Patient is focused on maintaining healthy teeth and overall oral hygiene. So, Dentist and patient obligations and duties must be fulfilled for both parties to benefit from the smart contract. Patients must achieve the best possible oral hygiene with the help of the Dentacare mobile app, and dentists restore and maintain their patients' teeth at their own expense with high-quality service and satisfaction. If patient and dentist missions are fulfilled, then monetary payments will be processed. This kind of motivation creates an environment where both parties overperform together to reach a common goal simultaneously as they benefit from it (Dentacoin Foundation, 2018). Following example between individual user X and dentist Y shows how this contract works:

User X wishes to get dental services from dentist Y, and the exchange will happen when X promises Y that payment in DCN will take place upon the fulfillment of services from Y. When Y has finished his commitment, a request by Y will be made, and the smart contract will carry out the request by means of transferring the DCNs from Xs' wallet into Y's wallet. The history of this transfer will be stored on the ledgers of both user X and dentist Y, and the balance for each account will be present in the contract state.

Finally, it is crucial to notice the benefits for either the Dentist or Patient on this process. The Dentist gets paid for prevention and better care, receives additional monthly income in DCN, and builds solid relations with his patient. On the other hand, patients receive lifelong preventive services, pay affordable monthly fees in DCN to reduce their dental costs, achieve better dental healthcare, earn rewards for reviews of the Dentist, surveys, and general usage of the Apps (Dentacoin Foundation, 2018).

Dental Health Database

Blockchain offers a brand-new model with the potential to enable secure lifetime medical record sharing with healthcare professionals. Blockchain electronic health care records have two main advantages: it eliminates the need of adding another organization to the process (the interaction is just between the patient and the healthcare professional); second, it adds considerably to a time-stamped, programmable ledger. That opens the door for intelligent control of record access without creating custom functionality for each vendor. This ledger also includes an audit trail (Maddux, 2017).

So, as part of the Dentacoin platform, this App will be a decentralized database of patients' overall medical records. Data will be highly reliable, protected, updatable, and accessible exclusively by patients or dentists upon given permission, generating value for the dental industry. Consequently, each patient activity will be rewarded with Dentacoin that could later be used for paying dental treatments. On the other hand, Dentists could consider Dentacoin as a financial investment, pay suppliers, or remunerate employees for their extraordinary performance in the workplace (Dentacoin Foundation, 2018).

To sum up, there are available and released five Apps: DentaVox Paid Surveys & dental stats; Dentacoin Trusted reviews; Dentacare Oral Health App; Dentacare (Jaws of Battle Game) and Dentacoin wallet. Additionally, will be upcoming soon: custom Dentacoin Hub App for dentists; Dental Health Database and Integrated Practice Management Software (Dentacoin Foundation, 2020).

WHAT IS NEXT FOR DENTACOIN IN BLOCKCHAIN-BASED HEALTHCARE

It is thought that blockchain can lead to radical changes in many sectors and impacting the economy, including the health economy. A blockchain for health would need to protect technological solutions for three main elements: scalability, access security, data privacy, data provenance, availability, and security as well as privacy.

The exciting part of this technology in the healthcare area is the blockchain's potential to allow the safe registration of the lifetime patient, sharing among the dispersed health providers. The disruptive effect that blockchain is expected to create in the healthcare area will arise from a common shared database that professionals can access from an electronic medical system, eliminating an undesired central intermediary and a single point of failure (Justinia, 2019). There are four existing health problems that Blockchain can solve:

- Patient-centric approach;
- Privacy and access;
- Information integrity;
- Cost integrity.

Dentacoin provides a great model for blockchain in healthcare. This novel platform is the first and the only solution that supports the dental community by creating solutions that aim to improve the quality of dental care across the world. Dentacoin numbers of users and partners are growing each day, and that is their primary focus. Therefore, structuring a well-designed plan is a crucial aspect for increasing membership and boosting its value.

Recent and upcoming features and concepts are the release of the Dentacoin Hub for Dentists, the Multiplayer option for the Dentacare: Jaws of Battle App and the alpha versions of the Dental Health Database, DentaVox App, and the concept of new software for the Dentacoin practices (Dentacoin Foundation, 2018).

It is considered essential to mention that the Dentacoin Token is already traded on some international exchange platforms. Also, the first partner dental clinics such as LifDental (based in New York), Dental on Flinders (in Melbourne, Australia); Dentech Dental Care (Pure, India); Content (Budapest, Hungary); F3T Dental Clinic (London, UK); Bredent (located in Germany); Swiss Dentaprime (Varna, Bulgaria) have implemented Dentacoin as a valid method of payment and as a basis of their Patient

Loyalty Program which rewards patients for sending feedback, writing reviews and making recommendations (Ostapenko, 2018).

Dentacoin Foundation has a strategic partnerships with Arklign (an end-to-end digital lab partner based in California), Ecodent, a dental laboratory in New York, PCP Dental Recruitment, in London, as other partners. Dentacoin Foundation announced a strategic partnership with Dentaprime, considered one of the major private dental clinics in Europe. As already mentioned, SWISS Dentaprime was the pioneer location of the chain and the first dental clinic to accept payments using Dentacoin. Now three years later, 80% of the clinical patients use their DCN tokens to pay for part of their dental bills and receive a discount for doing so.

The increasing devotion to become the best clinical care provider, such as implant restorations, exceptional patient care at affordable prices, and top-notch technology, naturally drove them towards Dentacoin and placed them among the first operation businesses to heavily integrate blockchain tools in their systems. The aim of this partnership between Dentacoin Foundation and Dentaprime is to closely integrate some additional processes into the clinic's workflow (Kraeva, 2020):

- Daily use of Dentacoin hub mobile app: a prototype version of the public Dentacoin hub app that gives access to patients to all relevant Dentacoin apps, their wallet, and other essential clinic resources.
- Daily use of employee bonus app: an app that encourages Dentaprime team members to achieve the company goals and have a healthier lifestyle. All exemplary achievements will be rewarded in DCN.

It is also important to point out the participation in dental industry conferences and summits like the IDS in Cologne, because this kind of marketing helps reach new dental practitioners, suppliers, and manufacturers (J. Grenzebach, 2020). Dentacoin Foundation aims to reach 10% of market share on a 25-year distance. This value was based on the number of Dentacoin wallets created. In the dental industry, 10% of the market share means approximately 600 million patients and 200 000 dentists using the Dentacoin shared value technology (Dentacoin Foundation, 2018).

CONCLUSION

Blockchain technology can offer long-term benefits such as improved cash flow, lower transaction costs, reduced settlement times, asset provenance, native asset creation, and creating new models of trust. Using a blockchain can eliminate the need for central authorities when making transactions. Thus, the potential of this technology to completely change economic transactions has aroused the interest of many people, such as economists, strategists, and healthcare providers.

The promising applications in healthcare include health information exchange, the battle against prescription drug frauds, the share of patient data, and health insurance. Dentacoin gives the opportunity to significantly reduce industry-specific costs, lead to economies of scale, and provide services that will improve the quality of life of people from lower-income groups. Therefore, Dentacoin places a premium on global dental healthcare by using blockchain technology. This system also ensures security, ease, and trust in transactions and confidentiality and immutability of data through various applications and online content to promote better dental healthcare and reward users with DCN tokens. By leaving quality reviews on the Dentacoin platform, they will earn DCN coins as a reward. This fund can be used as actual means of payment within the Dentacoin dental network dealing with all Dentacoin Ecosystem benefits. In addition, surveys are also offered to increase quality feedback to dental providers. On the other hand, patients can purchase DCN coins with "Fiat" currency on specific secure online platforms. In general, Healthcoins can help people realize that while it may be "expensive" at first, the benefits will emerge in the long run.

Despite the potential benefits of blockchain for various industries, many challenges remain overtaken, such as the size and volume of clinical data, information privacy concerns, and security issues.

In the banking area, blockchain use cases have been very successful, and to date, there are many use cases, pilot projects using blockchain technology to improve healthcare provision. In the future, we hope that these studies can help demonstrate the true potential for blockchain to influence a pragmatic shift in healthcare delivery.

An industry-specific cryptocurrency, such as Dentacoin, can provide both a customer-centric and an industry-centric solution. The primary purpose is to improve dental care worldwide and make it affordable by reducing the costs and increasing the benefits for all participants. As more and more people earn Dentacoin (DCN) and use them in various ways, the value of the cryptocurrency is expected to rise, which gives more freedom and trust to the Dentacoin Community. Indeed, the idea behind Dentacoin is a revolutionary technology, and it is thought that it will only be a matter of time before it reaches all areas of the healthcare industry.

ACKNOWLEDGMENT

This research received no specific grant from any funding agency in the public, commercial, or not-for-profit sectors.

REFERENCES

Abu Bakar, N., Rosbi, S., & Uzaki, K. (2017). Cryptocurrency Framework Diagnostics from Islamic Finance Perspective: A New Insight of Bitcoin System Transaction. *International Journal of Management Science and Business Administration*, 4(1), 19–28. doi:10.18775/ijmsba.1849-5664-5419.2014.41.1003

Atzei, N., Bartoletti, M., & Cimoli, T. (2017). A survey of attacks on Ethereum smart contracts. *Universit`a Degli Studi Di Cagliari, 10204 LNCS*(July), 164–186. doi:10.1007/978-3-662-54455-6_8

Barreiro-Gomez, J., & Tembine, H. (2019). Blockchain token economics: A mean-field-type game perspective. *IEEE Access: Practical Innovations, Open Solutions*, 7, 64603–64613. doi:10.1109/ACCESS.2019.2917517

Beck, R., Müller-Bloch, C., & King, J. L. (2018). Governance in the blockchain economy: A framework and research agenda. *Journal of the Association for Information Systems*, 19(10), 1020–1034. doi:10.17705/1jais.00518

Bennett, B. (2017). *Healthcoin - blockchain-enabled platform for diabetes prevention.* Retrieved January 29, 2021, from https://blockchainhealthcarereview.com/healthcoin-blockchain-enabled-platform-for-diabetes-prevention/

ClinicAll Healthcare. (2019, April 24). *Cryptocurrency In Healthcare: Gold Rush Or Bad News?* Medium. https://clinicallhealthcare.medium.com/cryptocurrency-in-healthcare-gold-rush-or-bad-news-889e73cd9142

Dapp, M. M. (2018). Toward a sustainable circular economy powered by community-based incentive systems. In *Business Transformation through Blockchain* (Vol. 2, pp. 153–181). Springer International Publishing., doi:10.1007/978-3-319-99058-3_6

Dentacoin Foundation. (2018). *Dentacoin: The Blockchain Solution for the Global Dental Industry. Whitepaper.* Retrieved from https://dentacoin.com/%0Ahttps://dentacoin.com/web/white-paper/Whitepaper-en1.pdf

Dentacoin Foundation. (2020). Dentacoin - The Blockchain Solution for Better Oral Health. Retrieved January 29, 2021, from https://dentacoin.com/assets/uploads/dentacoin-company-introduction.pdf

Dentacoin Foundation. (2021). *Dentists.* Retrieved January 30, 2021, from https://dentacoin.com/dentists

Dentacoin Team. (2019). *8 Use Cases for Your Dentacoin (DCN) Tokens.* Retrieved January 30, 2021, from https://blog.dentacoin.com/what-is-dentacoin-8-use-cases/

Engelhardt, M. A. (2017). Hitching Healthcare to the Chain: An Introduction to Blockchain Technology in the Healthcare Sector. *Technology Innovation Management Review, 7*(10), 22–34. doi:10.22215/timreview/1111

Frankenfield, J. (2020). *Cryptocurrency.* Retrieved January 29, 2021, from https://www.investopedia.com/terms/c/cryptocurrency.asp

Ghosh, J. (2019). The Blockchain: Opportunities for Research in Information Systems and Information Technology. *Journal of Global Information Technology Management, 22*(4), 235–242. doi:10.1080/1097198X.2019.1679954

Grenzebach, J. (2020). *Dentacoin Foundation is the future of the dental industry.* Retrieved January 30, 2021, from https://aspioneer.com/dentacoin-foundation-is-the-future-of-the-dental-industry/

Grenzebach, P. (2017). *Dentacoin: Transforming the Dental Industry with Blockchain.* Retrieved January 30, 2021, from https://blockchain.cioreview.com/vendor/2017/dentacoin

Justinia, T. (2019). Blockchain technologies: Opportunities for solving real-world problems in healthcare and biomedical sciences. *Acta Informatica Medica, 27*(4), 284–291. doi:10.5455/aim.2019.27.284-291 PMID:32055097

Kraeva, D. (2020). *Dentacoin Announces Partnership With Europe's Largest Dental Clinic.* Retrieved January 30, 2021, from https://blog.dentacoin.com/dentacoin-dentaprime-partnership-with-europe-largest-dental-clinic/

Maddux, D. (2017). *Cybersecurity and Blockchain in Health Care.* Retrieved January 29, 2021, from https://acumenmd.com/blog/cybersecurity-and-blockchain-in-health-care/

Mearian, L. (2019). *What is blockchain? The complete guide.* Retrieved January 29, 2021, from https://www.computerworld.com/article/3191077/what-is-blockchain-the-complete-guide.html

Nel, L. (2018, March 5). *Beginner's Guide to Dentacoin.* Retrieved January 30, 2021, from https://blockonomi.com/dentacoin-guide/

Ostapenko, G. F. (2018). Creating a Platform Based Business Model In Dental Industry. *Intern. Journal of Profess. Bus. Review, 4*(1), 106. doi:10.26668/businessreview/2019.v4i1.106

Prado, J. (2017). *O que é blockchain?* Retrieved January 29, 2021, from https://tecnoblog.net/227293/como-funciona-blockchain-bitcoin/

Royal, J., & Voigt, K. (2017). *What is cryptocurrency? Guide for beginners.* Retrieved January 29, 2021, from https://cointelegraph.com/bitcoin-for-beginners/what-are-cryptocurrencies

TyN Magazine. (2020). *How healthcare is entering the world of cryptocurrency.* Retrieved January 29, 2021, from https://www.tynmagazine.com/how-healthcare-is-entering-the-world-of-cryptocurrency/

UNECE. (2019). *Blockchain in Trade Facilitation. Whitepaper.* Retrieved from www.unece.org/cefact

Yassine, M., Alazab, M., & Romdhani, I. (2020). *Blockchain for Cybersecurity and Privacy.* Blockchain for Cybersecurity and Privacy. doi:10.1201/9780429324932

Yoo, S. (2020). How to design the token reinforcement based on token economy for blockchain model. *International Journal of Advanced Culture Technology, 8*(1), 157–164.

Chapter 13
Blockchain Pharma:
A Prospective Overview

Francisco Ribeiro de Sousa

ISEG, Lisbon School of Economics and Management, University of Lisbon, Portugal

ABSTRACT

Blockchain, a distributed ledger technology (DLT) that sustained the creation of the first digital currency, Bitcoin, crosses many business areas, including healthcare, to promise better economic solutions. Blockchain generalized implementation is already a reality in Estonia, perhaps the most digitally advanced country globally, with proven healthcare results for its citizens. From a pharmaceutical industry perspective, blockchain offers solutions as diverse as the structuring of clinical trial protocols, the traceability of medicines along the supply chain, and intellectual property rights. Additionally, the DLT's cryptographic protocol, whose main characteristics are immutability, consensus, security, and transparency, may support both the web's decentralization and the transition to a Semantic Web, which is recognized by many as highly recommended.

INTRODUCTION

"The physician patient relationship is forever changing. Now more than ever with the rise of access to data" David Schanger, CEO of Progyny

This chapter's primary purpose is to address the impact of digitalization on health systems and the pharmaceutical industry, emphasizing blockchain technology (BT).

BT aggravates the dilemma between data centralization and the original vision of a decentralized internet, namely because it brings to the Internet the required trust to transact value in the absence of intermediaries.

Throughout this chapter, the aim is to examine the eventual shift towards a health system where the patient is the legitimate owner of their medical records. Initiatives will be presented where the patient can profit from sharing their medical records, such as the partnership between a genomic sequencing company and a biopharmaceutical company interested in developing biological drugs (Grishin, 2019).

DOI: 10.4018/978-1-7998-7363-1.ch013

As it will be seen, Estonia, the most digital country globally, stands out as an example of the modernization of health systems. Using BT, these technological advances have allowed the implementation of an innovative alert system for drug interactions (Kõnd & Lillevâli, 2019).

BT's versatility can be demonstrated by the growth of many solutions serving the most diverse business areas. This chapter discusses blockchain's structural characteristics (immutability, transparency, and security) that it is thought will justify its wide use by the pharmaceutical industry. In the pursuit of greater process rationality and simplification, blockchain is applied in diverse areas as supply chain, clinical trials, and R&D (Premkumar & Shrimati, 2020).

Counterfeit drugs are a severe problem at the supply chain level. Ways to more effectively trace the drugs from their origin to the final consumer are discussed (Clark & Burstall, 2018). The authors will present existing solutions that allow the end consumer to verify provenance and authenticity using a smartphone app (Saxena et al., 2020).

Clinical trials will also be discussed, considering that their current form raises doubts about outcomes' reproducibility. In this sense, existent options are presented, including smart contracts to make study protocols more transparent (Benchoufi & Ravaud, 2017).

Finally, it will be observed how BT can play a crucial role in R&D, notably in protecting intellectual property rights.

BACKGROUND

Blockchain, a distributed ledger technology (DLT) popularized in 2009 by Satoshi Nakamoto while creating "Bitcoin" cryptocurrency, is the basis of a progressive digital revolution. The exact semantics of the word "blockchain" helps to understand its meaning: "block" represents a unit that contains encrypted information, which is in turn inserted into a "chain" that represents a database (Yaga et al., 2018). However, a blockchain differs from a common database in the way information is structured: each new piece of information is encrypted and inserted into a block until it is filled (these have a limited storage capacity), at which point it is submitted to a validation process carried out by different network participants (nodes); the block is aggregated to the end of the existing chain, in case it is consensually validated, ensuring a chronological order (Conway, 2020).

Cryptography is an integral and inseparable element of BT, guaranteeing the ledger's immutability, the security of transactions, and the safeguarding of players' identities. Cryptography can be defined as a method of ensuring a communication process's privacy and integrity by converting plaintext (standard text) into a ciphertext (random sequence of characters) using a mathematical algorithm, thus preventing outsiders from accessing private information. Two types of cryptography are essentially used in BT: asymmetric cryptography and hash function. In asymmetric cryptography, a public key (which can be openly shared) and a private key (which must be kept a secret) is used to encrypt and decrypt the ciphertext. The sender uses his private key and the recipient's public key to encrypt the text, and then the recipient uses his private key and the sender's public key to decrypt the text, thus resulting in a highly secure process. In turn, the hash function is a type of encryption that uses a mathematical algorithm to convert any information into a fixed-size string of characters. This type of one-way encryption means that it is impossible to retrieve the plaintext through the ciphertext. A given input always corresponds to the same output, and any change in that same input significantly changes the output, a determining characteristic for data integrity checking (Pasala et al., 2020).

In BT, a hash function is used to process information to be inserted into a block. Any small change in the information contained in any block generates a different hash, making the data tampering easily detectable, as shown in Figure 1.

Figure 1. The blockchain adulteration
Source: (author's work)

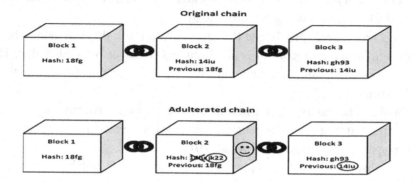

In the end, the blockchain works as a vast peer-to-peer (P2P), public and decentralized database, where all the records and events (contained in "blocks") are found in a chronologically ordered way. Events can only be updated with most users' consensus, and information cannot be erased, both factors that contribute to the transparency and traceability of this network (Bhowmik & Feng, 2017).

There are essentially three types of blockchains when it comes to privacy: public (or permission-less) - those in which anyone in the World can participate or use to view transactions, are therefore the most transparent (this is the case of Bitcoin); private (or permissioned) - those owned and controlled by a single organization; Consortium-based - those in which several organizations participate but access to which is restricted (Underwood, 2016).

Several advantages have been appointed to BT, such as ease of use, security, transparency, and decentralization (Mettler & Hsg, 2016). This security arises from the blockchain protocol, which is based on immutability and consensus, where the adulteration of a block prevents its connection to other blocks. Consensus between a majority of different users is required for data validation. Users are noti-fied in case of any adulteration to any block, having the power to deny it and preventing the adulterated blockchain to progress. The blockchain will then be returned to a previous state where all blocks are still chained together. A network of nodes is responsible for validating the chronological order at which requests, transactions, and information have been executed, modified, or created. The absence of an entity to "arbitrate" the transactions requires great trust in the network, which arises from the immutability recognized in the consensus protocol (Marbouh et al., 2020). Another element that adds confidence to blockchain transactions is the private keys, allocated to each node (participant in the network) and used to create a digital signature to sign each transaction. This way, data ownership is granted (Zheng et al., 2017). Besides, decentralization has been recognized as another of the advantages of blockchain since it operates as a P2P network with multiple spread copies of the same transactions without relying on a single database, meaning it is entirely decentralized. In practice, what this may mean is that even if some nodes are down, the system can still be running, and data is kept as usual (Saxena et al., 2020).

Inevitably, BT is not free of criticism, and, therefore, it is worth mentioning some of its features often pointed out as being less favorable. The storage capacity of each block is limited, as it is the number of blocks created at a time, creating doubts regarding scalability. Processing large volumes of information requires high computational power, resulting in high energy consumption. The privacy of public blockchains is also called into question because anyone can see the information. Besides, data, once entered into the blockchain, cannot be deleted, raising concerns on the compliance with RDGP policies (Golosova & Romanovs, 2018).

The Semantic Web (SW), also known as Web 3.0, is a step forward in the Internet's evolutionary process. It is thought that SW, whose purpose is to make information understandable and processable by both machines and humans, will be an essential tool to support modern medicine. This technology has taken the attention of the World Wide Web inventor himself, Tim Berners Lee, as it will be seen. The contextualization of information is of particular importance for researchers, whose challenge often involves filtering large amounts of dispersed information. The SW allows interoperability between different sources of information and relates it in order to generate knowledge. According to Tim Berners Lee, ontologies, which form the basis of SW, can be defined as "a text or a file that defines the relationship between elements" (Karami & Rahimi, 2019). BT can be combined with the Semantic Web to carry out data nodes' storage in a decentralized and secure manner. Also, BT makes the information reliable by the immutability inscribed in its protocol; that is, it guarantees that the information is not modified and allows to verify its provenance (Cano-Benito J., Cimmino A., 2019).

BT's growth and success could be consummated with the transition from the current Web to a decentralized web, a need recognized by many, including Tim Berners Lee. Nowadays, the Internet works in a mostly centralized way and controlled by big technological giants like Google, YouTube, or Facebook. Roughly, all these giants end up holding gigantic and centralized personal databases where they gather the information collected from millions of their users (Yeung et al., 2009). As a response to the need for a paradigm shift, proposals have emerged that allow users greater control of their data through decentralization, such as the Solid project, with promising applications in the health sector.

The progress of the BT and its attractiveness as a disruptive technology has been leveraged by the simultaneous development of other technological tools that complement it and enrich its potential. "Ethereum", launched in 2015 with collective funding, has been considered as a second-generation blockchain platform, which enables users to create customized decentralized applications ("DAPPS"). Besides, Ethereum allows creating "smart contracts," which are digital and auto executable contracts that dispense human intervention after the signature. As in any other contract, rules, benefits, penalties, and actions are defined and agreed upon, but unlike a traditional contract, a smart contract can obtain information, process it, and take the appropriate actions according to the agreed premises. Blockchain is the infrastructure that allows to run, store and verify smart contracts (Bocek et al., 2017). However, smart contracts would not be able to access data outside the network without a complementary tool called "oracles," which provide reliable and verified external data. "Tokens" are DLT's essential elements, as transferable value units, representing digital assets that can be used within a project's ecosystem, serving a specific purpose. Most of the tokens have been used in fundraising to help democratize access to capital through the so-called 'crowdfunding.' According to the CMVM of Portugal, "[crowdfunding] is a form of fundraising by entities or individuals, who intend to finance specific activities or projects, through their registration on electronic platforms, from which they raise investment from one or several individual investors." One of the most comprehensive examples of the use of tokens is the "Initial Coin Offerings (ICOs)," which consists of the sale to the public of a predefined number of digital tokens by a company with a promise of advantageous terms for the initial investors/clients (Y. Chen, 2018). Blockchain is also being applied to manage devices equipped with the "Internet of things" (IoT), a concept that refers to the digital interconnection between daily life physical objects and the Internet. The incorporation of low-cost technologies such as sensors, RFID (Radio Frequency Identification), QR codes, or electronic tags has given the most diverse everyday objects the possibility of connecting to the Internet, allowing the creation of relevant inputs for users or companies that manage the activities in which these objects are involved (Premkumar & Shrimati, 2020).

While blockchains have emerged in the context of financial applications, non-financial application areas are of interest. The "modus operandi" of this technology brings numerous advantages to the business world, streamlining processes, facilitating trade, reducing costs, increasing security, and, above all, boosting confidence among people and organizations (Y. Chen, 2018).

It is quite clear that BT is transforming the business world and many well-known companies are good examples of it. Technology giant Siemens, which takes a large share of the European energy market, has acquired a start-up, "LO3", which develops P2P systems to distribute, sell, and purchase energy. The aim is to create micro-energy networks managed by BT called "Exergy." The World's largest bank, the Bank of China, is investing heavily in this type of solution to create its own digital currency. In turn, Amazon has a service, "Amazon Managed Blockchain" (part of AWS), to create and manage customized blockchain networks, i.e., at the scale of each business.

With the increasing restructuring of the global economic tissue based on blockchain solutions, it is expected that by 2030 this technology could generate an annual turnover of around $3 trillion (Costello, 2019).

In the healthcare sector, there are several areas in which BT could add value. Enhancing patient health data management at both public and private institution levels is one way to significantly improve the speed and quality of health care. In the United States, a start-up called "Gem" moves towards facilitating access to medical information by health providers to minimize medical negligence and benefit the patient. However, other types of solutions put the patient in full possession of his or her health data by allowing safe storage of information such as heart rate, blood pressure, or sleeping habits, and by giving them the power to sell such data for research purposes, such as the Swiss app "Healthbank." It becomes clear how patient empowerment in healthcare rides alongside digitalization (Mettler & Hsg, 2016).

The pharmaceutical industry is the largest global player in healthcare systems, with several public and private stakeholders working to supply medicines on a large scale. It is also a growing sector and is willing to invest in BT to ensure the safety, efficacy, and quality of its latest product, the drug (Premkumar & Shrimati, 2020).

Implementing blockchain based-solutions depends on each business area's perspective to respond to each sector's challenges and requirements. For example, the pharmaceutical industry is a highly regulated sector, so it is necessary to ensure that all legal requirements and internal compliance standards are met. Regulatory issues emerged as a central concern to adopting blockchain for pharmaceutical companies' respondents in a 2019 survey from Deloitte (Deloitte, 2020). Because it is inviolable, BT can play a decisive role in demonstrating the authenticity and integrity of the data to be submitted to the authorities, which translates into greater protection for companies, but also in safeguarding public health by increasing confidence in companies' data management systems (Steinwandter & Herwig, 2019).

In the pharmaceutical industry, blockchain's growth is being enforced above all by improving data security, traceability, and transparency. Clinical trials and supply chain are both leading candidates for this kind of solution in the healthcare sector. Regarding R&D, blockchain solution seems to provide the ideal solution to safeguard Intellectual Property (IP) once it can provide a timestamp, proof of content, identity, and immutability (Shute, 2017).

Emerging technologies such as IoT and BT will favor a progressive digitalization of the healthcare system, which is expected to evolve towards a more rational healthcare provision with increasingly personalized and comfortable treatments for patients. Medical devices equipped with sensors capable of measuring physiological parameters such as body temperature, biomarkers, respiration, and even emotions will allow for earlier, simple, perhaps accurate diagnoses of diseases. In this sense, the pharmaceutical industry might have to adjust medicines' manufacture, leaving mass production (where doses are fixed) to start producing according to each individual's needs (Nørfeldt et al., 2019).

Decentralization in Healthcare

Internet design is decentralizing in nature and has introduced a new element in the ancestral tension and power struggle between centralizing and decentralizing forces, which involves control and establishing trust. However, despite initial hopes, current Internet functionality depends on only a few companies (Amazon, Apple, Facebook, Google, and Microsoft) which concentrate most user data and effectively control the Internet (Lopez et al., 2019), being in these technological colossuses that the users must rely mostly.

Sir Tim Berners-Lee, often referred to as the father of the World Wide Web (Gurstein, 2011), disapproves of this direction given to the Internet. Seeing his creation move so far away from the initial purposes, he presented his proposal to correct the current centralizing direction of the Internet and ensure the respective decentralization (Hageman et al., 2020).

"The vision I have for the Web is about anything being potentially connected with anything (…) inventing the World Wide Web involved my growing realization that there was a power in arranging ideas in an unconstrained, web-like way". (…) The very fact that it provides connection, content, and context is the basis for our ability to amalgamate data from myriad sources to provide the raw material for big data and predictive analytic solutions that would have been improbable just twenty years ago (Hageman et al., 2020).

To achieve his decentralized view of the Internet, Berners-Lee considers that users' control of personal data is an unavoidable premise.

As stated in Buyle et al. (2019), "the key concept is that people can choose where they store their personal data, which build upon the principles of decentralization." (p 2). While adding recognition that "blockchain is regularly referred to in this context as a solution for the management of personal data" (p.2), it is also pointed out that the "immutability character of Blockchain which implies that data cannot be deleted, might be a challenge in the context of article 17 of the GDPR that gives people the right to erase their personal data" (p. 3). This immutability is referred to as a challenge that can be perceived to be insurmountable in the face of General Data Protection Regulation (GDPR), a legal framework provided by the European Commission to empower individuals to control their personal information (Buyle et al., 2019). The authors consider, however, that such immutability will not prevent personal data from being managed with a guarantee of privacy, since each person's data can be recorded in a blockchain never to be known by third parties (Nakamoto & Bitcoin, 2008) unless of course, that person decides to transmit it to such third parties. It will then be impossible to delete the data from these people's memory (with or without GDPR). This guarantee of privacy happens thanks to the possibilities of data encryption offered by BT. For example, the "hash" function, a key element of the BT (Nakamoto & Bitcoin, 2008), makes it impossible, in practice, to reverse the data encoded by data holders. This function works as a "one-way trap door that allows mapping of an arbitrary input to an arbitrary output. The input to hash functions can vary in length; however, the generated output is of a fixed length" (Murtaza et al., 2019). Still another cryptographic technique, homomorphic cryptography, already allows data to be operated without it being known, although in this particular case, such possibilities "are still not efficient enough for real-time applications"(Moore et al., 2014).

It should be noted that Sir Tim Berners-Lee decided to take a different approach towards Internet decentralization by proposing the SOLID ecosystem. So, instead of separating people's identities from their data, which is now also possible because "metadata such as patient identity, visit ID, provider ID or payer ID, can be kept on a Blockchain, but the actual records should be stored in a separate universal health cloud" (Karafiloski & Mishev, 2017), Berners-Lee has embarked on separating data from their applications, "providing people with their personal data pod, in which they can store data independently of the applications that they or others use to access that data. [Hence] People can decide at a granular level which actors and applications can read from or write to" (Buyle et al., 2019). The Solid ecosystem provides an answer by proposing a personal data pod for every citizen, such that all of their public and private data remains in one place. Instead of moving data between A and D, each of the agencies asks for permission to view a highly specific part of the data. That way, data does not have to be moved around, and GDPR compliance can be assessed automatically for every single data request. The key concept is that people can choose where they store their data, which builds upon decentralization principles (Buyle et al., 2019).

Although still in the experimental phase, Solid technology is already being tested in Greater Manchester with the expectation of helping patients with dementia, for whom it is imperative to overcome the increased difficulty in managing their medical information (Cellan-Jones, 2020). From the patient's perspective, Solid provides greater autonomy in managing their medical records. From health professionals' perspective, there is less concern about data protection policies because they can access their patients' medical information with their consent. The system also allows patients' health data to be gathered regardless of where they come from and ensures that healthcare providers have consensual and uniform access to that information, which represents an unbureaucratic, simplified and secure solution for storing and sharing electronic medical records. Besides, the Solid ecosystem character associated with the possibility of an eclectic interaction with health and fitness applications may in the future provide relevant information on individual habits and behaviors with an impact on people's health, something neglected until now (Bingham, 2019). With this in mind, Jason Paulos, a master student at MIT has developed an app called Solid Health, with the purpose to gather information on users' physical activity and health collected through their wearable devices like smartwatches and archive it in a single format, in Solid Pods (Personal Online Data Stores) (Paulos, 2020).

The Semantic Web (SW) concept is based on ontologies' use to relate information by adding meaning and context. The Semantic Web's ultimate goal is to take advantage of the enormous amount of information available on the Web and interconnect it in a logical way of generating knowledge. Standardized languages such as Resource Description Framework (RDF) and Web Ontology Language (OWL) have been developed that support the idea that it is possible to present information in the form of a signifier and give it a meaning. The World Wide Web Consortium (W3C) has created a task force, LODD (linking open drug data), dedicated to the health area, focusing on collaborative drug development (H. Chen

& Xie, 2010). An example of this is the Gene Ontology project, which seeks to characterize genes from three distinct domains: molecular function, cellular components, and biological processes. Each of these domains reflects a particular side of the gene and integrates a series of related concepts; that is, each of these domains translates a complex structure composed of terms/concepts that can be perceived as data nodes (Kanza & Frey, 2019). BT can be combined with the Semantic Web to carry out data nodes' storage in a decentralized and secure manner. Also, blockchain makes the information reliable by the immutability inscribed in its protocol; that is, it guarantees that the information is not modified and allows to verify its provenance (Cano-Benito J., Cimmino A., 2019).

The Estonian Case

Estonia, one of the most advanced societies in the World in digital terms, where 99% of government services are online, has created a blockchain solution for managing its population's medical records (e-Estonia, 2020). The 1.3 million Estonians can quickly and unbureaucratically access their medical records without compromising data integrity and security. This is corroborated by the information published on the official e-Estonia website, where one can read:

With KSI Blockchain deployed in Estonian government networks, history cannot be rewritten by anybody, and the authenticity of the electronic data can be mathematically proven. It means that no-one – not hackers, not system administrators, and not even government itself – can manipulate the data and get away with that. (e-Estonia, 2020).

Estonian citizens benefit from a highly digitized and uncomplicated healthcare system where their healthcare data integration takes place in a unique and easily accessible (with citizen ID) database. This system also brings many advantages for health professionals by allowing easy access to patients' history, regardless of where they have previously received medical support. Besides, medical prescriptions are electronic, saving paper and avoiding unnecessary visits to the doctor since patients can remotely request a renewal of their prescription for their usual medication. In addition to the electronic prescriptions database, the software has been developed to alert doctors to the possibility of drug interactions or contraindications with the patient's usual medication. With this software's use, the government estimates that about 15 to 17% of prescriptions are changed at the time of prescribing, thanks to system alerts (Kõnd & Lilleväli, 2019).

According to Estonian Health and Labor Minister Riina Sikkut, the digitalization of the health system, supported by BT, is justified not only by the economic advantages but also by the increased quality of medical care provided to citizens, leveraging the transition from curative medicine to a more desirable preventive medicine (Healtheuropa.EU, 2019).

The digitalization of medicine may change the current paradigm of pharmaceuticals production based on the traditional indiscriminate and large-scale production of fixed-dose batches to a personalized and rational production where the dose is adjusted according to the needs of a specific patient. This concept can materialize through the use of serialized drugs via blockchain; that is, for each product, a unique record is created in the production unit, which after being validated and introduced into a blockchain becomes immutable. IoT will also allow for other features such as tracing the product, creating a history/chronology of the patient's medication, or even measuring the patient's physiological parameters (currently, there are already smart devices that measure, e.g., heartbeats). To meet the futuristic but realistic scenario of a digital medicine ecosystem, an app called MedBlockChain, was created to gather all the information with medical relevance in one place in favor of the patient. With the patient's permission, the doctor can use this information to entail a machine learning-oriented diagnosis (Nørfeldt et al., 2019). It is thought that these new possibilities and digital functionalities, due to increasing technological sophistication, reveal the need for consistent protection of patients' privacy and citizens' rights in general.

Supply-Chain

The supply chain supports a company's needs in creating and developing its products (SGS, 2020). Conceptually, it can be defined as a system of organizations, people, activities, information, and resources involved in transporting products or services from suppliers to customers. The success of a business is strictly related to the sustainable management of this structure.

Because of its unquestionable importance regarding pharmaceutical products' integrity, the pharma supply chain is the subject of great scrutiny and must comply with strict GDP (Good Distribution Practices).

GDP is essentially a set of standards covering all activities related to the distribution of medicines and constitutes a quality system to which wholesale distributors are bound to ensure the quality and integrity of medicines throughout its circuit. The GDP certification demonstrates the commitment to quality and regulatory requirements in all aspects of the service and is a significant goal for any drug distributor (SGS, 2020). According to the European Medicines Agency (EMA), compliance with GDP ensures: that medicines in the supply chain are authorized per European legislation; that storage conditions (such as temperature and humidity) are maintained throughout the circuit including transport; that cross-contamination is avoided; that delivery times are satisfactory; and that adequate product rotation takes place (EMA, 2020).

Supply-chains are a central piece of the pharmaceutical industry as they are involved in supplying raw materials to deliver the final product to the end-user (patient). As it is easy to imagine, a few actors are involved in this logistic network with several responsibilities: raw material supplier is responsible for addressing manufacturer's orders while recording quantities and technical specifications; manufacturers have to manage customers' orders, and additionally record quantities and technical specifications; carriers assume responsibility during transport; retailers carry out shopping, and also record quantity, quality, and technical specifications; consumers verify quality and specifications, effect shopping, and communicate information to the regulator; regulator evaluates quality and safety, and is also responsible for monitoring transport operations, as well as transactions. Such a vast and complex structure brings several difficulties, such as traceability, counterfeiting, excessive paperwork, inefficient processes, delays, and high costs (Settanni et al., 2017).

As described above, the supply chain's complex logistic network arouses several concerns, but perhaps the most worrying are counterfeit products. The black market for pharmaceuticals is a business that generates annual revenues of approximately 200 billion USD (Behner et al., 2020), and which entails perverse consequences that could culminate in the death of patients, either because of the lack of active ingredients or due to the presence of harmful ingredients. The problem is so severe that in 2019, a European Directive (2011/62/EU, "Falsified Medicines Directive") came into force in order to establish measures to protect the distribution chain from the entry of falsified medicinal products, with the ultimate goal of achieving a higher level of safety and traceability of the packaging of medicinal products circulating on the European market. Among the measures imposed by this EU Directive, the manufacturers are now obliged to place on the packaging of medicinal products information enabling them to be identified in a serialized manner, i.e., there is no longer an identification of the packaging exclusively by batch, but also an identification by unit (each packaging contains its own unique identification code: called "UDI code"). The unique identifier provides mandatory information about the product, namely, serial number, product code, expiration date, and a batch/lot number, in the form of a readable data matrix barcode. Manufacturers upload the unique identifiers to a European Medicines Verification System (EMVS) and, when the medicines are shipped to their point of sale, will be transferred into national verification systems. Pharmacies throughout the European Union have been equipped with barcode scanning equipment, allowing pharmacists to confirm a product's provenance before dispensing it to a patient. In the United States, similar legislation will enter into force by 2023, The Drug Supply Chain Security Act (DSCSA), which also requires implementing a system allowing traceability and serialization of medicines (Behner et al., 2020). Although these new serialization systems offer much greater security than in the past, where medicines were identified only by a single bar code common to all units belonging to the same batch, there are some concerns regarding the implementation solutions. In Europe's case, the system is in place in the hands of a centralized entity, meaning the information is linked to a single source of information, such as a website. Therefore, although it makes counterfeiting more complicated, the system is more liable to attacks, corruption, and copying (Clark & Burstall, 2018).

A future solution to overcome problems related to counterfeiting, further increase compliance, and meet regulatory requirements in the pharma supply chain could use a DLT such as blockchain. One of the advantages of this technology is that it allows different parties to verify transactions and not change records independently afterward. Furthermore, beyond the basic traceability applications, IoT devices running in blockchain could also assist in cold chain monitoring, ensuring that pharmaceuticals comply with temperature requirements in their passage through the supply chain (Clark & Burstall, 2018).

In a supply-chain scenario with blockchain, the manufacturer starts to identify each product in its origin through a unique hash that works as its ID until it reaches the final consumer. All participants in the supply chain (including manufacturer, packager, distributor, and doctor) have a digital key by which they are known, and all of them can follow the product in real-time (Haq & Muselemu, 2018).

Pharmaceutical recall, the process of retrieving defective products, often represent logistic challenges for companies to address. Being a procedure that directly involves the final consumer, any inefficiency may have harmful repercussions on the company's reputation. Although those companies want to avoid costly product recalls (due to operational effort and associated costs), these are often unavoidable and a lesser evil when consumer safety may be at risk. There are already proposals using BT that enable open-source management of the product recall process, where different stakeholders have access to a single, transparent, monitorable, and immutable record. The use of smart-contract clarifies and ensures compliance with all the operational steps of the recall and all the steps inherent to the investigation that usually follows this type of occurrence and any CAPA (Corrective And Preventing Actions) to adopt (Wu & Lin, 2019). In the path of serialization, the multinational SAP, launched a blockchain solution for the pharma supply chain. However, unlike in the current European system, the data matrix information is processed by an algorithm and converted into a hash (64-digit chain of letters and numbers that cannot be changed) to be inserted into the blockchain it becomes forever traceable (Schmitz, 2019).

The disruption brought by BT to the pharmaceutical sector is perfectly noticeable in the supply-chain, where it has made possible cooperation projects that were once unthinkable, such as the emergence of platforms shared by competing companies without the fear of revealing sensitive information, since the privacy reserve can be guaranteed by the agreed protocol (McCauley, 2020). In the United States, a project called MediLedger was born, which already counts with several well-known companies of the pharmaceutical industry such as Gilead, Abbvie, and Pfizer that are looking for a common strategy to address supply-chain vulnerabilities. One of the vulnerabilities that companies try to overcome is the verification of the authenticity of the returned products, a process that is known to be difficult and time consuming due to the difficulty of sharing information among the different stakeholders. Another of the project's objectives is the monitoring of products throughout the distribution chain, which makes it possible to audit the conditions to which any product has been subjected; in essence, the products will be equipped with a system resembling an aircraft's black box. In addition, efforts are also being made to simplify and streamline payment processes between partners, easier access to information, and greater security. In the end, these companies looked for a common strategy for better supply-chain operability based on a single source of truth (Mediledger, 2020).

In Frankfurt, a group of researchers created a blockchain-based solution, the LifeCrypter, to improve integrity, traceability, and transparency to the global drug supply chain. This group of researchers developed a mobile app that allows end-users to know there were no deviations throughout the product's trade circuit; this happens because a smart contract and a blockchain ensure that all necessary steps are accomplished (Schöner et al., 2017).

With recourse to AWS (an Amazon's service referred to in the introduction), an app called "PharmaCrypt" has been created to improve the supply chain. The platform allows developing a smart-contract where products can be registered and transferred between the various network players without losing track. By scanning the product with the "PharmaCrypt" app on the smartphone, both patients and dispensaries will be sure of the drug's provenance (Saxena et al., 2020).

IBM has developed a blockchain solution that aims to address managing suppliers and their qualifications, working as a digital passport. The solution called "Trust Your Supplier" claims several advantages: it allows speeding up (by about 70%) the process of onboarding suppliers through the creation of an immutable record with detailed information about them; it allows reducing costs (by about 50%) related to the acquisition of new suppliers; it allows easy and fast access to all the register associated with the supplier's performance, namely reviews and evaluations of other clients; it allows access to validated information because there are third parties that validate the supplier's record; and finally, it allows the sharing of relevant information about suppliers (IBM, 2020).

BT has been an integral part of logistics solutions for vaccines against COVID-19. The vaccine from Pfizer Inc and BioNTech, for example, must be sent and stored at shallow temperatures (-60°C to -80°C) or on dry ice, and can only remain at refrigerator temperatures (2°C to 8°C) up to five days. Therefore, strict cold chain monitoring plays a significant role in ensuring the quality, safety, and efficacy of vaccines during administration. Two English hospitals, Stratford-upon-Avon and Warwick, monitor the vaccines since their origin, thanks to the technology provided by the partnership between the company Hedera Hasgraph and Everyware (Wilson, 2021). Everyware uses sensors to monitor equipment in real-time, while Hedera is a blockchain consortium backed by Google and IBM. Hedera Hasgraph uses other DLT protocol than blockchain. In Hedera Hasgraph's protocol, directed acyclic graph (DAG), the data are directly linked to each other instead of first being aggregated into a block (Kahn, 2021).

Clinical Trials

Clinical trials are studies intended to find new and better ways to prevent, diagnose, treat, and control diseases and their symptoms. They can also focus on improving the quality of life and sense of well-being of patients. Clinical trials are usually sponsored by pharmaceutical companies interested in the approval of the new molecules they are developing. Most of the time, the sponsor is in charge of preparing the protocol for a clinical trial, consisting of a plan explaining how the trial will work, what will be done, and why. Essential information in a protocol includes the number of participants, eligibility criteria, what tests patients will get and how often, what type of data will be collected, and detailed information about the treatment plan.

Clinical trials are usually conducted in phases. Potential new drugs and treatments are tested in the laboratory (pre-clinical trials) before being administered to patients. Faced with the possibility of helping to treat a specific disease, they are tested in Phase I trials (firsts tests in humans, where usually a small number of healthy volunteers are tested) to assess the drug's safety profile. If successful, the drug is used in Phase II trials (performed on patients with the disease in question) to access the appropriate dose and efficacy, and then in Phase III trials (performed in a large population) to validate safety, interactions, and adverse effects in a larger scale. Phase IV trials test drugs that are already approved (CUF academic center, 2020).

Clinical trials play a crucial role in clinical investigation by studying the effects of new drugs on humans. The demand for innovative drugs and their importance for patients waiting for them requires mechanisms to speed up the generally slow clinical trials. This speed can be achieved through BT, which allows the data to be recorded in real-time as soon as it becomes available. Clinical trials' truthfulness and transparency are essential requirements for people to trust new drugs' safety and efficacy (Glover & Hermans, 2017). Some authors state that the vast majority of clinical trials are not reproducible and that the outcomes are, therefore, unreliable. Various factors, including errors, accidental loss of data, misconduct, or fraud, compromise clinical research quality (Ioannidis, 2005).

One of the problematic aspects of clinical trials has been the recruitment of patients, which compromises its course and may precipitate their early termination and affect the conclusions of the study. Among the causes identified for the poor adherence to clinical trials are the lack of patient's awareness, difficulty in understanding complex protocols, and lack of confidence in the study itself (Zhuang et al., 2020). BT may represent a future model to surpass the mentioned problems by ensuring a decentralized, secure tracking system for any data interactions that could occur in the context of clinical trials. A determinant aspect of BT in the scope of clinical trials, is that it ensures that events are tracked in their correct chronological order, preventing a later reconstruction analysis, thus providing a significant contribution to the inviolability historicity of data (Nugent et al., 2016).

"Smart contracts," a BT associated tool, could provide more transparency and truthfulness to clinical trials while preventing a posteriori reconstruction or beautification of data. Clinical trials are composed of several steps performed sequentially. Smart contracts can function as deterministic programs ensuring that the different steps of a clinical trial are completed so that each step depends on its predecessor's execution; this is possible because every piece of information introduced in the blockchain has a timestamp. Smart contracts are tools that dictate the self-execution of a protocol by complying with its clauses. In a clinical trial, numerous steps can initially be defined in the form of smart contract clauses. In the context of a clinical trial, an example of a smart contract' clause could include only patients who have submitted their informed consent. The protocol would not allow further data to be entered and the trial to progress without all patients included in the study having submitted their informed consent (Benchoufi & Ravaud, 2017). When talking about clinical trials, it is necessary to know that patients are at the center of the equation since their data will be aggregated and analyzed to formulate research hypotheses. Therefore, studies rely on patients' consent for the assessment of their clinical data. However, several barriers may inhibit patients from sharing their data. Medical data collection is often an inconvenient and time-consuming process: patients might have to collect data from various sources asking doctors and medical centers/hospitals. The process is inconvenient and covered by bureaucracy, such as manually filling out forms. This aspect is aggravated by medical information being frequently dispersed across different organizations such as hospitals, doctors, and insurance companies, each with different IT systems and little interoperability. Besides, medical information exposes intimate aspects of people, and therefore, their sharing is often viewed reluctantly by patients, who feel that their privacy may be compromised. Finally, limited accessibility and knowledge of clinical research opportunities may prevent patients from participating in clinical trials. Usually, patients are indicated to clinical trials where their doctors are involved, with the risk that such clinical trial does not suit them most. Traditional solutions have not addressed the problems mentioned, and BT might be a game-changer improving data sharing between patients and investigators, offering a solution to more easily aggregate health data in a trusted, secure, automated, and error-free way. These can be the results of a smart contract between patient and health care stakeholders. This way, patients would be able to gather and have possession of their medical information more efficiently, having the power to decide what to share and how. BT gives patients greater autonomy and decision-making power (Baara et al., 2020).

One of the existing blockchain solutions supporting clinical trials is BlockTrial, a digital interface that allows users to run smart contracts operating on the Ethereum network. Naturally, BlockTrial is a consortium-based blockchain where only authorized clinical trial stakeholders can act. The BlokTrial solution features two types of smart contracts. One is tailored and applied to the patient (Patient SC), and the other is tailored and applicable to the researcher (Research SC). The Patient SC controls patient involvement and the granting of permissions. The Research SC allows researchers to request and receive feedback through the trial database. This entire data management process for the clinical trial is carried out using BlockTrial's Web app. Patients who wish to participate in the clinical trial must first register through the web app, where they provide their informed consent and autonomously manage the permissions, wish to grant researchers access to their data. In turn, researchers can then apply filters and access the information they need with the certainty that it is consent (Maslove et al., 2018).

Research and Development

Research and development (R&D) are involved in the earlier stages of drug discovery representing pharmaceutical innovation's very essence. Each new molecule developed by a pharmaceutical company with the potential to reach the market is considered a valuable resource that must be patented to ensure the protection of intellectual property. The protection of intellectual property is crucial to a company's future (pwc Israel, 2020).

Intellectual property is an attribution of a legal right to the market's exclusive exploitation resulting from intellectual creations born of the human spirit. Market exclusivity is essential for companies in the pharmaceutical industry because it makes it possible to recover all the investment associated with the lengthy process of developing and bringing to market a new medicinal product. The average time from pre-clinical trials to a new drug's approval is 12 years, with costs around $1 billion in the US (Norman, 2016).

The traditional process of patenting a molecule is complicated, non-transparent, time-consuming because of the bureaucracy involved, and costly, sometimes hindering its access to entities with less financial capacity, such as universities. Blockchain entails the ability to track the entire life cycle of a right, with the possibility to address confidentiality concerns. Also, it allows for smoother intellectual property rights audits. Besides, smart-contracts can serve as a facilitating element in establishing agreements between companies for the transaction of intellectual property rights (Pascal Asselot, 2020). The preciousness of intellectual property and the insecurities surrounding existing data management systems mean that there are currently significant barriers to the sharing of information, which could in many cases contribute to speeding up research and become beneficial not only for business but also for society as a whole. Take, for example, the case of epidemic outbreaks, where the scientific community's rapid and assertive response can become vital. The lack of confidence in data protection leads to a latent reluctance on pharmaceutical companies to share scientific information at the early stages of research, which often hampers international cooperation. A clear example of a lack of cooperation dates to 2005, when the Indonesian government refused to share samples of the H5N1 virus because of concerns about a future vaccine's suitability. According to the Nagoya Protocol, the Indonesian government's position prevented the investigation from progressing in the absence of consent. Furthermore, Competition between laboratories can lead to fragmentation of intellectual property, with lengthy and costly legal proceedings to determine the legitimate owner of the innovation, which every company wants to avoid (Norman, 2016).

A private blockchain seems to be the ideal solution to overcome barriers, reserve data privacy, and safeguard intellectual property. This technology can meet all the requirements relating to the protection of a patent's data and, if necessary, of proving its possession employing a series of features. For instance, it can provide timestamp (indicating time of creation), proof of content (the content by the time of creation), identity (ensure who created the electronic record through the existence of a private key/digital signature), and immutability (guaranty that records were not changed, which is inherent to the blockchain protocol) (van der Waal et al., 2020). A recent example of successful cooperation in new drug research is the partnership between Nebula Genomics and biopharmaceutical company EMD Serono (a Merck subsidiary). The core business of Nebula Genomics is genomic sequencing, usually done to private individuals who are curious about their genetic origins or propensity to develop specific pathologies. EMD Serono is a biopharmaceutical company interested in the development of biological drugs. In the partnership between the two companies, patients have the power to make a profit by providing their data, which anonymously enter the blockchain to become accessible to researchers, thus contributing to scientific research progress (Grishin, 2019).

CONCLUSION

Blockchain is a disruptive technology that is gradually being implemented on a global scale by several organizations. The need for a decentralized system without intermediaries has triggered the expansion of these digital phenomena, representing significant economic and social transformations. Digital tokens, smart contracts, and IoT are modern tools with growing interest for many companies, which emerged alongside BT. In the business world, streamlining processes, facilitating trade, reducing costs, increasing security, and, above all, boosting confidence among people and organizations are primary goals to which blockchain can respond.

The Web and the Semantic Web development could be an opportunity to emerge decentralized innovative symbioses due to BT, which guarantees security in information storage through its consensus and immutability protocol. Sir Tim Berners-Lee took the initiative to address the need for a decentralized Internet by proposing the SOLID ecosystem, where patients can save and control their medical records in "personal online data stores." Solutions like this open doors to the decentralization of medical records and health systems with greater interoperability between the various stakeholders. The patient is the primary beneficiary by receiving more personalized and more convenient health care.

Pharmaceutical Industry is a growing sector willing to invest in BT to ensure its products' safety, efficacy, and quality. Clinical trials, Supply chain, and R&D are areas where the technology is already being implemented with promising results.

In supply-chain, the recognized need to combat counterfeit drugs' threat has led to adopting essential measures such as the serialization of products. However, the process falls on a centralized entity, raising two significant concerns: a centralized entity is more likely to be corrupted; if the centralized entity is the target of some computer attack or simply if the servers are down, the information is no longer accessible and can be irreversibly adulterated. The concerns mentioned are surmountable by the use of blockchain. It enables a highly secure and decentralized record (with several copies spread among multiple nodes of the network), working as a single source of truth.

Blockchain can add confidence in clinical trial outcomes since it prevents later reconstruction of the records. Besides, smart contracts could be put in place to ensure the accomplishment of protocols. Furthermore, patient data protection is no longer a concern with blockchain because all the data can be anonymized.

Research and development (R&D) are involved in the earlier stages of drug discovery representing pharmaceutical innovation's essence. BT can provide timestamps, proof of content, identity, and immutability, all the requirements to protect a patent.

A recent example of successful R&D cooperation happens between Nebula Genomics and EMD Serono. Patients can profit by making it anonymous their blockchain data, which can then be accessible to researchers, thus contributing to scientific research progress.

In short, it is essential to note that blockchain is at the epicenter of a progressive digital revolution, on which many companies are already betting. Blockchain's operating principles and various advantages constitute an added value for the Pharmaceutical Industry. BT is changing the supply chain, clinical trials, and research, offering more transparency, traceability, and security.

REFERENCES

Baara, M., Lipset, C., Kudumala, A., Fox, J., & Israel, A. (2020). *Blockchain opportunities for patient data donation & clinical research.* https://www2.deloitte.com/content/dam/Deloitte/us/Documents/process-and-operations/us-cons-blockchain-opportunities-patient-data-donation-clinical-research.pdf

Behner, P., Hecht, M.-L., & Wahl, F. (2020). *Fighting counterfeit pharmaceuticals & New defenses for an underestimated — and growing — menace.* https://www.strategyand.pwc.com/gx/en/insights/2017/fighting-counterfeit-pharmaceuticals/fighting-counterfeit-pharmaceuticals.pdf

Bhowmik, D., & Feng, T. (2017). The multimedia blockchain: A distributed and tamper-proof media transaction framework. *22nd International Conference on Digital Signal Processing (DSP),* 1–5. 10.1109/ICDSP.2017.8096051

Bingham, J. (2019). *How The Decentralized Web Will Drive Innovation In The Healthcare Industry.* Janeiro Digital. https://www.healthitoutcomes.com/doc/how-the-decentralized-web-will-drive-innovation-in-the-healthcare-industry-0001

Bocek, T. B., Rodrigues, B., Strasser, T., & Stiller, B. (2017). Blockchains Everywhere - A Use-case of Blockchains in the Pharma Supply-Chain. *2017 IFIP/IEEE International Symposium on Integrated Network Management (IM2017)*. 10.23919/INM.2017.7987376

Cano-Benito, J., & Cimmino, A. (2019). *G.-C. R.* Towards Blockchain and Semantic Web.

Cellan-Jones, R. (2020). *NHS data: Can web creator Sir Tim Berners-Lee fix it?* https://www.bbc.com/news/technology-54871705

Chen, H., & Xie, G. (2010). The use of web ontology languages and other semantic web tools in drug discovery. *Expert Opinion on Drug Discovery*, *5*(5), 413–423. doi:10.1517/17460441003762709 PMID:22823127

Chen, Y. (2018). Blockchain tokens and the potential democratization of entrepreneurship and innovation. *Business Horizons*, *61*(4), 567–575. doi:10.1016/j.bushor.2018.03.006

Clark, B., & Burstall, R. (2018). Blockchain, IP and the pharma industry-how distributed ledger technologies can help secure the pharma supply chain. Journal of Intellectual Property Law and Practice, 13(7).

Conway, L. (2020). *Blockchain Explained*. Investopedia. https://www.investopedia.com/terms/b/blockchain.asp

Costello, K. (2019). *Rapid Evolution of the Blockchain Platform Market*. https://www.gartner.com/en/newsroom/press-releases/2019-07-03-gartner-predicts-90--of-current-enterprise-blockchain

CUF academic center. (2020). *Cuf.pt*. https://www.cuf.pt/cuf-academic-center/investigacao

Deloitte. (2020). *5 Blockchain Trends for 2020*. https://www2.deloitte.com/content/dam/Deloitte/ie/Documents/Consulting/Blockchain-Trends-2020-report.pdf

e-estonia. (2020). *KSI Blockchain*. https://e-estonia.com/solutions/security-and-safety/ksi-blockchain/

EMA. (2020). *Good distribution practice*. https://www.ema.europa.eu/en/human-regulatory/post-authorisation/compliance/good-distribution-practice

Golosova, J., & Romanovs, A. (2018). The Advantages and Disadvantages of the Blockchain Technology. In *2018 IEEE 6th Workshop on Advances in Information, Electronic and Electrical Engineering (AIEEE)*. IEEE.

Gurstein, M. (2011). Open data: Empowering the empowered or effective data use for everyone? *First Monday*, *16*(2).

Hageman, J. R., Allen, K., Anderson, T., & Goldstein, M. (2020). Clinical Pearl: The Clinical Utility of the 'World Wide Web'with Historical Perspective from Tim Berners-Lee's Book 'Weaving the Web.' *TODAY Peer Reviewed Research. News and Information*, *15*(10), 122.

Haq, I., & Muselemu, O. (2018). Blockchain Technology in Pharmaceutical Industry to Prevent Counterfeit Drugs. *International Journal of Computers and Applications*, *180*(25), 8–12.

Healtheuropa.eu. (2019). *Health Europa*. Learning from the Estonian E-Health System. https://www.healtheuropa.eu/estonian-e-health-system/89750/

IBM. (2020). *Trust Your Supplier Solution Transforms Supplier Management.* https://www.ibm.com/blockchain/solutions/trust-your-supplier

Ioannidis, J. P. A. (2005). Why most published research findings are false. In Getting to Good: Research Integrity in the Biomedical Sciences (Vol. 2, Issue 8). Academic Press.

Kanza, S., & Frey, J. G. (2019). A new wave of innovation in Semantic web tools for drug discovery. In Expert Opinion on Drug Discovery. Academic Press.

Kõnd, K., & Lillevāli, A. (2019). E-Prescription success in Estonia: The journey from paper to pharmacogenomics. *Eurohealth (London), 25*(2), 18–19.

Lopez, P. G., Montresor, A., & Datta, A. (2019). Please, do not decentralize the Internet with (permissionless) blockchains! *2019 IEEE 39th International Conference on Distributed Computing Systems (ICDCS)*, 1901–1911.

Marbouh, D., Abbasi, T., Maasmi, F., Omar, I. A., Debe, M. S., Salah, K., Jayaraman, R., & Ellahham, S. (2020). Blockchain for COVID-19: Review, Opportunities, and a Trusted Tracking System. *Arabian Journal for Science and Engineering*, 1–17.

Maslove, D. M., Klein, J., Brohman, K., & Martin, P. (2018). Using Blockchain Technology to Manage Clinical Trials Data : A Proof-of-Concept Study. *JMIR Medical Informatics, 6*(4), 1–7.

McCauley, A. (2020). Why Big Pharma Is Betting on Blockchain. *Harvard Business Review.*

Mettler, M., & Hsg, M. A. (2016). Blockchain Technology in Healthcare The Revolution Starts Here. In *2016 IEEE 18th International Conference on e-Health Networking, Applications and Services, Healthcom.* IEEE.

Nakamoto, S. (2008). *A peer-to-peer electronic cash system.* Bitcoin. https://bitcoin.org/bitcoin.pdf

Nørfeldt, L., Bøtker, J., Edinger, M., Genina, N., & Rantanen, J. (2019). Cryptopharmaceuticals : Increasing the Safety of Medication by a Blockchain of Pharmaceutical Products. *Journal of Pharmaceutical Sciences, 108*, 2838–2841.

Nugent, T., Upton, D., & Cimpoesu, M. (2016). Improving data transparency in clinical trials using blockchain smart contracts. *F1000 Research, 5*, 1–4.

Paulos, J. (2020). *Investigating Decentralized Management of Health and Fitness Data.* Academic Press.

Premkumar, A., & Shrimati, C. (2020). Application of Blockchain and IoT towards Pharmaceutical Industry. *2020 6th International Conference on Advanced Computing & Communication Systems (ICACCS)*, 729–733.

pwc Israel. (2020). https://www.pwc.com/il/en/pharmaceuticals/intellectual-property-protection.html

Saxena, N., Thomas, I., Gope, P., Burnap, P., & Kumar, N. (2020). PharmaCrypt: Blockchain for Critical Pharmaceutical Industry to Counterfeit Drugs. *Computer, 53*(7), 29–44.

Schöner, M., Kourouklis, D., Sandner, P., Gonzalez, E., & Förster, J. (2017). Blockchain Technology in the Pharmaceutical Industry. *FSBC Working Paper,* 1–9.

Settanni, E., Harrington, T. S., & Srai, J. S. (2017). Pharmaceutical supply chain models: A synthesis from a systems view of operations research. *Operations Research Perspectives*, *4*, 74–95.

SGS. (2020). *Good Distribution Practices (GDP) Certification For Pharmaceutical Industry*. https://www.sgs.com/en/life-sciences/audit-certification-and-verification/quality/good-distribution-practices-gdp-certification-for-pharmaceutical-industry

Shute, R. (2017). *Blockchain Technology in Drug Discovery: Use-Cases in R&D*. Drug Discovery World.

Steinwandter, V., & Herwig, C. (2019). Provable data integrity in the pharmaceutical industry based on version control systems and the blockchain. *PDA Journal of Pharmaceutical Science and Technology*.

Underwood, S. (2016). Blockchain beyond bitcoin. *Communications of the ACM*, *59*(11), 15–17.

Van Norman, G. A. (2016). Drugs, Devices, and the FDA: Part 1: An Overview of Approval Processes for Drugs. *JACC. Basic to Translational Science*, *1*(3).

Wilson, T. (2021). *British hospitals use blockchain to track COVID-19 vaccines*. https://www.reuters.com/article/health-coronavirus-blockchain/british-hospitals-use-blockchain-to-track-covid-19-vaccines-idUSL4N2JQ3FD

Yeung, C. A., Liccardi, I., Lu, K., Seneviratne, O., & Berners-lee, T. (2009). Decentralization : The Future of Online Social Networking. In *W3C Workshop on the Future of Social Networking Position Papers* (Vol. 2). Academic Press.

Zheng, Z., Xie, S., Dai, H., Chen, X., & Wang, H. (2017). An Overview of Blockchain Technology: Architecture, Consensus, and Future Trends. *2017 IEEE International Congress on Big Data (BigData Congress)*, 557–564.

Zhuang, Y., Sheets, L. R., Shae, Z., Chen, Y.-W., Tsai, J. J. P., & Shyu, C.-R. (2020). Applying Blockchain Technology to Enhance Clinical Trial Recruitment. *AMIA ... Annual Symposium Proceedings - AMIA Symposium. AMIA Symposium*, *2019*, 1276–1285.

Compilation of References

Aarvik, P. (2020). *Blockchain as an anti-corruption tool. Case examples and introduction.* Academic Press.

Abdel-Basset, M., Chang, V., & Nabeeh, N. A. (2020). An intelligent framework using disruptive technologies for CO-VID-19 analysis. *Technological Forecasting and Social Change, 120431.* Advance online publication. doi:10.1016/j.techfore.2020.120431 PMID:33162617

Abu Bakar, N., Rosbi, S., & Uzaki, K. (2017). Cryptocurrency Framework Diagnostics from Islamic Finance Perspective: A New Insight of Bitcoin System Transaction. *International Journal of Management Science and Business Administration, 4*(1), 19–28. doi:10.18775/ijmsba.1849-5664-5419.2014.41.1003

Abu-elezz, I., Hassan, A., Nazeemudeen, A., Househ, M., & Abd-alrazaq, A. (2020). The benefits and threats of block-chain technology in healthcare: A scoping review. *International Journal of Medical Informatics, 142*(August), 104246. doi:10.1016/j.ijmedinf.2020.104246 PMID:32828033

Adeodato, R., & Pournouri, S. (2020). Secure Implementation of E-Governance: A Case Study About Estonia. In *Cyber Defence in the Age of AI, Smart Societies and Augmented Humanity* (pp. 397–429). Springer. doi:10.1007/978-3-030-35746-7_18

Adiyatma, S. E., & Maharani, D. F. (2020). Cryptocurrency's Control in the Misuse of Money Laundering Acts as an Effort to Maintain the Resilience and Security of the State. *Lex Scientia Law Review, 4*(1), 70–82. doi:10.15294/lesrev.v4i1.38257

Adnan, K., & Akbar, R. (2019). An analytical study of information extraction from unstructured and multidimensional big data. *Journal of Big Data, 6*(1), 91. Advance online publication. doi:10.118640537-019-0254-8

Agbo, C., Mahmoud, Q., & Eklund, J. (2019). Blockchain Technology in Healthcare: A Systematic Review. *Health Care, 7*(2), 56. doi:10.3390/healthcare7020056 PMID:30987333

Agrawal, A., Catalini, C., & Goldfarb, A. (2014). Some simple economics of crowdfunding. *Innovation Policy and the Economy, 14*, 63–97. Advance online publication. doi:10.1086/674021

Ahluwalia, S., Mahto, R. V., & Guerrero, M. (2020). Blockchain technology and startup financing: A transaction cost economics perspective. *Technological Forecasting and Social Change, 151*, 119854. doi:10.1016/j.techfore.2019.119854

AICPA. (2020). *Privacy Risk Management.* Available online at: https://www.aicpa.org/interestareas/informationtechnology/resources/privacy-risk-management.html

Akhtar, Z. (2019, November). From Blockchain to Hashgraph: Distributed Ledger Technologies in the Wild. In *2019 International Conference on Electrical, Electronics and Computer Engineering (UPCON)* (pp. 1-6). IEEE. 10.1109/UPCON47278.2019.8980029

Al Mamun, M., Uddin, G. S., Suleman, M. T., & Kang, S. H. (2020). Geopolitical risk, uncertainty and Bitcoin investment. *Physica A, 540*, 123107. doi:10.1016/j.physa.2019.123107

Albayati, H., Kim, S. K., & Rho, J. J. (2020). Accepting financial transactions using blockchain technology and cryptocurrency: A customer perspective approach. *Technology in Society, 62*, 101320. Advance online publication. doi:10.1016/j.techsoc.2020.101320

Alcazar, C. V. (2017). Data you can trust. *Air and Space Power Journal, 31*(2), 91–101.

Alexandru, I. (2018). *Comparative administrative law issues regarding central and local government*. Societatea de Stiinte Juridice si Administrative.

Alfieri, E. (2019). *Cryptocurrencies and market efficiency. Business administration*. Université Grenoble Alpes.

Alharam, A. K., & El-Madany, W. (2017). The Effects of Cyber-Security on Healthcare Industry. *IEEE GCC Conference and Exhibition GCCCE*.

Ali Sina User, I. A. (2020). The inevitable digitalization of the globe and the steps that are bringing us there. *New Europe*. https://www.neweurope.eu/article/the-inevitable-digitalization-of-the-globe-and-the-steps-that-are-bringing-us-there/

Ali, F., Aloqaily, M., Alfandi, O., & Ozkasap, O. (2020). *Peer-to-Peer Blockchain based Energy Trading*. arXiv preprint arXiv:2001.00746.

Aligica, P. D., & Tarko, V. (2012). Polycentricity: From Polanyi to Ostrom, and beyond. *Governance: An International Journal of Policy, Administration and Institutions, 25*(2), 237–262. doi:10.1111/j.1468-0491.2011.01550.x

Ali, R., & Narula, N. (2020). *Redesigning digital money: What can we learn from a decade of cryptocurrencies. Digital Currency Iniative (DCI)*. MIT Media Lab.

Allan, K., & Mortensen, J. (2020). Legal Identity Documenting in Disasters: Perpetuating Systems of Injustice. In Natural Hazards and Disaster Justice (pp. 261-278). Palgrave Macmillan.

Alleman, J. (2018). Threat of Internet Platforms: Facebook, Google, etc. In *29th European Regional Conference of the International Telecommunications Society (ITS): "Towards a Digital Future: Turning Technology into Markets?"*. Trento, Italy: International Telecommunications Society (ITS).

Allen, S., Čapkun, S., Eyal, I., Fanti, G., Ford, B. A., Grimmelmann, J., & Zhang, F. (2020). *Design Choices for Central Bank Digital Currency: Policy and Technical Considerations (No. w27634)*. National Bureau of Economic Research. doi:10.3386/w27634

Almasoud, A. S., Eljazzar, M. M., & Hussain, F. (2018). Toward a self-learned smart contracts. *Proceedings - 2018 IEEE 15th International Conference on e-Business Engineering, ICEBE 2018*, 269-273. 10.1109/ICEBE.2018.00051

Almeida, R. J. F. D. (2017). *Generation Y: an analysis of millennials' skills, perceptions, values and expectations against the promise (s) of the Gen-Y City project* (Doctoral dissertation). Universidade de Coimbra.

Almeida, M. (1982). *Catálogo geral de cédulas de Portugal / Low emergency paper Money of Portugal*. Sociedade Portuguesa de Numismática.

Al-Omari, A., Rabaan, A. A., Salih, S., Al-Tawfiq, J. A., & Memish, Z. A. (2019). MERS coronavirus outbreak: Implications for emerging viral infections. *Diagnostic Microbiology and Infectious Disease, 93*(3), 265–285. Advance online publication. doi:10.1016/j.diagmicrobio.2018.10.011 PMID:30413355

Alpay, L. L., Henkemans, O. B., Otten, W., Rovekamp, T. A. J. M., & Dumay, A. C. M. (2010). E-health Applications and Services for Patient Empowerment: Directions for Best Practices in The Netherlands. *Telemedicine Journal and e-Health, 16*(7), 787–791. doi:10.1089/tmj.2009.0156 PMID:20815745

Altcointoday. (2017). *Bitcoin and Ethereum vs Visa and PayPal – Transactions per second - Altcoin Today*. Altcointoday.

Amend, J., Kaiser, J., Uhlig, L., Urbach, N., & Völter, F. (2021). *What Do We Really Need? A Systematic Literature Review of the Requirements for Blockchain-based E-government Services*. Academic Press.

AmetranoF. M. (2016). Hayek money: The cryptocurrency price stability solution. *Available at* SSRN 2425270.

Ammous, S. (2018). *The bitcoin standard: the decentralized alternative to central banking*. John Wiley & Sons.

Anderson, C. (2009). *Free: The future of a radical price*. Random House.

Andolfatto, D., & Spewak, A. (2019). Whither the price of bitcoin? *Economic Synopses*, (1), 1–2.

Angeletti, F., Chatzigiannakis, I., & Vitaletti, A. (2017). The role of blockchain and IoT in recruiting participants for digital clinical trials. *2017 25th International Conference on Software, Telecommunications and Computer Networks (SoftCOM)*, 1–5. 10.23919/SOFTCOM.2017.8115590

Angst, C. M., & Agarwal, R. (2009). Adoption of electronic health records in the presence of privacy concerns: The elaboration likelihood model and Individual Persuasion. *Management Information Systems Quarterly, 33*(2), 339–370. doi:10.2307/20650295

AnteL. (2021). How Elon Musk's Twitter Activity Moves Cryptocurrency Markets. *Available at* SSRN 3778844.

Antonopoulos, A. M. (2016). *The internet of money* (Vol. 1). Merkle Bloom LLC.

Antonopoulos, A. M. (2016). *The Internet of Money* (Vol. 1). Merkle Bloom LLC.

Antonopoulos, A. M. (2017). *Mastering Bitcoin: Programming the open blockchain*. O'Reilly Media, Inc.

Antonopoulos, A. M. (2017). *The Internet of Money: Volume Two*. Merkle Bloom LLC.

Apis, D., & Benligiray, B. (2020). *Decentralized APIs for Web 3.0*. Academic Press.

Applebaum, A. (2012). Iron curtain: the crushing of Eastern Europe 1944-56. Penguin UK.

Ardo, A. A., & Zamani, E. D. (2019, April). Mobile phone for financial inclusiveness and empowerment: a case study of anchor borrowers programme. In *Proceedings of 2019 UK Academy for Information Systems International Conference*. AIS.

Aristotle. (2004). *Nicomachean Ethics* (R. Crisp, Trans.). Cambridge University Press. doi:10.1017/CBO9781139600514

Arslanian, H., Fischer, F., Arslanian, H., & Fischer, F. (2019). Blockchain As an Enabling Technology. In The Future of Finance. doi:10.1007/978-3-030-14533-0_10

Atlam, H. F., Alenezi, A., Alassafi, M. O., & Wills, G. B. (2018). Blockchain with Internet of Things: Benefits, Challenges, and Future Directions. *International Journal of Intelligent Systems and Applications, 10*(6), 40–48. doi:10.5815/ijisa.2018.06.05

Atzei, N., Bartoletti, M., & Cimoli, T. (2017). A survey of attacks on Ethereum smart contracts. *Universit`a Degli Studi Di Cagliari, 10204 LNCS*(July), 164–186. doi:10.1007/978-3-662-54455-6_8

AtzoriM. (2015). Blockchain technology and decentralized governance: Is the state still necessary? Available at SSRN 2709713. doi:10.2139srn.2709713

Avital, M. (2018). Peer Review: Toward a Blockchain-enabled Market-based Ecosystem. *Peer Review : Toward a Blockchain-enabled Market-based Ecosystem, 42*, 646–653. Advance online publication. doi:10.17705/1CAIS.04228

Ayed, A. B. (2017). A conceptual secure blockchain-based electronic voting system. *Int. J. Netw. Secur. Its Appl., 9*, 1–9.

Aysan, A. F., Demir, E., Gozgor, G., & Lau, C. K. M. (2019). Effects of the geopolitical risks on Bitcoin returns and volatility. *Research in International Business and Finance, 47*, 511–518. doi:10.1016/j.ribaf.2018.09.011

Azati. (2020). *How Much Does It Cost To Develop Blockchain In 2020.* Azati. https://azati.ai/how-much-does-it-cost-to-blockchain/

Baara, M., Lipset, C., Kudumala, A., Fox, J., & Israel, A. (2020). *Blockchain opportunities for patient data donation & clinical research.* https://www2.deloitte.com/content/dam/Deloitte/us/Documents/process-and-operations/us-cons-blockchain-opportunities-patient-data-donation-clinical-research.pdf

Baird, L. (2016). *The swirlds hashgraph consensus algorithm: Fair, fast, byzantine fault tolerance.* Swirlds Tech Reports SWIRLDS-TR-2016-01, Tech. Rep.

Baird, L., Harmon, M., & Madsen, P. (2018). *Hedera: A governing council & public hashgraph network.* The trust layer of the internet, whitepaper, 1, 1-97.

Bakarich, K. M., Castonguay, J. J., & O'Brien, P. E. (2020). The Use of Blockchains to Enhance Sustainability Reporting and Assurance. *Accounting Perspectives, 19*(4), 389–412. doi:10.1111/1911-3838.12241

Bao, J., He, D., Luo, M., & Choo, K. K. R. (2020). A survey of blockchain applications in the energy sector. *IEEE Systems Journal*, 1–12. doi:10.1109/JSYST.2020.2998791

Baran, P. (1964). On distributed communications networks. *IEEE Transactions on Communications Systems, 12*(1), 1–9. doi:10.1109/TCOM.1964.1088883

Barański, S., Szymański, J., Sobecki, A., Gil, D., & Mora, H. (2020). Practical I-Voting on Stellar Blockchain. *Applied Sciences (Basel, Switzerland), 10*(21), 7606. doi:10.3390/app10217606

Barki, A., & Gouget, A. (2020). *Achieving privacy and accountability in traceable digital currency.* Cryptology ePrint Archive, Report 2020/1565.

Barnes, A., Brake, C., & Perry, T. (2016). *Digital Voting with the use of Blockchain Technology.* Team Plymouth Pioneers – Plymouth University.

Barnes, S. B. (2006). A privacy paradox: Social networking in the united states. *First Monday, 11*(9). Advance online publication. doi:10.5210/fm.v11i9.1394

Barreiro-Gomez, J., & Tembine, H. (2019). Blockchain token economics: A mean-field-type game perspective. *IEEE Access: Practical Innovations, Open Solutions, 7*, 64603–64613. doi:10.1109/ACCESS.2019.2917517

Barth, S., & De Jong, M. D. (2017). The privacy paradox–Investigating discrepancies between expressed privacy concerns and actual online behavior–A systematic literature review. *Telematics and Informatics, 34*(7), 1038–1058. doi:10.1016/j.tele.2017.04.013

Bate, R. (2017). *India's dodgy pharmacy. AEI Paper & Studies.* COVB.

Baudier, P., Kondrateva, G., Ammi, C., & Seulliet, E. (2021). Peace engineering: The contribution of blockchain systems to the e-voting process. *Technological Forecasting and Social Change, 162*, 120397. doi:10.1016/j.techfore.2020.120397 PMID:33071364

BBC. (2018). *Singapore personal data hack hits 1.5m, health authority says*. BBC News. Retrieved Feb 25th 2021 from https://www.bbc.com/news/world-asia-44900507

Becker, C. (2020). *Financial services powered by Ethereum smart contracts grow exponentially*. Investec. https://www.investec.com/en_za/focus/innovation/financial-services-powered-by-ethereum-smart-contracts-grow-exponentially-in-2020.html

Beck, R., Müller-Bloch, C., & King, J. L. (2018). Governance in the blockchain economy: A framework and research agenda. *Journal of the Association for Information Systems*, *19*(10), 1020–1034. doi:10.17705/1jais.00518

Beever, J., McDaniel, R., & Stanlick, N. A. (2019). *Understanding Digital Ethics: Cases and Contexts*. Routledge. doi:10.4324/9781315282138

Behner, P., Hecht, M.-L., & Wahl, F. (2020). *Fighting counterfeit pharmaceuticals & New defenses for an underestimated —and growing—menace*. https://www.strategyand.pwc.com/gx/en/insights/2017/fighting-counterfeit-pharmaceuticals/fighting-counterfeit-pharmaceuticals.pdf

Beller, J. (2020). Economic Media: Crypto and the Myth of Total Liquidity. *Australian Humanities Review*, *66*, 215–225.

Bellini, E., Iraqi, Y., & Damiani, E. (2020). Blockchain-based distributed trust and reputation management systems: A survey. *IEEE Access: Practical Innovations, Open Solutions*, *8*, 21127–21151. doi:10.1109/ACCESS.2020.2969820

Benchoufi, M., & Ravaud, P. (2017). Blockchain technology for improving clinical research quality. In Trials (Vol. 18, Issue 1, p. 335). BioMed Central Ltd. doi:10.118613063-017-2035-z

Benchoufi, M., Altman, D., & Ravaud, P. (2019). From Clinical Trials to Highly Trustable Clinical Trials: Blockchain in Clinical Trials, a Game Changer for Improving Transparency? *Frontiers in Blockchain*, *2*, 23. doi:10.3389/fbloc.2019.00023

Benchoufi, M., Porcher, R., & Ravaud, P. (2018). Blockchain protocols in clinical trials: Transparency and traceability of consent. *F1000 Research*, *6*, 66. doi:10.12688/f1000research.10531.5 PMID:29167732

Bencsik, A., Jakubik, M., & Juhasz, T. (2020). The Economic Consequences of Trust and Distrust in Knowledge-Intensive Organizations. *Journal of Competitiveness*, *12*(3), 28–46. doi:10.7441/joc.2020.03.02

Bengio, Y., Ippolito, D., Janda, R., Jarvie, M., Prud'homme, B., Rousseau, J. F., ... Yu, Y. W. (2020). Inherent privacy limitations of decentralized contact tracing apps. *Journal of the American Medical Informatics Association: JAMIA*. Advance online publication. doi:10.1093/jamia/ocaa153 PMID:32584990

Benhabib, S. (1997). Between Facts and Norms: Contributions to a Discourse Theory of Law and Democracy. *The American Political Science Review*, *91*(3), 725–726. doi:10.2307/2952099

Beniiche, A. (2020). *A study of blockchain oracles*. arXiv preprint arXiv:2004.07140.

Benítez-Martínez, F. L., Hurtado-Torres, M. V., & Romero-Frías, E. (2021). A neural blockchain for a tokenizable e-Participation model. *Neurocomputing*, *423*, 703–712. doi:10.1016/j.neucom.2020.03.116

Bennett, B. (2017). *Healthcoin - blockchain-enabled platform for diabetes prevention*. Retrieved January 29, 2021, from https://blockchainhealthcarereview.com/healthcoin-blockchain-enabled-platform-for-diabetes-prevention/

Berg, A. (2020). The Identity, Fungibility and Anonymity of Money. *Economic Papers: A Journal of Applied Economics and Policy*, *39*(2), 104-117.

Berg, C., Davidson, S., & Potts, J. (2018). *Beyond money crypto currencies.pdf*. Scribd. https://www.scribd.com/document/426669100/Beyond-money-crypto-currencies-pdf

BergC.DavidsonS.PottsJ. (2017). Blockchains industrialise trust. Available at SSRN 3074070.

Berg, C., Davidson, S., & Potts, J. (2019). BT as economic infrastructure: Revisiting the electronic markets hypothesis. *Frontiers in Blockchain, 2*, 22. doi:10.3389/fbloc.2019.00022

Bergeron, J., Nguyen, A., Alt, C., Brewster, N., Krohn, T., Luong, V., ... Moss-Pultz, S. (2020). Simulating patient matching to clinical trials using a property rights blockchain. *Digital Medicine, 6*(1), 44. doi:10.4103/digm.digm_30_19

Bernabe, J. B., Canovas, J. L., Hernandez-Ramos, J. L., Moreno, R. T., & Skarmeta, A. (2019). Privacy-preserving solutions for Blockchain: Review and challenges. *IEEE Access: Practical Innovations, Open Solutions, 7*, 164908–164940. doi:10.1109/ACCESS.2019.2950872

Berners-Lee, T. Fielding, R. & Frystyk, H. (1996). *Hypertext transfer protocol--HTTP/1.0*. Academic Press.

Berry, P. (2020). Troubleshooting algorithms: A book review of Weapons of Math Destruction by Cathy O'Neil. *The McMaster Journal of Communication, 12*(2), 91–96. doi:10.15173/mjc.v12i2.2450

Berwick, D. M. (2020). Choices for the "new normal". *Journal of the American Medical Association, 323*(21), 2125–2126. doi:10.1001/jama.2020.6949 PMID:32364589

Bhowmik, D., & Feng, T. (2017). The multimedia blockchain: A distributed and tamper-proof media transaction framework. *22nd International Conference on Digital Signal Processing (DSP)*, 1–5. 10.1109/ICDSP.2017.8096051

Bhushan, B. (2018). Historical evolution of magnetic data storage devices and related conferences. Microsystem Technologies. doi:10.100700542-018-4133-6

Bhutani, A., & Wadhwani, P. (2017). *Blockchain Technology Market 2019-2025 | Global Report*. https://www.gminsights.com/industry-analysis/blockchain-technology-market

Bichler, S., & Nitzan, J. (2021). *Corporate Power and the Future of US Capitalism*. Real-World Economics Review Blog.

Biersteker, T. J., & Weber, C. (2011). The social construction of state sovereignty. In State Sovereignty as Social Construct. doi:10.1017/CBO9780511598685.001

Bindseil, U. (2019). Central Bank Digital Currency: Financial System Implications and Control. *International Journal of Political Economy, 48*(4), 303–335. doi:10.1080/08911916.2019.1693160

Bingham, J. (2019). *How The Decentralized Web Will Drive Innovation In The Healthcare Industry*. Janeiro Digital. https://www.healthitoutcomes.com/doc/how-the-decentralized-web-will-drive-innovation-in-the-healthcare-industry-0001

Birch, D. (2020). *Digital Currency Revolution*. Centre for the Study.

Bisbal, J., & Berry, D. (2011). An Analysis Framework for Electronic Health Record Systems Interoperation and Collaboration in Shared Healthcare. *Methods of Information in Medicine, 50*(2), 180–189. doi:10.3414/ME09-01-0002 PMID:19936438

Bjercke, B., & Finlow-Bates, K. (2020). *Decoupling Bitcoins from Their Transaction History Using the Coinbase Transaction*. Academic Press.

Bland, R. (2012). From Gordian III to the Gallic Empire (AD 238-274). In W Metcalf (Ed.), *The Oxford Handbook of Greek and Roman Coinage* (pp. 514-537). Oxford University Press. https://doi:10.1093/oxfordhb/9780195305746.013.0029

Blaustein, A. P. (1987). Our Most Important Export: The Influence of the United States Constitution Abroad. *Conn. J. Int'l L., 3*, 15.

Bleier, A., Goldfarb, A., & Tuckerc, C. (2020). Consumer privacy and the future of data-based innovation and marketing. *International Journal of Research in Marketing*, *37*(3), 466–480. doi:10.1016/j.ijresmar.2020.03.006

Blockchain and the General Data Protection Regulation Can distributed ledgers be squared with European data protection law? (n.d.). doi:10.2861/535

Blue, A. (2020). Evaluating Estonian E-residency as a tool of soft power. *Place Branding and Public Diplomacy*, 1–9. doi:10.105741254-020-00182-3

Blumenthal, D., & Tavenner, M. (2010). The "Meaningful Use" Regulation for Electronic Health Records. *The New England Journal of Medicine*, *363*(6), 501–504. doi:10.1056/NEJMp1006114 PMID:20647183

Bocek, T. B., Rodrigues, B., Strasser, T., & Stiller, B. (2017). Blockchains Everywhere - A Use-case of Blockchains in the Pharma Supply-Chain. *2017 IFIP/IEEE International Symposium on Integrated Network Management (IM2017)*. 10.23919/INM.2017.7987376

Boettke, P. J., & Prychitko, D. (2011). 1985: A defining year in the history of modern Austrian economics. *The Review of Austrian Economics*, *24*(2), 129–139. doi:10.100711138-011-0142-8

Bopearachchi, O. (2017). Achaemenids and Mauryas: Emergence of coins and plastic art in India. In A. Patel & T. Daryaee (Eds.), *India and Iran in the Longue Durée* (pp. 15–47). UCI Indian Centre for Persian Studies.

Bostock, S., & Steptoe, A. (2012). Association between low functional health literacy and mortality in older adults: longitudinal cohort study. *BMJ*, *344*(3), e1602–e1602. doi:10.1136/bmj.e1602

Bot, B. M., Suver, C., Neto, E. C., Kellen, M., Klein, A., Bare, C., Doerr, M., Pratap, A., Wilbanks, J., Dorsey, E. R., Friend, S. H., & Trister, A. D. (2016). The mPower study, Parkinson disease mobile data collected using ResearchKit. *Scientific Data*, *3*(1), 160011. Advance online publication. doi:10.1038data.2016.11 PMID:26938265

Bouri, E., Gupta, R., & Vo, X. V. (2020). Jumps in Geopolitical Risk and the Cryptocurrency Market: The Singularity of Bitcoin. *Defence and Peace Economics*, 1–12. doi:10.1080/10242694.2020.1848285

Bram, J. T., Warwick-Clark, B., Obeysekare, E., & Mehta, K. (2015). Utilization and Monetization of Healthcare Data in Developing Countries. *Big Data*, *3*(2), 59–66. doi:10.1089/big.2014.0053 PMID:26487984

Bransbourg, G. (2011). *Fides et pecunia numerate*. Chartalism and metallism in the Roman World. Part 1: The Republic. *American Journal of Numismatics*, *2*(23), 87–152.

BreastWeCan. (n.d.). *Crowdsourcing earlier detection of breast cancer from patient imaging*. https://www.breastwecan.org/

Breen, M. (2018, May 2). An *Introduction to district0x: A Network of Decentralized Communities*. CryptoSlate. https://cryptoslate.com/district0x/

Breslin, S. (2021). *China Risen?: Studying Chinese Global Power*. Policy Press. doi:10.2307/j.ctv1gm00k4

Brinks, V. (2019). 'And Since I Knew About the Possibilities There…': The Role of Open Creative Labs in User Innovation Processes. *Tijdschrift voor Economische en Sociale Geografie*, *110*(4), 381–394. doi:10.1111/tesg.12353

Brito, J., Shadab, H., & Castillo, A. (2014). Bitcoin financial regulation: Securities, derivatives, prediction markets, and gambling. *Colum. Sci. & Tech. L. Rev.*, *16*, 144. doi:10.2139srn.2423461

Brown, D. W., Burton, A., Gacic-Dobo, M., Karimov, R. I., Vandelaer, J., & Okwo-Bele, J. (2011). A mid-term assessment of progress towards the immunization coverage goal of the Global Immunization Vision and Strategy (GIVS). In BMC Public Health (Vol. 11). doi:10.1186/1471-2458-11-806

Brown, I., & Korff, D. (2009). Terrorism and the proportionality of internet surveillance. *European Journal of Criminology*, *6*(2), 119–134. doi:10.1177/1477370808100541

Bruland, K., & Mowery, D. C. (2004). *Innovation through time*. Georgia Institute of Technology.

Brummer, C., & Yadav, Y. (2018). Fintech and the innovation trilemma. *Geological Journal*, *107*, 235.

Bucherer, E., & Uckelmann, D. (2011). Architecting the Internet of Things. *Architecting the Internet of Things*. doi:10.1007/978-3-642-19157-2_10

Buckley, R. P., Arner, D. W., Zetzsche, D. A., Didenko, A. N., & Van Romburg, L. J. (2021). Sovereign digital currencies: Reshaping the design of money and payments systems. *Journal of Payments Strategy & Systems*, *15*(1), 7–22.

Buiter, W. H. (2007). *Seigniorage* (No. w12919). National Bureau of Economic Research.

Burnett, A., Amandry, M., & Ripollès, P. P. (1992). Roman Provincial Coinage (vol. 1). British Museum Press / Bibliothèque nationale de France.

Busygina, I., Filippov, M., & Taukebaeva, E. (2018). To decentralize or to continue on the centralization track: The cases of authoritarian regimes in Russia and Kazakhstan. *Journal of Eurasian Studies, 9*(1), 61-71.

Buterin, V. (2013). A next-generation smart contract and decentralized application platform. *Etherum*, 1–36.

Buterin, V. (2014). *A next generation smart contract & decentralized application platform*. Academic Press.

Buterin, V. (2014). *A next-generation smart contract and decentralized application platform*. Retrieved from http://buyxpr.com/build/pdfs/EthereumWhitePaper.pdf

Buterin, V. (2017). *Introduction to Cryptoeconomics*. Paper presented to Ethereum Foundation.

Buterin, V. (2014). DAOs, DACs, DAs and more: An incomplete terminology guide. *Ethereum Blog*, *6*, 2014.

Butt, S. A., Pappel, I., & Õunapuu, E. (2020, November). Potential for Increasing the ICT Adaption and Identifying Technology Readiness in the Silver Economy: Case of Estonia. In *International Conference on Electronic Governance and Open Society: Challenges in Eurasia* (pp. 139-155). Springer.

Buyle, R., Taelman, R., Mostaert, K., Joris, G., Mannens, E., Verborgh, R., & Berners-Lee, T. (2019). *Streamlining governmental processes by putting citizens in control of their personal data*. Academic Press.

Buyle, R., Taelman, R., Mostaert, K., Joris, G., Mannens, E., Verborgh, R., & Berners-Lee, T. (2019, November). Streamlining governmental processes by putting citizens in control of their personal data. In *International Conference on Electronic Governance and Open Society: Challenges in Eurasia* (pp. 346-359). Springer.

Çabuk, U. C., Adiguzel, E., & Karaarslan, E. (2020). *A survey on feasibility and suitability of blockchain techniques for the e-voting systems*. arXiv preprint arXiv:2002.07175.

Cachin, C. (2016). *Architecture of the hyperledger blockchain fabric*. https://pdfs.semanticscholar.org/f852/c5f3fe-649f8a17ded391df0796677a59927f.pdf

Cadwalladr, C., & Graham-Harrison, E. (2018). Revealed: 50 million Facebook profiles harvested for Cambridge Analytica in major data breach. *The Guardian, 17*, 22.

Calcaterra, C., & Kaal, W. A. (2021). The Importance of Reputation for the Evolution of Decentralization. In *Decentralization-Technology's Impact On Organizational And Societal Structure*. DeGruyter Publishers.

Campione, T. (2019). *The Blockchain Case: Can we trust the intermediary of trust?* PwC. https://blog.pwc.lu/blockchain-case-trust-the-intermediary-of-trust/

Campo, M. (2010). Producción i circulación de moneda falsa a la Península Ibèrica (s. IV aC – I dC). In M. Campo (Ed.), *Falsificació i manipulació de la moneda. XIV Curs d'Història monetària d'Hispània* (pp. 23–39). MNAC – Gabinet Numismatic de Catalunya.

Cano-Benito, J., & Cimmino, A. (2019). *G.-C. R.* Towards Blockchain and Semantic Web.

Cao, S., Lyu, H., & Xu, X. (2020). InsurTech development: Evidence from chinese media reports. *Technological Forecasting and Social Change*, *161*, 120277. Advance online publication. doi:10.1016/j.techfore.2020.120277

CareChain. (n.d.). *A joint effort to establish blockchain infrastructure and personal data management for health.* https://www.carechain.io/

Carter, S. (2018). *Timestamping Smart Ledgers: Comparable, Universal, Traceable, Immune.* Timestamping Smart Ledgers-Long Finance.

Casey, M. J., & Vigna, P. (2018). In blockchain we trust. *MIT's Technology Review*, *121*(3), 10–16.

Castells, M. (2011). *The rise of the network society* (Vol. 12). John Wiley & Sons.

Castells, M. (2014). The impact of the internet on society: A global perspective. *Change*, *19*, 127–148.

Catalini, C., & Gans, J. S. (2016). Some Simple Economics of the Blockchain. SSRN *Electronic Journal*. doi:10.2139srn.2874598

Cawthorn, D. M., Kennaugh, A., & Ferreira, S. M. (2020). The future of sustainability in the context of COVID-19. *Ambio*, 1–10. PMID:33289053

Cellan-Jones, R. (2020). *NHS data: Can web creator Sir Tim Berners-Lee fix it?* https://www.bbc.com/news/technology-54871705

Chahrour, M., Assi, S., Bejjani, M., Nasrallah, A. A., Salhab, H., Fares, M. Y., & Khachfe, H. H. (2020). A Bibliometric Analysis of COVID-19 Research Activity: A Call for Increased Output. *Cureus*. Advance online publication. doi:10.7759/cureus.7357 PMID:32328369

Chambers, C. (2019). Money+ markets: Blockchain isn't just a new technology, it is a political disrupter that takes away the state's monopoly on money. try as they might, governments won't be able to legislate it away. *Engineering & Technology*, *14*(7/8), 13–13.

Chamola, V., Hassija, V., Gupta, V., & Guizani, M. (2020). A comprehensive review of the COVID-19 pandemic and the role of IoT, drones, AI, blockchain, and 5G in managing its impact. *IEEE Access: Practical Innovations, Open Solutions*, *8*, 90225–90265. doi:10.1109/ACCESS.2020.2992341

Chan, Y. F. Y., Wang, P., Rogers, L., Tignor, N., Zweig, M., Hershman, S. G., Genes, N., Scott, E. R., Krock, E., Badgeley, M., Edgar, R., Violante, S., Wright, R., Powell, C. A., Dudley, J. T., & Schadt, E. E. (2017). The Asthma Mobile Health Study, a large-scale clinical observational study using ResearchKit. *Nature Biotechnology*, *35*(4), 354–362. doi:10.1038/nbt.3826 PMID:28288104

Chattu, V. K., Nanda, A., Chattu, S. K., Kadri, S. M., & Knight, A. W. (2019). The emerging role of blockchain technology applications in routine disease surveillance systems to strengthen global health security. In Big Data and Cognitive Computing (Vol. 3, Issue 2, pp. 1–10). MDPI AG. doi:10.3390/bdcc3020025

Chen & Jarrel. (2019). Blockchain in Healthcare: A Patient-Centered Model. *Biomedical Journal of Scientific & Technical Research, 20*(3), 15017–15022. PMID:31565696

Chen, S., Shi, R., Ren, Z., Yan, J., Shi, Y., & Zhang, J. (2017). A blockchain-based supply chain quality management framework. *Proceedings - 14th IEEE International Conference on E-Business Engineering, ICEBE 2017 - Including 13th Workshop on Service-Oriented Applications, Integration and Collaboration, SOAIC 207*, 172-176. 10.1109/ICEBE.2017.34

Cheng, V. C. C., Lau, S. K. P., Woo, P. C. Y., & Yuen, K. Y. (2007). Severe Acute Respiratory Syndrome Coronavirus as an Agent of Emerging and Reemerging Infection. *Clinical Microbiology Reviews, 20*(4), 660–694. Advance online publication. doi:10.1128/CMR.00023-07 PMID:17934078

Chen, H., & Xie, G. (2010). The use of web ontology languages and other semantic web tools in drug discovery. *Expert Opinion on Drug Discovery, 5*(5), 413–423. doi:10.1517/17460441003762709 PMID:22823127

Chen, J. (2017). Can online social networks foster young adults' civic engagement? *Telematics and Informatics, 34*(5), 487–497. doi:10.1016/j.tele.2016.09.013

Chen, Q., & Lambright, J. (2016). Towards Realizing a Self-Protecting Healthcare Information System. *Proceedings International Computer Software and Applications Conference.* 10.1109/COMPSAC.2016.264

Chen, Y. (2018). Blockchain tokens and the potential democratization of entrepreneurship and innovation. *Business Horizons, 61*(4), 567–575. doi:10.1016/j.bushor.2018.03.006

Chen, Y., & Bellavitis, C. (2020). Blockchain disruption and decentralized finance: The rise of decentralized business models. *Journal of Business Venturing Insights, 13*, e00151. doi:10.1016/j.jbvi.2019.e00151

Chen, Y., Mao, Z., & Qiu, J. L. (2018). *Super-Sticky Design and Everyday Cultures', Super-Sticky Wechat and Chinese Society.* Emerald Publishing Limited. doi:10.1108/9781787430914

Choi, D. H., & Seo, T. S. (2021). Development of an open peer review system using blockchain and reviewer recommendation technologies. *Science Editing, 8*(1), 104–111. doi:10.6087/kcse.237

Choi, M. K., Yeun, C. Y., & Seong, P. H. (2020). A Novel Monitoring System for the Data Integrity of Reactor Protection System Using Blockchain Technology. *IEEE Access: Practical Innovations, Open Solutions, 8*, 118732–118740. doi:10.1109/ACCESS.2020.3005134

Choudhury, O., Fairoza, N., Sylla, I., & Das, A. (2019). A Blockchain Framework for Managing and Monitoring Data in Multi-Site Clinical Trials. *ArXiv*, 1–13.

Clark, B., & Burstall, R. (2018). Blockchain, IP and the pharma industry-how distributed ledger technologies can help secure the pharma supply chain. Journal of Intellectual Property Law and Practice, 13(7).

Clark, D. (1988, August). The design philosophy of the DARPA Internet protocols. In *Symposium proceedings on Communications architectures and protocols* (pp. 106-114) 10.1145/52324.52336

Clavin, J., Duan, S., Zhang, H., Janeja, V. P., Joshi, K. P., Yesha, Y., Erickson, L. C., & Li, J. D. (2020). Blockchains for Government: Use Cases and Challenges. *Digital Government: Research and Practice, 1*(3), 1–21. doi:10.1145/3427097

Clements, C. J., Nshimirimanda, D., & Gasasira, A. (2008). Using immunization delivery strategies to accelerate progress in Africa towards achieving the Millennium Development Goals. In Vaccine (Vol. 26, Issue 16). doi:10.1016/j.vaccine.2008.02.032

ClinicAll Healthcare. (2019, April 24). *Cryptocurrency In Healthcare: Gold Rush Or Bad News?* Medium. https://clinicallhealthcare.medium.com/cryptocurrency-in-healthcare-gold-rush-or-bad-news-889e73cd9142

Coase, R. H. (1991). *The nature of the firm (1937). The Nature of the Firm.* Origins, Evolution, and Development.

Coase, R. H. (1993). *The nature of the firm: origins, evolution, and development.* Oxford University Press.

Cochoy, F., Hagberg, J., & Niklas, S. (2017). *Digitalizing Consumption: How devices shape consumer culture. Publisher.* Routledge. doi:10.4324/9781315647883

CoinDesk. (2021). *Bitcoin.* Www.Coindesk.Com. https://www.coindesk.com/price/bitcoin

CoinDesk. (n.d.). *Bitcoin.* Retrieved January 22, 2021, from https://www.coindesk.com/price/bitcoin

CoinMarketCap. (2020a). *Ethereum.* https://coinmarketcap.com/currencies/ethereum/

CoinMarketCap. (2020b). *yearn.finance.* https://coinmarketcap.com/currencies/yearn-finance/

Cointelegraph. (2018, February 13). *What is DAO and how it works.* https://cointelegraph.com/ethereum-for-beginners/what-is-dao

Colhoun, H. M., McKeigue, P. M., & Smith, G. D. (2003). Problems of reporting genetic associations with complex outcomes. *Lancet, 361*(9360), 865–872. doi:10.1016/S0140-6736(03)12715-8 PMID:12642066

Commission, E. (2004). e-Health - making healthcare better for European citizens: An action plan for a European e-Health Area. Brussels: European Commission

Cong, L. W., & He, Z. (2019). Blockchain Disruption and Smart Contracts. Review of Financial Studies. doi:10.1093/rfs/hhz007

Conway, L. (2020). *Blockchain Explained.* Investopedia. https://www.investopedia.com/terms/b/blockchain.asp

Conway, D., & Garimella, K. (2020). Enhancing Trust in Business Ecosystems With Blockchain Technology. *IEEE Engineering Management Review, 48*(1), 24–30. doi:10.1109/EMR.2020.2970387

Coorevits, P., Sundgren, M., Klein, G. O., Bahr, A., Claerhout, B., Daniel, C., Dugas, M., Dupont, D., Schmidt, A., Singleton, P., De Moor, G., & Kalra, D. (2013). Electronic health records: New opportunities for clinical research. *Journal of Internal Medicine, 274*(6), 547–560. doi:10.1111/joim.12119 PMID:23952476

Cordeiro, J. L. (2003). Different Monetary Systems: Costs and Benefits to Whom? *Revista Venezolana de Análisis de Coyuntura, 9*(1), 107–140.

Costello, K. (2019). *Rapid Evolution of the Blockchain Platform Market.* https://www.gartner.com/en/newsroom/press-releases/2019-07-03-gartner-predicts-90--of-current-enterprise-blockchain

Cribb, J. (2003). The origins of the Indian coinage tradition. *South Asian Studies, 19*(1), 1–19. doi:10.1080/02666030.2003.9628617

CryptoSlate. (2020). https://cryptoslate.com/cryptos/healthcare/

Cryptowerk. (2018). *Using Blockchains and IoT to Record Clinical Trial Data.* Retrieved January 22, 2021, from https://cryptowerk.com/blockchains-iot-clinical-trial-data

CUF academic center. (2020). *Cuf.pt.* https://www.cuf.pt/cuf-academic-center/investigacao

Cuneta, M. (2017). *The Big Bitcoin Battle: What I Found Out About Bitcoin VS BCash.* Hackernoon. https://medium.com/hackernoon/the-big-bitcoin-battle-what-i-found-out-about-bitcoin-vs-bcash-d9ebca8d370e

Cunningham, S. (2010). Joseph A. Schumpeter, Capitalism, socialism, and democracy. *International Journal of Cultural Policy, 16*(1), 20–22. doi:10.1080/10286630902807278

Curry, E. (2016). The big data value chain: Definitions, concepts, and theoretical approaches. In New Horizons for a Data-Driven Economy: A Roadmap for Usage and Exploitation of Big Data in Europe. doi:10.1007/978-3-319-21569-3_3

D'Andrea, R., & O'Dwyer, J. P. (2017). Can editors save peer review from peer reviewers? *PLoS One, 12*(10), e0186111. Advance online publication. doi:10.1371/journal.pone.0186111 PMID:29016678

Dahlman, C. J. (1979). The problem of externality. *The Journal of Law & Economics, 22*(1), 141–162.

Dai, H., Young Phd, P., Js, T., Md, D., Gong, G., Kang Phd, M., Krumholz, H. M., Sm, M. D., Schulz, W. L., & Jiang, L. (2018). *TrialChain: A Blockchain-Based Platform to Validate Data Integrity in Large, Biomedical Research Studies.* https://github.com/ComputationalHealth/TrialChain

Dai, C. (2020). DEX: A DApp for the Decentralized Marketplace. In *Blockchain and Crypt Currency* (pp. 95–106). Springer. doi:10.1007/978-981-15-3376-1_6

Dalton, G. (1982). Barter. *Journal of Economic Issues, 16*(1), 181–190.

Dalton, G. (1982). Barter. *Journal of Economic Issues, 16*(1), 181–190. doi:10.1080/00213624.1982.11503968

Dapp, M. M. (2019). Toward a Sustainable Circular Economy Powered by Community-Based Incentive Systems. In *Business Transformation through Blockchain* (pp. 153–181). Palgrave Macmillan. doi:10.1007/978-3-319-99058-3_6

Darlington III, J. K. (2014). *The future of Bitcoin: mapping the global adoption of world's largest cryptocurrency through benefit analysis.* Academic Press.

Datta, P., & Chatterjee, S. (2008). The economics and psychology of consumer trust in intermediaries in electronic markets: The EM-Trust Framework. *European Journal of Information Systems, 17*(1), 12–28. doi:10.1057/palgrave.ejis.3000729

DavidsonS.De FilippiP.PottsJ. (2016). Disrupting governance: The new institutional economics of distributed ledger technology. Available at SSRN 2811995. doi:10.2139srn.2811995

DavidsonS.De FilippiP.PottsJ. (2016). *Economics of blockchain.* Available at SSRN 2744751.

Davidson, S., De Filippi, P., & Potts, J. (2017). Blockchains and the economic institutions of capitalism. *Journal of Institutional Economics, 14*(4), 639–658. doi:10.1017/S1744137417000200

DavidsonS.NovakM.PottsJ. (2018). The cost of trust: a pilot study. Available at SSRN 3218761.

Davis, J. (2015). *7 Largest Data Breaches of 2015.* Healthcare IT News.

Davis, T. C., Holcombe, R. F., Berkel, H. J., Pramanik, S., & Divers, S. G. (1998). Informed consent for clinical trials: A comparative study of standard versus simplified forms. *Journal of the National Cancer Institute, 90*(9), 668–674. Advance online publication. doi:10.1093/jnci/90.9.668 PMID:9586663

De Beauclair, I. (1963). The Stone Money of Yap Island. *Bulletin of the Institute of Ethnology, Academia Sinica, 16*, 147–160.

De Beauclair, I. (1971). Studies on Botel Tobago, and Yap. In *Asian Folklore and Social Life Monographs, edited by Lou Tsu-k'uang* (pp. 183–203). Orient Cultural Service.

De Callataÿ, F. (2013). White gold: An enigmatic start to Greek coinage. *American Numismatic Society Magazine, 12*(2), 7–17.

de Diego, S., Gonçalves, C., Lage, O., Mansell, J., Kontoulis, M., Moustakidis, S., Guerra, B., & Liapis, A. (2019). Blockchain-Based Threat Registry Platform. *2019 IEEE 10th Annual Information Technology, Electronics and Mobile Communication Conference (IEMCON)*, 892–898. 10.1109/IEMCON.2019.8936249

De Filippi, P. (2016). The interplay between decentralization and privacy: the case of blockchain technologies. *Journal of Peer Production*.

De Filippi, P., Mannan, M., & Reijers, W. (2020). Blockchain as a confidence machine: The problem of trust & challenges of governance. *Technology in Society*, *62*, 1–24. doi:10.1016/j.techsoc.2020.101284

de Graaf, T. J. (2019). From old to new: From internet to smart contracts and from people to smart contracts. *Computer Law & Security Review*, *35*(5), 105322. Advance online publication. doi:10.1016/j.clsr.2019.04.005

De Montjoye, Y. A., Radaelli, L., Singh, V. K., & Pentland, A. S. (2015). Unique in the shopping mall: On the reidentifiability of credit card metadata. *Science*, *347*(6221), 536–539. doi:10.1126cience.1256297 PMID:25635097

De Oliveira Rodrigues, D. (2021). Marketing-Mix Metamorphosis and New Trusted Business Practices. In *Competitive Drivers for Improving Future Business Performance* (pp. 46–66). IGI Global. doi:10.4018/978-1-7998-1843-4.ch004

De Roover, R. (1953). *L'Évolution de la lettre de change XIVe-XVIIIe siècles*. Librairie Armand Colin.

Degeling, C., Chen, G., Gilbert, G. L., Brookes, V., Thai, T., Wilson, A., & Johnson, J. (2020). Changes in public preferences for technologically enhanced surveillance following the COVID-19 pandemic: A discrete choice experiment. *BMJ Open*, *10*(11), e041592. doi:10.1136/bmjopen-2020-041592 PMID:33208337

Dehaye, P. O., & Reardon, J. (2020, November). Proximity Tracing in an Ecosystem of Surveillance Capitalism. In *Proceedings of the 19th Workshop on Privacy in the Electronic Society* (pp. 191-203). 10.1145/3411497.3420219

Deloitte. (2020). *5 Blockchain Trends for 2020*. https://www2.deloitte.com/content/dam/Deloitte/ie/Documents/Consulting/Blockchain-Trends-2020-report.pdf

Deloitte. (2020). *Intelligent drug discovery About the Deloitte Centre for Health Solutions*. Author.

DeMartino, I. (2018). *The Bitcoin Guidebook: How to Obtain, Invest, and Spend the World's First Decentralized Cryptocurrency*. Simon and Schuster.

Dentacoin Foundation. (2018). *Dentacoin: The Blockchain Solution for the Global Dental Industry. Whitepaper*. Retrieved from https://dentacoin.com/%0Ahttps://dentacoin.com/web/white-paper/Whitepaper-en1.pdf

Dentacoin Foundation. (2020). Dentacoin - The Blockchain Solution for Better Oral Health. Retrieved January 29, 2021, from https://dentacoin.com/assets/uploads/dentacoin-company-introduction.pdf

Dentacoin Foundation. (2021). *Dentists*. Retrieved January 30, 2021, from https://dentacoin.com/dentists

Dentacoin Team. (2019). *8 Use Cases for Your Dentacoin (DCN) Tokens*. Retrieved January 30, 2021, from https://blog.dentacoin.com/what-is-dentacoin-8-use-cases/

Denzel, M. A. (2014). Monetary and financial innovations in Flanders, Antwerp, London and Hamburg: fifteenth to eighteenth century. In P. Bernholz & R. Vaubel (Eds.), Explaining monetary and financial innovation: a historical analysis (pp. 252-282). Springer. doi:10.1007/978-3-319-06109-2_10

Dewing, M. (2021). Combining Social & Legal Constructions: Constitutional Reformations for the Future. *FAU Undergraduate Law Journal*, 57-79.

Dhanalakshmi, S., & Babu, G. C. (2019). An Examination Of Big Data And Blockchain Technology. *International Journal of Innovative Technology and Exploring Engineering*, 8(11), 2278–3075. doi:10.35940/ijitee.K2497.0981119

Dhinakaran, K., Raj, P. B. H., & Vinod, D. (2021). A Secure Electronic Voting System Using Blockchain Technology. In *Proceedings of the Second International Conference on Information Management and Machine Intelligence* (pp. 307-313). Springer. 10.1007/978-981-15-9689-6_34

Didenko, A. N., Zetzsche, D. A., Arner, D. W., & Buckley, R. P. (2020). *After Libra, Digital Yuan and COVID-19: Central Bank Digital Currencies and the New World of Money and Payment Systems*. Academic Press.

Dierksmeier, C., & Seele, P. (2018). Cryptocurrencies and business ethics. *Journal of Business Ethics*, 152(1), 1–14. doi:10.100710551-016-3298-0 PMID:30930508

Diffie, W., & Hellman, M. (1976). New directions in cryptography. *IEEE Transactions on Information Theory*, 22(6), 644–654. doi:10.1109/TIT.1976.1055638

Dijkman, R. M., Sprenkels, B., Peeters, T., & Janssen, A. (2015). Business models for the Internet of Things. *International Journal of Information Management*, 35(6), 672–678. doi:10.1016/j.ijinfomgt.2015.07.008

DiMasi, J. A., Grabowski, H. G., & Hansen, R. W. (2016). Innovation in the pharmaceutical industry: New estimates of R&D costs. *Journal of Health Economics*, 47, 20–33. doi:10.1016/j.jhealeco.2016.01.012 PMID:26928437

Dinh, T. N., & Thai, M. T. (2018). AI and Blockchain: A Disruptive Integration. *Computer*, 51(9), 48–53. doi:10.1109/MC.2018.3620971

District0x. (2020). *An Introduction To Decentralization. District0x Education Portal*. https://education.district0x.io/general-topics/what-is-decentralization/introduction/

Dixon, C. (2018). *Why Decentralization Matters*. https://medium.com/s/story/why-decentralization-matters-5e3f79f7638e

Drescher, D. (2017). Blockchain basics: A non-technical introduction in 25 steps. In Blockchain Basics: A Non-Technical Introduction in 25 Steps. doi:10.1007/978-1-4842-2604-9

Drosatos, G., & Kaldoudi, E. (2019). Blockchain Applications in the Biomedical Domain: A Scoping Review. *Computational and Structural Biotechnology Journal*, 17, 229–240. doi:10.1016/j.csbj.2019.01.010 PMID:30847041

Drutarovska, J. (2015). The Linkage between Speculation and Derivatives' Trading Society. Academic Press.

Ducci, F. (2020). *Natural Monopolies in Digital Platform Markets*. Cambridge University Press. doi:10.1017/9781108867528

Dula, C., & Chuen, L. K. D. (2018). Reshaping the financial order. Handbook of blockchain, digital finance, and inclusion, volume 1: Cryptocurrency, FinTech, InsurTech, and regulation (pp. 1-18) doi:10.1016/B978-0-12-810441-5.00001-4

Dumas, J. G., Jimenez-Garcès, S., & Şoiman, F. (2021, March). Blockchain technology and crypto-assets market analysis: vulnerabilities and risk assessment. The 12th International Multi-Conference on Complexity, Informatics and Cybernetics: IMCIC 2021.

Dunbar, R. (2010). *How many friends does one person need? Dunbar's number and other evolutionary quirks*. Faber & Faber.

Dush, L. (2015). When writing becomes content. *College Composition and Communication*, 173–196.

Dwyer, R. (2017). *Code! = Law: Explorations of the Blockchain as a Mode of Algorithmic Governance*. Retrieved from https://www.academia.edu/34734732/Code_Law_Explorations_of_the_Blockchain_as_a_Mode_of_Algorithmic_Governance

Dwyer, R. (2017). *Code! = Law: Explorations of the Blockchain as a Mode of Algorithmic Governance.* Retrieved March 23, 2021, from https://www.academia.edu/34734732/Code_Law_Explorations_of_the_Blockchain_as_a_Mode_of_Algorithmic_Governance

Dzieduszycka-Suinat, S., Murray, J., Kiniry, J., Zimmerman, D., Wagner, D., Robinson, P., Foltzer, A., & Morina, S. (2015). *The Future of Voting End-to-End – Verifiable Internet Voting. Specification and Feasibility Assessment Study.* U.S. Vote Foundation. https://usvotefoundation-drupal.s3.amazonaws.com/prod/E2EVIV_full_report.pdf

Ebadi, E., Yajam, H., & Akhaee, M. (2020, September). Improvements on Easypaysy: The Bitcoin's Layer-2 Accounts Protocol. In *2020 17th International ISC Conference on Information Security and Cryptology (ISCISC)* (pp. 54-59). IEEE.

Ebner, N. (2017). Negotiation is changing. *J. Disp. Resol., 99.*

Echarte Fernández, M. Á., Náñez Alonso, S. L., Jorge-Vázquez, J., & Reier Forradellas, R. F. (2021). Central Banks' Monetary Policy in the Face of the COVID-19 Economic Crisis: Monetary Stimulus and the Emergence of CBDCs. *Sustainability, 13*(8), 4242. doi:10.3390u13084242

Economist. (2015). The promise of the blockchain: The trust machine'. *The Economist, 31,* 27.

Economist, T. (2015). The promise of the blockchain: The trust machine'. *The economist, 31,* 27.

Edwood, F. (2020). *Cryptocurrency On-Ramps and Off-Ramps, Explained.* Cointelegraph. https://cointelegraph.com/explained/cryptocurrency-on-ramps-and-off-ramps-explained

e-estonia. (2020). *KSI Blockchain.* https://e-estonia.com/solutions/security-and-safety/ksi-blockchain/

e-estonia. (n.d.). *Healthcare.* https://e-estonia.com/solutions/healthcare/

Eiglier, P., & Langeard, E. (1987). *La servuction: stratégie et managment.* Ediscience.

Eikmanns, B. C. (2018). *Blockchain: Proposition of a new and sustainable macroeconomic system.* Frankfurt School, Blockchain Center.

Einaste, T. (2018). *Blockchain and healthcare: the Estonian experience—e-Estonia.* https://eestonia.com/blockchain-healthcare-estonian-experience/

Eisner, D. A. (2018). Reproducibility of science: Fraud, impact factors and carelessness. *Journal of Molecular and Cellular Cardiology.* doi:10.1016/j.yjmcc.2017.10.009

Elflein, J. (2017). Projected distribution of healthcare blockchain adoption worldwide 2017-2025. *Statista Website.* https://www.statista.com/statistics/759208/healthcare-blockchain-adoption-rate-in-health-apps-worldwide/

Elisa, N., Yang, L., Li, H., Chao, F., & Naik, N. (2019). Consortium blockchain for security and privacy-preserving in E-government systems. *Proceedings of the International Conference on Electronic Business (ICEB),* 99-107.

Elliott, C. E. (2020). The role of money in the economies of Ancient Greece and Rome. In S. Battilossi, Y. Cassis & K. Yago (Eds.), Handbook of the History of Money and Currency (pp. 67-86). Springer. doi:10.1007/978-981-13-0596-2_46

El-Mousa, F. (2018). *GDPR Privacy Implications for the Internet of Things.* https://www.researchgate.net/publication/331991225

EMA. (2020). *Good distribution practice.* https://www.ema.europa.eu/en/human-regulatory/post-authorisation/compliance/good-distribution-practice

Emmer, T. (2020, June). *Virtual Hearing - Inclusive Banking During a Pandemic: Using FedAccounts and Digital Tools to Improve Delivery of Stimulus Payments*. US House Committee on Financial Services. https://financialservices.house.gov/calendar/eventsingle.aspx?EventID=406617

Engelhardt, M. A. (2017). Hitching Healthcare to the Chain: An Introduction to Blockchain Technology in the Healthcare Sector. *Technology Innovation Management Review*, 7(10), 22–34. doi:10.22215/timreview/1111

Entriken, Evans, & Sachs. (2018). *ERC-721 Non-Fungible Token Standard*. Retrieved from https://eips.ethereum.org/EIPS/eip-721

Enyinda, C. I., & Tolliver, D. (2009). Taking Counterfeits out of the Pharmaceutical Supply Chain in Nigeria: Leveraging Multilayer Mitigation Approach. *Journal of African Business*, 10(2), 218–234. Advance online publication. doi:10.1080/15228910903187957

Erikson, E. H. (1982). *The life cycle completed*. W. W. Norton & Company.

Esposito, C., De Santis, A., Tortora, G., Chang, H., & Choo, K. K. R. (2018). Blockchain: A Panacea for Healthcare Cloud-Based Data Security and Privacy? *IEEE Cloud Computing*, 5(1), 31–37. doi:10.1109/MCC.2018.011791712

Ethereum. (2020). *Home*. https://ethereum.org/en/

Ethical IoT, GDPR, Personal Data, and Maintaining Consumer Trust. (n.d.). Retrieved April 17, 2021, from https://www.aeris.com/news/post/ethical-iot-gdpr-personal-data-and-maintaining-consumer-trust/

Etwaru, R. (2017). *Blockchain: Trust Companies: Every Company Is at Risk of Being Disrupted by a Trusted Version of Itself*. Dog Ear Publishing.

EUblockchain. (2019). *Feeling good: Healthcare data and the blockchain*. https://www.eublockchainforum.eu/news/feeling-good-healthcare-data-and-blockchain

European Parliament. (2001). EU Clinical Directive 2001/20/EC of the European Parliament and of the Council of 4 April 2001 on the approximation of the laws, regulations, and administrative provisions of the Member States relating to the implementation of good clinical practice. *Official Journal of the European Communities*.

Euzenat, J., & Rousset, M. C. (2020). Semantic web. In *A Guided Tour of Artificial Intelligence Research* (pp. 181–207). Springer. doi:10.1007/978-3-030-06170-8_6

Faber, N. R., & Hadders, H. (2016, June). Towards a blockchain enabled social contract for sustainability, Creating a fair and just operating system for humanity. In *Proceedings of the First International Conference on New Business Models, Toulouse, France* (pp. 16-17). Academic Press.

Faber, B., Michelet, G. C., Weidmann, N., Mukkamala, R. R., & Vatrapu, R. (2019, January). BPDIMS: a blockchain-based personal data and identity management system. In *Proceedings of the 52nd Hawaii International Conference on System Sciences*. 10.24251/HICSS.2019.821

Fanelli, D. (2009). How many scientists fabricate and falsify research? A systematic review and meta-analysis of survey data. *PLoS ONE*. doi:10.1371/journal.pone.0005738

Fanelli, D. (2012). Negative results are disappearing from most disciplines and countries. *Scientometrics*. doi:10.100711192-011-0494-7

Fang, H. S. A. (2021). *Commercially Successful Blockchain Healthcare Projects: A Scoping Review*. Blockchain in Healthcare Today.

Faridi, O. (2020). *12 Billion in Decentralized Application (dApp) Transactions Processed during Q2 2020, with Ethereum (ETH) Accounting for 82% of "Created Value": Report*. Crowded Media Group.

Faroukhi, A. Z., El Alaoui, I., Gahi, Y., & Amine, A. (2020). Big data monetization throughout Big Data Value Chain: A comprehensive review. *Journal of Big Data*, 7(1), 1–22. doi:10.118640537-019-0281-5

Farringer, D. R. (2019). Maybe If We Turn It Off and Then Turn It Back On Again? Exploring Health Care Reform as a Means to Curb Cyber Attacks. *The Journal of Law, Medicine & Ethics*, 47(4, SUPPL), 91–102. doi:10.1177/1073110519898046 PMID:31955693

FDA & CDER. (2020). *Conduct of Clinical Trials of Medical Products During the COVID-19 Public Health Emergency Guidance for Industry, Investigators, and Institutional Review Boards Preface Public Comment*. https://www.fda.gov/regulatory-

Federal Reserve System. (2020, October 6). *Federal Reserve Board - Currency Print Orders*. https://www.federalreserve.gov/paymentsystems/coin_currency_orders.htm

Feilmayr, C., & Wolfram, W. (2016). An Analysis of Ontologies and Their Success Factors for Application to Business. *Data & Knowledge Engineering*, 101, 1–23. doi:10.1016/j.datak.2015.11.003

Feldstein, S. (2019). The road to digital unfreedom: How artificial intelligence is reshaping repression. *Journal of Democracy*, 30(1), 40–52. doi:10.1353/jod.2019.0003

Fenwick, M., & Vermeulen, E. P. (2019). Technology and corporate governance: Blockchain, crypto, and artificial intelligence. *Tex. J. Bus. L.*, 48, 1.

Ferguson, N. (2008). *The ascent of money: A financial history of the world*. Penguin.

Ferrer-Gomila, J., Francisca Hinarejos, M., & Isern-Deyà, A.-P. (2019). A fair contract signing protocol with blockchain support. *Electronic Commerce Research and Applications*, 36, 100869. Advance online publication. doi:10.1016/j.elerap.2019.100869

Finck, M. (2018). Blockchains and Data Protection in the European Union. *European Data Protection Law Review*. doi:10.21552/edpl/2018/1/6

Finck, M. (2019). Blockchain and the General Data Protection Regulation : can distributed ledgers be squared with European data protection law? European Parliament.

Fisher, R., Ury, W., & Patton, B. (1991). Getting to yes: Negotiating agreement without giving in (No. 158.5). FIS. CIMMYT.

Fisher, R., Ury, W. L., & Patton, B. (2011). *Getting to yes: Negotiating agreement without giving in*. Penguin.

Fitzpatrick, S. M., & Diveley, B. (2004). Interisland exchange in Micronesia: a case of monumental proportions. *Voyages of discovery: The archaeology of islands*, 129-146.

Fitzpatrick, S. (2004a). Banking on Stone Money. For the Yapese of Micronesia, a disk of sculpted limestone could buy just about anything. *Archaeology*, 19–23. https://www.researchgate.net/profile/Scott-Fitzpatrick/publication/255687068_Banking_on_Stone_Money/links/0c9605202df58df571000000/Banking-on-Stone-Money.pdf

Fitzpatrick, S. M., & Diveley, B. D. (2004). Interisland Exchange in Micronesia: A Case of Monumental Proportions. In S. M. Fitzpatrick (Ed.), *Voyages of Discovery: The Archaeology of Islands* (pp. 129–146). Praeger.

Fitzpatrick, S. M., & McKeon, S. (2020). Banking on Stone Money: Ancient Antecedents to Bitcoin. *Economic Anthropology*, 7(1), 7–21. doi:10.1002ea2.12154

Flew, T. (2005). Creative Commons and the creative industries. *Media and Arts Law Review, 10*(4), 257–264.

Fliphodl, F. (2018, November 22). *Social Media Alternatives Series, EP. 1: What You NEED to Know.* Fliphodl. https://www.fliphodl.com/social-media-alternatives-series-ep-1-what-you-need-to-know/

Floridi, L. (2018). Artificial intelligence, deepfakes and a future of ectypes. *Philosophy & Technology, 31*(3), 317–321. doi:10.100713347-018-0325-3

Fogel, D. B. (2018). Factors associated with clinical trials that fail and opportunities for improving the likelihood of success: A review. *Contemporary Clinical Trials Communications, 11*, 156–164. https://doi.org/10.1016/j.conctc.2018.08.001

Fousekis, P., & Grigoriadis, V. (2021). Directional predictability between returns and volume in cryptocurrencies markets. *Studies in Economics and Finance, ahead-of-print*(ahead-of-print). Advance online publication. doi:10.1108/SEF-08-2020-0318

Frankenfield, J. (2020). *Cryptocurrency.* Retrieved January 29, 2021, from https://www.investopedia.com/terms/c/cryptocurrency.asp

Fraser, H. S. f., & Blaya, J. (2010). Implementing medical information systems in developing countries, what works and what doesn't. *AMIA ... Annual Symposium Proceedings / AMIA Symposium. AMIA Symposium, 2010.*

Freitas, C. (2020). *How many cryptocurrencies are there?* Currency.Com. https://currency.com/how-many-cryptocurrencies-are-there

French, D. E. (2009). *Early speculative bubbles and increases in the supply of money.* Ludwig von Mises Institute.

Friedman, M. (1991). *The Island of Stone Money.* Hoover Institution, Stanford University.

Fritsch, F., Emmett, J., Friedman, E., Kranjc, R., Manski, S. G., Zargham, M., & Bauwens, M. (2021). Challenges and Approaches to Scaling the Global Commons. *Frontiers in Blockchain, 4*, 9. doi:10.3389/fbloc.2021.578721

Frizzo-Barker, J., Chow-White, P. A., Adams, P. R., Mentanko, J., Ha, D., & Green, S. (2020). Blockchain as a disruptive technology for business: A systematic review. *International Journal of Information Management, 51*, 102029. doi:10.1016/j.ijinfomgt.2019.10.014

Fukuyama, F. (1995). *Trust: The social virtues and the creation of prosperity.* Free Press.

Fulmer, C. A., & Gelfand, M. J. (2012). At what level (and in whom) we trust: Trust across multiple organizational levels. *Journal of Management, 38*(4), 1167–1230. doi:10.1177/0149206312439327

Furness, W. H. III. (1910). *The Island of Stone Money, Uap of the Carolines.* J. B. Lippincott.

Fusco, A., Dicuonzo, G., Dell'atti, V., & Tatullo, M. (2020). Blockchain in healthcare: Insights on COVID-19. *International Journal of Environmental Research and Public Health, 17*(19), 1–12. doi:10.3390/ijerph17197167 PMID:33007951

Gabardi, W. (2001). Contemporary models of democracy. *Polity, 33*(4), 547–568. doi:10.2307/3235516

Gadoury, V., & Élie, R. (1990). *Monnaies de nécessité françaises, 1789-1990.* Éditions Victor Gadoury.

Galloway, S. (2017). *The four: the hidden DNA of Amazon, Apple, Facebook and Google.* Random House.

Gammon, K. (2018). Experimenting with blockchain: Can one technology boost both data integrity and patients' pocketbooks? *Nature Medicine, 24*(4), 378–381. https://doi.org/10.1038/nm0418-378

Gandy, O. H. Jr. (2010). Engaging rational discrimination: Exploring reasons for placing regulatory constraints on decision support systems. *Ethics and Information Technology, 12*(1), 29–42. doi:10.100710676-009-9198-6

Garcia-Rivadulla, S. (2016). Personalization vs. privacy: An inevitable trade-off? *IFLA Journal*, *42*(3), 227–238. doi:10.1177/0340035216662890

Garrison, R. W., & Kirzner, I. M. (1989). Friedrich August von Hayek. In *The Invisible Hand* (pp. 119–130). Palgrave Macmillan. doi:10.1007/978-1-349-20313-0_14

Gartner. (2019). *Data Monetization - Gartner Information Technology Glossary*. Gartner IT Glossary. https://www.gartner.com/en/information-technology/glossary/data-monetization

Gassner, U. M. (2018). *Blockchain in EU e-health - blocked by the barrier of data protection?* Compliance Elliance Journal.

GDPR. (2018). *General data protection regulation (GDPR)*. Intersoft Consulting.

Gefenas, E., Cekanauskaite, A., Lekstutiene, J., & Lukaseviciene, V. (2017). Application challenges of the new EU Clinical Trials Regulation. In European Journal of Clinical Pharmacology (Vol. 73, Issue 7, pp. 795–798). Springer Verlag. doi:10.100700228-017-2267-6

General Data Protection Regulation (GDPR) – Official Legal Text. (n.d.). Retrieved April 17, 2021, from https://gdpr-info.eu/

George, S. L., & Buyse, M. (2015). Data fraud in clinical trials. *Clinical Investigation*, *5*(2), 161–173. doi:10.4155/cli.14.116 PMID:25729561

Gerard, D. (2020). *Libra Shrugged: How Facebook Tried to Take Over the Money*. David Gerard.

Gerba, E., & Rubio, M. (2019). *Virtual money: how much do cryptocurrencies alter the fundamental functions of money?* (PE 642.360). European Parliament. https://www.europarl.europa.eu/cmsdata/190132/PE%20642.360%20LSE%20final%20publication-original.pdf

Ghabri, Y., Guesmi, K., & Zantour, A. (2020). Bitcoin and liquidity risk diversification. *Finance Research Letters*, 101679.

Ghaiti, K. (2021). *The Volatility of Bitcoin, Bitcoin Cash, Litecoin, Dogecoin and Ethereum* (Doctoral dissertation). Université d'Ottawa/University of Ottawa.

Gheorghiu, B., & Hagens, S. (2017). Use and Maturity of Electronic Patient Portals. *Studies in Health Technology and Informatics*, *234*, 136–141. PMID:28186030

Ghosh, D. (2019). *A New Digital Social Contract to Encourage Internet Competition*. Antitrust Chronicle.

Ghosh, J. (2019). The Blockchain: Opportunities for Research in Information Systems and Information Technology. *Journal of Global Information Technology Management*, *22*(4), 235–242. doi:10.1080/1097198X.2019.1679954

Gibbons, R. (2001). Trust in social structures: Hobbes and Coase meet repeated games. *Trust in Society, 2*, 332-353.

Giovannini, A. (1975). Athenian currency in the late fifth and early fourth century B.C. *Greek, Roman and Byzantine Studies*, *16*(2), 185–195.

Gipp, B., & Meuschke, N. (2009). *Decentralized Trusted Timestamping using the Crypto Currency Bitcoin Trusted Timestamping*. Academic Press.

GkillasK.LonginF. (2018). Is Bitcoin the new digital gold? Evidence from extreme price movements in financial markets. SSRN. Available at https://papers. ssrn. com/sol3/papers. cfm doi:10.2139srn.3245571

Glover, D. G., & Hermans, J. (2017). Improving the Traceability of the Clinical Trial Supply Chain | Applied Clinical Trials Online. *Applied Clinical Trials*, *26*(12). https://www.appliedclinicaltrialsonline.com/view/improving-traceability-clinical-trial-supply-chain

Goeg, K. R., Cornet, R., & Andersen, S. K. (2015). Clustering clinical models from local electronic health records based on semantic similarity. *Journal of Biomedical Informatics*, *54*, 294–304. doi:10.1016/j.jbi.2014.12.015 PMID:25557885

Goldacre, B., DeVito, N., Heneghan, C., Irving, F., & Bmj, S. B. (2018). undefined. (2018). Compliance with requirement to report results on the EU Clinical Trials Register: Cohort study and web resource. *BMJ (Clinical Research Ed.)*, *362*. https://www.bmj.com/content/362/bmj.k3218

Goldberg, D. (2009). The Massachusetts paper money of 1690. *The Journal of Economic History*, *69*(4), 1092–1106. doi:10.1017/S0022050709001399

Goldberg, D. (2012). The tax-foundation theory of fiat money. *Economic Theory*, *50*(2), 489–497. doi:10.100700199-010-0564-8

Goldberg, S. C. (2020). Trust and reliance. In J. Simon (Ed.), *The Routledge handbook of trust and philosophy* (pp. 97–108). Routledge. doi:10.4324/9781315542294-8

Goldwater, J. (2016). The use of a blockchain to foster the development of patient-reported outcome measures. In *ONC/NIST Use of Blockchain for Healthcare and Research Workshop*. Gaithersburg, MD: ONC/NIST.

Golosova, J., & Romanovs, A. (2018). The Advantages and Disadvantages of the Blockchain Technology. In *2018 IEEE 6th Workshop on Advances in Information, Electronic and Electrical Engineering (AIEEE)*. IEEE.

Gordon, N. P., & Hornbrook, M. C. (2016). Differences in Access to and Preferences for Using Patient Portals and Other eHealth Technologies Based on Race, Ethnicity, and Age: A Database and Survey Study of Seniors in a Large Health Plan. *Journal of Medical Internet Research*, *18*(3), e50–e50. doi:10.2196/jmir.5105 PMID:26944212

Gordon, W. J., & Catalini, C. (2018). Blockchain Technology for Healthcare: Facilitating the Transition to Patient-Driven Interoperability. *Computational and Structural Biotechnology Journal*, *16*, 224–230. doi:10.1016/j.csbj.2018.06.003 PMID:30069284

Goss, A. K. (2007). Codifying a commons: Copyright, copyleft, and the Creative Commons project. Chi.-. *Kent L. Rev.*, *82*, 963.

Graeber, D. (2011). *Debt: the first 5,000 years*. Melville House Printing.

Grant, J. M. (2014). *Is Bitcoin Money? Implications for Bitcoin derivatives regulation and security interest treatment of bitcoins under article 9 of the uniform commercial code*. Implications for Bitcoin Derivatives Regulation and Security Interest Treatment of Bitcoins Under Article 9.

Greenberg, A. (2011). Crypto currency. Forbes.

Greif, A. (2006). Family structure, institutions, and growth: The origins and implications of western corporations. *The American Economic Review*, *96*(2), 308–312. Advance online publication. doi:10.1257/000282806777212602

Greitens, S. C. (2020). Surveillance, Security, & Democracy in a Post-COVID World. *International Organization*, *74*(S1), E169–E190. doi:10.1017/S0020818320000417

Grenzebach, J. (2020). *Dentacoin Foundation is the future of the dental industry*. Retrieved January 30, 2021, from https://aspioneer.com/dentacoin-foundation-is-the-future-of-the-dental-industry/

Grenzebach, P. (2017). *Dentacoin: Transforming the Dental Industry with Blockchain*. Retrieved January 30, 2021, from https://blockchain.cioreview.com/vendor/2017/dentacoin

Grossman, L. A. (2014). The rise of the empowered consumer: In recent decades, the FDA has allowed people to take a more active role in their health care. *Regulation*, (4), 34.

Grover, P., Kar, A. K., Janssen, M., & Ilavarasan, P. V. (2019). Perceived usefulness, ease of use and user acceptance of blockchain technology for digital transactions–insights from user-generated content on Twitter. *Enterprise Information Systems, 13*(6), 771–800. doi:10.1080/17517575.2019.1599446

Günzel-Jensen, F. & Holm, A. B. (2015). Freemium Business Models as the Foundation for Growing an E-Business Venture: A Multiple Case Study of Industry Leaders. *Journal of Entrepreneurship, Management and Innovation, 10.*

Gupta, A. (2013). Fraud and misconduct in clinical research: A concern. *Perspectives in Clinical Research, 4*(2), 144. doi:10.4103/2229-3485.111800 PMID:23833741

Gurguc, Z., & Knottenbelt, W. (2018). *Cryptocurrencies: overcoming barriers to trust and adoption.* eToro.

Gurstein, M. (2011). Open data: Empowering the empowered or effective data use for everyone? *First Monday, 16*(2).

Habermann, B., Broome, M., Pryor, E. R., & Ziner, K. W. (2010). Research Coordinators' Experiences With Scientific Misconduct and Research Integrity. *Nursing Research, 59*(1), 51–57. https://doi.org/10.1097/NNR.0b013e3181c3b9f2

Habermas, J., & Rehg, W. (1997). *Contributions to a discourse theory of law and democracy.* Polity Press.

Haber, S., & Stornetta, W. S. (1991). How to Time-Stamp a Digital Document. In *LNCS* (Vol. 537). Springer-Verlag.

Haber, S., & Stornetta, W. S. (1991). How to time-stamp a digital document. *Journal of Cryptology, 3*(2), 99–111. https://doi.org/10.1007/BF00196791

Hacker, P., & Petkova, B. (2016). Reining in the Big Promise of Big Data: Transparency, Inequality, and New Regulatory Frontiers. SSRN *Electronic Journal.* doi:10.2139srn.2773527

Hageman, J. R., Allen, K., Anderson, T., & Goldstein, M. (2020). Clinical Pearl: The Clinical Utility of the 'World Wide Web'with Historical Perspective from Tim Berners-Lee's Book 'Weaving the Web.' *TODAY Peer Reviewed Research. News and Information, 15*(10), 122.

Hamel, G. (2000). *Leading the revolution.* Harvard Business School Press.

Haneem, F., Bakar, H. A., Kama, N., Mat, N. Z. N., Ghazali, R., & Mahmood, Y. (2020). *Recent Progress of Blockchain Initiatives in Government.* Academic Press.

Haq, I., & Muselemu, O. (2018). Blockchain Technology in Pharmaceutical Industry to Prevent Counterfeit Drugs. *International Journal of Computers and Applications, 180*(25), 8–12.

Harari. (2020). *The world after coronavirus.* https://www.ft.com/content/19d90308-6858-11ea-a3c9-1fe6fedcca75

Harari, Y. N. (2014). *Sapiens: a brief history of mankind* (Y. N. Harari, J. Purcell, & H. Watzman, Trans.). Vintage Books.

Hardy, K., & Maurushat, A. (2017). Opening up government data for Big Data analysis and public benefit. *Computer Law & Security Review, 33*(1), 30–37. doi:10.1016/j.clsr.2016.11.003

Harel, T. O., Jameson, J. K., & Maoz, I. (2020). The Normalization of Hatred: Identity, Affective Polarization, and Dehumanization on Facebook in the Context of Intractable Political Conflict. *Social Media + Society, 6*(2). doi:10.1177/2056305120913983

Harford, T. (2019). *How important will blockchain be to the world's economy?* BBC News. https://www.bbc.com/news/business-48526666

Harrison, M. (2018). *Decentralizing the International Monetary System: An Assessment of Regulatory Structures for Cryptocurrencies in the Age of Digital Finance.* Academic Press.

Hartel, P., Homoliak, I., & Reijsbergen, D. (2019). An Empirical Study Into the Success of Listed Smart Contracts in Ethereum. *IEEE Access: Practical Innovations, Open Solutions*, *7*, 177539–177555. doi:10.1109/ACCESS.2019.2957284

Hart, W., Albarracín, D., Eagly, A. H., Brechan, I., Lindberg, M. J., & Merrill, L. (2009). Feeling validated versus being correct: A meta-analysis of selective exposure to information. *Psychological Bulletin*, *135*(4), 555–588. doi:10.1037/a0015701 PMID:19586162

Hasan, H. R., & Salah, K. (2019). Combating deepfake videos using blockchain and smart contracts. *IEEE Access: Practical Innovations, Open Solutions*, *7*, 41596–41606. doi:10.1109/ACCESS.2019.2905689

Hasan, H. R., Salah, K., Jayaraman, R., Arshad, J., & Omar, M. (2020). Blockchain-Based Solution for COVID-19 Digital Medical Passports and Immunity Certificates. *IEEE Access: Practical Innovations, Open Solutions*, *8*, 222093–222108. doi:10.1109/ACCESS.2020.3043350

Hassan, M. U., Rehmani, M. H., & Chen, J. (2019). Differential privacy techniques for cyber physical systems: A survey. *IEEE Communications Surveys and Tutorials*, *22*(1), 746–789. doi:10.1109/COMST.2019.2944748

Hasselgren, A., Kralevska, K., Gligoroski, D., Pedersen, S. A., & Faxvaag, A. (2020). Blockchain healthcare and health sciences—A scoping review. *International Journal of Medical Informatics*, *134*, 104040. doi:10.1016/j.ijmedinf.2019.104040 PMID:31865055

Hassine, M. B., Kmimech, M., Hellani, H., & Sliman, L. (2020, September). Toward a Mixed Tangle-Blockchain Architecture. In *Knowledge Innovation Through Intelligent Software Methodologies, Tools and Techniques: Proceedings of the 19th International Conference on New Trends in Intelligent Software Methodologies, Tools and Techniques (SoMeT_20)* (Vol. 327, p. 221). IOS Press.

Hau, Y. S., & Chang, M. C. (2020). Healthcare Information Technology Convergence to Effectively Cope with the COVID-19 crisis. *Health Policy and Technology*. Advance online publication. doi:10.1016/j.hlpt.2020.10.010 PMID:33163353

Hawlitschek, F., Notheisen, B., & Teubner, T. (2020). A 2020 perspective on "The limits of trust-free systems: A literature review on blockchain technology and trust in the sharing economy". *Electronic Commerce Research and Applications*, *40*, 100935. Advance online publication. doi:10.1016/j.elerap.2020.100935

Hayek, F. (1990), Denationalisation of Money-The Argument Refined. An Analysis of the Theory and Practice of Concurrent Currencies (3rd ed.). Academic Press.

Hayek, F. (1944). The road to serfdom. London. *George Routledge & Sons*, *67*, 84.

Hayek, F. (1976). *Denationalization of money*. Institute of Economic Affairs.

Hayek, F. A. (1976). *Denationalisation of money*. Ludwig von Mises Institute.

Hayes, A. S. (2017). Cryptocurrency value formation: An empirical study leading to a cost of production model for valuing bitcoin. *Telematics and Informatics*, *34*(7), 1308–1321. doi:10.1016/j.tele.2016.05.005

Hayrinen, K., Saranto, K., & Nykanen, P. (2008). Definition, structure, content, use and impacts of electronic health records: A review of the research literature. *International Journal of Medical Informatics*, *77*(5), 291–304. doi:10.1016/j.ijmedinf.2007.09.001 PMID:17951106

Healtheuropa.eu. (2019). *Health Europa*. Learning from the Estonian E-Health System. https://www.healtheuropa.eu/estonian-e-health-system/89750/

Heiberg, S., Krips, K., & Willemson, J. (2020). Planning the next steps for Estonian Internet voting. *E-Vote-ID*, *2020*, 82.

Heiss, J., Eberhardt, J., & Tai, S. (2019, July). From oracles to trustworthy data on-chaining systems. In *2019 IEEE International Conference on Blockchain (Blockchain)* (pp. 496-503). IEEE. 10.1109/Blockchain.2019.00075

HelbingD. (2014). *Qualified money-a better financial system for the future.* Available at SSRN 2526022 doi:10.2139srn.2526022

Helbing, D. (2017). From remote-controlled to self-controlled citizens. *The European Physical Journal. Special Topics, 226*(2), 313–320. doi:10.1140/epjst/e2016-60372-1

Heller, B. N. (2017). Estonia, the Digital Republic. *New Yorker (New York, N.Y.),* 1–25. https://www.newyorker.com/magazine/2017/12/18/estonia-the-digital-republic

HendricksonJ.HoganT.LutherW. (2015). The political economy of bitcoin. SSRN.

Heston, T. (2017). *A case study in blockchain healthcare innovation.* Academic Press.

Hill, N. S., Preston, I. R., & Roberts, K. E. (2008). Patients with Pulmonary Arterial Hypertension in Clinical Trials: Who Are They? *Proceedings of the American Thoracic Society, 5*(5), 603–609. https://doi.org/10.1513/pats.200803-032SK

Hill, T. P. (1977). On goods and services. *Review of Income and Wealth, 23*(4), 315–338. Advance online publication. doi:10.1111/j.1475-4991.1977.tb00021.x

Hirano, T., Motohashi, T., Okumura, K., Takajo, K., Kuroki, T., Ichikawa, D., Matsuoka, Y., Ochi, E., & Ueno, T. (2020). Data validation and verification using blockchain in a clinical trial for breast cancer: Regulatory sandbox. *Journal of Medical Internet Research, 22*(6), e18938. doi:10.2196/18938 PMID:32340974

Hirst, M., Harrison, J., & Mazepa, P. (2014). *Communication and new media: From broadcast to narrowcast.* Oxford University Press.

Hjálmarsson, F. Þ., Hreiðarsson, G. K., Hamdaqa, M., & Hjálmt'ysson, G. (2018). Blockchain-based e-voting system. *Proceedings of the 2018 IEEE 11th International Conference on Cloud Computing (CLOUD),* 983–986. 10.1109/CLOUD.2018.00151

Hobbes, T. (1914). *Leviathan.* Dent.

Hoberman, S., & Safari, O. R. M. C. (2018a). *Blockchain Explanation, Usage, and Impact.* Technics Publications. https://library.villanova.edu/Find/Record/2246337/Description

Hoberman, S., & Safari, O. R. M. C. (2018b). Blockchainopoly: How Blockchain Changes the Rules of the Game. Technics Publications.

Holochain.org. (2020). *What is Holochain?* https://developer.holochain.org/docs/what-is-holochain/

Hopkins, J. C., III, Prasad, B., Jameson, H. R., & Rangan, G. (2019). *U.S. Patent No. 10,521,780.* Washington, DC: U.S. Patent and Trademark Office.

Hosely, M. (2020). *Retention in Clinical Trials – Keeping Patients on Protocols.* Academic Press.

House of Commons Science and Technology Committee. (2018). *Research integrity: clinical trials transparency Tenth Report of Session 2017-19 Report, together with formal minutes relating to the report.* www.parliament.uk/science

Howgego, C. (1992). The supply and use of money in the Roman World 200 B.C. to A.D. 300. *Journal of Roman Studies, 82,* 1–31. doi:10.2307/301282

Hoxtell, W., & Nonhoff, D. (2019). *Internet Governance: Past, Present and Future.* Konrad Adenauer Stiftung. https://www.gppi.net/media/Internet-Governance-Past-Present-and-Future.pdf

Hsieh, K., & Li, E. Y. (2017). Progress of fintech industry from venture capital point of view. *Proceedings of the International Conference on Electronic Business (ICEB)*, 303-307.

Hsieh, M., Chung, M., & Chi, Y. (2016). A probability model for analysis of attacks on blockchain. *Proceedings of the International Conference on Electronic Business (ICEB)*, 352-355.

Hu, J., Deng, J., Gao, N., & Qian, J. (2020). Application architecture of product information traceability based on blockchain technology and a lightweight secure collaborative computing scheme. *Proceedings - 2020 International Conference on E-Commerce and Internet Technology, ECIT 2020*, 335-340. 10.1109/ECIT50008.2020.00084

Huang, G. K. J., & Chiang, K. -. (2017). RegTech evolution: The TrustChain. *Proceedings of the International Conference on Electronic Business (ICEB)*, 308-311.

Hudson, M. (2020). Origins of Money and Interest: Palatial Credit, Not Barter. In. S. Battilossi, Y. Cassis & K. Yago (Eds.), Handbook of the History of Money and Currency (pp. 45-65). Springer. doi:10.1007/978-981-13-0596-2_1

Hu, H., Wen, Y., Chua, T. S., & Li, X. (2014). Toward scalable systems for big data analytics: A technology tutorial. *IEEE Access: Practical Innovations, Open Solutions*, 2, 652–687. Advance online publication. doi:10.1109/ACCESS.2014.2332453

Hülsemann, P., & Tumasjan, A. (2019). *Walk this Way!* Incentive Structures of Different Token Designs for Blockchain-Based Applications.

Humer, C., & Finkle, J. (2014). *Your medical record is worth more to hackers than your credit card*. Philly.Com.

Humphrey, C. (1985). Barter and Economic Disintegration. *Man*, 20(1), 48–72. doi:10.2307/2802221

Hurlburt, G. F., & Voas, J. (2011). Storytelling: From cave art to digital media. *IT Professional*, 13(5), 4–7. doi:10.1109/MITP.2011.87

Hussien, H. M., Yasin, S. M., Udzir, S. N. I., Zaidan, A. A., & Zaidan, B. B. (2019). A Systematic Review for Enabling of Develop a Blockchain Technology in Healthcare Application: Taxonomy, Substantially Analysis, Motivations, Challenges, Recommendations and Future Direction. *Journal of Medical Systems*, 43(10), 320. Advance online publication. doi:10.100710916-019-1445-8 PMID:31522262

Hyduchack. (2020). *API Tools Offer Easier KYC/AML Compliance*. Aver. https://medium.com/goaver/api-tools-offer-easier-kyc-aml-compliance-e852a0c52902

Iansiti, M., & Lakhani, K. R. (2017). The truth about blockchain. Harvard Business Review.

IBM. (2020). *Trust Your Supplier Solution Transforms Supplier Management*. https://www.ibm.com/blockchain/solutions/trust-your-supplier

IEEE SA Beyond Standards. (2018). *Leveraging Blockchain for Clinical Trials/Research*. Available at: https://beyondstandards.ieee.org/leveraging-blockchain-clinical-trials-research/

IMI. (2020). *PharmaLedger selects use cases to advance adoption of blockchain in healthcare*. https://www.imi.europa.eu/news-events/newsroom/pharmaledger-selects-use-cases-advance-adoption-blockchain-healthcare

Ingham, G. (1996). Money is a social relation. *Review of Social Economy*. doi:10.1080/00346769600000031

Ingham, G. (2013). *The nature of money*. John Wiley & Sons.

Insight, A. (2021, May 30). *Digital Currency v/s Cryptocurrency: Brief Overview for Beginners*. Retrieved May 30, 2021, from https://www.analyticsinsight.net/digital-currency-v-s-cryptocurrency-brief-overview-for-beginners/

Insights, L. (2020, June 12). *Congressman argues for permissionless digital dollar to demonstrate U.S. values.* Ledger Insights - Enterprise Blockchain. https://www.ledgerinsights.com/digital-dollar-congress-permissionless/

Institute of Medicine (US) Forum on Drug Discovery Development and Translation. (2010). Transforming Clinical Research in the United States: Challenges and Opportunities. In *Medical Journal of Malaysia* (Vol. 62, Issue 4). National Academies Press (US). https://www.ncbi.nlm.nih.gov/books/NBK50888/

Ioannidis, J. P. A. (2005). Why most published research findings are false. In Getting to Good: Research Integrity in the Biomedical Sciences (Vol. 2, Issue 8). Academic Press.

Ioannidis, J. P. A. (2005). Why Most Published Research Findings Are False. *PLoS Medicine*, *2*(8), e124. doi:10.1371/journal.pmed.0020124 PMID:16060722

Ioannidis, J. P. A. (2005). Why most published research findings are false. *PLoS Medicine*, *2*(8), e124–e124. https://doi.org/10.1371/journal.pmed.0020124

IrresbergerF.JohnK.SalehF. (2020). The Public Blockchain Ecosystem: An Empirical Analysis. Available at SSRN. doi:10.2139srn.3592849

Islam, A. K. M. N., Mäntymäki, M., & Turunen, M. (2019). Why do blockchains split? an actor-network perspective on bitcoin splits. *Technological Forecasting and Social Change*, *148*, 119743. Advance online publication. doi:10.1016/j.techfore.2019.119743

Ismail, L., Materwala, H., Karduck, A. P., & Adem, A. (2020). Requirements of Health Data Management Systems for Biomedical Care and Research: Scoping Review [Review]. *Journal of Medical Internet Research*, *22*(7), 16. doi:10.2196/17508

Ivan on Tech. (2020). *A Closer Look - What is Yearn Finance and YFI?* Ivan on Tech Academy.

Iwamoto, K. (2021, February 15). *China's New Year digital yuan tests hasten Asia e-currency race.* Nikkei Asia. https://asia.nikkei.com/Spotlight/Asia-Insight/China-s-New-Year-digital-yuan-tests-hasten-Asia-e-currency-race

JaccardG. (2018). Smart contracts and the role of law. Available at SSRN 3099885. doi:10.2139srn.3099885

Jacobovitz, O. (2016). *Blockchain for identity management.* The Lynne and William Frankel Center for Computer Science Department of Computer Science. Ben-Gurion University.

JainD. (2020). The Economics of Cryptocurrencies-Why Does It Work? Available at SSRN 3644159.

Jamil, F., Hang, L., Kim, K., & Kim, D. (2019). A Novel Medical Blockchain Model for Drug Supply Chain Integrity Management in a Smart Hospital. *Electronics (Basel)*, *8*(5), 505. doi:10.3390/electronics8050505

Jeffries, D. (2021, May 21). *Dan Jeffries: It's 2031. This Is the World That Crypto Created.* Retrieved May 22, 2021, from https://www.coindesk.com/its-2031-this-is-the-world-that-crypto-created

Jemel, M., & Serhrouchni, A. (2017). Decentralized access control mechanism with temporal dimension based on blockchain. *Proceedings - 14th IEEE International Conference on E-Business Engineering, ICEBE 2017 - Including 13th Workshop on Service-Oriented Applications, Integration and Collaboration, SOAIC 207*, 177-182. Retrieved from www.scopus.com doi:10.1109/ICEBE.2017.35

Jensen, J. L. (2020). *The Medieval Internet: Power, politics and participation in the digital age.* Emerald Group Publishing.

Jensen, T., Hedman, J., & Henningsson, S. (2019). How tradelens delivers business value with blockchain technology. *MIS Quarterly Executive*, *18*(4), 221–243. doi:10.17705/2msqe.00018

Jha, P. (2021, May 14). *Guaranty Escrow to Accept Dogecoin Payment For Real Estate Purchases*. Retrieved May 14, 2021, from https://coingape.com/guaranty-escrow-to-accept-dogecoin-payment-for-real-estate-purchases/amp/

Jim Sergent. (2020). *Apple is first $2 trillion US company. What that would look like in iPhones*. USA Today. https://eu.usatoday.com/in-depth/money/2020/08/19/apple-2-trillion-company-worth-what-looks-like-iphones/3353398001/

Jordanova, M., & Lievens, F. (2011). *Global Telemedicine and eHealth (A synopsis). E-Health and Bioengineering Conference*. EHB.

Jørgensen, R. F. (2020). The right to privacy under pressure. *Nordicom Review, 37*(s1), 165–170. doi:10.1515/nor-2016-0030

Joshi, R. (2020). *How Can Blockchain Be Implemented in the Life Sciences Ecosystem?* Technology Networks. https://www.technologynetworks.com/informatics/articles/how-can-blockchain-be-implemented-in-the-life-sciences-ecosystem-330614

Kabi, O. R., & Franqueira, V. N. L. (2019). *Blockchain-based distributed marketplace*. doi:10.1007/978-3-030-04849-5_17

Kakinuma, Y. (2014). The emergence and spread of coins in China from the Spring and Autumn Period to the Warring States Period. In P. Bernholz & R. Vaubel (Eds.), *Explaining monetary and financial innovation: a historical analysis* (pp. 79–126). Springer. doi:10.1007/978-3-319-06109-2_5

Kalla, A., Hewa, T., Mishra, R. A., Ylianttila, M., & Liyanage, M. (2020). The Role of Blockchain to Fight Against COVID-19. *IEEE Engineering Management Review, 48*(3), 85–96. Advance online publication. doi:10.1109/EMR.2020.3014052

Kamel Boulos, M. N., Wilson, J. T., & Clauson, K. A. (2018). Geospatial blockchain: Promises, challenges, and scenarios in health and healthcare. *International Journal of Health Geographics, 17*(1), 25. doi:10.118612942-018-0144-x

Kanza, S., & Frey, J. G. (2019). A new wave of innovation in Semantic web tools for drug discovery. In Expert Opinion on Drug Discovery. Academic Press.

Kapassa, E., Touloupos, M., Kyriazis, D., & Themistocleous, M. (2020). *A smart distributed marketplace*. doi:10.1007/978-3-030-44322-1_34

Karafiloski, E., & Mishev, A. (2017, July). Blockchain solutions for big data challenges: A literature review. In *IEEE EUROCON 2017-17th International Conference on Smart Technologies* (pp. 763-768). IEEE. 10.1109/EUROCON.2017.8011213

Kassab, M. H., DeFranco, J., Malas, T., Laplante, P., Destefanis, G., & Graciano Neto, V. V. (2019). Exploring Research in Blockchain for Healthcare and a Roadmap for the Future. *IEEE Transactions on Emerging Topics in Computing, 6750*(c), 1–16. doi:10.1109/TETC.2019.2936881

Kathuria, S., Grover, A., Perego, V. M. E., Mattoo, A., & Banerjee, P. (2019). *Understanding E-Commerce*. World Bank Group.

Katzenbach, C., & Ulbricht, L. (2019). Algorithmic Governance. *Internet Policy Review, 8*(4), 1–18. doi:10.14763/2019.4.1424

Kauffman, S. A. (1993). *The origins of order: Self-organization and selection in evolution*. Oxford University Press.

Kehoe, L., O'Connell, N., Andrzejewski, D., Gindner, K., & Dalal, D. (2017). *When two chains combine Supply chain meets blockchain*. https://www2.deloitte.com/tr/en/pages/technology/articles/when-two-chains-combine.html

Keller, T., & Kessler, N. (2018). Yet another blockchain use case-the label chain. *Proceedings - 2018 IEEE 15th International Conference on e-Business Engineering, ICEBE 2018*, 187-194. 10.1109/ICEBE.2018.00037

Kellner, D. M., & Durham, M. G. (2001). Adventures in media and cultural studies: Introducing the keyworks. *Media and cultural studies: Keyworks*, 1-29.

Kethineni, S., & Cao, Y. (2020). The rise in popularity of cryptocurrency and associated criminal activity. *International Criminal Justice Review*, 30(3), 325–344. doi:10.1177/1057567719827051

Kewell, B., Adams, R., & Parry, G. (2017). Blockchain for good? *Strategic Change*, 26(5), 429–437. doi:10.1002/jsc.2143

Keynes, J. M. (1915). The Island of Stone Money. *Economic Journal (London)*, 25(98), 281–283. doi:10.2307/2222196

Khan, M. A. U. D., Uddin, M. F., & Gupta, N. (2014). Seven V's of Big Data understanding Big Data to extract value. *Proceedings of the 2014 Zone 1 Conference of the American Society for Engineering Education - "Engineering Education: Industry Involvement and Interdisciplinary Trends", ASEE Zone 1 2014.* 10.1109/ASEEZone1.2014.6820689

Khare, R. (2003). *Extending the REpresentational State Transfer REST Architectural Style for Decentralized Systems* (Doctoral dissertation). University of California, Irvine.

Khare, R., & Taylor, R. N. (2004, May). Extending the representational state transfer (rest) architectural style for decentralized systems. In *Proceedings. 26th International Conference on Software Engineering* (pp. 428-437). IEEE.

Khezr, S., Moniruzzaman, M., Yassine, A., & Benlamri, R. (2019). Blockchain technology in healthcare: A comprehensive review and directions for future research. *Applied Sciences (Basel, Switzerland)*, 9(9), 1736. doi:10.3390/app9091736

Khezr, S., Moniruzzaman, M., Yassine, A., & Benlamri, R. (2019). Blockchain Technology in Healthcare: A Comprehensive Review and Directions for Future Research. *Applied Sciences (Basel, Switzerland)*, 9, 1736. https://doi.org/10.3390/app9091736

KiffJ.AlwazirJ.DavidovicS.FariasA.KhanA.KhiaonarongT.ZhouP. (2020). A survey of research on retail central bank digital currency. Available at SSRN 3639760.

Kim, S. (2020). *Fractional Ownership*. Democratization and Bubble Formation - The Impact of Blockchain Enabled Asset Tokenization.

Kim, Y. S., & Lee, J. W. (2011). Corruption and Government Roles: Causes, Economic Effects, and Scope. *Korea and the World Economy*, 12(3), 513–553.

King, P. W. (2009). *Climbing Maslow's pyramid*. Troubador Publishing Ltd.

Kirillova, E., Bogdan, V. V., Filippov, P., Tkachev, V., & Zulfugarzade, T. (2020). The Main Features of Blockchain Technologies Classification. *COMPUSOFT: An International Journal of Advanced Computer Technology*, 9(10), 3900–3905.

Knittel, M. L., & Wash, R. (2019, May). How "True Bitcoiners" work on reddit to maintain bitcoin. In *Extended Abstracts of the 2019 CHI Conference on Human Factors in Computing Systems* (pp. 1-6). ACM.

Kohn, M. (2020). Money, trade, and payments in Preindustrial Europe. In S. Battilossi, Y. Cassis & K. Yago (Eds.), Handbook of the History of Money and Currency (pp. 223-244). Springer. doi:10.1007/978-981-13-0596-2_15

Kolias, C., Kambourakis, G., Stavrou, A., & Voas, J. (2017). DDoS in the IoT: Mirai and other botnets. *Computer*, 50(7), 80–84. doi:10.1109/MC.2017.201

Kõnd, K., & Lilleväli, A. (2019). E-Prescription success in Estonia: The journey from paper to pharmacogenomics. *Eurohealth (London)*, 25(2), 18–19.

Konst, S., & Wätjen, D. (2000). *Sichere Log-Dateien auf Grundlage kryptographisch verketteter Einträge*. http://publikationsserver.tu-braunschweig.de/get/64933

Kotler, P. (1999). *Marketing management: The millennium edition* (Vol. 199). Prentice Hall.

Kotler, P., Kartajaya, H., & Setiawan, I. (2016). *Marketing 4.0: Moving from traditional to digital*. John Wiley & Sons.

Koufakis, A., Chatzakou, D., Meditskos, G., Tsikrika, T., Vrochidis, S., & Kompatsiaris, I. (2020). *Invited keynote on IOT4SAFE 2020: Semantic Web Technologies in Fighting Crime and Terrorism: The CONNEXIONs Approach*. Academic Press.

Kouzinopoulos, C. S., Giannoutakis, K. M., Votis, K., Tzovaras, D., Collen, A., Nijdam, N. A., Konstantas, D., Spathoulas, G., Pandey, P., & Katsikas, S. (2018, September 14). Implementing a Forms of Consent Smart Contract on an IoT-based Blockchain to promote user trust. *2018 IEEE (SMC) International Conference on Innovations in Intelligent Systems and Applications, INISTA 2018*. 10.1109/INISTA.2018.8466268

Kraeva, D. (2020). *Dentacoin Announces Partnership With Europe's Largest Dental Clinic*. Retrieved January 30, 2021, from https://blog.dentacoin.com/dentacoin-dentaprime-partnership-with-europe-largest-dental-clinic/

Krafft, P. M., & Donovan, J. (2020). Disinformation by design: The use of evidence collages and platform filtering in a media manipulation campaign. *Political Communication*, *37*(2), 194–214. doi:10.1080/10584609.2019.1686094

Kranzberg, M. (1986). Technology and History:" Kranzberg's Laws. *Technology and Culture*, *27*(3), 544–560. doi:10.2307/3105385

Kravchenko, P. (2018). *Blockchain doesn't Eliminate Intermediaries and Never Will — It's a Fact*. Coinspeaker. https://www.coinspeaker.com/blockchain-doesnt-eliminate-intermediaries-and-never-will-its-a-fact/

Krawiec, R. J., Housman, D., White, M., Filipova, M., Quarre, F., Barr, D., Nesbitt, A., Fedosova, K., Killmeyer, J., Israel, A., & Tsai, L. (2017). *Blockchain: Opportunities for Health Care*. Academic Press.

Krieger, J. L., Neil, J. M., Strekalova, Y. A., & Sarge, M. A. (2017). Linguistic Strategies for Improving Informed Consent in Clinical Trials Among Low Health Literacy Patients. *Journal of the National Cancer Institute*, *109*(3), djw233. https://doi.org/10.1093/jnci/djw233

Krittanawong, C., Rogers, A. J., Aydar, M., Choi, E., Johnson, K. W., Wang, Z., & Narayan, S. M. (2020). Integrating blockchain technology with artificial intelligence for cardiovascular medicine. *Nature Reviews. Cardiology*, *17*(1), 1–3. https://doi.org/10.1038/s41569-019-0294-y

Kroll, J. a, Davey, I. C., & Felten, E. W. (2013). The Economics of Bitcoin Mining, or Bitcoin in the Presence of Adversaries. *The Twelfth Workshop on the Economics of Information Security (WEIS 2013)*.

Kroll, J. (1976). Aristophanes' *ponera chalkia*: A reply. *Greek, Roman and Byzantine Studies*, *17*(4), 329–341.

Kroll, J. (2012). The monetary background of early coinage. In W. Metcalf (Ed.), *The Oxford Handbook of Greek and Roman Coinage* (pp. 33–42). Oxford University Press., doi:10.1093/oxfordhb/9780195305746.013.0003

Kruijff, J. T., & Weigand, H. (2018, February). An introduction to Commitment Based Smart Contracts using Reaction-RuleML. In VMBO (pp. 149-157). Academic Press.

Kshetri, N. (2017). Can blockchain strengthen the internet of things? *IT Professional*, *19*(4), 68–72. doi:10.1109/MITP.2017.3051335

Kshetri, N., & Voas, J. (2018). Blockchain-enabled e-voting. *IEEE Software*, *35*(4), 95–99. doi:10.1109/MS.2018.2801546

Kugler, P., & Straumann, T. (2020). International monetary regimes: the Bretton Woods system. In S. Battilossi, Y. Cassis & K. Yago (Eds.), Handbook of the History of Money and Currency (pp. 665-685). Springer. doi:10.1007/978-981-13-0596-2_25

Kumar, S., & Pundir, A. K. (2020). *Blockchain–Internet of things (IoT) Enabled Pharmaceutical Supply Chain for COVID-19.* Academic Press.

Kuo, C. D. L., Guo, L., & Wang, Y. (2017). Cryptocurrency: A New Investment Opportunity? *The Journal of Alternative Investments, 20*(3), 16–40. doi:10.3905/jai.2018.20.3.016

Kuperberg, M. (2019). Blockchain-based identity management: A survey from the enterprise and ecosystem perspective. *IEEE Transactions on Engineering Management, 67*(4), 1008–1027. doi:10.1109/TEM.2019.2926471

Kurihara, Y. (2021). *Has the Price of Bitcoin changed during COVID-19?* Academic Press.

Lafaurie, J. (1981). *Les assignats et les papiers-monnaies émis par l'État au XVIIIe siècle.* Le Leopard d'Or.

Lamport, L. (1998). The Part-Time Parliament. *ACM Transactions on Computer Systems.* doi:10.1145/279227.279229

Lamport, L., Shostak, R., & Pease, M. (2019). The Byzantine generals problem. In Concurrency: The Works of Leslie Lamport (pp. 203-226). Academic Press.

Lan, R., Upadhyaya, G., Tse, S., & Zamani, M. (2021). *Horizon: A Gas-Efficient, Trustless Bridge for Cross-Chain Transactions.* arXiv preprint arXiv:2101.06000.

Landemore, H. (2012). *Democratic reason: Politics, collective intelligence, and the rule of the many.* Princeton University Press.

Lane, F. C., & Mueller, R. C. (1987). Coins and moneys of account. In F. C. Lane & R. C. Mueller (Eds.) Money and banking in medieval Renaissance Venice (Vol. 1). The John Hopkins University Press.

Langfred, C. W. (2004). Too much of a good thing? Negative effects of high trust and individual autonomy in self-managing teams. *Academy of Management Journal, 47*(3), 385–399. doi:10.5465/20159588

Lannoye, V. (2020). *The History of Money for Understanding Economics.* Vincent Lannoye.

Lascaux, A. (2014). Money, trust and hierarchies: Understanding the foundations for placing confidence in complex economic institutions. *Journal of Economic Issues, 46*(1), 75–100. doi:10.2753/JEI0021-3624460103

Laure, A., & Linn, M. B. K. (2016). Blockchain For Health Data and Its Potential Use in Health IT and Health Care Related Research. *ONC/NIST Use of Blockchain for Healthcare and Research Workshop,* 1–10. 10.5455/aim.2019.27.284-291

Laurent, P. (2017). *Continuous interconnected supply chain Using Blockchain & Internet-of-Things in supply chain traceability.* Academic Press.

Leach, M., MacGregor, H., Scoones, I., & Wilkinson, A. (2020). Post-pandemic transformations: How and why COVID-19 requires us to rethink development. *World Development, 138,* 105233. doi:10.1016/j.worlddev.2020.105233 PMID:33100478

Lecarme, L. (2019). *What Is the Early Adopters Advantage in Crypto?* The Startup. https://medium.com/swlh/what-is-the-early-adopters-advantage-in-crypto-4ee18984f707

Lee, J. Y. (2019). A decentralized token economy: How blockchain and cryptocurrency can revolutionize business. *Business Horizons.* doi:10.1016/j.bushor.2019.08.003

Lee, J., Yoo, B., & Jang, M. (2019). *Is a blockchain-based game a game for fun, or is it a tool for speculation? an empirical analysis of player behavior in crypokitties.* doi:10.1007/978-3-030-22784-5_14

Leeming, G., Cunningham, J., & Ainsworth, J. (2019). A Ledger of Me: Personalizing Healthcare Using Blockchain Technology. *Frontiers in Medicine.* doi:10.3389/fmed.2019.00171

Leiner, B. M., Cerf, V. G., Clark, D. D., Kahn, R. E., Kleinrock, L., Lynch, D. C., ... Wolff, S. (2009). A brief history of the Internet. *Computer Communication Review, 39*(5), 22–31.

Leonard, D., & Treiblmaier, H. (2019). Can cryptocurrencies help to pave the way to a more sustainable economy? Questioning the economic growth paradigm. In *Business transformation through Blockchain* (pp. 183–205). Palgrave Macmillan. doi:10.1007/978-3-319-99058-3_7

Lesser, M. L., & Haanstra, J. W. (2000). Random-Access Memory Accounting Machine. I. System organization of the IBM 305. *IBM Journal of Research and Development*. doi:10.1147/JRD.2000.5389196

Lessig, L. (2015). *De ja vu all over again*. Talk given at Sydney Blockchain workshop.

Lewicki, R. J., McAllister, D. J., & Bies, R. J. (1998). Trust and distrust: New relationships and realities. *Academy of Management Review, 23*(3), 438–458. doi:10.5465/amr.1998.926620

Lewis, A. (2015). *A Gentle Introduction to Digital Tokens*. Bits on Blocks. https://bitsonblocks.net/2015/09/28/a-gentle-introduction-to-digital-tokens

Lewis, A. (2015). *A gentle introduction to digital tokens*. https://bitsonblocks.net/2015/09/28/a-gentleintroduction-to-digital-tokens/

Li, G. (2008). *Economic sense of Metcalfe's Law*. Academic Press.

Li, Q., Xu, M., Fang, M., Yang, M., & Guo, Y. (2019). A conceptual framework for data property protection based on blockchain. *Proceedings of the International Conference on Electronic Business (ICEB),* 501-505.

Li, S. (2018). An author-centered media blockchain ecosystem. *Proceedings - 2018 IEEE 15th International Conference on e-Business Engineering, ICEBE 2018,* 201-206. 10.1109/ICEBE.2018.00039

Li, Y. (2019). Emerging blockchain-based applications and techniques. In Service Oriented Computing and Applications. doi:10.100711761-019-00281-x

Li, Y., Liang, X., Zhu, X., & Wu, B. (2018). A blockchain-based autonomous credit system. *Proceedings - 2018 IEEE 15th International Conference on e-Business Engineering, ICEBE 2018,* 178-186. 10.1109/ICEBE.2018.00036

Li, Y., Xue, S., Liang, X., & Zhu, X. (2017). I2I: A balanced ecommerce model with creditworthiness cloud. *Proceedings - 14th IEEE International Conference on E-Business Engineering, ICEBE 2017 - Including 13th Workshop on Service-Oriented Applications, Integration and Collaboration, SOAIC 207,* 150-158. 10.1109/ICEBE.2017.31

Liang, Y. C. (2020). Blockchain for dynamic spectrum management. In *Signals and Communication Technology* (pp. 121–146). Springer. doi:10.1007/978-981-15-0776-2_5

Lindley, J., Coulton, P., Akmal, H. A., Hay, D., Van Kleek, M., Cannizzaro, S., & Binns, R. (2019). *The Little Book of*. Academic Press.

Linn, L. A., & Koo, M. B. (2016). *Blockchain For Health Data and Its Potential Use in Health IT and Health Care Related Research*. Academic Press.

Liquid. (2020). *Bitcoin price history & future of the fastest-growing asset class*. Beginner Guide. https://blog.liquid.com/bitcoin-price-history

Liu, J., Li, X., Ye, L., Zhang, H., Du, X., & Guizani, M. (2018a, December). BPDS: A blockchain based privacy-preserving data sharing for electronic medical records. In *2018 IEEE Global Communications Conference (GLOBECOM)* (pp. 1-6). IEEE.

Liu, L., Piao, C., Jiang, X., & Zheng, L. (2018). Research on governmental data sharing based on local differential privacy approach. *Proceedings - 2018 IEEE 15th International Conference on e-Business Engineering, ICEBE 2018,* 39-45. 10.1109/ICEBE.2018.00017

Liu, J., Li, B., Chen, L., Hou, M., Xiang, F., & Wang, P. (2018, June). A data storage method based on blockchain for decentralization DNS. In *2018 IEEE Third International Conference on Data Science in Cyberspace (DSC)* (pp. 189-196). IEEE.

Liu, J., Li, X., Ye, L., Zhang, H., Du, X., & Guizani, M. (2018, December). BPDS: A blockchain based privacy-preserving data sharing for electronic medical records. In *2018 IEEE Global Communications Conference (GLOBECOM)* (pp. 1-6). IEEE. 10.1109/GLOCOM.2018.8647713

Liu, T., Cui, Z., Du, H., & Wu, Z. (2021). Privacy-Preserving and Verifiable Electronic Voting Scheme Based on Smart Contract of Blockchain. *International Journal of Network Security, 23*(2), 296–304.

Livingston, D., Sivaram, V., Freeman, M., & Fiege, M. (2018). *Applying blockchain technology to electric power systems.* Academic Press.

Lopes, J., Pereira, J. L., & Varajão, J. (2019). *Blockchain based E-voting system: a proposal.* Academic Press.

Lopez, P. G., Montresor, A., & Datta, A. (2019). Please, do not decentralize the Internet with (permissionless) blockchains! *2019 IEEE 39th International Conference on Distributed Computing Systems (ICDCS),* 1901–1911.

Lopez, P. G., Montresor, A., & Datta, A. (2019, July). Please, do not decentralize the Internet with (permissionless) blockchains! In *2019 IEEE 39th International Conference on Distributed Computing Systems (ICDCS)* (pp. 1901-1911). IEEE.

Lopez, R. S. (1976). *The commercial revolution of the Middle Ages.* Cambridge University Press.

Lorne, F. T., Daram, S., Frantz, R., Kumar, N., Mohammed, A., & Muley, A. (2018). Blockchain Economics and Marketing. *Journal of Computer and Communications, 6*(12), 107–117.

Lo, S. K., Xu, X., Staples, M., & Yao, L. (2020). Reliability analysis for blockchain oracles R. *Computers & Electrical Engineering, 83*(10658), 2.

Lotti, L. (2019). The Art of Tokenization: Blockchain Affordances and the Invention of Future Milieus. *Media Theory, 3*(1), 287–320.

Lowry, P. B., Schuetzler, R., Giboney, J. S., & Gregory, T. (2015). Is trust always better than distrust? The potential value of distrust in newer virtual teams engaged in short-term decision-making. *Group Decision and Negotiation, 24*(4), 723–752. doi:10.100710726-014-9410-x

Lo Y. C. (2017). Blockchain and bitcoin: technological breakthrough or the latest tulip price bubble? Available at SSRN 3198530. doi:10.2139srn.3198530

Lu, C., Batista, D., Hamouda, H., & Lemieux, V. (2020). Consumers' Intention to Adopt Blockchain-based Personal Health Records (PHR) and Data Sharing: Focus-group Study (Preprint). *JMIR Formative Research, 4*(11), e21995. Advance online publication. doi:10.2196/21995 PMID:33151149

Luhmann, N. (1988). Familiarity, confidence, trust: Problems and alternatives. In D. Gambetta (Ed.), *Trust: Making and breaking cooperative relations* (pp. 94–107). Basil Blackwell.

Lusa, A. (2020a). *Covid-19: Portugal já fez 3,2 milhões de testes e "app" de rastreio soma 2,4 milhões de 'downloads.'* https://www.lusa.pt/article/S8LuGAwMQ7SQaypC08jvETMSZM5iuSI1/covid-19-portugal-já-fez-3-2-milhões-de-testes-e-app-de-rastreio-soma-2-4-milhões-de-downloads

Lusa, A. (2020b). StayAway Covid obrigatória abre "graves questões" de privacidade. *RTP Notícias - Economia*. https://www.rtp.pt/noticias/economia/stayaway-covid-obrigatoria-abregraves-questoes-de-privacidade_n1267109

Lu, Y., & Pan, J. (2020). Capturing Clicks: How the Chinese Government Uses Clickbait to Compete for Visibility. *Political Communication*, 1–32. doi:10.1080/10584609.2020.1765914

Lyon, D. (2014). Surveillance, Snowden, and Big Data: Capacities, consequences, critique. *Big Data & Society*, *1*(2). Advance online publication. doi:10.1177/2053951714541861

Mack, E. (2021, May 14). *Wow, much value: Dogecoin seals New England real estate deal*. Retrieved May 14, 2021, from https://www.cnet.com/google-amp/news/wow-much-value-dogecoin-seals-new-england-real-estate-deal/

Mack, C. A. (2011). Fifty years of Moore's law. *IEEE Transactions on Semiconductor Manufacturing*, *24*(2), 202–207. doi:10.1109/TSM.2010.2096437

Mackey, T. K., Kuo, T. T., Gummadi, B., Clauson, K. A., Church, G., Grishin, D., Obbad, K., Barkovich, R., & Palombini, M. (2019). "Fit-for-purpose?" - Challenges and opportunities for applications of blockchain technology in the future of healthcare. *BMC Medicine*, *17*(1), 1–17. doi:10.118612916-019-1296-7 PMID:30914045

Maddux, D. (2017). *Cybersecurity and Blockchain in Health Care*. Retrieved January 29, 2021, from https://acumenmd.com/blog/cybersecurity-and-blockchain-in-health-care/

Magyar, G. (2017, November). Blockchain: Solving the privacy and research availability tradeoff for EHR data: A new disruptive technology in health data management. In *2017 IEEE 30th Neumann Colloquium (NC)* (pp. 135-140). IEEE.

Maher, M. E., & Andersson, T. (2005). Corporate Governance: Effects on Firm Performance and Economic Growth. SSRN *Electronic Journal*. doi:10.2139srn.218490

Mainelli, M. (2017). Blockchain could help us reclaim control of our personal data. *Harvard Business Review Digital Articles*, 2-5.

Makridakis, S., & Christodoulou, K. (2019). Blockchain: Current challenges and future prospects/applications. In Future Internet (Vol. 11, Issue 12). MDPI AG. doi:10.3390/fi11120258

Mamoshina, P., Ojomoko, L., Yanovich, Y., & Ostrovski, A. (2018). *Converging blockchain and next-generation artificial intelligence technologies to decentralize and accelerate biomedical research and healthcare Converging blockchain and next-generation artificial intelligence technologies to decentralize and accelerate*. doi:10.18632/oncotarget.22345

Mamun, M. A., Bhuiyan, A. I., & Manzar, M. D. (2020). The first COVID-19 infanticide-suicide case: Financial crisis and fear of COVID-19 infection are the causative factors. *Asian Journal of Psychiatry*, *54*, 102365. doi:10.1016/j.ajp.2020.102365 PMID:33271687

Mangus, S. M., Jones, E., Folse, J. A. G., & Sridhar, S. (2020). The interplay between business and personal trust on relationship performance in conditions of market turbulence. *Journal of the Academy of Marketing Science*, *48*(6), 1138–1155. doi:10.100711747-020-00722-6

Manovich, L. (2002). *The Language of New Media*. MIT.

Manovich, L. (2013). *Software Takes Command*. Bloomsbury Academic.

Marbouh, D., Abbasi, T., Maasmi, F., Omar, I. A., Debe, M. S., Salah, K., Jayaraman, R., & Ellahham, S. (2020). Blockchain for COVID-19: Review, Opportunities, and a Trusted Tracking System. In Arabian Journal for Science and Engineering (p. 1). Springer Science and Business Media Deutschland GmbH. doi:10.100713369-020-04950-4

Marbouh, D., Abbasi, T., Maasmi, F., Omar, I. A., Debe, M. S., Salah, K., Jayaraman, R., & Ellahham, S. (2020). Blockchain for COVID-19: Review, Opportunities, and a Trusted Tracking System. *Arabian Journal for Science and Engineering*, 1–17.

Markham, K. (2018). *A practical guide to the general data protection regulation (GDPR)*. Law Brief Publishing, Ltd.

Marten, R., & Kai, S. (2017). A blockchain research framework–What we (don't) know, where we go from here, and how we will get there. *Business & Information Systems Engineering*, *59*(6), 385–409. doi:10.100712599-017-0506-0

Martin & Murphy. (2017). The role of data privacy in marketing. *Journal of the Academy of Marketing Science, 45*(2), 135-155.

Martinelli, E. (2017). *The Politics of Bitcoin*. http://www.brunoleonimedia.it/public/Mises2018/Papers/Mises2018-Paper_Martinelli.pdf

Martin, F. (2013). *The Unauthorised Biography*. Random House.

Martin, K. (2019). Designing Ethical Algorithms. *MIS Quarterly Executive, 18*(2).

Martins, P. (2018). *Introdução à Blockchain*. FCA-Editora de Informática, Lda.

Marturano, A. (2002). The role of metaethics and the future of computer ethics. *Ethics and Information Technology, 4*(1), 71–78.

Maslove, D. M., Klein, J., Brohman, K., & Martin, P. (2018). Using Blockchain Technology to Manage Clinical Trials Data : A Proof-of-Concept Study. *JMIR Medical Informatics, 6*(4), 1–7.

Maslove, D. M., Klein, J., Brohman, K., & Martin, P. (2018). Using Blockchain Technology to Manage Clinical Trials Data: A Proof-of-Concept Study. *JMIR Medical Informatics, 6*(4), e11949. doi:10.2196/11949 PMID:30578196

Maslow, A. H. (1943). A theory of human motivation. *Psychological Review, 50*(4), 370–396. doi:10.1037/h0054346

Maslow, A. H. (1943). A Theory of Human Motivation. *Psychological Review, 50*, 370–396.

Massey, R., Dalal, D., & Dakshinamoorthy, A. (2017). *Initial coin offering: A new paradigm*. Deloitte. Available at https:// www2.deloitte.com/content/dam/Deloitte/us/Documents/ process-and-operations/us-cons-new-paradigm.pdf

Matseshe, L. K., Arasa, R., & Yohannes, T. H. (2017). *The Moderating Effect Of Decision-Maker On The Relationship Between Strategy And Organizational Structure*. Academic Press.

Mattke, J., Maier, C., & Reis, L. (2020, June). Is cryptocurrency money? Three empirical studies analyzing medium of exchange, store of value and unit of account. In *Proceedings of the 2020 on Computers and People Research Conference* (pp. 26-35). 10.1145/3378539.3393859

Maxmen, A. (2018). AI researchers embrace Bitcoin technology to share medical data. *Nature, 555*(7696), 293–294. https://doi.org/10.1038/d41586-018-02641-7

Mayer, R. C., Davis, J. H., & Schoorman, F. D. (1995). An integrative model of organizational trust. *Academy of Management Review, 20*(3), 709–734. doi:10.5465/amr.1995.9508080335

Mazlan, A. A., Daud, S. M., Sam, S. M., Abas, H., Rasid, S. Z. A., & Yusof, M. F. (2020). Scalability Challenges in Healthcare Blockchain System-A Systematic Review. *IEEE Access*. doi:10.1109/ACCESS.2020.2969230

McCauley, A. (2020). Why Big Pharma Is Betting on Blockchain. *Harvard Business Review*.

McDermott, D. S., Kamerer, J. L., & Birk, A. T. (2019). Electronic Health Records- A Literature Review of Cyber Threats and Security Measures. *International Journal of Cyber Research and Education, 1*(2), 42–49. doi:10.4018/IJCRE.2019070104

McIntosh, R. (2021, May 12). *While Tesla Decides on Dogecoin, FNTX Users Can Buy Condos with DOGE.* Retrieved May 13, 2021, from https://www.financemagnates.com/cryptocurrency/news/while-tesla-decides-on-dogecoin-fntx-users-can-buy-condos-with-doge/?tg=1620799861

McKee, M., Karanikolos, M., Belcher, P., & Stuckler, D. (2012). Austerity: A failed experiment on the people of Europe. *Clinical Medicine, 12*(4), 346–350. doi:10.7861/clinmedicine.12-4-346 PMID:22930881

McLeod, C. (2020). Trust. In E. N. Zalta (Ed.), *Stanford Encyclopedia of Philosophy.* Retrieved March 1, 2021, from https://plato.stanford.edu/archives/fall2020/entries/trust/

McLuhan, M., & McLuhan, M. A. (1994). *Understanding media: The extensions of man.* MIT Press.

McLuhan, M., & Powers, B. R. (1989). *The Global Village: Transformations in World, Life and Media in the 21st Century.* Oxford University Press.

Mearian, L. (2019). *What is blockchain? The complete guide.* Retrieved January 29, 2021, from https://www.computerworld.com/article/3191077/what-is-blockchain-the-complete-guide.html

Medtronic. (2020). Blockchain in healthcare - Meaningful innovation. *Medtronic website.* https://www.medtronic.com/us-en/transforming-healthcare/meaningful-innovation/science-behind-healthcare/blockchain-in-healthcare.html

Meier, P., Beinke, J. H., Fitte, C., & Teuteberg, F. (2020). Generating design knowledge for blockchain-based access control to personal health records. *Information Systems and e-Business Management,* ●●●, 1–29.

Mello, M. M., Lieou, V., & Goodman, S. N. (2018). Clinical Trial Participants' Views of the Risks and Benefits of Data Sharing. *The New England Journal of Medicine, 378*(23), 2202–2211. https://doi.org/10.1056/NEJMsa1713258

Menachemi, N., & Collum. (2011). Benefits and drawbacks of electronic health record systems. *Risk Management and Healthcare Policy, 47,* 47. Advance online publication. doi:10.2147/RMHP.S12985 PMID:22312227

Mengelkamp, E., Notheisen, B., Beer, C., Dauer, D., & Weinhardt, C. (2018). "A blockchain-based smart grid: Towards sustainable local energy markets," Comput. Sci.-. *Research for Development, 33*(1-2), 207–214.

Merkle, R. C. (1990). *One Way Hash Functions and DES.,* doi:10.1007/0-387-34805-0_40

Mertes, T. (2002). Wall Street. *Amass, 12*(2), 80.

Metaxiotis, K., Ptochos, D., & Psarras, J. (2004). E-health in the new millennium: A research and practice agenda. *International Journal of Electronic Healthcare, 1*(2), 165–175. doi:10.1504/IJEH.2004.005865 PMID:18048218

Metcalfe, B. (1995). Metcalfe's law: A network becomes more valuable as it reaches more users. *InfoWorld, 17*(40), 53–54.

Metcalfe, B. (2013). Metcalfe's law after 40 years of Ethernet. *IEEE Computer, 46*(12), 26–31. doi:10.1109/MC.2013.374

Metsallik, J., Ross, P., Draheim, D., & Piho, G. (2018). Ten Years of the e-Health System in Estonia. CEUR Workshop Proceedings.

Mettler, M. (2016). Blockchain technology in healthcare: The revolution starts here. *2016 IEEE 18th International Conference on E-Health Networking, Applications and Services (Healthcom),* 1–3. doi:10.1109/HealthCom.2016.7749510

Mettler, M., & Hsg, M. A. (2016). Blockchain Technology in Healthcare The Revolution Starts Here. In *2016 IEEE 18th International Conference on e-Health Networking, Applications and Services, Healthcom.* IEEE.

Meunier, S. (2018). Blockchain 101: What is Blockchain and How Does This Revolutionary Technology Work? What is Blockchain and How Does This Revolutionary Technology Work? In *Transforming Climate Finance and Green Investment with Blockchains*. Elsevier Inc. doi:10.1016/B978-0-12-814447-3.00003-3

Mik, E. (2017). Smart contracts: Terminology, technical limitations and real world complexity. *Law, Innovation and Technology*, *9*(2), 269–300. doi:10.1080/17579961.2017.1378468

Milberg, S. J., Smith, H. J., & Burke, S. J. (2000). Information privacy: Corporate management and national regulation. *Organization Science*, *11*(1), 35–57. doi:10.1287/orsc.11.1.35.12567

Mirchandani, P. (2020). Health Care Supply Chains: COVID-19 Challenges and Pressing Actions. In Annals of internal medicine (Vol. 173, Issue 4, pp. 300–301). NLM (Medline). doi:10.7326/M20-1326

Mittal, S. (2012). *Is bitcoin money? bitcoin and alternate theories of money*. Bitcoin and Alternate Theories of Money.

Mittal, A. (2013). Trustworthiness of Big Data. *International Journal of Computers and Applications*, *80*(9), 35–40. Advance online publication. doi:10.5120/13892-1835

Mollick, E. (2006). Establishing Moore's law. *IEEE Annals of the History of Computing*, *28*(3), 62–75. doi:10.1109/MAHC.2006.45

Moniruzzaman, M., Chowdhury, F., & Ferdous, M. S. (2020, February). Examining Usability Issues in Blockchain-Based Cryptocurrency Wallets. In *International Conference on Cyber Security and Computer Science* (pp. 631-643). Springer. 10.1007/978-3-030-52856-0_50

Monkiewicz, J. (2020). New Finance: In Search for Analytical Framework. Academic Press.

Monrat, A. A., Schelén, O., & Andersson, K. (2019). A Survey of Blockchain From the Perspectives of Applications, Challenges, and Opportunities. *IEEE Access: Practical Innovations, Open Solutions*, *7*, 117134–117151. doi:10.1109/ACCESS.2019.2936094

Monroe, A. (1923). *Monetary Theory before Adam Smith* (Vol. 25). Harvard University Press. doi:10.4159/harvard.9780674183438

Moore, C., O'Neill, M., O'Sullivan, E., Doröz, Y., & Sunar, B. (2014, June). Practical homomorphic encryption: A survey. In *2014 IEEE International Symposium on Circuits and Systems (ISCAS)* (pp. 2792-2795). IEEE.

Moore, G. E. (1998). Cramming More Components Onto Integrated Circuits. *Proceedings of the IEEE*, *86*(1), 82–85. https://doi.org/10.1109/JPROC.1998.658762

Moreno, J. (n.d.). *Blockchain for Life Sciences*. https://www.capgemini.com/de-de/service/blockchain-for-life-sciences/#nutzung-von-blockchains-fuer-die-einwilligungserklaerung-in-klinischen-studien

Morgan, G. (2009). *Globalization, multinationals and institutional diversity*. Academic Press.

Morley-Fletcher, E. (2017). MHMD: My health, my data. *CEUR Workshop Proceedings*, 1810.

Moro Visconti, R., Larocca, A., & Marconi, M. (2017). Big Data-Driven Value Chains and Digital Platforms: From Value Co-Creation to Monetization. SSRN *Electronic Journal*. doi:10.2139srn.2903799

Morris, D., Solon, L., Simpson, J., Read, O., & Abel, J. (2020). *Tech powered healthcare: a strategic approach to implementing technology in health and care*. PricewaterhouseCoopers.

Morrow, M. J., & Zarrebini, M. (2019). Blockchain and the Tokenization of the Individual: Societal Implications. *Future Internet*, *11*(10), 220.

Möser, M., Böhme, R., & Breuker, D. (2014, March). Towards risk scoring of Bitcoin transactions. In *International Conference on Financial Cryptography and Data Security* (pp. 16-32). Springer.

Mouial-Bassilana, E., Restrepo, D., & Colombani, L. (2018). Le déséquilibre significatif dans les contrats commerciaux: nouvel outil de lutte contre les GAFA. *Actualité juridique. Contrat, 471.*

Mueller, L., Glarner, A., Linder, T., Meyer, S. D., Furrer, A., Gschwend, C., & Henschel, P. (2018). *Conceptual Framework for Legal and Risk Assessment of Crypto Tokens.* Academic Press.

Mueller, R. C. (1997). The Venetian money market: Banks, panics, and the public debt, 1200-1500. In F. C. Lane & R. C. Mueller (Eds.), Money and banking in medieval Renaissance Venice (Vol. 2). The John Hopkins University Press.

Muller, M., Janczura, J. A., & Ruppel, P. (2020). DeCoCo: Blockchain-based decentralized compensation of digital content purchases. *2nd Conference on Blockchain Research and Applications for Innovative Networks and Services,* 152-159. Retrieved from www.scopus.com doi:10.1109/BRAINS49436.2020.9223299

Mulligan, A., Hall, L., & Raphael, E. (2013). Peer review in a changing world: An international study measuring the attitudes of researchers. *Journal of the American Society for Information Science and Technology.* doi:10.1002/asi.22798

Murphy, A. E. (1997). *John Law: economic theorist and policy-maker.* Clarendon Press. doi:10.1093/019828649X.001.0001

Muthe, K. B., Sharma, K., & Sri, K. E. N. (2020, November). A Blockchain Based Decentralized Computing And NFT Infrastructure For Game Networks. In *2020 Second International Conference on Blockchain Computing and Applications (BCCA)* (pp. 73-77). IEEE.

Muzzy, E. (2018). *CryptoKitties Isn't About the Cats.* Retrieved from https://medium.com/@everett.muzzy/cryptokitties-isnt-about-the-cats-aef47bcde92d

Muzzy, E. (2018, October 9). *CryptoKitties Isn't About the Cats - Everett Muzzy.* Retrieved April 27, 2021, from https://medium.com/@everett.muzzy/cryptokitties-isnt-about-the-cats-aef47bcde92d

MX Technologies Inc. (2016). *Checks, Balances, and Bitcoin: The Genius of the Blockchain.* Retrieved from https://www.mx.com/moneysummit/checks-balances-and-bitcoin-the-genius-of-the-blockchain/

MyHealthMyData. (2016a). *A New Paradigm in Healthcare Data Privacy and Security.* http://www.myhealthmydata.eu/

MyHealthMyData. (2016b). *Consortium.* http://www.myhealthmydata.eu/consortium/

Nagasubramanian, G., Sakthivel, R. K., Patan, R., Gandomi, A. H., Sankayya, M., & Balusamy, B. (2020). Securing e-health records using keyless signature infrastructure blockchain technology in the cloud. *Neural Computing & Applications, 32*(3), 639–647. doi:10.100700521-018-3915-1

Nagori, V. (2021). "Aarogya Setu": The mobile application that monitors and mitigates the risks of COVID-19 pandemic spread in India. *Journal of Information Technology Teaching Cases.* doi:10.1177/2043886920985863

Nakamoto, S. (2008). *A peer-to-peer electronic cash system.* Bitcoin. https://bitcoin.org/bitcoin.pdf

Nakamoto, S. (2008). *Bitcoin: A peer-to-peer electronic cash system* [White paper]. https://bitcoin.org/bitcoin.pdf

Nakamoto, S. (2008). *Bitcoin: A Peer-to-Peer Electronic Cash System.* www.bitcoin.org

Nakamoto, S. (2008). *Bitcoin: A Peer-to-Peer Electronic Cash System.* Www.Bitcoin.Org doi:10.1162/ARTL_a_00247

Nakamoto, S. (2009). *Bitcoin: A Peer-to-Peer Electronic Cash System.* Cryptography Mailing List. Https://Metzdowd.Com

Nakamoto, S. (2009). *Bitcoin: A Peer-to-Peer Electronic Cash System.* Https://Metzdowd.Com

Nakamura, Y., Zhang, Y., Sasabe, M., & Kasahara, S. (2020). Exploiting smart contracts for capability-based access control in the Internet of Things. *Sensors (Basel)*, *20*(6), 1793.

Nakamura, Y., Zhang, Y., Sasabe, M., & Kasahara, S. (2020). Exploiting Smart Contracts for Capability-Based Access Control in the Internet of Things. *Sensors (Basel)*, *20*(6), 1793. doi:10.339020061793 PMID:32213888

Namasudra, S., Deka, G. C., Johri, P., Hosseinpour, M., & Gandomi, A. H. (2020). The Revolution of Blockchain: State-of-the-Art and Research Challenges. *Archives of Computational Methods in Engineering*. Advance online publication. doi:10.100711831-020-09426-0

Nandi, S., Sarkis, J., Hervani, A. A., & Helms, M. M. (2021). Redesigning Supply Chains using Blockchain-Enabled Circular Economy and COVID-19 Experiences. *Sustainable Production and Consumption*, *27*, 10–22. doi:10.1016/j.spc.2020.10.019 PMID:33102671

Náñez Alonso, S. L., Jorge-Vazquez, J., & Reier Forradellas, R. F. (2021). Central Banks Digital Currency: Detection of Optimal Countries for the Implementation of a CBDC and the Implication for Payment Industry Open Innovation. *Journal of Open Innovation*, *7*(1), 72. doi:10.3390/joitmc7010072

Narayan, R., & Tidström, A. (2020). Tokenizing coopetition in a blockchain for a transition to circular economy. *Journal of Cleaner Production*, *263*, 121437.

NathG. V. (2020). *Cryptocurrency and Privacy-An Introduction to the Interface*. Available at SSRN 3658459. doi:10.2139srn.3658459

Naudet, L. B. (2021). *Regard sur les conséquences des mutations organiques de la monnaie dans la manifestation des conflits armés depuis l'éclatement du système de Bretton-Woods*. Academic Press.

Negroponte, N. (1995). *Being Digital–A Book (P) review*. Wired.com, 3.

Neitz, M. B. (2019). The Influencers: Facebook's Libra, Public Blockchains, and the Ethical Considerations of Centralization. *NCJL & Tech.*, *21*, 41.

Nel, L. (2018, March 5). *Beginner's Guide to Dentacoin*. Retrieved January 30, 2021, from https://blockonomi.com/dentacoin-guide/

Nofer, M., Gomber, P., Hinz, O., & Schiereck, D. (2017). Blockchain. *Business & Information Systems Engineering*, *59*(3), 183–187. https://doi.org/10.1007/s12599-017-0467-3

Nørfeldt, L., Bøtker, J., Edinger, M., Genina, N., & Rantanen, J. (2019). Cryptopharmaceuticals : Increasing the Safety of Medication by a Blockchain of Pharmaceutical Products. *Journal of Pharmaceutical Sciences*, *108*, 2838–2841.

Norta, A. (2016, November). Designing a smart-contract application layer for transacting decentralized autonomous organizations. In *International Conference on Advances in Computing and Data Sciences* (pp. 595-604). Springer.

Noura, M., Atiquzzaman, M., & Gaedke, M. (2019). Interoperability in Internet of Things: Taxonomies and Open Challenges. *Mobile Networks and Applications*, *24*(3), 796–809. doi:10.100711036-018-1089-9

Noyen, K., Volland, D., Wörner, D., & Fleisch, E. (2014). *When money learns to fly: Towards sensing as a service application using bitcoin*. arXiv preprint arXiv:1409.5841

Noyen, K., Volland, D., Wörner, D., & Fleisch, E. (2014). *When money learns to fly: Towards sensing as a service applications using bitcoin*. arXiv preprint arXiv:1409.5841

Nugent, T., Upton, D., & Cimpoesu, M. (2016). Improving data transparency in clinical trials using blockchain smart contracts. *F1000 Research*, *5*, 1–4.

NugentT.UptonD.CimpoesuM. (2016). Improving data transparency in clinical trials using blockchain smart contracts. *F1000Research, 5*. doi:10.12688/f1000research.9756.1

O'Neil, C. (2017). How can we stop algorithms telling lies? *The Guardian*, 7-16.

Officer, L. H. (2020). International monetary regimes: the gold standard. In S. Battilossi, Y. Cassis & K. Yago (Ed.), Handbook of the History of Money and Currency (pp. 599-631). Springer. doi:10.1007/978-981-13-0596-2_23

Omar, I. A., Jayaraman, R., Salah, K., Simsekler, M. C. E., Yaqoob, I., & Ellahham, S. (2020). Ensuring protocol compliance and data transparency in clinical trials using Blockchain smart contracts. *BMC Medical Research Methodology*, *20*(1), 224. doi:10.118612874-020-01109-5 PMID:32894068

Omar, I. A., Jayaraman, R., Salah, K., Yaqoob, I., & Ellahham, S. (2020). Applications of Blockchain Technology in Clinical Trials: Review and Open Challenges. *Arabian Journal for Science and Engineering*. Advance online publication. doi:10.100713369-020-04989-3

Orléan, A. (2008). Crise de la souveraineté et crise de la monnaie: l'hyperinflation allemande des années 1920. In B. Théret (Ed.), La monnaie dévoilée par ses crises, vol. 2, Crises monétaires en Russie et en Allemagne au XXe siècle. Éditions de l'EHESS.

Osborn, C. Y., Mayberry, L. S., Wallston, K. A., Johnson, K. B., & Elasy, T. A. (2013). Understanding Patient Portal Use: Implications for Medication Management. *Journal of Medical Internet Research*, *15*(7), 204–215. doi:10.2196/jmir.2589 PMID:23823974

Ostapenko, G. F. (2018). Creating a Platform Based Business Model In Dental Industry. *Intern. Journal of Profess. Bus. Review*, *4*(1), 106. doi:10.26668/businessreview/2019.v4i1.106

Overview, D. A. O. (2020). *A List of Ethereum's Top DAOs and DAO Structures*. DeFi Rate. https://defirate.com/daos/

Paik, H. Y., Xu, X., Bandara, H. D., Lee, S. U., & Lo, S. K. (2019). Analysis of data management in blockchain-based systems: From architecture to governance. *IEEE Access: Practical Innovations, Open Solutions*, *7*, 186091–186107. doi:10.1109/ACCESS.2019.2961404

Pandey, P., & Litoriya, R. (2020). Securing and authenticating healthcare records through blockchain technology. *Cryptologia*, *44*(4), 341–356. doi:10.1080/01611194.2019.1706060

Pane, J., Verhamme, K. M. C., Shrum, L., Rebollo, I., & Sturkenboom, M. C. J. M. (2020). Blockchain technology applications to postmarket surveillance of medical devices. *Expert Review of Medical Devices*, *17*(10), 1–10. doi:10.1080/17434440.2020.1825073 PMID:32954855

Park, Y. R., Lee, E., Na, W., Park, S., Lee, Y., & Lee, J. H. (2019). Is blockchain technology suitable for managing personal health records? Mixed-methods study to test feasibility. *Journal of Medical Internet Research*, *21*(2), e12533. doi:10.2196/12533 PMID:30735142

Parliament, E. (2014). *Regulation (EU) No 536/2014 of the European Parliament and the Council*. Official Journal of the European Union.

Passinsky, A. (2021). Should Bitcoin Be Classified as Money? *Journal of Social Ontology*.

Pasuthip, P., & Yang, S. (2020). *Central Bank Digital Currency: Promises and Risks*.

Pasuthip, P., & Yang, S. (2020). *Central Bank Digital Currency: Promises and Risks*. Academic Press.

Paulos, J. (2020). *Investigating Decentralized Management of Health and Fitness Data*. Academic Press.

Peng, X. Z., Zhang, J. Q., Zhang, S. B., Wan, W. N., Chen, H., & Xia, J. Y. (2021). A Secure Signcryption Scheme for Electronic Health Records Sharing in Blockchain. *Computer Systems Science and Engineering*, *37*(2), 265–281. doi:10.32604/csse.2021.014557

Perera, C., Zaslavsky, A., Christen, P., & Georgakopoulos, D. (2014). Sensing as a service model for smart cities supported by internet of things. *Transactions on Emerging Telecommunications Technologies*, *25*(1), 81–93. doi:10.1002/ett.2704

Perez, S. (2018, June 20). *Does a Blockchain Need a Token? The Startup*. Retrieved February 20, 2021, from https://medium.com/swlh/does-a-blockchain-need-a-token-66c894d566fb

Peters, M. A. Green, B. & Yang, H. (2020). *Cryptocurrencies, China's sovereign digital currency (DCEP) and the US dollar system*. Academic Press.

Peters, G. W., & Panayi, E. (2016). Understanding modern banking ledgers through blockchain technologies: Future of transaction processing and smart contracts on the internet of money. In *Banking beyond banks and money* (pp. 239–278). Springer. doi:10.1007/978-3-319-42448-4_13

Peters, S., & Bilton, D. (2018). 'Right-Touch' trust: Thoughts on trust in healthcare. In R. H. Searle, A. I. Nienaber, & S. B. Sitkin (Eds.), *The Routledge companion to trust*. Routledge.

Petracca, F., Ciani, O., Cucciniello, M., & Tarricone, R. (2020). Harnessing Digital Health Technologies During and After the COVID-19 Pandemic: Context Matters. *Journal of Medical Internet Research*, *22*(12), e21815. Advance online publication. doi:10.2196/21815 PMID:33351777

Petre, A., & Haï, N. (2018). Opportunités et enjeux de la technologie blockchain dans le secteur de la santé. *Medecine Sciences*, *34*(10), 852–856. doi:10.1051/medsci/2018204 PMID:30451661

Petrescu, M., & Krishen, A. S. (2020). The dilemma of social media algorithms and analytics. *J Market Anal*, *8*, 187–188. https://doi.org/10.1057/s41270-020-00094-4

Pham, H. L., Tran, T. H., & Nakashima, Y. (2018, December). A Secure Remote Healthcare System for Hospital Using Blockchain Smart Contract. *2018 IEEE Globecom Workshops (GC Wkshps)*. doi:10.1109/GLOCOMW.2018.8644164

Piscini, E., Dalton, D., & Kehoe, L. (2017). *Blockchain & Cyber Security. Let's Discuss*. https://www2.deloitte.com/tr/en/pages/technology-media-and-telecommunications/articles/blockchain-and-cyber.html

Plumptre, T. (2006). *"How Good is our Board?" How Board Evaluations Can*. Policy.

Pocher, N. (2019). The Internet of Money between Anonymity and Publicity: Legal Challenges of Distributed Ledger Technologies in the Crypto Financial Landscape. In *JURIX*. Doctoral Consortium.

Pomeranz, K. (2001). *The World's First Corporations*. The Globalist. https://www.theglobalist.com/the-worlds-first-corporations/

Poovey, M. (1998). *A history of the modern fact: Problems of knowledge in the sciences of wealth and society*. University of Chicago Press. doi:10.7208/chicago/9780226675183.001.0001

Power, D. J., & Phillips-Wren, G. (2011). Impact of social media and Web 2.0 on decision-making. *Journal of Decision Systems*, *20*(3), 249–261.

Prado, J. (2017). *O que é blockchain?* Retrieved January 29, 2021, from https://tecnoblog.net/227293/como-funciona-blockchain-bitcoin/

Premkumar, A., & Shrimati, C. (2020). Application of Blockchain and IoT towards Pharmaceutical Industry. *2020 6th International Conference on Advanced Computing & Communication Systems (ICACCS)*, 729–733.

Prinz, A. (1999). Money in the real and the virtual world: E-money, c-money and the demand for cb-money. *NETNOMICS: Economic Research and Electronic Networking, 1*(1), 11–35. doi:10.1023/A:1011441519577

Priyadharshini, A., Prasad, M., Raj, R. J. S., & Geetha, S. (2021). An Authenticated E-Voting System Using Biometrics and Blockchain. In *Intelligence in Big Data Technologies—Beyond the Hype* (pp. 535–542). Springer. doi:10.1007/978-981-15-5285-4_53

pwc Israel. (2020). https://www.pwc.com/il/en/pharmaceuticals/intellectual-property-protection.html

PwC Portugal. (2019). *Ensaios Clínicos em Portugal*. Author.

PwC. (2018). A Prescription for Blockchain and Healthcare: Reinvent or be Reinvented. *PriceWaterhouseCoopers*, 19. www.pwc.com/us/en/health-industries.html%0A©

Qadah, G. Z. (2005). Requirements, design and implementation of an e-voting system. *Proceedings of the IADIS International Conference on Applied Computing*, 405–409.

Qian, Y. (2019). Central Bank Digital Currency: optimization of the currency system and its issuance design. *China Economic Journal, 12*(1), 1-15.

Qiang, X. (2019). The road to digital unfreedom: President xi's surveillance state. *Journal of Democracy, 30*(1), 53–67. doi:10.1353/jod.2019.0004

Qin, K., & Gervais, A. (2018). *An overview of blockchain scalability, interoperability and sustainability*. Hochschule Luzern Imperial College London Liquidity Network.

Quinn, S., & Roberds, W. (2008). The evolution of the check as a means of payment: A historical survey. *Economic Review (Kansas City, Mo.), 93*(4), 1–28.

Quinn, S., & Roberds, W. (2014). The Bank of Amsterdam through the lens of monetary competition. In P. Bernholz & R. Vaubel (Eds.), *Explaining monetary and financial innovation: a historical analysis* (pp. 283–300). Springer. doi:10.1007/978-3-319-06109-2_11

R3. (2020a, September 16). *How "public-permissioned" blockchains are not an oxymoron*. https://www.r3.com/blog/how-public-permissioned-blockchains-are-not-an-oxymoron-2/

R3. (2020b, October 30). *Should we already be using blockchain as a voting system for elections?* Corda. https://www.corda.net/blog/should-we-already-be-using-blockchain-as-a-voting-system-for-elections/

Radanović, I., & Likić, R. (2018). Opportunities for Use of Blockchain Technology in Medicine. *Applied Health Economics and Health Policy, 16*(5), 583–590. doi:10.100740258-018-0412-8 PMID:30022440

Rajapashe, M., Adnan, M., Dissanayaka, A., Guneratne, D., & Abeywardena, K. (2020). Multi-Format Document Verification System. *American Scientific Research Journal for Engineering, Technology, and Sciences, 74*(2), 48–60.

Ramachandran, M., Chowdhury, N., Third, A., Domingue, J., Quick, K., & Bachler, M. (2020, April). Towards Complete Decentralised Verification of Data with Confidentiality: Different ways to connect Solid Pods and Blockchain. In *Companion Proceedings of the Web Conference 2020* (pp. 645-649). Academic Press.

Rao & Jain. (2019). *Improving Integrated Clinical Trial Management Systems through Blockchain*. Genetic Engineering & Biotechnology News. https://www.genengnews.com/insights/improving-integrated-clinical-trial-management-systems-through-blockchain/

Rao, R., & Jain, H. (2019). Improving Integrated Clinical Trial Management Systems through Blockchain. *Genetic Engineering & Biotechnology News*.

Rath, M. (2019, November). A review of Artificial Intelligence Emerging technologies and challenges in Block Chain Technology. In *2019 International Conference on Smart Systems and Inventive Technology (ICSSIT)* (pp. 1031-1035). IEEE. 10.1109/ICSSIT46314.2019.8987807

Ray, P. P., Dash, D., Salah, K., & Kumar, N. (2020). Blockchain for IoT-Based Healthcare: Background, Consensus, Platforms, and Use Cases. *IEEE Systems Journal*.

Regner, F. Urbach, N. & Schweizer, A. (2019). *NFTs in Practice–Non-Fungible Tokens as Core Component of a Blockchain-based Event Ticketing Application*. Academic Press.

Regner, F., Urbach, N., & Schweizer, A. (2019). *NFTs in Practice–Non-Fungible Tokens as Core Component of a Blockchain-based Event Ticketing Application*. Academic Press.

ReinersL. (2020). *Cryptocurrency and the State: An Unholy Alliance*. Available at SSRN 3682724.

Reisenwitz, C. (2014). Smart contracts promise for the Poor. *Bitcoin Mag*. https://bitcoinmagazine.com/articles/smart-propertys-promise-poor-1390852097/

Resnik, D. B., & Shamoo, A. E. (2017). Reproducibility and Research Integrity. *Accountability in Research*. doi:10.10 80/08989621.2016.1257387

Reyna, A., Martín, C., Chen, J., Soler, E., & Díaz, M. (2018). On blockchain and its integration with IoT. Challenges and opportunities. *Future Generation Computer Systems*, *88*, 173–190. Advance online publication. doi:10.1016/j.future.2018.05.046

RFID Journal. (n.d.). Retrieved January 22, 2021, from https://www.rfidjournal.com/

Rho, M. J., Yoon, K. H., Kim, H. S., & Choi, I. Y. (2015). Users' perception on telemedicine service: A comparative study of public healthcare and private healthcare. *Multimedia Tools and Applications*, *74*(7), 2483–2497. doi:10.100711042-014-1966-6

Rikap, C., & Lundvall, B. Å. (2020). Big tech, knowledge predation and the implications for development. *Innovation and Development*, 1-28.

Robinson, K. G. (Ed.). (2004). General conclusions and reflections. In J. Needham, Science and civilisation in China (vol. 7.2). Cambridge University Press.

Rodrigues, D. (2012). Cyberethics of Business Social Networking. In E-Marketing: Concepts, Methodologies, Tools, and Applications (pp. 756-780). IGI Global.

Rodrigues, D. (2020, October 29). *The Dangerous Business Model of Social Networks*. Observador. https://observador.pt/opiniao/o-perigoso-modelo-de-negocio-das-redes-sociais/

Roman-Belmonte, J. M., De la Corte-Rodriguez, H., & Rodriguez-Merchan, E. C. (2018). How blockchain technology can change medicine. In Postgraduate Medicine (Vol. 130, Issue 4, pp. 420–427). Taylor and Francis Inc. doi:10.1080/00325481.2018.1472996

Romano, D., & Schmid, G. (2017). *Beyond Bitcoin: A Critical Look at Blockchain-Based Systems*. Cryptography. doi:10.3390/cryptography1020015

Romer, P. (2002). When should we use intellectual property rights? *The American Economic Review*, *92*(2), 213–216.

Rooney, D., & Chavan, M. (2017). Globalization/internationalization. The International Encyclopedia of Organizational Communication, 1-15.

Rooney, L., Rimpiläinen, S., Morrison, C., & Nielsen, S. L. (2019). *Review of emerging trends in digital health and care.* A report by the Digital Health and Care Institute.

Rosário, A. T., Fernandes, F., Raimundo, R. G., & Cruz, R. N. (2021). Determinants of Nascent Entrepreneurship Development. In A. Carrizo Moreira & J. G. Dantas (Eds.), *Handbook of Research on Nascent Entrepreneurship and Creating New Ventures* (pp. 172–193). IGI Global. doi:10.4018/978-1-7998-4826-4.ch008

Rosário, A., & Cruz, R. (2019). Determinants of Innovation in Digital Marketing, Innovation Policy and Trends in the Digital Age. *Journal of Reviews on Global Economics*, *8*, 1722–1731. doi:10.6000/1929-7092.2019.08.154

Rosbach, M., & Andersen, J. S. (2017). Patient-experienced burden of treatment in patients with multimorbidity – A systematic review of qualitative data. *PLoS One*, *12*(6), e0179916. https://doi.org/10.1371/journal.pone.0179916

Rotich, J. K., Hannan, T. J., Smith, F. E., Bii, J., Odero, W. W., Vu, N., Mamlin, B. W., Mamlin, J. J., Einterz, R. M., & Tierney, W. M. (2003). Installing and implementing a computer-based patient record system in sub-saharan Africa: The Mosoriot Medical Record System. *Journal of the American Medical Informatics Association: JAMIA*, *10*(4), 295–303. Advance online publication. doi:10.1197/jamia.M1301 PMID:12668697

Rowe, F., Ngwenyama, O., & Richet, J. L. (2020). Contact-tracing apps and alienation in the age of COVID-19. *European Journal of Information Systems*, 1–18.

Royal, J., & Voigt, K. (2017). *What is cryptocurrency? Guide for beginners.* Retrieved January 29, 2021, from https://cointelegraph.com/bitcoin-for-beginners/what-are-cryptocurrencies

Rybarczyk, R., Armstrong, D., & Fabiano, A. (2021, May). *20210513 Galaxy Digital Mining - On Bitcoin Energy Consumption.* Retrieved June 1, 2021, from https://docsend.com/view/adwmdeeyfvqwecj2

Sacavém, A., Cruz, R., Sousa, M., & Rosário, A. (2019). An integrative literature review on leadership models for innovative organizations, innovation policy and trends in the digital age. *Journal of Reviews on Global Economics*, *8*, 1741–1751. doi:10.6000/1929-7092.2019.08.156

Sadia, K., Masuduzzaman, M., Paul, R. K., & Islam, A. (2019). *Blockchain Based Secured E-voting by Using the Assistance of Smart Contract.* arXiv:1910.13635.

Sadowski, J. (2020). *Too smart: How digital capitalism is extracting data, controlling our lives, and taking over the world.* MIT Press. doi:10.7551/mitpress/12240.001.0001

Safiullin, M., Savelichev, M., Elshin, L., & Moiseev, V. (2020). *Increasing stability of economy through supply chain management and the circular economy.* Electronic archive of the Kazan Federal University. https://dspace.kpfu.ru/xmlui/handle/net/163214

Safko, L. (2010). *The social media bible: tactics, tools, and strategies for business success.* John Wiley & Sons.

Saiedi, E., Broström, A., & Ruiz, F. (2020). Global drivers of cryptocurrency infrastructure adoption. *Small Business Economics*. Advance online publication. doi:10.100711187-019-00309-8

Salah, K., Alfalasi, A., & Alfalasi, M. (2019, April). A Blockchain-based System for Online Consumer Reviews. In *IEEE INFOCOM 2019-IEEE Conference on Computer Communications Workshops (INFOCOM WKSHPS)* (pp. 853-858). IEEE. 10.1109/INFOCOMW.2019.8845186

Salber, P. R. (2002). The role of purchasers in the clinical research enterprise.). . *Journal of Investigative Medicine*, *50*(3). doi:10.2310/6650.2002.33429

Salem, A. O., Safeia, M. T. A., & Siam, S. M. (2008). *Report of Blockchain Techniques and Applications.* Academic Press.

Santos Rutschman, A. (2018). *Healthcare Blockchain Infrastructure: a Comparative Approach.* Academic Press.

Sanz Bas, D. (2020). Hayek and the cryptocurrency revolution. *Iberian Journal of the History of Economic Thought,* 7(1), 15–28. doi:10.5209/ijhe.69403

Satia, M. C. (2017). Global challenges in conducting clinical trials. *Journal of Clinical Trials.* https://www.longdom.org/proceedings/global-challenges-in-conducting-clinical-trials-56064.html

Savelyev, A. (2017). Contract law 2.0: 'Smart'contracts as the beginning of the end of classic contract law. *Information & Communications Technology Law,* 26(2), 116–134. doi:10.1080/13600834.2017.1301036

Savelyev, A. (2018). Copyright in the blockchain era: Promises and challenges. *Computer Law & Security Review,* 34(3), 550–561.

Saxena, N., Thomas, I., Gope, P., Burnap, P., & Kumar, N. (2020). PharmaCrypt: Blockchain for Critical Pharmaceutical Industry to Counterfeit Drugs. *Computer,* 53(7), 29–44.

Sayeed, S., & Marco-Gisbert, H. (2019). Assessing blockchain consensus and security mechanisms against the 51% attack. *Applied Sciences (Basel, Switzerland),* 9(9), 1788.

Schaller, R. R. (1997). Moore's law: Past, present and future. *IEEE Spectrum,* 34(6), 52–59. doi:10.1109/6.591665

Schaps, D. M. (2004). *The invention of coinage and the monetization of Ancient Greece.* The University of Michigan Press. doi:10.3998/mpub.17760

Schneier, B. (2007). Applied Cryptography: Protocols, Algorithms, and Source Code in C (2nd ed.). John Wiley & Sons, Inc.

Schneier, B. (2012). *Liars and outliers: enabling the trust that society needs to thrive.* John Wiley & Sons.

Schöner, M., Kourouklis, D., Sandner, P., Gonzalez, E., & Förster, J. (2017). Blockchain Technology in the Pharmaceutical Industry. *FSBC Working Paper,* 1–9.

Schoorman, F. D., Mayer, R. C., & Davis, J. H. (2007). An integrative model of organizational trust: Past, present, and future. *Academy of Management Review,* 32(2), 344–354. doi:10.5465/amr.2007.24348410

Schulz, K. F., Altman, D. C., & Moher, D. (2010). CONSORT 2010 Statement: Updated guidelines for reporting parallel group randomised trials. *Italian Journal of Public Health.* doi:10.4178/epih/e2014029

Schumpeter, J. A. (1942). *Capitalism, socialism and democracy.* Routledge.

Scott-Briggs, A. (2018, January 12). *Introduction to Decentralized Autonomous Organization.* TechBullion. https://techbullion.com/introduction-decentralized-autonomous-organization/

Sedlmeir, J., Buhl, H. U., Fridgen, G., & Keller, R. (2020). The energy consumption of blockchain technology: Beyond myth. *Business & Information Systems Engineering,* 62(6), 599–608. doi:10.100712599-020-00656-x

Settanni, E., Harrington, T. S., & Srai, J. S. (2017). Pharmaceutical supply chain models: A synthesis from a systems view of operations research. *Operations Research Perspectives,* 4, 74–95.

Sfetcu, N. (2019, February 17). *Blockchain Design and Modelling.* SetThings. https://www.setthings.com/en/blockchain-design-and-modelling/

SFOX. (2018a). *From Crowdfunded Blockchain to ICO Machine: An Ethereum Price History.* SFOX Inc.

SFOX. (2018b). *Miners, Developers, and Users: The Checks and Balances of Bitcoin.* https://www.sfox.com/blog/miners-developers-and-users-the-checks-and-balances-of-bitcoin/

SGS. (2020). *Good Distribution Practices (GDP) Certification For Pharmaceutical Industry.* https://www.sgs.com/en/life-sciences/audit-certification-and-verification/quality/good-distribution-practices-gdp-certification-for-pharmaceutical-industry

Shae, Z., & Tsai, J. J. P. (2017). On the Design of a Blockchain Platform for Clinical Trial and Precision Medicine. *Proceedings - International Conference on Distributed Computing Systems*, 1972–1980. 10.1109/ICDCS.2017.61

Sharma, P., Jindal, R., & Borah, M. D. (2020). Blockchain technology for cloud storage: A systematic literature review. *ACM Computing Surveys*, *53*(4), 1–32. doi:10.1145/3403954

Shermin, V. (2017). Disrupting governance with blockchains and smart contracts. *Strategic Change*, *26*(5), 499–509. doi:10.1002/jsc.2150

Shirky, C. (2008). *Here comes everybody: The power of organizing without organizations.* Penguin.

Shovlin, A., Ghen, M., Simpson, P., & Mehta, K. (2013). Challenges facing medical data digitization in low-resource contexts. *Proceedings of the 3rd IEEE Global Humanitarian Technology Conference, GHTC 2013.* 10.1109/GHTC.2013.6713713

Shrestha, A. K., Vassileva, J., & Deters, R. (2020). A Blockchain Platform for User Data Sharing Ensuring User Control and Incentives. *Frontiers in Blockchain, 3*(October), 1–22. doi:10.3389/fbloc.2020.497985

Shute, R. (2017). *Blockchain Technology in Drug Discovery: Use-Cases in R&D.* Drug Discovery World.

Sims, A. (2020). Blockchain and Decentralised Autonomous Organizations (DAOs): The Evolution of Companies? SSRN *Electronic Journal.* doi:10.2139srn.3524674

Slawotsky, J. (2020). US Financial Hegemony: The Digital Yuan and Risks of Dollar De-Weaponization. *Fordham Int'l LJ*, *44*, 39.

SMA. (2018, November). *FLIPHODL.* https://www.fliphodl.com/social-media-alternatives-series-ep-1-what-you-need-to-know/

Smetanin, S., Ometov, A., Komarov, M., Masek, P., & Koucheryavy, Y. (2020). Blockchain evaluation approaches: State-of-the-art and future perspective. *Sensors (Switzerland)*, *20*(12), 1–20. doi:10.339020123358 PMID:32545719

Smith, A. (1937). *The wealth of nations.* Academic Press. (Original publication 1776)

Smith, A. (1989). Of the Origin and Use of Money. In General Equilibrium Models of Monetary Economies (pp. 47-53). Academic Press.

Smith, K. (2019). *Ethereum losing share as dapp developers choose other networks.* Brave New Coin.

Snyder, H. (2019). Literature review as a research methodology: An overview and guidelines. *Journal of Business Research*, *104*, 333–339. doi:10.1016/j.jbusres.2019.07.039

Somerville, I., & Wood, E. (2008). Business ethics, public relations and corporate social responsibility. In *The public relations handbook* (pp. 143–160). Routledge.

Son, W., & Sheikh, N. J. (2018). Assessment of electronic authentication policies using multi-stakeholder multi-criteria hierarchical decision modeling. *PICMET 2018 - Portland International Conference on Management of Engineering and Technology: Managing Technological Entrepreneurship: The Engine for Economic Growth, Proceedings.* 10.23919/PICMET.2018.8481798

Sosnovik, V., & Goga, O. (2021). *Understanding the Complexity of Detecting Political Ads.* arXiv preprint arXiv:2103.00822.

Soto Cabezas, M. G., Munayco Escate, C. V., Escalante Maldonado, O., Valencia Torres, E., Arica Gutiérrez, J., & Yagui Moscoso, M. J. A. (2020). Perfil epidemiológico de la tuberculosis extensivamente resistente en el Perú, 2013-2015. *Revista Panamericana de Salud Pública, 44*, 1. Advance online publication. doi:10.26633/RPSP.2020.29 PMID:32973891

Specter, M. A., Koppel, J., & Weitzner, D. (2020). *The Ballot is Busted Before the Blockchain: A Security Analysis of Voatz, the First Internet Voting Application Used in U.S. Federal Elections.* Available online: https: //www.usenix.org/system/files/sec20-specter.pdf

Spufford, P. (1988). *Money and its use in medieval Europe.* Cambridge University Press. doi:10.1017/CBO9780511583544

Srinivasan, P. (2017, November 9). *Healthcare Blockchain: How smart contracts could revolutionize care delivery.* Prolifics.

Srivastava, A., Jain, P., Hazela, B., Asthana, P., & Rizvi, S. W. A. (2021). Application of Fog Computing, Internet of Things, and Blockchain Technology in Healthcare Industry. In *Fog Computing for Healthcare 4.0 Environments* (pp. 563–591). Springer. doi:10.1007/978-3-030-46197-3_22

Starr, R. M. (1989). The structure of exchange in barter and monetary economies. In *General Equilibrium Models of Monetary Economies* (pp. 129–143). Academic Press. doi:10.1016/B978-0-12-663970-4.50014-1

Steinwandter, V., & Herwig, C. (2019). Provable data integrity in the pharmaceutical industry based on version control systems and the blockchain. *PDA Journal of Pharmaceutical Science and Technology.*

Stroukal, D. (2018). Can bitcoin become money? Its money functions and the regression theorem. *International Journal of Business and Management, 6*(1), 36–53. doi:10.20472/BM.2018.6.1.004

Su, L., & Wang, H. (2020). Supply chain finance research in digital bulk commodities service platform based on blockchain. *Proceedings - 2020 International Conference on E-Commerce and Internet Technology, ECIT 2020*, 341-344. 10.1109/ECIT50008.2020.00085

Sung, H. (2020). Can online courts promote access to justice? A case study of the internet courts in China. *Computer Law & Security Review, 39*, 105461. Advance online publication. doi:10.1016/j.clsr.2020.105461

Sunstein, C. R. (2009). *Going to extremes: How like minds unite and divide.* Oxford University Press.

Sunyaev, A. (2020). Distributed ledger technology. In *Internet Computing* (pp. 265–299). Springer. doi:10.1007/978-3-030-34957-8_9

Supranee, S., & Rotchanakitumnuai, S. (2017). The acceptance of the application of blockchain technology in the supply chain process of the Thai automotive industry. *Proceedings of the International Conference on Electronic Business (ICEB)*, 252-257.

Surowiecki, J. (2005). *The wisdom of crowds.* Anchor.

Swan, M. (2015). Blockchain: Blueprint for a new economy. In Climate Change 2013 - The Physical Science Basis.

Swan, M. (2015). *Blockchain: Blueprint for a new economy.* O'Reilly Media, Inc.

Sweeney, L. (2015). Only you, your doctor, and many others may know. *Technology Science, 2015092903*(9), 29.

Szabo, N. (1997). Formalizing and Securing Relationships on Public Networks. *First Monday, 2*(9). Advance online publication. doi:10.5210/fm.v2i9.548

Szabo, N. (2002). *The Origins of Money (No. 0211005).* University Library of Munich.

Szabo, N., & The, I. (2015). Smart Contracts. *Building Blocks for Digital Markets., c*, 1–11.

Takabatake, Y., Kotani, D., & Okabe, Y. (2016). An anonymous distributed electronic voting system using Zerocoin. *IEICE Technical Report, 116*(282), 127–131.

Tam, K. P. (2021). The new normal of social psychology in the face of the COVID-19 pandemic: Insights and advice from leaders in the field. *Asian Journal of Social Psychology, 24*(1), 8.

Tandon, A., Dhir, A., Islam, N., & Mäntymäki, M. (2020). Blockchain in healthcare: A systematic literature review, synthesizing framework and future research agenda. *Computers in Industry, 122*, 103290. Advance online publication. doi:10.1016/j.compind.2020.103290

Tan, L., Tivey, D., Kopunic, H., Babidge, W., Langley, S., & Maddern, G. (2020). Part 2: Blockchain technology in health care. *ANZ Journal of Surgery, 90*(12), 2415–2419. doi:10.1111/ans.16455 PMID:33236489

Tanner, A. (2017). *Strengthening protection of patient medical data*. The Century Foundation.

Tanner, A. (2016). For Sale: Your Medical Records. *Scientific American, 314*(2), 26–27. Retrieved November 30, 2020, from https://www.scientificamerican.com/article/how-data-brokers-make-money-off-your-medical-records/

Taplin, J. (2017). *Move fast and break things: How Facebook, Google, and Amazon have cornered culture and what it means for all of us*. Pan Macmillan.

Tapscott, A., & Tapscott, D. (2007). *How blockchain is changing finance* [White paper]. Harvard business review. https://hbr.org/2017/03/how-blockchain-is-changing-finance

Tapscott, D. (1997). *Growing Up Digital: The Rise of the Net Generation*. Harvard Business Press.

Tapscott, D., & Euchner, J. (2019). Blockchain and the Internet of Value: An Interview with Don Tapscott Don Tapscott talks with Jim Euchner about blockchain, the Internet of value, and the next Internet revolution. *Research Technology Management, 62*(1), 12–19. doi:10.1080/08956308.2019.1541711

Tapscott, D., & Euchner, J. (2019). Blockchain and the IoV: An Interview with Don Tapscott Don Tapscott talks with Jim Euchner about blockchain, the IoV, and the next Internet revolution. *Research Technology Management, 62*(1), 12–19.

Tapscott, D., & Tapscott, A. (2016). *Blockchain revolution: how the technology behind bitcoin is changing money, business, and the world*. Penguin.

Tardi, C. (2020). *Decentralized Market*. Investopedia. https://www.investopedia.com/terms/d/decentralizedmarket.asp

Tavares, J., & Oliveira, T. (2016a). Electronic Health Record Patient Portal Adoption by Health Care Consumers: An Acceptance Model and Survey. *Journal of Medical Internet Research, 18*(3), e49. doi:10.2196/jmir.5069 PMID:26935646

Tavares, J., & Oliveira, T. (2016b). Electronic Health Record Portals Definition and Usage. In C.-C. Maria Manuela, M. Isabel Maria, M. Ricardo, & R. Rui (Eds.), *Encyclopedia of E-Health and Telemedicine* (pp. 555–562). IGI Global. doi:10.4018/978-1-4666-9978-6.ch043

Tavares, J., & Oliveira, T. (2017). Electronic Health Record Portal Adoption: A cross country analysis. *BMC Medical Informatics and Decision Making, 17*(1), 1–17. doi:10.118612911-017-0482-9 PMID:28679423

Tavares, J., & Oliveira, T. (2018). New Integrated Model Approach to Understand the Factors That Drive Electronic Health Record Portal Adoption: Cross-Sectional National Survey. *Journal of Medical Internet Research, 20*(11), e11032. doi:10.2196/11032 PMID:30455169

Team, C. E. (2019). *What are Communication APIs and why are they needed?* CEQUENS. https://www.cequens.com/story-hub/what-are-communication-apis-and-why-are-they-needed

Telugunta, R., & Choudhary, S. (2020). *Internet of Things (IOT) in Healthcare Market Size, and Growth 2027.* https://www.alliedmarketresearch.com/iot-healthcare-market

Temin, P. (2013). *The Roman market economy.* Princeton University Press.

Tennant, J. P., Dugan, J. M., Graziotin, D., Jacques, D. C., Waldner, F., Mietchen, D., Elkhatib, Y., Collister, B. L., Pikas, C. K., Crick, T., Masuzzo, P., Caravaggi, A., Berg, D. R., Niemeyer, K. E., Ross-Hellauer, T., Mannheimer, S., Rigling, L., Katz, D. S., Greshake Tzovaras, B., … Colomb, J. (2017). A multi-disciplinary perspective on emergent and future innovations in peer review. *F1000Research*. doi:10.12688/f1000research.12037.3

Tennant, L. (2017). *Improving the Anonymity of the IOTA Cryptocurrency.* Academic Press.

Thagapsov, A., & Kozlovskiy, M. (2020). Bitcoin as Money. *Economic Analysis*.

Thagard, P. (2019). *Mind-society: From brains to social sciences and professions.* Oxford University Press. doi:10.1093/oso/9780190678722.001.0001

Thierry, F. (1997). Monnaies chinoises, vol. I – L'Antiquité préimpériale. Bibliothèque nationale de France.

Thierry, F. (2001). La fiduciarité idéale à l'épreuve des couts de production: Quelques éléments sur la contradiction fondamentale de la monnaie en Chine. *Revue Numismatique*, *6*(157), 131–152. doi:10.3406/numi.2001.2323

Thorneycroft, R. (2020). *The Role of APIs in Modern Commerce.* Profound. https://www.profound.works/digital-transformation/application-programming-interfaces-for-headless-ecommerce/

Thornhill, J. (2021) The tech platforms are not entirely to blame for Washington unrest: knee-jerk reactions in the wake of the storming of Capitol Hill could have unintended consequences. *Financial Times.* Available at: https://www.ft.com/content/ef64b160-5f01-404a-bb39-d013fde808ca

Tingström, B. (1986). *Plate money: the world's largest currency.* Royal Coin Cabinet.

Toffler, A., & Alvin, T. (1980). *The third wave* (Vol. 484). Bantam books.

Tom Lyons, L. C. (2020). *Blockchain use cases in healthcare.* Academic Press.

Tomescu, A., & Devadas, S. (2017). Catena: Efficient Non-equivocation via Bitcoin. *Proceedings - IEEE Symposium on Security and Privacy.* 10.1109/SP.2017.19

Tonin, P., Gosselet, N., Halle, E., & Henrion, M. (2018). Ideal oil and protein crops–what are users ideotypes, from the farmer to the consumer? *OCL*, *25*(6), D605. doi:10.1051/ocl/2018060

Torraco, R. J. (2005). Writing integrative literature reviews: Guidelines and examples. *Human Resource Development Review*, *4*(3), 356–367. doi:10.1177/1534484305278283

Transformation, T. C. (2010). Corporations in the Modern Era. *Tuitt, 2006*, 280–332.

Trials4us. (2020a). *Clinical Trials - C19040 Cohort 4.* https://www.trials4us.co.uk/ongoing-clinical-trials/caucasian-type-2-diabetic-male-and-female-patients-aged-18-to-65-c19040-part-1/

Trials4us. (2020b). *Clinical Trials - C19048 Cohort 2.* https://www.trials4us.co.uk/ongoing-clinical-trials/male-and-female-patients-with-wilson-disease-c19048/

Troshchinskiy, P. V. (2021, February). Main Directions of Digitalization in China. In *International Scientific and Practical Conference "Russia 2020-a new reality: economy and society" (ISPCR 2020)* (pp. 451-454). Atlantis Press.

Truong, N. B., Um, T. W., Zhou, B., & Lee, G. M. (2018, May). Strengthening the blockchain-based IoV with trust. In *2018 IEEE International Conference on Communications (ICC)* (pp. 1-7). IEEE.

Tunis, S., Korn, A., & Ommaya, A. (2002). Definitions of Clinical Research and Components of the Enterprise. In *The Role of Purchasers and Payers in the Clinical Research Enterprise: (p. Appendix V)*. National Academies Press. https://www.ncbi.nlm.nih.gov/books/NBK220717/

Turi, A. N. (2020). Currency Under the Web 3.0 Economy. In Technologies for Modern Digital Entrepreneurship (pp. 155-186). Apress.

Turkanović, M., Hölbl, M., Košič, K., Heričko, M., & Kamišalić, A. (2018). EduCTX: A blockchain-based higher education credit platform. *IEEE Access: Practical Innovations, Open Solutions*, 6, 5112–5127.

Turner, A. B., McCombie, S., & Uhlmann, A. J. (2020). Analysis techniques for illicit Bitcoin transactions. *Frontiers of Computer Science*, 2, 53.

Tuwiner, J. (2020). *What is Bitcoin Mining and How Does it Work?* Buy Bitcoin Worldwide. https://www.buybitcoinworldwide.com/mining/

Twesige, R. (2015). *A simple explanation of Bitcoin and Block Chain technology*. Academic Press.

Twesige, R. (2015). *A simple explanation of Bitcoin and Block Chain technology*. https://www.researchgate.net/profile/Richard-Twesige 2/publication/270287317_Bitcoin_A_simple_explanation_of_Bitcoin_and_Block_Chain_technology_JANUARY_2015_RICHARD_LEE_TWESIGE/links/54a7836f0cf267bdb90a0ee6/Bitcoin-A-simple-explanation-of-Bitcoin-and-Block-Chain-technology-JANUARY-2015-RICHARD-LEE-TWESIGE.pdf

TyN Magazine. (2020). *How healthcare is entering the world of cryptocurrency*. Retrieved January 29, 2021, from https://www.tynmagazine.com/how-healthcare-is-entering-the-world-of-cryptocurrency/

U.S. Food & Drug. (2020). *What Are the Different Types of Clinical Research?* https://www.fda.gov/patients/clinical-trials-what-patients-need-know/what-are-different-types-clinical-research

Underwood, S. (2016). Blockchain beyond bitcoin. *Communications of the ACM*, 59(11), 15–17.

UNECE. (2019). *Blockchain in Trade Facilitation. Whitepaper*. Retrieved from www.unece.org/cefact

United Nations General Assembly. (1948). Universal declaration of human rights. United Nations.

Urgo, A. K., Lestan, M., & Khoriaty, A. (2017, September 17). *A cooperative of decentralized marketplaces and communities*. Powered by Ethereum, Aragon, and IPFS. District0x. https://district0x.io/docs/district0x-whitepaper.pdf

Valério, N. (2007). From the first Portuguese bank to the Bank of Portugal's role as central bank. In N. Valério (Ed.), *History of the Portuguese banking system* (Vol. 1). Banco de Portugal.

Van De Mieroop, M. (1997). *The ancient Mesopotamian city*. Clarendon Press.

Van De Mieroop, M. (2014). Silver as a financial tool in ancient Egypt and Mesopotamia. In P. Bernholz & R. Vaubel (Eds.), *Explaining monetary and financial innovation: a historical analysis* (pp. 17–29). Springer. doi:10.1007/978-3-319-06109-2_2

van den Hoven, J., Pouwelse, J., Helbing, D., & Klauser, S. (2019). The blockchain age: Awareness, empowerment and coordination. In *Towards digital enlightenment* (pp. 163–166). Springer. doi:10.1007/978-3-319-90869-4_13

Van der Aalst, W., Hinz, O., & Weinhardt, C. (2019). *Big digital platforms*. Academic Press.

Van der Meer, T. G., Hameleers, M., & Kroon, A. C. (2020). Crafting our own biased media diets: The effects of confirmation, source, and negativity bias on selective attendance to online news. *Mass Communication & Society, 23*(6), 937–967.

van der Waal, M. B., dos S. Ribeiro, C., Ma, M., Haringhuizen, G. B., Claassen, E., & van de Burgwal, L. H. M. (2020). Blockchain-facilitated sharing to advance outbreak R&D. *Science, 368*(6492), 719–721. doi:10.1126cience.aba1355

van Dorn, A. (2020). COVID-19 and readjusting clinical trials. *Lancet, 396*(10250), 523–524. doi:10.1016/S0140-6736(20)31787-6 PMID:32828180

Van Nieuwkerk, M. (2009). How a city bank became a world-famous bank. In M. van Nieuwkerk (Ed.), *The Bank of Amsterdam: on the origins of central banking* (pp. 12–27). De Nederlandsche Bank / Sonsbeek Publishers.

Van Norman, G. A. (2016). Drugs, Devices, and the FDA: Part 1: An Overview of Approval Processes for Drugs. *JACC. Basic to Translational Science, 1*(3).

Vandenbroucke, J. P. (2004). When are observational studies as credible as randomised trials? *Lancet, 363*(9422), 1728–1731. https://doi.org/10.1016/S0140-6736(04)16261-2

Vassiliadis, S., Papadopoulos, P., Rangoussi, M., Konieczny, T., & Gralewski, J. (2017). Bitcoin value analysis based on cross-correlations. *Journal of Internet Banking and Commerce, 22*(S7), 1.

Vazirani, A. A., O'Donoghue, O., Brindley, D., & Meinert, E. (2020). Blockchain vehicles for efficient medical record management. *NPJ Digital Medicine, 3*(1), 1–5. doi:10.103841746-019-0211-0 PMID:31934645

Veblen, T. (1899). Mr. Cummings's Strictures on The Theory of the Leisure Class. *Journal of Political Economy, 8*(1), 106–117. doi:10.1086/250640

Veitas, V., & Weinbaum, D. (2017). Living cognitive society: A 'digital'world of views. *Technological Forecasting and Social Change, 114*, 16–26. doi:10.1016/j.techfore.2016.05.002

Verde, F., Stanzione, A., Romeo, V., Cuocolo, R., Maurea, S., & Brunetti, A. (2019). Could Blockchain Technology Empower Patients, Improve Education, and Boost Research in Radiology Departments? An Open Question for Future Applications. In Journal of Digital Imaging (Vol. 32, Issue 6, pp. 1112–1115). Springer New York LLC. doi:10.100710278-019-00246-8

Vergne, J. P. (2020). *Decentralized vs. Distributed Organization: A Framework for the Future of Blockchain and Machine Learning and for Avoiding Digital Platform Dystopia.* Academic Press.

Vergne, J. P. (2020). Decentralized vs. Distributed Organization: A Framework for the Future of Blockchain and Machine Learning and for Avoiding Digital Platform Dystopia. *Distributed Organization: A Framework for the Future of Blockchain and Machine Learning and for Avoiding Digital Platform Dystopia.*

Viriyasitavat, W., da Xu, L., Bi, Z., & Pungpapong, V. (2019). Blockchain and Internet of Things for Modern Business Process in Digital Economy—The State of the Art. *IEEE Transactions on Computational Social Systems, 6*(6), 1420–1432. doi:10.1109/TCSS.2019.2919325

Visconti, R. M. (2020). Blockchain Valuation: IoV and Smart Transactions. In The Valuation of Digital Intangibles (pp. 401-422). Palgrave Macmillan.

Voatz. (2021, February 4). *Voatz Response to Researchers' Flawed Report.* Voatz. https://voatz.com/2020/02/13/voatz-response-to-researchers-flawed-report/

Vo-Cao-Thuy, L., Cao-Minh, K., Dang-Le-Bao, C., & Nguyen, T. A. (2019). Votereum: An Ethereum-Based E-Voting System. *Proceedings of the 2019 IEEE-RIVF International Conference on Computing and Communication Technologies (RIVF)*, 1–6.

Volety, T., Saini, S., McGhin, T., Liu, C. Z., & Choo, K. K. R. (2019). Cracking Bitcoin wallets: I want what you have in the wallets. *Future Generation Computer Systems*, *91*, 136–143. Advance online publication. doi:10.1016/j.future.2018.08.029

Von Glahn, R. (1996). *Fountain of fortune: money and monetary policy in China, 1000-1700*. University of California Press. doi:10.1525/9780520917453

Von Glahn, R. (2005). The origins of paper money in China. In W. N. Goetzmann & K. G. Rouwenhorst (Eds.), *The origins of value: financial innovations that created modern capital markets* (pp. 65–89). Oxford University Press.

Waldron, C. (2019). *Viability of the Usage of Blockchain Technology in Electronic Voting*. Academic Press.

Wang, J. (2021). *An In-depth Review of Privacy Concerns Raised by the COVID-19 Pandemic*. arXiv preprint arXiv:2101.10868.

Wang, W. (2020a). A SME credit evaluation system based on blockchain. *Proceedings - 2020 International Conference on E-Commerce and Internet Technology, ECIT 2020*, 248-251. 10.1109/ECIT50008.2020.00064

Wang, W. (2020b). Exploring personal credit evaluation model based on blockchain. *Proceedings - 2020 International Conference on E-Commerce and Internet Technology, ECIT 2020*, 163-166. 10.1109/ECIT50008.2020.00043

Wang, S., Ding, W., Li, J., Yuan, Y., Ouyang, L., & Wang, F. Y. (2019). Decentralized autonomous organizations: Concept, model, and applications. *IEEE Transactions on Computational Social Systems*, *6*(5), 870–878. doi:10.1109/TCSS.2019.2938190

Wanitcharakkhakul, L., & Rotchanakitumnuai, S. (2017). Blockchain technology acceptance in electronic medical record system. *Proceedings of the International Conference on Electronic Business (ICEB)*, 53-58.

Wattegama, D., Silva, P. S., Jayathilake, C. R., Elapatha, K., Abeywardena, K., & Kuruwitaarachchi, N. (2021). *"iSAY": Blockchain-based Intelligent Polling System for Legislative Assistance*. Academic Press.

Weatherford, J. (2009). *The history of money*. Currency.

Weber, M. (1958). *The Protestant Ethic and The Spirit of Capitalism*. Charles Scribner's Sons.

Weber, M. (1978). *Economy and society: An outline of interpretive sociology* (Vol. 1). Univ of California Press.

Weigmann, K. (2015). The ethics of global clinical trials. *EMBO Reports*. doi:10.15252/embr.201540398

Weil, K. E. (1985). PORTER, Competitive advantage, creating and sustaining superior performance. *Revista de Administração de Empresas*, *25*(2). doi:10.15900034-75901985000200009

Weinberg, B. (2019). *14 Major Real Use Cases of Blockchain in Healthcare | OpenLedger Insights*. https://openledger.info/insights/blockchain-healthcare-use-cases/

Weingart, S. N., Rind, D., Tofias, Z., & Sands, D. Z. (2006). Who uses the patient Internet portal? The PatientSite experience. *Journal of the American Medical Informatics Association: JAMIA*, *13*(1), 91–95. doi:10.1197/jamia.M1833 PMID:16221943

Wen, H. (2020). A study of the privacy of covid-19 contact tracing apps. *International Conference on Security and Privacy in Communication Networks*.

Werbach, K. (2018). *The blockchain and the new architecture of trust*. MIT Press.

Westerlund, M. (2019). The emergence of deepfake technology: A review. *Technology Innovation Management Review, 9*(11).

Wetterberg, G. (2009). *Money and power: From Stockholms Banco 1656 to Sveriges Riksbank today*. Sveriges Riksbank.

Wilczak, A. (2018). Between Consumerism and Deconsumption – Attitudes of Young People as a Challenge for Marketers. *Economic and Social Development: Book of Proceedings*, 297-305.

Wildman, N., Archer, A., Brouwer, H. M., & Cawston, A. (2019). *The ethics of data acquisition: Protecting Privacy and Autonomy While Harnessing the Potential of Big Data*. Academic Press.

Wilson, T. (2021). *British hospitals use blockchain to track COVID-19 vaccines*. https://www.reuters.com/article/health-coronavirus-blockchain/british-hospitals-use-blockchain-to-track-covid-19-vaccines-idUSL4N2JQ3FD

Wong, C. H., Siah, K. W., & Lo, A. W. (2019). Estimation of clinical trial success rates and related parameters. *Biostatistics (Oxford, England), 20*(2), 273–286. https://doi.org/10.1093/biostatistics/kxx069

Wong, D. R., Bhattacharya, S., & Butte, A. J. (2019). Prototype of running clinical trials in an untrustworthy environment using blockchain. *Nature Communications, 10*(1), 917. doi:10.103841467-019-08874-y PMID:30796226

Wood Gavin. (2014). *Ethereum: A Secure Decentralised Generalised Transaction Ledger*. Ethereum Project Yellow Paper.

Wood, G. (2014). Ethereum: A secure decentralised generalised transaction ledger. *Ethereum Project Yellow Paper, 151*(2014), 1-32.

Woods, D. (2013). How To Create A Moore's Law For Data. *Forbes*. https://www.forbes.com/sites/danwoods/2013/12/12/how-to-create-a-moores-law-for-data/?sh=22e2db0f44ca

Wray, L. R. (2015). *Modern money theory: a primer on macroeconomics for sovereign monetary systems* (2nd ed.). Palgrave Macmillan. doi:10.1057/9781137539922

Wright, T. (2020). *Blockchain App Used to Track COVID-19 Cases in Latin America*. https://cointelegraph.com/news/blockchain-app-used-to-track-covid-19-cases-in-latin-america

Wright. De Filippi, Primavera. (2015). Decentralized Blockchain Technology and the Rise of Lex Cryptographia, SSRN 1, 16 (Mar. 20, 2015)

Wu, B., & Li, Y. (2018). Design of evaluation system for digital education operational skill competition based on blockchain. *Proceedings - 2018 IEEE 15th International Conference on e-Business Engineering, ICEBE 2018*, 102-109. 10.1109/ICEBE.2018.00025

Wüst, K., & Gervais, A. (2018, June). Do you need a blockchain? In *2018 Crypto Valley Conference on Blockchain Technology (CVCBT)* (pp. 45-54). IEEE. 10.1109/CVCBT.2018.00011

Xie, C., & He, D. (2019). Design of traceability system for quality and safety of agricultural products in e-commerce based on blockchain technology. *Proceedings of the 7th International Symposium on Project Management, ISPM 2019*, 26-31.

Xie, C., & Xiao, X. (2020). Research on decision support system of E-commerce agricultural products based on blockchain. *Proceedings - 2020 International Conference on E-Commerce and Internet Technology, ECIT 2020*, 24-27. 10.1109/ECIT50008.2020.00013

Xu, X., Pautasso, C., Zhu, L., Gramoli, V., Ponomarev, A., Tran, A. B., & Chen, S. (2016, April). The blockchain as a software connector. In *2016 13th Working IEEE/IFIP Conference on Software Architecture (WICSA)* (pp. 182-191). IEEE. 10.1109/WICSA.2016.21

Xu, M., Chen, X., & Kou, G. (2019). A systematic review of blockchain. *Financial Innovation*, 5(1), 1–14. doi:10.118640854-019-0147-z

Yablonskaya, T. (2018, October 18). *Ethereum-Based Organization The DAO Launches and Raises Millions Worth of... Coinspeaker.* https://www.coinspeaker.com/dao-new-breath-of-blockchain-ethereum/

Yaeger, K., Martini, M., Rasouli, J., & Costa, A. (2019). Emerging BT solutions for modern healthcare infrastructure. *Journal of Scientific Innovation in Medicine*, 2(1).

Yaga, D., Mell, P., Roby, N., & Scarfone, K. (2019). *Blockchain technology overview.* arXiv preprint arXiv:1906.11078.

Yaji, S., Bangera, K., & Neelima, B. (2018). Privacy Preserving in Blockchain Based on Partial Homomorphic Encryption System for Ai Applications. *IEEE 25th International Conference on High Performance Computing Workshops (HiPCW)*, 81-85. doi: 10.1109/HiPCW.2018.8634280

Yang, X., Chen, Y., & Chen, X. (2019). Effective scheme against 51% attack on proof-of-work blockchain with history weighted information. *Proceedings - 2019 2nd IEEE International Conference on Blockchain, Blockchain 2019.* 10.1109/Blockchain.2019.00041

Yang, X., Yi, X., Nepal, S., Kelarev, A., & Han, F. (2020). Blockchain voting: Publicly verifiable online voting protocol without trusted tallying authorities. *Future Generation Computer Systems*, 112, 859–874. doi:10.1016/j.future.2020.06.051

Yassine, M., Alazab, M., & Romdhani, I. (2020). *Blockchain for Cybersecurity and Privacy.* Blockchain for Cybersecurity and Privacy. doi:10.1201/9780429324932

yearn.finance. (2021). *Introduction to Yearn.* https://docs.yearn.finance

Yermack, D. (2015). Is Bitcoin a Real Currency? An Economic Appraisal. In *Handbook of Digital Currency.* Bitcoin, Innovation, Financial Instruments, and Big Data; doi:10.1016/B978-0-12-802117-0.00002-3

Yeung, B., & Eichengreen, B. (2020). From Commodity to Fiat and Now to Crypto: What Does History Tell Us? *Digital Currency Economics and Policy.* doi:10.1142/9789811223785_0003

Yeung, C. A., Liccardi, I., Lu, K., Seneviratne, O., & Berners-lee, T. (2009). Decentralization : The Future of Online Social Networking. In *W3C Workshop on the Future of Social Networking Position Papers* (Vol. 2). Academic Press.

Yoo, S. (2020). How to design the token reinforcement based on token economy for blockchain model. *International Journal of Advanced Culture Technology*, 8(1), 157–164.

Young, S. (2018). Changing governance models by applying blockchain computing. *Catholic University Journal of Law and Technology*, 26(2), 87–128.

Young, S. (2018a). Enforcing constitutional rights through computer code. *Cath. UJL & Tech*, 26, 52.

Zaman, S., Khandaker, M. R., Khan, R. T., Tariq, F., & Wong, K. K. (2021). *Thinking Out of the Blocks: Holochain for Distributed Security in IoT Healthcare.* arXiv preprint arXiv:2103.01322.

Zaprutin, D. G., Nikiporets-Takigawa, G., Goncharov, V. V., Sekerin, V. D., & Gorokhova, A. E. (2020). Legal Practice in the Blockchain era. *Revista Gênero e Interdisciplinaridade, 1*(1).

Zaprutin, D. G., Nikiporets-Takigawa, G., Goncharov, V. V., Sekerin, V. D., & Gorokhova, A. E. (2020). Legal Practice in the Blockchain Era. *Revista Gênero e Interdisciplinaridade, 1*(1).

Zelmanovitz, L. (2011). Money: Origin and essence. *Criterio Libre*, 9(14), 65–90. doi:10.18041/1900-0642/criteriolibre.2011v9n14.1232

Zhai, S., Yang, Y., Li, J., Qiu, C., & Zhao, J. (2019). Research on the Application of Cryptography on the Blockchain. *Journal of Physics: Conference Series, 1168,* 032077.

Zhang, R., Xue, R., & Liu, L. (2019). Security and privacy on blockchain. *ACM Computing Surveys, 52*(3), 1–34.

Zhang, X. Z., Liu, J. J., & Xu, Z. W. (2015). Tencent and Facebook data validate Metcalfe's law. *Journal of Computer Science and Technology, 30*(2), 246–251. doi:10.100711390-015-1518-1

Zhao, J. L., Fan, S., & Yan, J. (2016). *Overview of business innovations and research opportunities in blockchain and introduction to the special issue.* Academic Press.

Zhao, S., & O'Mahony, D. (2020). Applying Blockchain Layer2 Technology to Mass E-Commerce. *IACR Cryptol. ePrint Arch., 2020,* 502.

Zhavoronkov, A., & Church, G. (2019). The Advent of Human Life Data Economics. *Trends in Molecular Medicine, 25*(7), 566–570. https://doi.org/10.1016/j.molmed.2019.05.002

Zheng, Z., Dai, H.-N., Tang, M., & Chen, X. (Eds.). (2020). *Blockchain and Trustworthy Systems: First International Conference, BlockSys 2019, Guangzhou, China, December 7–8, 2019, Proceedings.* Springer Nature.

Zheng, Z., Xie, S., Dai, H. N., Chen, X., & Wang, H. (2018). Blockchain challenges and opportunities: A survey. *International Journal of Web and Grid Services, 14*(4), 352–375. doi:10.1504/IJWGS.2018.095647

Zheng, Z., Xie, S., Dai, H., Chen, X., & Wang, H. (2017). An Overview of Blockchain Technology: Architecture, Consensus, and Future Trends. *2017 IEEE International Congress on Big Data (BigData Congress),* 557–564.

Zhuang, Y., Sheets, L. R., Shae, Z., Chen, Y. W., Tsai, J. J. P., & Shyu, C. R. (2019). Applying Blockchain Technology to Enhance Clinical Trial Recruitment. *AMIA ... Annual Symposium Proceedings. AMIA Symposium, 2019,* 1276–1285.

Zhuang, Yu., Sheets, L., Shae, Z., Tsai, J. J. P., & Shyu, C. R. (2018). Applying Blockchain Technology for Health Information Exchange and Persistent Monitoring for Clinical Trials. *AMIA ... Annual Symposium Proceedings. AMIA Symposium, 2018,* 1167–1175.

Zhuang, Y., Sheets, L. R., Shae, Z., Chen, Y.-W., Tsai, J. J. P., & Shyu, C.-R. (2020). Applying Blockchain Technology to Enhance Clinical Trial Recruitment. *AMIA ... Annual Symposium Proceedings - AMIA Symposium. AMIA Symposium, 2019,* 1276–1285.

Zimprich, S. (2019). *Data Protection and Blockchain - Security & Trust in Digital Services - Issues - dotmagazine.* https://www.dotmagazine.online/issues/security-trust-in-digital-services/data-protection-and-blockchain

Zwitter, A., & Hazenberg, J. (2020). Decentralized Network Governance: Blockchain Technology and the Future of Regulation. *Frontiers in Blockchain-Blockchain for Good, 3,* 12. doi:10.3389/fbloc.2020.00012

Zyskind, G., & Nathan, O. (2015, May). Decentralizing privacy: Using blockchain to protect personal data. In *2015 IEEE Security and Privacy Workshops* (pp. 180-184). IEEE.

About the Contributors

Dario de Oliveira Rodrigues received his Ph.D. in Management from the Lusíada University of Lisbon in 2012. Before that, he pioneered e-business activities in the pharmaceutical industry at the Portuguese subsidiary of the former German pharmaceutical multinational Schering AG. He is currently a Professor of Business and Administration and presents widely on the Blockchain's implications.

* * *

Ana Dias is a Sales Representative in a Medical Devices Company, MSc Nursing, Student Post Graduate Pharmaceutical Marketing and Business Development on ISEG.

Marta de-Melo-**Diogo** received her MSc degree in Pharmaceutical Sciences from the Faculty of Health Sciences of the University of Beira Interior in 2018. Since then, Marta works in Regulatory Affairs and Marketing in the cosmetics, medical devices, and pharmaceuticals industries.

João Fonseca-Gomes received his Ph.D. in Neurosciences from the Faculty of Medicine of the University of Lisbon in 2016. He also holds a degree in Biochemistry, and a Master in Neurosciences. João developed a potential drug for Alzheimer's disease, which is now under patent review. He is taking a post-graduate course in Pharmaceutical Marketing and Business Development in ISEG - Lisbon School of Economics & Management - University of Lisbon. Recently, João joined a consulting company, focusing on pharmaceutical and biotechnological areas on a European and Worldwide level.

Denise Francisco has an MSc in Microbiology, Instituto Superior Técnico, University of Lisbon, Degree in Biomedical Sciences, Faculty of Health Sciences, University of Beira Interior.

Andreia Robert **Lopes** received her MSc in Chemical and Biochemical Engineering from the NOVA University of Lisbon in 2008. She was the Lead Scientist of the Project "OPTIMED: Optimization of mono and biphasic microflows in medical devices for powder inhalation. Ref. PTDC/EME-MFE/103640" at the Faculty of Pharmacy of the University of Lisbon in 2013 and the Lead Scientist of the Project "Rotocork ADI FCOMP-01-0202-FEDER-021542" at the Technical Higher Institute of the University of Lisbon in 2014 Since 2017, she is the Lead Scientist in the field of ophthalmic and inhalation products at Hovione Farmaciencia.

Pedro Santana Lopes is a lawyer and a former Prime Minister of Portugal, ex-Mayor of Lisbon, and ex-President of Charity House and National Lotteries. He is the President of the Ricardo Espírito Santo Foundation.

Mitchell Amador Loureiro was born in Vancouver, Canada. He is the CEO of Immunefi, one of DeFi's leading cybersecurity projects protecting over $25 billion in user funds. Before founding Immunefi, Mitchell was best known taking making Sophia the Robot a worldwide sensation as the CMO of SingularityNET and as the VP of Marketing at Steemit. In addition, as a member of the rLoop Hyperloop team, he drove growth to the world's dominant web .pdf company and helped launch the largest user-owned open world, Decentraland.

Ângelo Miguel Nunes Luís is a 28 year old pharmacist. Currently he's an assistant pharmacist and has worked in pharmacy for the past three years. He graduated from the Faculty of Pharmacy at the University of Lisbon in 2016. He's currently frequenting the Pharmaceutical Marketing & Business Development course in ISEG - Lisbon School of Economics & Management, and he's one of the authors of the article "Data Security in Clinical Trials Using Blockchain Technology", that was written during the course as a proposed project of the discipline "New Models of Business in the Pharmaceutical Sector" taught by Prof. Dr. Dário Félix de Oliveira Rodrigues.

Bebiana Sá Moura is currently Head of Discovery at VectorB2B- Drug Developing Association. Being a native of Vila Nova de Gaia, she studied in University of Porto from where she received her B.S. in Biochemistry in 2007. She went on to do her M.S. in the Institute for Molecular and Cell Biology, in the Crystallography group, under the supervision of Sandra Macedo Ribeiro. In 2008 she was accepted in the GABBA program and moved to United States where she did her PhD at Mark Hochstrasser's laboratory at Yale University. There, Bebiana worked on the characterization of a novel protein, Ynl155w, involved in the ubiquitin-proteasome system. In 2014, she moved to Heidelberg and joined the Hurt lab where she worked on ribosome biogenesis. In 2017, she returned to Portugal, to Faculty of Medicine of University of Coimbra. As Science and Technology Manager, she was responsible for the submission of several healthcare projects to different funding agencies and saw through their implementation.

Pedro P. Nevado is a PhD in Management, Professor of Management Strategy, International Business, co-Director of postgraduate programs in International Business and Marketing at ISEG – Lisbon School of Economics & Management of Lisbon University. He also teaches and undertakes research into multinationals, subsidiary management and corporate and international strategies. He has also previous experience as a consultant to a number of corporations.

Ana Pêgo received her MSc from the Faculty of Pharmacy of the University of Lisbon in 2018. She is a Ph.D. student at the same institute and was awarded an FCT 2019 Call for Ph.D. Studentships.

Rafael Duarte Pinto received his MSc degree in Pharmaceutical Sciences from the Egas Moniz Higher Institute of Health Sciences in 2015. Currently, he is Community Pharmacist in Almada.

Inês G. Raposo started her path in the life sciences field as a Biomedical Research student at Universidade do Algarve. Her interest has then moved forward into the pharmaceutical sphere, having enrolled in a Specialization in Clinical Research and a master's degree in Biopharmaceutical Sciences at Faculdade de Farmácia da Universidade de Lisboa. During those years, Inês essentially worked as a researcher in the fields of regeneration, inflammation, and oncology focusing on genotyping and gene editing. Additionally, she was involved in the progress of several pharmaceutical products in the pipeline. Although her actual main activity is the pharmaceutical regulatory field, she is currently conducting a post-graduate course in Pharmaceutical Marketing and Business Development at ISEG Executive Education, where her knowledge has gotten deeper into the blockchain technology topic.

Francisco Ribeiro de Sousa received his MSc degree in Pharmaceutical Sciences from the Faculty of Pharmacy of the University of Lisbon in 2018. Currently, he is a Regulatory Affairs Specialist at GE Healthcare.

Albérico Travassos Rosário received his Ph.D. in Marketing and Strategy from the Universities of Aveiro (UA), Minho (UM), and Beira Interior (UBI) and is affiliated to the GOVCOPP research center of the University of Aveiro. He also holds an MSc in Marketing and is graduated in Marketing, Advertising, and Public Relations, from ISLA Campus Lisbon-European University | Laureate International Universities. Marketing Specialist and Assistant Professor at IADE-Faculty of Design, Technology, and Communication at the European University. Currently, he is a Visiting Professor at the Santarém Higher School of Management and Technology (ESGTS) of the Polytechnic Institute of Santarém. Marketing and strategy consultant for SMEs.

João Sequeira has a Degree of Mathematics Applied to Economics and Management, ISEG - Lisbon School of Economics & Management, Universidade de Lisboa.

Marta Silva is a graduate in veterinary medicine and about 8 years of experience managing sales and technical services in pharmaceutical industry.

Cátia Neves **Sousa** received her MSc in Clinical Psychology from the Faculty of Psychology of the University of Lisbon in 2010. Marketing passionate, she works with several companies and continues her studies attending a Graduate Academic and Professional Course.

Jorge Tavares received his MSc in Pharmaceutical Sciences from the Faculty of Pharmacy of the University of Lisbon in 2008. In addition, he received an MSc in Statistics and Information Management (2008) and a Ph.D. in Information Management from the NOVA University of Lisbon – NOVA IMS in 2018. Jorge has more than 20 years of experience in healthcare as a scientific researcher and working with multinational healthcare companies. He published several studies concerning eHealth, the adoption of EHR Patient Portals, and statistical modeling in healthcare.

João Pedro **Vieira** graduated in History from the Faculty of Social Sciences and Humanities of NOVA University and holds a specialization in Ancient History from the School of Arts and Humanities of Lisbon University. Currently, he works at the Bank of Portugal Museum (Money Museum) as the Curator of Coins and Paper Money.

Index

A

agency costs 120, 124, 158
Algorithmic Governance 106, 118, 136, 149, 151
API3 160, 167, 169
applicability 250-251, 254, 260, 262
artificial intelligence 8, 14, 26, 33-34, 92, 94, 107, 127, 139, 144, 149, 154, 183, 196-197, 251, 276, 285, 288-290, 298

B

Backdoor 158
Big Data 6, 34-35, 40, 94, 127, 139, 144, 152, 154, 172, 211, 214, 231, 238-239, 243-247, 249, 275, 317, 329
Bitcoin 3-4, 7, 13, 31, 37, 39, 43-44, 61-62, 64, 66-67, 69-71, 74-77, 81-84, 86-87, 96-101, 103-104, 106-108, 110-113, 115, 124-125, 130-132, 134, 140-144, 148-150, 153-156, 160-161, 163-166, 169-172, 188, 199-200, 216, 222, 229-230, 239, 247, 251, 265, 269, 271, 274-275, 279-280, 282, 284-286, 288, 293, 296, 298-299, 309, 312-314, 317-318, 328-329
block 5, 39, 83, 115, 121, 139, 142, 154, 160, 164-165, 199-202, 217, 221-222, 229-230, 251, 263, 271, 288, 294, 306, 313-315, 322
block explorers 160, 164-165
blockchain 1-7, 9-15, 17-18, 20-23, 25-41, 43-44, 46, 61-64, 67-71, 73-74, 77-81, 83, 85-93, 95, 97-100, 102-111, 113-127, 129-190, 194-195, 199-219, 221-237, 239, 241-248, 250-273, 275, 278-302, 304, 306-319, 321-329
Blockchain of Internet of Things 194, 204, 217
blockchain technology 1-3, 6, 9-10, 14-15, 25-26, 28-29, 34, 40, 61, 69, 73-74, 79-80, 85-86, 89-91, 97, 99, 102, 105-106, 114, 118-123, 126-127, 131, 134-135, 137, 139-141, 144-149, 151-152, 155-158, 161, 173-175, 177-188, 190, 201-203, 205-208, 211, 213-214, 216-219, 221, 223-224, 226, 228-237, 239, 241-248, 250-251, 253-254, 257-270, 272, 282, 285-290, 292-297, 299-301, 306, 308-310, 312, 327-329
Bockchain 173
business models 1, 3, 8-9, 16, 23-24, 32, 34, 79, 97, 133, 149, 173, 269, 271, 281, 283, 290, 300, 302

C

Chain Value 249
clinical data 6, 17, 19, 21-22, 27-28, 203, 207, 221, 228-229, 235, 241-242, 262, 269-270, 272, 275, 277, 280-281, 309, 323
clinical research 27, 207-209, 228-229, 231-237, 239, 242-243, 245-246, 248-249, 253, 257, 266, 269-275, 277, 279-283, 287, 290-291, 323-324, 326
clinical trial 17, 27, 207-208, 214, 217, 228, 234-237, 240-242, 245, 247-251, 253-254, 257-269, 273, 276, 281, 286-287, 312, 323-324, 326, 329
clinical trials 6, 13, 17, 27-28, 30, 32, 35, 207-210, 213-214, 216, 226, 229, 231-232, 234-237, 240, 243, 245-248, 250-251, 254-268, 270, 273, 278-281, 283-287, 295, 312-313, 316, 322-324, 326, 328
cloud 11, 92, 100, 114, 125-126, 150, 155, 180, 189, 196-197, 226, 273, 283, 288, 290, 318
coinage 43, 49-51, 59, 64-65, 67, 73, 100
commodity money 43, 57-58, 84, 116
confidence 1, 4, 22, 24, 26, 28, 43, 46, 52-54, 58-62, 64, 66, 77, 79-81, 118, 134, 139, 185, 187, 220, 230, 261-262, 271, 314, 316, 323, 325-326
consensus 1, 3, 19, 25, 29, 38, 41, 46-47, 61-62, 84, 87, 100, 103, 116, 118, 121, 123, 125, 130, 132, 138, 140, 142, 158, 161, 165, 186, 201, 204, 222-224, 229, 231, 252, 262-264, 271, 279, 295, 312, 314, 325, 329
content precision 1-2, 25-26, 29
core developers 29, 160, 164-165
COVID-19 6, 10, 33, 38-40, 69, 99, 102, 105, 110-

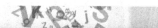
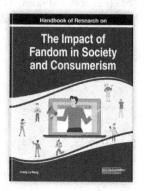
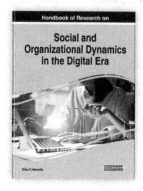
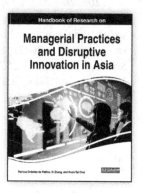
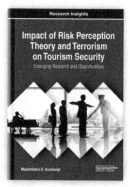
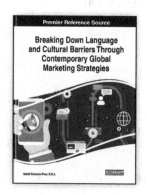
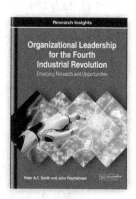
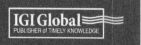

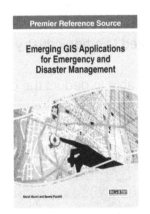
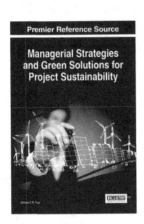
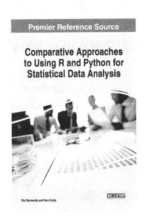
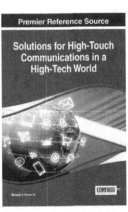

IGI Global Author Services

Providing a high-quality, affordable, and expeditious service, IGI Global's Author Services enable authors to streamline their publishing process, increase chance of acceptance, and adhere to IGI Global's publication standards.

Benefits of Author Services:

- **Professional Service:** All our editors, designers, and translators are experts in their field with years of experience and professional certifications.

- **Quality Guarantee & Certificate:** Each order is returned with a quality guarantee and certificate of professional completion.

- **Timeliness:** All editorial orders have a guaranteed return timeframe of 3-5 business days and translation orders are guaranteed in 7-10 business days.

- **Affordable Pricing:** IGI Global Author Services are competitively priced compared to other industry service providers.

- **APC Reimbursement:** IGI Global authors publishing Open Access (OA) will be able to deduct the cost of editing and other IGI Global author services from their OA APC publishing fee.

Author Services Offered:

English Language Copy Editing
Professional, native English language copy editors improve your manuscript's grammar, spelling, punctuation, terminology, semantics, consistency, flow, formatting, and more.

Scientific & Scholarly Editing
A Ph.D. level review for qualities such as originality and significance, interest to researchers, level of methodology and analysis, coverage of literature, organization, quality of writing, and strengths and weaknesses.

Figure, Table, Chart & Equation Conversions
Work with IGI Global's graphic designers before submission to enhance and design all figures and charts to IGI Global's specific standards for clarity.

Translation
Providing 70 language options, including Simplified and Traditional Chinese, Spanish, Arabic, German, French, and more.

Hear What the Experts Are Saying About IGI Global's Author Services

"Publishing with IGI Global has been **an amazing experience** for me for sharing my research. The **strong academic production** support ensures quality and timely completion." – **Prof. Margaret Niess, Oregon State University, USA**

"The service was **very fast, very thorough, and very helpful** in ensuring our chapter meets the criteria and requirements of the book's editors. I was **quite impressed and happy** with your service." – **Prof. Tom Brinthaupt, Middle Tennessee State University, USA**

Learn More or Get Started Here:

For Questions, Contact IGI Global's Customer Service Team at cust@igi-global.com or 717-533-8845

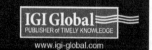
www.igi-global.com

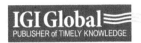

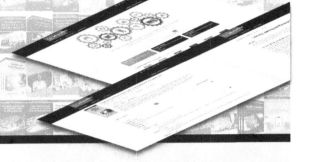

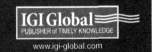